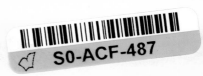

Neuro-Ophthalmology:

Clinical Signs and Symptoms

Neuro-Ophthalmology:

Clinical Signs and Symptoms

THOMAS J. WALSH, M.D.

Professor of Ophthalmology and Visual Science and Neurology
Yale School of Medicine
Consultant Neuro-Ophthalmology
U.S. Army, Walter Reed Hospital
Washington, D.C.

SECOND EDITION

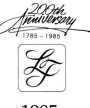

1985

Lea & Febiger · *Philadelphia*

Lea & Febiger
600 Washington Square
Philadelphia, PA 19106-4198
U.S.A.
(215) 922-1330

Library of Congress Cataloging in Publication Data

Walsh, Thomas J. (Thomas Joseph), 1931–
  Neuro-ophthalmology: clinical signs and symptoms.

  Includes bibliographies and index.
  1. Neuro-ophthalmology. I. Title. [DNLM: 1. Eye
Diseases—diagnosis. 2. Eye Manifestations.
3. Neurologic Manifestations. WW 141 W227n]
RE725.W34 1985   617.7'3   84-26103
ISBN 0-8121-0945-7

First Edition, 1978

PRINTED IN THE UNITED STATES OF AMERICA

Print No. 4   3   2   1

TO SALLY
  A basket of love for her understanding

Foreword to the First Edition

The dynamic nature of the subspecialty of neuro-ophthalmology, which encompasses not only the entire field of ophthalmology, but also the disciplines of neurology, neuro-surgery, and general medicine, continually challenges its practitioner with new knowledge. New concepts of disease, new diagnostic techniques, and new therapies gleaned from the literature and from the large personal clinical experience of Dr. Thomas Walsh form the basis for this new textbook.

The author of this book, a member of the faculty of Yale University Medical School, has had a wealth of experience in the field of neuro-ophthalmology. The style is unique. Instead of the usual method, beginning with the anatomy and followed by physiology, clinical diagnosis, pathology, and therapeutics, he has captioned most chapters with a single clinical sign and has incorporated these entities in detail. These titles are: papilledema, pupillary abnormalities, exophthalmos, ptosis, diplopia, blurred vision, gaze, headache, nystagmus, and field defects. Doctor Rothman has also written an excellent chapter, beautifully illustrated, on Radiology in Neuro-ophthalmology.

Dr. Robert B. Welch, retinal surgeon of Baltimore, wrote the chapter entitled Retinal Disease, concerned chiefly with the phakomatoses. Dr. Peter D. Williamson, neurologist, wrote the chapter on Facial Nerve Paralysis.

I feel greatly honored to have been asked by Doctor Walsh to prepare this brief Foreword to what promises to be a book well received by those interested in the neurologic aspects of ophthalmology. I am grateful not only for this, but for the diligence and concern that has led him to compile this most readable and valuable work.

ROBERT W. HOLLENHORST, M.D.
Professor of Ophthalmology
Mayo Graduate School of Medicine
Rochester, Minnesota

Foreword

In the past, and throughout the world, few medical doctors dedicated their professional lives to neuro-ophthalmology. The larger, mostly unexplored part of the visual pathway deserves more interest, and every medical doctor should be aware that a normal-looking posterior segment of the eye, with even 10/10 vision does not eliminate subclinical pathology in the neurologic domain, as decreased vision may be primarily due to motor as well as sensorial brain disorders. Younger colleagues should be educated with alert curiosity to apply interdisciplinary neuro-ophthalmologic strategies. Furthermore, correlation of the observed functional changes with the morphologic clinico-anatomic facts is one of the basic foundations of neuro-ophthalmology, formerly a noble intellectual art, recently more and more a separate clinical entity, confirmed by objective investigations.

Subjective and objective exploration, evaluation, and follow-up of visual loss and/or diplopia will define signs and symptoms that are not necessarily pathologic. If pathologic, the question arises as to whether the symptom is due to disease of the peripheral perception tissue of the eye or only related to nervous disease or to both. To properly evaluate the symptoms, sophisticated diagnostic equipment may be used, which means that the patient has to stay under the supervision of a medical team, taking care of and being concerned with the functional visual problem, unfortunately often ignored by the neurologist.

By misuse of diagnostic equipment, without proper evaluation of symptoms, without justified indications, without qualified interpretation, pitfalls are created that grow exponentially as the machinery and imaging techniques become more expensive and sophisticated. Ultimately, the patient's best protection is the doctor's sound clinical judgement and extensive knowledge. Even in the diagnosis of lesions far from the eye, the ophthalmologist has a critical role to play. Only the ophthalmologist is familiar enough with ocular and orbital causes of visual loss and/or diplopia to forestall a massive intracranial workup. Moreover, he has to be aware, more than his neurologist-colleagues, of nonstructural and structural intracranial mechanisms, resulting in symptoms that do not require major studies, at least in the short term and after neuro-ophthalmologic staff discussions.

Because the visual pathway appears as an important diagnostic tool for the neurologist, it is clear that the diagnosis and follow-up of brain diseases at this crossroad have to be assessed by clinicians with mixed interests: the ophthalmologist with broad neurologic insight, permanently in contact and discussion with the neurologist, neuroradiologist, neurosurgeon, and neuropathologist. Traditional disciplinary boundaries should be broken down and all these related disciplines should join under the neuro-ophthalmologic umbrella.

The respective textbooks of Frank Burton Walsh and his namesake, Thomas Walsh, from Yale University, match excellently. If the former may be considered a bible, the latter may be considered for the scientifically oriented practitioner a bible in a nutshell, containing an accurate message to all those interested in neuro-ophthalmology. The first edition was a newcomer; each chapter was dedicated to objective symptoms or subjective signs, discussing their correct evaluation and referring to their importance in routine and exceptional disease

entities, mentioning the anatomy and physiology necessary to understand the pathogenesis but omitting unnecessary historical stepping stones. Rapid extension of information has justified this new edition; therefore, the author focuses on the complexity of new syndromes while new levels of understanding of known diseases have been added.

This volume is not only a token and a symbol of the scientific authority and the clinical dedication of the author but a basic guide to students and medical scientists, in both the ophthalmologic and neurologic disciplines. Therefore, I feel honored and especially privileged to emphasize by this foreword the practical importance of this book.

With these convictions, I warmly recommend this comprehensive work to everyone interested and involved in this relatively new and fascinating field of learning. This book will deeply contribute to enrich the skills of those practicing neuro-ophthalmology, which means genuinely keen observation and experience matching extensive knowledge, combined with scientific erudition, intellectual capacities, and brain work.

ADOLPHE NEETENS, M.D., PH.D.
Chairman and Professor,
Institute of Ophthalmology,
University of Antwerp, U.I.A.
Dean of the Academic Hospital

Preface

Medical textbooks are of several types and purposes. Some are encyclopedias of a particular subject, and such books are excellent sources of reference. At the other end of the spectrum is the so-called introductory text, which frequently is so abbreviated that the physician is led only halfway toward an appropriate diagnosis. Between these two extremes, a gap exists in neuro-ophthalmic literature. What is required is a clinically useful textbook for the practicing as well as the resident ophthalmologist, and I have striven to fill that need in this book.

My focus has been on the practical application of well-accepted diagnostic techniques and the interpretation of clinically relevant information needed to form sound differential diagnoses. Since this textbook is intended for use in a clinical situation, I have assumed that the reader is familiar with the discipline of ophthalmology.

On that basis, I have covered the most important aspects of the field of ophthalmology succinctly, but sufficiently to enable the practitioner to determine an appropriate diagnosis and course of treatment. With respect to rare and unusual diseases, I have included only those that are especially critical to the patient's vision or to his general health.

As the title indicates, the book discusses neuro-ophthalmology in terms of its signs and symptoms. Thus, each chapter deals with either a symptom that leads the patient to seek medical attention or a sign that is demonstrated on physical examination. Each chapter has been written in the form of a monograph. Although this practice leads to some repetition, it permits the reader to research a sign or symptom by reference to one chapter and eliminates checking numerous page references in the index. For this reason also, cross references have been kept to a minimum. I believe that this format will give the physician who is less familiar with certain conditions a better chance of arriving at a correct diagnosis. Besides diagnoses, in each chapter I have suggested diagnostic tests and techniques that I have found particularly useful with the type of condition being discussed.

One of the essentials of having several co-authors in a textbook with this approach is that all contributors see the book and their subject in the same light as does the senior author in order to give the book a certain cohesiveness. I feel that my co-authors have achieved this while adding their own particular expertise in their subject of interest. Some of the chapters are also a basic review of laboratory subjects, such as radiology and electrodiagnosis. These chapters are meant to give the reader a firm grounding in what these tests can do for him in making a diagnosis and when they are likely to be employed.

Rather than covering ancillary data in depth in the text, I have supplied pertinent bibliographic references in order to facilitate further research by either those who seek additional evidence for the conclusions reached on a particular subject or those who would like to further explore a subject in the literature.

New Haven, Connecticut

THOMAS J. WALSH, M.D.

Acknowledgments

Despite a text's having one name as its author, many people vitally contribute to the final copy. It is difficult to be sure to thank each one in true measure, but I will try to make special mention of a few.

I particularly want to thank all my contributors, Dr. Melvin Alper, Dr. Charles Citrin, Dr. Nicholas Galloway, Dr. Rufus Howard, Dr. Patrick Lavin, Dr. Stephen Rothman, Dr. Robert Welch, Dr. Peter Williamson, and Dr. Jonathan Wirtschafter, who have not only produced superb works in the areas of their own expertise, but have done so in a style in keeping with my perception of the book. They also rearranged their own busy schedules to meet my deadlines and for this, too, I am grateful.

I would also like to thank Dr. Caleb Gonzalez for his contribution to the initial portion of the section on diplopia, and Dr. William Eckhardt for his contribution on the thyroid tests.

Several friends have kindly supplied me with illustrations that I felt were important to the text. These illustrations were supplied by Dr. Morton Goldberg, 13-5; Dr. Douglas McCrae, 14-1 and 14-2; Dr. Lee Jampol, 13-3 and 13-8A and B; and Lewis Craven, 13-4C.

I am grateful to Dr. Marvin Sears, Chairman of the Department of Ophthalmology and Visual Sciences, Dr. Gilbert Glaser, Chairman of the Department of Neurology, and Dr. William Collins, Chairman of the Department of Neuro-Surgery at Yale, who gave me the opportunity to see neuro-ophthalmic patients in their departments and allowed me to gain the experience to write this book.

Special thanks should go to Mrs. Irma Jury for her patience in typing the many versions of this text.

Contributors

Melvin G. Alper, M.D.
Clinical Professor of Ophthalmology
  and Neurological Surgery
George Washington University

Charles M. Citrin, M.D.
The Neurology Center
Clinical Associate Professor of Radiology
George Washington University Medical
  Center

Nicholas R. Galloway, M.D., F.R.C.S.
Consultant, Ophthalmic Surgeon and
  Clinical Teacher
University Hospital
Nottingham, England

Rufus O. Howard, M.D.
Clinical Professor of Ophthalmology
Yale School of Medicine

Patrick J.M. Lavin, M.D.
Assistant Professor, Neurology and
  Ophthalmology
Vanderbilt University School of Medicine
Director, Ocular Motility Laboratory
Vanderbilt University Medical Center

Stephen L.G. Rothman, M.D.
Medical Director
Multi-Planar Diagnostic Imaging, Inc.
Torrance, California

Robert B. Welch, M.D.
Associate Professor, Ophthalmology
  and Director Retina Service
Wilmer Ophthalmological Institute
Johns Hopkins Hospital

Peter D. Williamson, M.D.
Associate Professor, Neurology
Yale School of Medicine

Jonathan D. Wirtschafter, M.D.
Professor of Ophthalmology, Neurology,
  Neurosurgery
Director, Neuro-ophthalmology Orbital
  Plastic Service
University of Minnesota Medical School

Contents

Chapter 1

Neuro-Ophthalmologic History and Neurologic Examination

JONATHAN D. WIRTSCHAFTER

The patient who is referred for a neuro-ophthalmologic problem is different than most patients seen by either the ophthalmologist or the neurologist. For the ophthalmologist who is used to making a diagnosis by examination of a transparent organ, the neuro-ophthalmologic patient requires more investment of time and talent to obtain a better history and to arrange alternative and supplementary examinations. For the neurologist who is accustomed to emphasizing the history, the neuro-ophthalmologic patient requires the mastery of additional examination techniques and their interpretation. This eclectic and anecdotal chapter will highlight some of the aspects of the neuro-ophthalmologic history and nonocular neurologic examination. Some of the newer techniques will be mentioned briefly, but the details will be left for other chapters or reviews of the current medical literature.

PURPOSE OF THE HISTORY AND EXAMINATION

The examiner attempts to answer several questions during the neuro-ophthalmologic examination. The relationships of the questions are easily stated, but the answers may come in any order.

1. Does the patient have one or more organic or functional disorders?
2. What is the topographic localization of the organic lesions?
3. What is the etiology?

The neuro-ophthalmologist frequently is confronted by multiple diagnoses in the same patient. For example, the patient may not have reported the best visual acuity when tested, the patient may need a refraction to improve the acuity, a posterior subcapsular cataract may be interfering with vision when the patient is tested looking at a near visual acuity chart in bright illumination, there may be macular degeneration, and the patient may have alexia. When one or more problems occur along a single neurologic pathway, they are said to be *linearly localized*. Conversely, when the problem can be specified as occurring at only one location along a pathway, it is described as *point localized*. For example, a patient first identified as having a visual pathway lesion could have visual fields leading to point localization of a chiasmal

1

syndrome. One of the reasons for performing multiple examination procedures on the same patient is to avoid the risks of *faulty topographic localization and diagnosis.*

ANSWERING THE PATIENT'S CONCERNS

The patient's own diagnostic assessment, insight, and concerns are an important part of the neuro-ophthalmic agenda. In my experience, the final outcome of about one-third of neuro-ophthalmic workups is to reassure the patient that the problem is likely to be static or to improve spontaneously after some period of time. Moreover, it may be desirable to limit the further expenditure of health care resources on the problem. These issues cannot be approached unless the examiner knows if the patient is concerned about specific diagnostic possibilities such as brain tumor or multiple sclerosis. Alternatively, the patient may be concerned about the relationship of his symptom to a disease present in a relative or friend. There may be a medicolegal issue pending, and information should be specifically sought as to whether all litigation and disability claims have been settled or whether such action is pending or contemplated. In this regard, it is also important to establish in the medical record whether the patient is seeking consultation for medical care or because he has been referred by an attorney or insurance company.

HISTORY OF THE PRESENT ILLNESS

The importance of the history in the evaluation of the awake neurologic patient cannot be over-emphasized. Much of the examination can be omitted or minimized if the review of neurologic symptoms is negative and the patient is not deceiving, confused, nor suffering from loss of memory or intellectual ability. Conversely, objective examination techniques are required if the patient is not able to provide a good history or cooperate for various subjective tests.

Certain diagnoses can only be made by history. Migraine headaches are an example. Moreover, it is usually possible to use the patient's description to distinguish the flashing lights that may result from classic migraine (a cortical symptom), vitreous traction on the retina (a mechano-neural symptom), or amaurosis fugax (a neural transmission symptom). It is important to try to distinguish between symptoms of carotid artery stenosis or embolism and symptoms of vertebrobasilar artery stenosis because carotid artery disorders are more likely to require further differentiation as a prelude to surgery.

The multiplicity of the times of occurrence and types of past neurologic symptoms may cause you to suspect that the patient has multiple sclerosis. An ophthalmologist must remember to ask about urinary incontinence because this rivals paresthesias as one of the most frequent complaints of patients with multiple sclerosis.

Communicating With the Patient

The chief complaint and history of the present illness may need to be elicted more than once. If several problems exist, they should be identified separately and ranked in their importance to the patient. Not infrequently, you will have to teach the patient some fact and have him report after a subsequent attack of an episodic phenomenon. Examples of this include the differences between (1) the left eye and the left visual field of each eye, (2) monocular and binocular diplopia, (3) crossed and uncrossed diplopia, and (4) ghost, blurred, and doubled images. Sometimes you will want to give the patient a pinhole occluder to look through during an attack of blurring so that you will know whether this simple "universal lens" has relieved the symptom. You will frequently be frustrated by the patient ascribing different meanings to words than you would. Examples of this occur in the language used to describe headache. Patients may use the terms "migraine," or "sinus," to describe symptoms ultimately proved to be greater occipital neuralgia. The term "dizzy" may be used to mean "feeling faint or light-headed" or to mean "oscillopsia" or that "the environment appears to be moving." Oscillopsia and nystagmus can occur simultaneously or independently.

Onset and Recurrences of Symptoms

The onset of symptoms is of obvious importance in the evaluation of trauma, infection, and postinflammatory events. In addition to external events, time of day or the posture of the patient may be associated with the onset or the recurrence of a symptom. Certain events may be more likely to begin during sleep. It has been suggested that the cerebral blood flow may be decreased at night and lead to thrombosis, whereas embolism from an ulcerated plaque may occur more frequently during hours of greater activity. Postural changes at night may increase the cerebrospinal fluid pressure, giving rise to headaches. Patients with papilledema resulting from increased intracranial pressure will frequently report that they have transient obscurations of vision immediately after standing. A colloid cyst of the third ventricle may produce sudden headache, owing to increased cerebrospinal fluid pressure resulting from a ball-valve action at the aqueduct of Sylvius or the foramen of Monro. This symptom was precipitated recurrently in one of our patients when he crawled in the window of a married lady's apartment. Changes in head position may also contribute to many other neuro-ophthalmic symptoms, including paroxysmal positional vertigo, head pain associated with posterior fossa tumors, and the amplitude of intracranial bruits.

You must use caution in accepting the patient's interpretation of the mechanism or time of onset. The accidental covering of each eye may lead to the discovery of a long-standing condition that the patient believes has just begun. The sudden onset of bilateral blindness may result from an acute hemianopia in one hemifield in a patient with an unrecognized long-standing contralateral hemianopia.

Other events that seem to provoke recurrent symptoms also should be addressed. Fatigue may increase the symptoms of myasthenia gravis, and exercise and increased body temperature may produce visual loss or other neurologic symptoms in multiple sclerosis; this is known as the Uhthoff phenomenon. The relationship between menses and migraine should be probed.

Foods may play an important role as recurrent causes of headaches of several varieties. Migraine may be precipitated by alcohol in general and red wine in particular. Other foods associated with migraine include chocolate, hard cheeses, preserved meats, and sodium salts. Caffeine withdrawal and hypoglycemia are other dietary causes of headache.

Reading is blamed for many symptoms and you will need to examine the circumstances surrounding this activity in some detail. Try to determine what activities have been given up or are being performed less well as a result of the illness. It may be worth asking whether there are difficulties seeing the stairs (in patients with severe constriction of the visual field or vertical diplopia), using the rear-view mirror of an automobile (in diplopia), finding the curb or the bathroom in the dark (in retinal degenerations), or seeing the highway when driving in bright light (in the case of posterior subcapsular cataracts).

One of the most difficult symptoms to evaluate is loss of depth perception, especially of moving objects, such as baseballs or automobiles. It is much less frequent for patients to complain of loss of stereopsis when viewing small objects, but when they do so it is usually easy to find a cause related to loss of visual acuity in one or both eyes.

Try to get some external confirmation of the patient's assertions. Family members can report on unusual behavior such as appropriate responses to abnormally perceived visual stimuli, as occurs in Alzheimer's disease. For example, the patient may walk up to and try to straighten a door frame that is misperceived as warped. Old photographs of the patient can often be used to find unremembered ptosis or anisocoria.

Prior Radiologic and Electrophysiologic Examinations

Previously performed diagnostic studies are becoming increasingly important and confusing in the practice of neuro-ophthalmology. Unfortunately, many of the patients you see will report that they have had a computed tomographic or magnetic resonance scan and that the results were "normal." Do not be misled by this. Many of these scans never included the optic canals or the sellar region. The superior orbital fissure is 3 cm in height and is easily mistaken for the optic canal which is only 3 mm in height. In axial sections, the optic nerve will appear to be anterior to either of these structures. Unless you have confidence in the report and technique, it is best to review these scans yourself with a neuroradiologist before accepting them as normal. Scepticism may be justified concerning other past diagnostic studies. Significant differences exist in the information obtained from digital subtraction angiograms, which may provide adequate information about the extracranial circulation but insufficient information concerning the intracranial vessels. In cases where this information may be needed to plan surgery, a standard arteriogram may be required. While discussing past diagnostic studies, you should determine whether any problems occurred, such as allergic reactions to the intravenous contrast material.

It may be necessary to prompt the patient concerning various diagnostic studies they have had done and have forgotten or not understood. Many patients are not yet conversant with any of the electrodiagnostic tests except the electroencephalogram.

It may require some effort to determine whether the patient was examined for any of the evoked responses (visual, brainstem auditory, or somatosensory) or by electroretinography, electro-oculography, or electronystagmography.

Past and Present Medications

The response to prior treatment(s) may be of value in determining or ruling out various pathogenic mechanisms. This information may also tell when and to what extent the symptom bothers the patient. The medications presently used by the patient may provide etiologic clues because they may be the direct cause of the patient's symptoms or they may reveal a diagnosis not considered by the patient to be relevant to the neuro-opthalmic symptom. Examples of the latter include medications for hypertension, diabetes mellitus, or hypothyroidism following treatment for hyperthyroidism. Thus the patient who presents with diplopia from a restrictive myopathy may have once had a hyperthyroid condition and now may have Graves' disease. Of course, medications can cause dysfunction of the oculomotor system (nystagmus, paresis, impaired smooth pursuit movements, and dysmetria), ocular autonomic system (particularly affecting accommodation), and the afferent visual system (toxic optic neuropathies and retinopathies). The systemic effects of present ocular medications may also be considered, for example the asthma that can be produced by systemic absorption of beta-blockers. Fraunfelder and Grant have each compiled texts listing the ocular effects of systemic medications and the systemic effects of ocular medications.

Review of the Ocular History and Symptoms

The review of ocular history and symptoms is mandatory. Since most patients date their ocular problems from when they may have been examined for glasses, it may be best at least to record when they obtained their first and most recent lenses. The frequency, amount, and effectiveness of changes in the prescription can be helpful in the diagnosis of structural changes in the eye. Frequent changes of refraction suggest the diagnosis of diabetes mellitus. It is important to document when glasses ceased to fully correct the problem. It can be useful to obtain the prescription for the lenses from the patient, because sometimes it may not be appreciated that the patient is wearing a "hidden" progressive bifocal or a prism, either of which may explain diplopia. A high amount of astigmatic correction with an axis of more than 15° from the vertical or horizontal meridians may be associated with the "tilted disk syndrome" and a visual field defect spilling out of the superior temporal quadrant.

After obtaining the refraction history, one can ask about prior ocular surgery, patching for amblyopia, orthoptic exercises, topical eyedrops, and systemic medications for glaucoma or inflammation.

Transient Loss of Vision. Transient loss of vision is defined according to the time involved and the extent and depth of the loss. The transient obscurations of vision may last only a few seconds when they are caused by papilledema and increased intracranial pressure. Bilateral loss of vision with vertigo may last only a few seconds at a time with vertebrobasilar artery disease and hypotensive episodes. Monocular hypoperfusion episodes may last seconds to minutes and are often associated with the sensation that a curtain has come down before the affected eye. Emboli from the carotid artery and other sources usually obscure vision for 3 to 5 minutes at a time, while uniocular migraine may last 10 to 20 minutes. Classic ophthalmic migraine with a positive scotoma may last 20 to 30 minutes and is followed by a headache.

Qualitative Loss of Vision. Qualitative loss of vision is a frequent complaint in monocular optic neuropathies. The patient may report that objects appear less bright or colors less intense than they are with the opposite eye. Objective visual acuity may be normal, so that more subtle tests such as the determination of contrast sensitivity or the visual evoked potential are required to confirm the patient's subjective complaint. When qualitative loss of vision occurs in both eyes, the patient may complain of difficulty in recognizing faces or in driving at night.

Scotoma. As perceived by the patient, scotoma may be positive (that is, something perceived as dark and lying in the way of seeing the object) or negative (something perceived as bright or dazzling and lying in the way of seeing the object) or both (a frequent symptom in classic migraine). Negative scotomas are also called photopsias and are considered a formed hallucination. Frequently, positive or negative scotomas coexist. Patients may also report symptoms of teichopsia with a wall of fog or steamy and wavy lines separating them from the object of regard. When the patient reports a moving positive scotoma, its direction, velocity, and duration should be recorded. For example, patients with carotid artery stenosis may report a reversible curtain coming down from above.

Visual Field Defects. Visual field defects may be noted by the patient when they are binocular, large, or interfere with specific activities. A patient with a large visual field defect may be able to note and even be annoyed by a target moving within the defective field. This ability to recognize moving but not static targets is called statico-kinetic dissociation or the Riddoch phenomenon. Although it was first thought to be a specific characteristic of occipital lobe lesions, the phenomenon has been demonstrated throughout the retrobulbar visual pathway.

Photophobia. Photophobia is an aversion to light and depends on a combination of optic and trigeminal nerve stimuli. It does not occur in blind eyes. Irritation of the eyes, nasal mucous membrane, and structures at the base of the skull can all act as stimuli. Photophobia and photopsia have been reported to coexist in optic neuropathies.

Metamorphopsia. Metamorphopsia is a distortion of vision. The most common form is micropsia and occurs in macular disease. It does not change much from day to day. Refractive surgery of the cornea may also induce distortions. Rapidly changing distortions are usually caused by diffuse disorders of visual pathway.

Entoptic Phenomena. Entoptic phenomena are flashes of light that originate in the retina, probably from direct traction by the vitreous.

Hallucinations. Visual hallucinations are experiences that have no basis in external reality. The patient with an organic hallucination (e.g., a whiskey bottle tied to the leg) may respond appropriately (e.g., "cut the whiskey bottle off my leg"), whereas the patient with schizophrenia may not. Formed hallucinations usually result from disorders involving the temporal lobes of the brain, whereas unformed hallucinations reflect occipital and parietal lobe disorders.

Acquired Reading Difficulties. Acquired reading difficulties may result from visual field defects, specific and localized disorders involving alexia, or nonspecific loss of cerebral function.

Diplopia. Diplopia may vary with time or day or use of the eyes. The most valuable clue here may be the coexistence of ptosis, which strongly suggests myasthenia gravis. Most of the slowly progressive systemic or ocular myopathies are not associated with diplopia. It is critical to determine whether the diplopia is monocular (seen with one eye or each eye independently) or binocular. It used to be thought that most monocular diplopia was caused by psychogenic factors, with a few cases resulting from intraocular conditions such as a partially dislocated lens. Now it is recognized that most of these cases are caused by problems in the optical alignment of the cornea and lens and that the patients can be shown that monocular diplopia can be eliminated by the use of a pinhole occluder. Multiple pupils or a peripheral iridectomy will not produce a second image if a normal lens is properly located within the eye or if the patient is aphakic. Patients often have difficulty in distinguishing low degrees of diplopia as such and instead describe blurring of images. Binocular diplopia results from deviation of the visual axes of the two eyes. Horizontal and vertical diplopia may interact in ways that can distract attention from the main diagnosis. For instance, a patient who should complain of vertical diplopia owing to a paralysis of the superior oblique muscle may complain of a large amplitude secondary horizontal deviation. Only when the patient is given a horizontal prism is the true diagnosis made. Cyclodeviations may also be difficult to detect when taking the history or during the examination. It is even more difficult to detect such a problem when the examiner is not thinking about the possibility of a bilateral superior oblique paresis.

Neurologic History

The review of a neurologic history and symptoms can often be brief, but it is best to have a pattern to ensure completeness. A good approach is to ask about prior neurologic and psychiatric diagnoses, then the dysfunctions of the major structural and functional groups of the nervous system, and then about neurologic and psychiatric symptom complexes such as pain, headache, seizures, and abnormalities of mental function.

Review of Cranial Nerve Symptoms

The review of neuro-ophthalmologic symptoms begins with the cranial nerves. Loss of smell is sometimes a feature of olfactory groove meningiomas or other tumors extending into the prechiasmal region, but in neuro-ophthalmologic practice, anosmia most often follows severence of the *olfactory nerves* during surgical exploration of the region of the optic chiasm. Anosmia may result from severe head trauma in the syndrome of anosmia-ageusia or, more rarely, from tumors that invade the orbit.

Trigeminal nerve symptoms or dysfunctions are frequently important. The onset and severity of anesthesia or pain of the head or face should be explored. The patient may not be aware of corneal anesthesia, but may have blurred vision from minor corneal abrasions. Alternatively, the patient may complain of a red eye and conjunctival discharge, unaware that the cornea is being injured. Numbness and parasthesia occur more frequently than pain when the preganglionic portion of the trigeminal nerve is involved at the superior orbital fissure, the cavernous sinus, or Meckel's cave. Herpes zoster is the most common disorder of the gasserian ganglion and you should enquire whether the patient has had the characteristic vesicular rash.

Pain occurring when the eyes are moved is often associated with idiopathic or demyelinating types of optic neuritis, but you should be aware that inflammation of the ethmoid or other sinuses may also be associated with pain during ocular movements. In about 20% of cadavers, the ethmoid sinus mucosa is in direct contact with the dura of the optic nerve, so that impaired vision and painful ocular movements may occur for more than one reason.

The electric shock-like pain of trigeminal neuralgia usually results from vascular compression in the root entry zone at the lateral border of the pons. More rarely, it occurs from primary demyelinating disease or tumors in this region. Trigeminal neuralgia in young women is more likely to be the result of multiple sclerosis than a premature presentation of the idiopathic variety. Pain that is not typical for tic douloureux or that cannot be ascribed to an obvious peripheral cause should be described as "atypical facial neuralgia" with the implication that repeated examinations may be required to exclude tumors invading the skull.

It is also important to remember that the first division of the trigeminal nerve projects centrally to the second or possibly lower cervical levels through its descending tract and nucleus, so that misreferral of pain can extend anywhere from the neck to the eye. Irritation of sensory nerve roots in the neck can cause eye pain. Pain from intracranial vascular structures can also be referred to the eye. Common problems causing misreferral of pain to the eye are greater occipital neuralgia, intracranial tumors, temperomandibular joint and myofacial pain syndromes, and diseases of the paranasal sinuses. Although photophobia usually results from corneal irritation, it may result from stimulation anywhere within the trigeminal distribution, particularly the nasal mucosa and the dura in the parasellar region. The greater occipital nerve (derived from the second cervical level) can become a source of neuralgia that is frequently detected by getting the patient to point with one finger to the location of the pain. The patient makes a sweeping motion from the lateral portion of the orbit backward along the parietal bone. The patient may not connect the motion to the occipital bone, so that you will have to demonstrate the local sensitivity during the physical examination. Disease of the motor branch of the nerve can result in difficulty chewing. Myofacial pain syndrome is a benign problem related to chewing. Temporomandibular joint pain is often referred to the lower portion of the orbit.

The facial nerve may give rise to numerous ocular symptoms because of impaired closure of the eyelids. The history should focus on the onset of the facial palsy, the amount of any previous recovery of function, and the degree of further recovery that is anticipated. For example, surgery for an acoustic neuroma may traumatize but not sever the facial nerve, so that the neurosurgeon may have told the patient that further recovery is expected. This information could alter your treatment. In cases where the more proximal regions of the facial nerve may be involved, you might also ask whether sounds are abnormally loud in one ear (stapedius nerve paresis) or whether tear production is deficient in one eye (greater superficial petrosal nerve paresis). The combination of trigeminal and facial nerve dysfuntion is particularly dangerous for the cornea and may cause you to follow the patient more closely.

Depending on the patient's complaints, you may wish to ask about excessive and episodic closure of the eyelids as occurs in benign essential blepharospasm, which is usually bilateral, or in hemifacial spasm, which is usually unilateral. In blepharospasm, you will wish to know whether only the eyelids or more of the face is involved. In hemifacial spasm, you need to find out whether weakness, usually of the lower facial muscles, also exists that interferes with smiling, chewing, kissing, or whistling.

The eighth cranial nerve is composed of the acoustic and vestibular nerves. Symptoms involving both nerves suggest extra-axial problems within the temporal bone or at the pontocerebellar angle. Questions concerning hearing should concentrate on whether any loss is bilateral or unilateral, whether it came on gradually or suddenly, and whether it is progressive. Tinnitus (with or without vertigo) is not a common presenting symptom in neuro-ophthalmology because these patients usually enter the health care system at other points.

If patients have vertigo, you should determine whether it is postural (resulting from standing) or positional (resulting from a change in head position). Ask whether the vertigo persists or whether it quickly fatigues. In neurologic patients with unexplained blurred vision, you may wish to ask quetions directed toward an overactive vestibulo-ocular reflex. Patients with this problem may note that their vision is blurrier in an automobile while it is moving than when it is stopped. More-

over, these patients find that they can read the labels of goods on the shelves of a grocery store much better when they stand still than when they are walking.

The caudal cranial nerves and bulbar muscles can be considered as a group. Questions concerning taste sensation have a disappointing yield, but questions concerning chewing and swallowing can be rewarding. Patients with bulbar myopathies and neuropathies often report that attempts to swallow liquids may result in water coming out of the nose. Alternatively, patients may report that solid foods such as meat or a toasted peanut butter sandwich cannot be swallowed without additional liquids. The patient is not usually a good source of information about the volume and quality of his speech, and these questions are best addressed to family members.

Review of General Neurologic Symptoms

After reviewing the cranial nerve symptoms, the sensory, motor, and autonomic symptoms are reviewed. The sensory questions are directed toward numbness and parasthesia that may have been forgotten as well as current dysfunction. If positive answers are obtained, the follow-up questions seek to localize the symptom to the peripheral nerves, a spinal cord level, or a more rostral location. The patient is asked whether there is any focal or generalized weakness. Occasionally, you will want to ask about involuntary movements, myotonia, or fasciculations. More frequently, you will want to ask about incoordination or difficulty with gait or balance. Urinary incontinence was mentioned earlier as a frequent sign of multiple sclerosis, although it may occur in a wide variety of neurologic disorders such as normal pressure hydrocephalus. Changes in menses and in sexual drive and performance should be considered because of close proximity of the neuro-endocrine structures to the optic nerves, chiasm, and tracts.

Neurologic and Psychiatric Symptom Complexes

The neurologic questionnaire may conclude with a review of neurologic and psychiatric symptom complexes such as pain, headache, seizures, and abnormalities of mental function. You may already have an opinion about the patient's memory, intelligence, and affect. If not, you may wish to explore these subjects further by asking questions about falling performance in school, in business, or in homemaking. You will probably have to initiate questions concerning illusions, hallucinations, metamorphopsia and other complex visual problems. Patients are embarrassed to bring these topics up and may fail to do so. We have seen patients with Alzheimer's disease who have enough insight to recognize that people will think that they are mentally ill if they reveal the chaotic visual world they are experiencing.

Obtaining An Unedited Prior Medical History

The prior medical history is reviewed in the usual manner but guarding against the possibility that the patient is editing the history so as to omit information such as the previous removal of a tumor of the lung, breast, or neck. The general review of symptoms is routine except that you may concentrate on the symptoms of any particular diagnosis or syndrome that have come into consideration.

Family History

Frequently, the family history is not productive and can be confusing; for example, the large number of persons with a positive family history of migraine. When the family history is positive, however, it can help to make the diagnosis and define the prognosis. The minimum question strategy is to ascertain that the patient's parents are not related except by marriage and that no other person in the family has a similar illness. Frequently, you may need to contact the physicians caring for other family members, but it is best to examine the family yourself. You can often obtain a dilated fundus examination of the parents who have brought a child to your office. Ethnic history can be valuable; for example, progressive oculopharyngeal muscular dystrophy occurs most frequently in families of French-Canadian background.

Social and Occupational History

A patient's habitual use of alcohol can give rise to alcoholic optic neuropathy, cranial nerve palsies, nystagmus, and Wernicke's encephalopathy. We have found that it is well to over-estimate the amount of alcohol that the patient may consume and use that as a basis for questioning (i.e., "Do you buy more than one bottle of whiskey a week?"). A spouse may be helpful in confirming the patient's alcohol use, unless they drink in excess together. The interviewing technique called the "CAGE questions" are many times more sensitive than the best laboratory tests in the detection of chronic alcoholism. The questions are arranged in the following order to permit the use of the mnemonic CAGE. Have you (1) felt the need to Cut down drinking?; (2) ever felt Annoyed by criticism of drinking?; (3) had a Guilty feeling about drinking?; (4) ever taken a morning Eye-opener? You should record the amount of tobacco use, although the role of tobacco in tobacco-alcohol optic neuropathy is controversial. In considering the toxic-metabolic causes of neuro-ophthalmic disorders, it may be necessary to ask about the possibility of vitamin deficiency resulting from prior surgery or other disorders of the upper gastrointestinal tract. So-called "recreational drugs" may become a source of ocular problems when they are taken intravenously.

With the recognition of acquired immune deficiency disease (AIDS), you may need to expand the social history to include questions concerning sexual preferences and multiplicity of partners.

NONOCULAR ASPECTS OF THE PHYSICAL EXAMINATION

Examination of the Head, Face, and Neck

You will find it useful to have a system for examining the head, face, and neck. Observation may be all that is necessary, although palpation and auscultation may also be required. As you begin observation, be certain that you have considered all of the devices used to hide true condition of the head. Caps must be removed. Wigs may hide alopecia, surgical scars, abnormal skin, nevi, and inflamed temporal arteries. Hair dyes or tints may mask a white forelock. Cosmetics may cover the butterfly rash of the collagen vascular diseases or the port wine stain of Sturge-Weber syndrome. In tuberous sclerosis, cosmetics may cover flat depigmented spots or elevated lesions such as the more common erythematous angiofibromas and the less common maculopapular fibromas. Lipstick may disguise the signs of Sturge-Weber syndrome, Osler-Weber-Rendu syndrome, or neurofibromatosis. Unopened lips may cover what would otherwise be obvious findings of the buccal surface, gums, teeth, and tongue in a number of neuro-ophthalmologic disorders. A high collar may hide a thickened sternocleidomastoid which turns the head in torticollis or an overacting trapezius muscle which may tilt the head in dystonia. A long neck has been noted in mental retardation syndromes, a short neck occurs as a result of malformation of the cervical vertebrae, and a webbed neck is a characteristic of Turner syndrome. A simple necklace may mask the scar of thyroid surgery or a scar that would explain a Horner syndrome. Also look for scars where tags of skin may have been removed from the external ear.

The shape and symmetry of the head can be noted, particularly with regard to the vertical midfacial line. The other important vertical lines are those through the medial and lateral canthi. The medial intercanthal distance is normally one third of the outer canthal distance. If it varies from this, hypotelorism or hypertelorism may be present and associated with a neurologic syndrome. The distance between the medial and lateral canthi is short in the fetal alcohol syndrome.

Traditionally, the face has been divided into three segments by horizontal lines at the level of the medial canthi and by diagonal lines passing from the corners of the mouth to the aural points where the most anterior portion of the upper ear connects with the face. The upper segment includes the cranium, and the lower segment includes the face. With the recent emphasis on the embryology of the neural crest-derived mesoderm, some authorities now describe the face as developing in two portions: a medial portion derived from the frontonasal process and a lateral portion derived from the branchial clefts. The medial aspects of the orbits and nose and the central portion of the upper lip arise from the neural crest.

Abnormalities of the configuration of the cranial vault can result from primary or secondary suture abnormalities. Increased intracranial pressure is the major cause of visual loss in such patients. Microcephaly and macrocephaly are recognized first by measuring the skull circumference. In the infant referred for apparent blindness, simple transillumination of the skull in a darkened room may diagnose loss of substance as occurs in hydranencephaly or congenital occlusion of the middle cerebral arteries.

Excessive amounts of hair in the eyebrows, synophrys, and excessive frontal hair are seen in infants with chromosomal and metabolic disorders. Premature frontal balding occurs in myotonic dystrophy.

The eyes, nose, and ears are the major features of the middle face. The tilt of the lid fissures is controlled by the relative growth of the first branchial arch laterally to the frontonasal process medially. Thus, the A-shaped tilt or antimongoloid slant of the eyelids frequently occurs when development of the first branchial arch is defective.

Proptosis may be bilateral or unilateral and is measured with an exophthalmometer. Enophthalmos is usually unilateral. Sometimes, an abnormally large or small globe can simulate proptosis or enophthalmos. One clue to this may be the diameter of the cornea or a high refractive error. Ultrasonography can measure the axial length of the globe without radiation to the patient. Palpation of the orbit may reveal tenderness, bony depressions, masses, crepitus, or pulsation. Palpation lateral to the orbit can be used to recognize enlarged preauricular nodes or salivary glands.

Abnormalities (particularly widening) of the proximal portion of the nose are associated with many important neuro-ophthalmologic diagnoses. You may conclude that the ears are low set if the aural points are below a line through the medial canthi and if the lowest aspects of the ear are below the bottom of the nose when the patient is viewed from the front. Such patients are likely to have developmental abnormalities of the first branchial arch. Large ear lobules occur in the mucopolysaccharidoses.

Abnormalities of the lip and palate are the most important congenital abnormalities of the lower facial segment. Their association with severe neurologic abnormalities, such as optic nerve hypoplasia, is highest if the nose is also involved and least if there is a small midline defect. Tenting of the upper lip occurs in long-standing bilateral facial weakness, as in the Möbius syndrome, and pursed lips occur in myotonic dystrophy, perhaps as an effort to keep the mouth closed. The bibliography includes several sources that are useful for identifying specific syndromes of the head, face, and mouth.

The neck may be inspected and palpated for evidence of enlargement of the thyroid gland and lymph nodes or for other abnormalities.

Auscultation of the carotid arteries or of the head may be performed. When you attempt to confirm the presence of a bruit it is best to have the patient assume the position in which he hears it. To avoid the artifact induced by movement of the eyes or eyelids, have the patient close both eyes, place the bell of the stethoscope gently over one eye, and then have the patient open the other eye. You will then be able to recognize when eye movement occurs.

Examination of the "Other" Cranial Nerves

It is difficult to make a strict division between the ophthalmologic and non-ophthalmologic portion of the neuro-ophthalmologic examination; however, it is helpful to list those aspects that may not be covered in the routine ophthalmologic examination. For example, I find it convenient to keep a packet of instant coffee in my "neurology drawer." It can easily be brought out, smelled, and replaced.

If your office routine calls for most return patients to have their vision and intraocular pressure measured prior to "routine" dilatation of the pupil, you will have to make allowances for the neuro-ophthalmologic examination. The pupils should be checked for an afferent pupillary defect, accommodation and near visual acuity may need to be determined, and corneal sensation must be tested before mydriatic, cycloplegic, and anesthetic solutions are instilled.

Trigeminal Nerve. An esthesiometer is rarely required for quantitative testing of the corneal reflex. What is most important is to avoid a response to threat rather than to corneal pain. First, place the cotton fiber on the perilimbal conjunctiva and then drag it across the limbus. The nasal response to a tickle with a cotton swab is a useful way to confirm assymmetry of trigeminal nerve function. Unilateral depression of the nasolacrimal reflex has been reported to be the only physical sign in some cases of meningioma of the temporal fossa.

Each of the three divisions of the trigeminal nerve is tested for pin and touch; and the responses are recorded, if necessary, on a diagram of the face. It is sometimes useful to test for sensation of the infraorbital nerve by lifting the lip and touching the gingiva above the canine tooth with the broken wooden portion of a cotton tip applicator. This will also allow you to identify and get above the margin of any dentures the patient may have. I find it much easier to confirm anesthesia here than on a swollen lip in a patient who has sustained an orbital floor fracture and other facial trauma. I have not found the oculo-pupillary reflex of constriction or dilatation followed by constriction to be useful in evaluating the afferent pathway. Although the corneo-mandibular reflex may occur in 10% of normal subjects, patients with supranuclear paralysis of the trigeminal nerves may have a brisk corneo-mandibular reflex of movement of the mandible away from the side of stimulation.

Chronic peripheral trigeminal weakness can produce flattening of the face above and below the zygomatic arch, while acute unilateral motor paralysis can be detected by deviation of the jaw towards the paralyzed side.

Electrophysiologic testing of the blink reflex is rarely indicated. Exceptions may include the need to confirm subjective anesthesia or to decide whether a problem is inside or outside of the brain stem (intra-axial or extra-axial). The test is performed by recording the electromyogram bilaterally from the orbicularis oculi muscles, following a unilateral stimulus given alternately to each side of the face. Normally, there will be an early, monosynaptic ipsilateral reflex and a late, polysynaptic bilateral reflex.

Facial Nerve. The function of the facial nerve fibers distal to the stylomastoid foramen can be determined by inspection. During the taking of the history, the functions of the superior and inferior groups of the facial muscles can be observed. The superior group is involved in movements of the eyebrows, forehead, scalp, and ears, whereas the inferior group is involved in smiling and other movements of the lips. Flattening of the nasolabial fold is characteristic of facial nerve weakness. The intermediate group of muscles that are responsible for tightly squeezing the eyelids must be specifically tested in the awake patient. With tight squeezing, the bases of the eyelashes should become hidden or "buried." The patient should be able to overcome the examiner's gentle effort to force the lids open. If one of the groups appears weak, you should compare the relative strength of all three groups on both the ipsilateral and contralateral sides of the face. The patient should then be asked to elevate the eyebrows, to wrinkle the nose, to show the teeth, and to whistle. In some patients with impaired cerebral functions, you may need to look for an infranuclear paresis by using a glabellar tap to test the orbicularis oculi reflex. Supranuclear palsies may dissociate the voluntary from the involuntary action of the facial muscles; thus, the nasolabial fold may be flat except when the patient is induced to smile.

Localization and electrophysiologic studies are important in the management of an idiopathic, total, or progressive Bell's palsy. Three tests can localize the problem satisfactorily in most cases. A Schirmer's test revealing a unilateral absence of reflex tear production localizes lesions proximal to the geniculate ganglion because the greater superficial petrosal nerve leaves the facial nerve at the ganglion and the bend between the horizontal and vertical portions of the facial canal. Crocodile tears or gustatory lacrimation results from misregeneration of the facial nerve following proximal lesions.

The stapedius reflex is used to test the function of the stapedius nerve, which arises just distal to the junction of the horizontal and top of the vertical portion of the facial canal. This is tested with a tympanometer in which fluid is placed in the ear and the pressure measured. A loud noise is made to provoke the stapedius reflex, and the small movement of the tympanic membrane results in a change in the pressure recorded by the tympanometer. If the stapedius reflex persists, the problem is distal to the pyramidal eminence of the mastoid bone. The clinical symptom of an absence of the stapedius reflex is the impression that sounds are too loud on the affected side. Patients with hemifacial spasm may also report relating to nonreflex stimulation of the stapedius nerve.

The third test for facial function is electrophysiologic. It involves bipolar stimulation of the facial nerve at the stylomastoid foramen. If the threshold for muscle contraction is 3.5 mamp higher on the side of the facial palsy than on the opposite side, surgical decompression of the facial canal is often performed. Usually, the loss of responsiveness to electrical testing for more than 48 hours makes it unlikely that there will be a complete recovery of function without synkinesis. Unless contraindicated, steroids are generally used in the cases of Bell's palsy that do not require surgical decompression.

One can test the function of the chorda tympani nerve to reveal the status of the facial nerve in about the middle of the vertical portion of the facial canal. Because this test is subjective, it is not as frequently used as the tests listed above. This nerve provides taste sensation to the anterior two thirds of the tongue. Cannulation of the ducts from the submandibular glands can be used to compare the reflex secretion of each side following stimulation with lemon juice.

Pain and sensory loss may accompany facial paralysis from all causes. It is important to remember that tumors invading the base of the skull can involve the cranial nerves. The cutaneous distribution of the sensory fibers of the facial nerve is represented by the Ramsay Hunt syndrome of geniculate herpes zoster. The vesicles may appear within and behind the opening of the external auditory canal on the external ear. They may also be seen on the tympanic membrane and on a small patch of skin above the tip of the mastoid.

Chronic, recurrent unilateral or bilateral swelling of the face and facial palsy occur in an idiopathic condition known as Melkersson syndrome.

Observation of abnormal movements in the distribution of the facial nerve reveals several patterns. The most frequent and least troublesome is known as benign facial myokymia. It tends to occur when a person is tired and primarily involves the eyelids. Occasionally, waves of incoordinated contractions are seen passing over the face in a more serious facial myokymia associated with pontine disorders. In recent years, it has been shown that hemifacial spasm is frequently caused by compression of the proximal portions of the facial nerve by vascular loops, particularly of the anterior inferior cerebellar artery. This produces progressive weakness of the facial nerve together with the episodic spasm. In advanced cases, the patient cannot keep food out of the buccal region, and cannot whistle or kiss. Benign essential blepharospasm and its more severe counterpart involving the entire face, the Breughel syndrome, seem to be caused by disorders of the basal ganglia and are similar to drug-induced tardive dyskinesia. There is increased interest in these disorders, partially resulting from improvements in medical and surgical therapy.

Vestibuloacoustic Nerve. The *vestibuloacoustic nerve* has two divisions, which share the proximal portion of the internal auditory canal with the facial nerve. Thus, any patient with facial nerve findings should at least have a minimal examination of hearing function and at most have formal audiometry and electronystagmography.

Hearing. Hearing is more easily examined than vestibular function. A tuning fork is used to determine whether the patient has equal hearing in each ear. The C tuning fork is used. It is preferable to use the 512-Hz tuning fork to the 256-Hz tuning fork, which can be felt to vibrate as well as to be heard. The Weber test is used to determine whether one ear has impaired bone conduction from the tympanic membrane to the cochlea or whether one ear has impaired perception owing to abnormalities of cochlear apparatus and nerve. The vibrating tuning fork is placed in the center of the forehead, and the patient indicates the ear that hears best. The louder sound is heard on the affected side in conductive deafness and on the unaffected side in perceptive deafness. In the Rinne test, the vibrating tuning fork is placed against the mastoid process until the patient no longer hears it; it is then placed in air near the ear, where it should be heard about twice as long, unless the patient has conductive deafness. Other tests of hearing require an audiologist.

Vestibular Function. Vestibular function testing is performed for different purposes. For example, caloric stimulation can be used to demonstrate unilateral vestibular nerve dysfunction, if it is assumed that the brain stem and ocular motor system are intact, or to demonstrate brain stem function, assuming the vestibular nerve is intact. The details of these tests will not be described here except to point out that irrigation of the external auditory canal in a patient with a basilar skull fracture and blood in the canal may contribute to intracranial infection. Irrigation should not be performed when there is a defect in the tympanic membrane.

The other tests of vestibulo-ocular function that I perform most often are (1) observation of spontaneous nystagmus with Frenzel's (+ 30 Diopter) spectacles; (2) determination of whether the patient can use the smooth pursuit system to visually suppress the vestibulo-ocular reflex; and (3) demonstration of positional and postural nystagmus. The Frenzel lenses are used primarily when nystagmus is suspected but cannot be observed owing to visual suppression. The ophthalmoscope is an al-

ternative way to observe spontaneous nystagmus. The examiner focuses the light on the optic disk and has the patient use the opposite eye to look at a target. The opposite eye is then covered and the spontaneous movements of the first eye can be observed as magnified by the ophthalmoscope.

The vestibulo-ocular reflex is tested by placing the patient in an examining chair that can rotate or in a wheel chair. The patient is given a fixation target suspended about 25 cm in front of his eyes and arranged so that it will rotate with his head. A metal coat hanger may be compressed so that it will fit around the head and a piece of tape placed over the hook which is bent at right angles to its usual position. The tape makes the wire of the tip thick enough to constitute an easily seen target. The vestibulo-oculo reflex is induced by rotating the patient about 30° to one side, waiting at least 5 seconds and then rotating him in the opposite direction. The patient should be able to keep his eyes on the target. If there were no target moving with the head and the vestibulo-ocular reflex (VOR) gain were normal, the eyes would move an equal amount opposite the direction of the head movement. Disorders of the vestibulocerebellar connections increase VOR gain in the horizontal plane, whereas disorders of the median longitudinal fasciculus decrease VOR gain in the vertical plane. Thus, if a patient shakes his head faster than once per second while attempting to read a near vision chart, he may lose several lines of acuity. This test must be done with both horizontal and vertical head shaking. It requires an electronystagmography laboratory to measure VOR gain, but the 2 tests described can tell whether vision stimuli can cancel out the gain.

Positional nystagmus is tested using the Barany-Nylen maneuver, having the patient sitting on an examining table. The head is turned 45° toward the right shoulder and rapidly guided over the edge of the table so that the head hangs at a 45° angle from the table and the eyes are observed. Frenzel lenses may be used. Nystagmus may appear after a 10-second latent period. While the patient gazes toward the down-turned ear, predominantly rotary eye movements will result; while the patient gazes toward the upturned ear, predominantly vertical movements occur. Repeated testing usually fatigues the nystagmus in benign paroxysmal positional vertigo, which seems to be caused by dysfunction of the posterior semicircular canal. Failure to fatigue may indicate a posterior fossa lesion. The test must also be performed with the head turned left. Postural nystagmus may be observed when the patient suddenly rises from a recumbent position to a sitting or standing position.

Bony fistulas of the semicircular canals can produce oculomotor symptoms. The response to auditory stimuli is known as Tullio's phenomenon; the response to air pressure is known as Hennebert's sign.

Tests of vestibulospinal function may also test the cerebellar systems and the spinal tracts. The tests I can perform conveniently in an office setting include (1) the Romberg test (performed with the shoes off, feet together, and the eyes closed), (2) walking toward a target (for convenience, I follow this with the tandem walk test), and (3) a past pointing test. The past pointing test consists of requesting that the patient's finger be repeatedly moved between the examiner's finger and the patient's nose. The examiner's finger is kept at arm's length and is moved into each direction of gaze.

Caudal Cranial Nerves. The neuro-ophthalmologic examination may include an assessment of the caudal cranial nerves. It is not practical to test taste sensation on the posterior third of the tongue. The pharyngeal motor functions of the glossopharyngeal and vagus nerves are tested primarily by observing for deviation of the uvula to one side while the patient attempts to say "ah," or by demonstating loss of the gag reflex. Bilateral vagal paralysis is accompanied by loss of speech and difficulty swallowing. The distinction between a bulbar (infranuclear) palsy and a pseudobulbar (supranuclear) palsy is made on the basis of the absence or presence of a gag reflex.

The laryngeal function of the vagus nerve is best demonstrated by direct laryngoscopy, which should be performed if the patient is hoarse. There is a small sensory representation in the external auditory canal and auricular concha. Loss of vagus function may cause a tachycardia not responsive to carotid sinus compression or the oculocardiac reflex.

The accessory nerve supplies both the sternocleidomastoid and the upper portion of the trapezius muscles. Both muscles are affected by lesions at the jugular foramen, but the most common injuries to the nerve occur more distally and spare the sternocleidomastoid.

The hypoglossal nerves supply the tongue muscles. Obvious atrophy of one side of the tongue follows hypoglossal-facial anastomoses. More subtle bilateral involvements occur in disorders of the cranial base or in syringobulbia.

Examination of Muscles, Motor Functions, and Reflexes

It is not my goal in this chapter to describe a complete neurologic examination, but to describe what I actually do with some patients. If I am concerned about a myopathy, I will look carefully at the gag reflex for loss of function of the pharyngeal muscles. There may be a droopy appearance without sharp angles. I would then look for weakness of the neck and proximal muscles of the arms and legs. The hands are inspected for atrophy and tested for strength. If myotonic dystrophy is suspected, you will want to test for percussion myotonia of the thenar eminence. The calves and the feet can be inspected while examining the deep tendon reflexes. The plantar reflex is examined and recorded. The heel-shin test of coordination may be conveniently performed at this point. The examination is adjusted and motor milestones recorded if the patient is an infant.

Examination of Sensation

A basic examination of touch, pin, and vibratory sensations can be performed while the patient has his shoes and stockings removed. Grafesthesia can also be tested.

Examination of Mental Functions

By this point in the examination, you should have a good grasp of the patient's mental function and should record any abnormalities. Formal testing of orientation, memory, or ability to calculate is rarely needed. You may want to ask again about recurrent ideas or abnormal sensory experiences.

General Observations

Although you may wish to refer the patient for a "complete physical examination," you may wish to selectively pursue a few leads at this time. I have found that some of the most rewarding efforts include (1) looking at prior photographs of the patient, (2) completely undressing infants to look for other congenital abnormalities, (3) examining the skin and nails, (4) listening for cardiac murmurs, and (5) observing the patient suspected of malingering after he believes that the examination is completed.

BIBLIOGRAPHY

Aronson, A.E. (ed.): Clinical Examinations in Neurology; by Members of the Department of Neurology and the Department of Physiology and Biophysics; Mayo Clinic, 4th Ed. Philadelphia, W.B. Saunders, 1976.

Dyken, P.R., and Miller, M.D.: Facial Features of Neurologic Syndromes. St. Louis, C.V. Mosby, 1980.

Ewing, J.A.: Detecting alcoholism: The CAGE questionnaire. J. Am. Med. Assoc. 252:1905, 1984.

Fraunfelder, F.T.: Drug-induced Ocular Side Effects and Drug Interactions, 2nd Ed. Philadelphia, Lea & Febiger, 1982.

Gorlin, R.J., and Pindborg, J.J.: Syndromes of the Head and Neck, 2nd Ed. New York, McGraw-Hill, 1976.

Grant, W.M.: Toxicology of the Eye: Drugs, Chemicals, Plants, Venoms, 2nd Ed. Springfield, IL, Charles C Thomas, 1974.

Hammerschlag, S.B., Hesselink, J.R., and Weber, A.L.: Computed Tomography of the Eye and Orbit. Norwalk, CT, Appleton-Century-Crofts, 1983.

Karp, J.S.: Functional disease in neuro-ophthalmology. Int. Ophthalmol. Clin. 17(1):157, 1977.

Leigh, R.J., and Zee, D.S.: The Neurology of Eye Movement. Philadelphia, F.A. Davis, 1983.

Newman, N.M.: The prechiasmal afferent visual pathways. Int. Ophthalmol. Clin. 17(1):27, 1977.

Safron, A.B., Kline, L.B., and Glaser, J.S.: Positive visual phenomenon in optic nerve and chiasmal disease: photopsias and photophobia.In Neuro-ophthalmology. Edited by J.S. Glaser. St. Louis, C.V. Mosby, 1980.

Samil, M., and Jannetta, P.J. (eds.): The Cranial Nerves. Berlin, Springer-Verlag, 1981.

Wirtschafter, J.D., and Taylor, S.: Computed Tomography: An Atlas for Ophthalmologists. San Francisco, American Academy of Ophthalmology, 1982.

Chapter 2

Papilledema

THOMAS J. WALSH

In this chapter, the term papilledema is used to describe disc edema associated with increased intracranial pressure. The term papillitis is used to describe inflammations of the optic nerve associated with a decrease in vision or field. All other swellings of the disc are referred to as disc edema.

Ophthalmologists are frequently asked whether a disc is edematous and, if it is, whether the cause of the edema is increased intracranial pressure. The decision to call a disc edematous often is based on the presence of a combination of signs rather than on any one specific sign. To illustrate, a disc may be blurred (owing to drusen) and have a flame-shaped hemorrhage associated with it. The association of drusen and hemorrhage is recognized although rare, and a diagnosis of papilledema should not be made merely because hemorrhage is present. Frequently, a disc may be grossly edematous but not because of increased intracranial pressure—hemorrhage and marked nerve-head edema may be seen in cases of severe hypertension or venous occlusive disease.

Thus, it is the responsibility of the ophthalmologist to decide first whether the signs are of true papilledema or of pseudopapilledema and then whether a diagnostic workup is indicated. If he diagnoses the condition as disc edema, the ophthalmologist must then decide whether it is secondary to increased intracranial pressure or to one of the other conditions that give a similar appearance. This last decision is as important as the first ones since certain tests are pertinent to specific diagnoses and mistakes may cause delay in instituting proper treatment or may cause the patient to undergo unnecessary, expensive, or dangerous tests.

FUNDUS SIGNS OF PAPILLEDEMA

Hyperemia

This disorder is caused by capillary dilatation in the nerve head. The age of the patient must be taken into consideration since the color of the disc varies with age. In the infant, the disc frequently is pale and hyperemia is more easily seen, whereas in the young or middle-aged adult, the disc is frequently pink to hyperemic in appearance. In the person 70 years of age or older, the disc color is more waxy, and hyperemia is more noticeable when it occurs. Hyperopic discs look more hyperemic, whereas myopic discs appear paler, particularly in the temporal sector.

17

Venous Distention

An impression of an increase in diameter of the retinal veins may be spurious. If the observer uses only the arteriovenous ratio as an index, he is assuming that the arterial size is normal; however, the arteriovenous ratio may be increased because of decreased arterial size, such as in hypertension. Venous distention may also be seen in conditions that cause increased venous pressure and slowing or swelling of the blood column. If these signs are present, consideration should be given to the possibility of diabetes, dysproteinemias, glaucoma, or vascular shunts with increased venous pressure, as in carotid cavernous sinus fistula.

Retinal veins may be enlarged because of increased shunting of blood, as in arteriovenous fistula in the orbit or the cavernous sinus. If either type of fistula is present, bruits or pulsations of the globe may be present. The pulsations of the globe may not be easily seen on external inspection, but they can be readily observed if the fundus is examined with an ophthalmoscope. The subtle pulsation is manifested by a sharpness and then blurring of focus of the retina that is synchronous with the pulse at the wrist.

In diagnosing diabetes, a formal glucose tolerance test must be performed, not just a random blood glucose evaluation. A carotid cavernous sinus fistula has the clinical signs of ocular bruits, pulsations of the globe, ophthalmoplegia, hypalgesia of the first division of the fifth cranial nerve, and evidence of venous distention of the lids, orbit (exophthalmos), and external surfaces of the globe.

Filling in of the Optic Cup

Since the presence or absence of a cup, as well as its size, varies from patient to patient, its absence is difficult to ascribe to edema unless the patient's cup size was determined in a previous examination. The fundus contact lens is of little value in distinguishing between absence of the cup and filling in of the cup by edema.

Blurring of Disc Margin

This sign is more difficult to detect in the hyperopic eye than in the myopic eye, in which a choroidal pigment line frequently demarcates the disc margin; however, blurring always begins on the nasal margin. If the temporal margin is more blurred, a local process, such as juxtapapillary choroiditis or a tumor, should be suspected. Since the degree of blurring may look much different with the indirect ophthalmoscope than with the direct one, both instruments should be used in the evaluation.

Paton's Lines

Recognition of Paton's lines (Plate 2-IA) is difficult only because it is a subtle sign that will probably be missed if the observer does not specifically check for it. It is one of the surest signs of true disc edema. The lines appear only on the temporal side of the disc and are in a vertical direction concentric with the disc. As the disc swells, a slight displacement of the retina away from the temporal edge of the disc occurs, causing the retina to fold on itself, or corrugate. This folding, in turn, causes a variation of the reflection from the internal limiting membrane, which is seen as Paton's lines. As the edema increases, this area becomes edematous and Paton's lines are no longer seen. Any cause of edema can produce Paton's lines, so that their presence signifies only edema. It is not seen with such entities as drusen of the nerve head. The appearance of horizontal lines in the macula, on the other hand, signifies tumors of the muscle cone, thyroid disease, or brawny scleritis.

Edema may also spread from the disc along the arcuate fibers, making them more prominent. This appearance is not a clear-cut sign of edema; it may be seen also in cases of mild myelination of the fibers, which is difficult to differentiate from edema.

Spontaneous Venous Pulse

Many people do not have a spontaneous venous pulse at times, an absence that is frequently normal. It has been shown experimentally, however, that, when the spinal fluid pressure reaches 200 mm of spinal fluid or water, the venous pulse disappears. It has been my experience that this is a reliable sign. Other investigators, such as Williamson-Noble, Hayreh, and Levin, have evaluated this concept and found it to be not only experimentally but clinically valid. The most recent clinical review of the subject was by Levin who reviewed 33 patients with increased intracranial pressure. Van Uitert and Eisenstadt in commenting on Levin's experience disagree that the presence of a venous pulse rules out significantly increased intracranial pressure. In their comments they site 4 cases of their own in which there was a spontaneous venous pulse at the same time as they measured a significantly increased intracranial pressure. All previous reports of such an occurrence have been anecdotal and not supported by simultaneous fundus observation and spinal fluid pressure measurements. No test in medicine is perfect or without exceptions; however, given the surrounding clinical facts, the presence of venous pulse is one more piece of evidence to support the clinical diagnosis of no significantly increased intracranial pressure above 200 mm of spinal fluid. It is a clinical sign that has been valuable to me over the years and I will continue to use it in my evaluation of a swollen disc.

Although some observers consider a light touch to bring out the pulse valid, I do not think it advisable since it might introduce a significant error. Since the lightness of the touch is an unknown quantity and since intraocular pressure is measured in millimeters of mercury and not of water, the touch introduces an error of 13.5 to 1 for each millimeter of digital increase in ocular pressure. A collapsing of the vein, even if incomplete, is the sign to be observed (rather than a moving of the vessel caused by adjacent arterial pulsations). Collapsing of the vein is best seen deep in the disc or as the vein crosses the disc margin.

Deflection of Vessels

The location of vessels coming off the disc into the vitreous and then back to the level of the retina is not an unusual anomaly. It does not represent papilledema because the disc can be seen at a different level from the elevated vessels. The presence of vessels elevated by a swollen disc, however, suggests papilledema.

Hemorrhages and Exudates

The presence or absence of hemorrhages does not indicate either the cause or severity of the edema. If the hemorrhages are caused by increased intracranial pressure, their quantity does not change the gravity of the condition. A small number of hemorrhages should not provide a sense of security.

Certain types or locations of hemorrhages and exudates, however, may be of diagnostic help. Disc edema associated with hemorrhages and exudates that are not only located at the posterior pole but also found all the way out to the equator suggest hypertension rather than papilledema. Exudate in the macular, such as a macular star, has no etiologic significance but denotes chronicity (Plate 2-IB). If hemorrhage is an overwhelming feature and the veins are engorged, central retinal vein obstruction is more likely. Hemorrhage located in the subhyaloid area, particularly over the disc or macula, suggests a subarachnoid hemorrhage such as results from a ruptured cerebral aneurysm (Fig. 2–1).

Hemorrhages with white centers are called Roth's spots. They suggest septic embolization, leukemia, lupus erythematosus, or pernicious anemia.

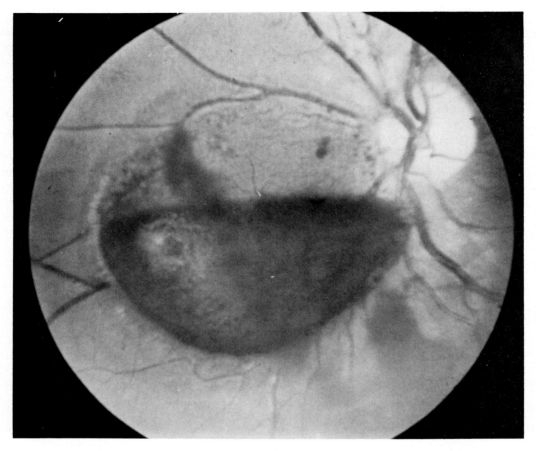

Fig. 2–1. Preretinal hemorrhage. The hemorrhage is preretinal, accounting for the disappearance of the superficial retinal vessels as they approach it.

Vision Changes

The rule is that disc edema with a loss of vision signifies optic neuritis and that papilledema with normal vision signifies increased intracranial pressure, but this rule does not always hold. Occasionally, optic neuritis occurs with good visual acuity. One of the signs of optic neuritis is the afferent pupillary defect (Marcus Gunn pupillary escape phenomenon), which indicates damage to the conduction system. Axial optic neuritis with a central scotoma and full peripheral field is the common defect, but field defects with good visual acuity can also occur.

Loss of acuity can occur with papille-dema or disc edema from any cause when hemorrhages occur in the macula, as in hypertension, or in the subhyaloid area, with subarachnoid hemorrhages. Long-standing increased intracranial pressure may cause decompensation of the optic nerve, with resulting loss of acuity. This decompensation is one complication of prolonged pseudotumor cerebri and one of the principal reasons for surgical intervention when medical therapy fails.

Cells in the Vitreous Humor

In cases of papillitis or of retrobulbar optic neuritis in close proximity to the globe, cells can occasionally be seen in front of the disc. This phenomenon is detected only with the fundus contact lens and is rarely seen even when expected. Cells can appear in the vitreous humor as a result of other inflammatory conditons, but they are not as discrete or as localized as in papillitis or retrobulbar optic neuritis.

Height of the Disc Edema

The referring physician frequently requests information about the height of the disc edema. Unfortunately, the information causes more problems than it solves because of the misplaced emphasis that some people put, for example, on 1 diopter of elevation as opposed to 5 diopters, as if the urgency regarding hospitalization and diagnostic tests varied with the height of the edema. Once the diagnosis of papilledema is made, prompt hospitalization and evaluation are mandatory, because of the increased intracranial pressure.

When measuring the degree of disc edema, the observer measures from the highest part of the edematous disc down to the normal nonedematous retina. The difference in dioptic power is read on the ophthalmoscope. If one is to record disc edema in millimeters of elevation, 2 diopters of disc elevation denote 1 mm of elevation in the phakic person, and 3 diopters of disc elevation denote 1 mm of elevation in an aphakic person.

Optociliary Shunt Vessels

Optociliary shunt vessels in association with poor vision or blindness and pale disc edema are highly suggestive of the diagnosis of anterior optic nerve sheath meningioma. They have also been reported in association with optic disc drusen, central retinal vein obstruction, arachnoid cysts, gliomas, and coloboma of the optic nerve.

The reason for the development of venous shunt vessels may be increased pressure in the optic nerve sheath. The relationship of pressure in the sheath to disc edema was shown by Hayreh in his experimental work on monkeys. When he incised 1 optic nerve sheath in monkeys with

increased intracranial pressure, the disc edema resolved only on that side. The other side maintained the papilledema when the intracranial pressure was maintained at pre-operative levels. A clinical report on 2 patients by Perlmutter seems to support this finding. These 2 patients had pseudotumor cerebri and developed optociliary shunt vessels. In 1 of the patients, 1 optic nerve was decompressed; within 3 days, the disc edema disappeared and the shunt vessels were markedly reduced. This is in keeping with the results in the monkey experiments by Hayreh.

NONFUNDUS SIGNS OF PAPILLEDEMA
Enlargement of the Blind Spot

Measuring the blind spot may be difficult either because the patient may not be fully conscious or because it is the first field examination of a neuro-ophthalmologic patient, who may be frightened or confused and thus not completely cooperative. The blind spot may even be enlarged before any gross evidence of edema of the disc appears. Enlargement of the blind spot is not an entirely dependable sign of early papilledema since the enlargement in itself may not be pathologic, as can be seen in patients who are slow responders or who want to be extra sure of their observations. The pathologic cause of the enlargement is twofold: (1) the slight displacement of the retina away from the disc, which also causes Paton's lines, and (2) a slight serous detachment of the retina away from the choriocapillaris, causing a relative scotoma of the overlying sensory retina.

Transient Obscurations

The patient with transient obscurations frequently does not mention them. Transient obscurations differ from amaurosis fugax in duration. Transient obscurations last 10 to 15 seconds and are often mistakenly ascribed to other causes, such as dirty eyeglasses or tears. By the time the patient wipes his glasses or clears the tears from his eye, the phenomenon is over. The physician should ask the patient whether he has episodes of bilateral blurring or graying out of vision. The cause of this symptom is obscure, but its significance is not. It is always related to increased intracranial pressure, and not to any other cause of disc edema. During the blurring episodes, no visible fundus change occurs. Increasing obscurations are a forewarning of decompensation of the optic nerve, which may lead to blindness.

Pupillary Abnormalities

When disease affects the conducting mechanism of one optic nerve, the afferent pupillary defect may be present. It may be caused by optic neuritis, vascular disease of the optic nerve, tumor, or any other optic nerve lesion.

Increased intracranial pressure, on the other hand, causes no direct pupillary signs. Supratentorial masses, however, as they encroach on the tentorial notch, compress the third cranial nerve and cause pupillary abnormalities. The abnormality may vary from a slightly dilated and/or sluggish pupil, at one end of the spectrum, to a fixed maximally dilated pupil, at the other.

In supratentorial tumor herniation, an ipsilateral pupillary abnormality is often associated with contralateral motor signs owing to cerebral peduncle compression. Occasionally, the pupillary and motor signs are ipsilateral, owing to cross-compression of the other cerebral peduncle, producing a Kernohan notch syndrome. This syndrome sometimes causes confusion in determining on which side the lesion is located. A good rule of thumb is to trust the pupil to point out the appropriate side.

Lateral Rectus Muscle Weakness

A frank lateral rectus muscle weakness is a helpful sign of increased intracranial pressure. The sign of divergence insuffi-

ciency, or increasing esophoria at distance, is equally important. If a decision concerning a papilledema cannot be made, measure and record the patient's muscle balance for distance. Ask the patient to return in a week, and, at his next visit, repeat the test. A significant shift toward the esophoric side suggests a lateral rectus muscle weakness. This change may be from an exophoria to a zero measurement or from zero or esophoria to a marked esophoria measurement.

The onset of apparent bilateral symmetric lateral rectus muscle weakness may signal the syndrome of divergence paralysis rather than increased intracranial pressure. The clinical feature that suggests the first diagnosis is the complete symmetry of the measurements in all fields of gaze and full ductions. Evidence is increasing that divergence paralysis is a variation of bilateral sixth nerve paresis rather than supranuclear involvement of a divergence center. In children, however, a bilateral sixth cranial nerve weakness may reflect an intrinsic pontine tumor, such as a glioma. The strabismus in this condition is not concomitant and ductions are not full.

State of Consciousness

The patient's level of consciousness is a nonspecific sign. Consciousness may be altered in any disease that affects cerebral metabolism, a category that includes most causes of increased intracranial pressure, with the notable exception of pseudotumor cerebri. Significantly increased intracranial pressure, however, does not always cause changes in consciousness, whereas hypertensive encephalopathy frequently does.

Headache

This symptom is also nonspecific. It can be related to increased intracranial pressure, or it can be a symptom of associated tension or anxiety. One feature of headache, however, is specific to increased intracranial pressure. When the intracranial pressure is increased, such as with Valsalva

PLATE 2–I

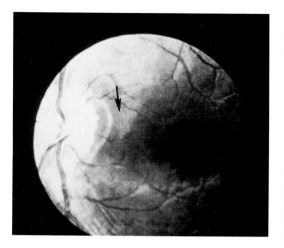

Fig. A. Paton's lines. The lines appear as several concentric reflexes seen on the temporal side of the disc and extending considerably above and below it.

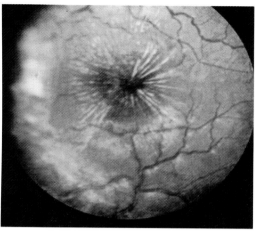

Fig. B. Macular star. Denotes long-standing increased intracranial pressure and not any one cause.

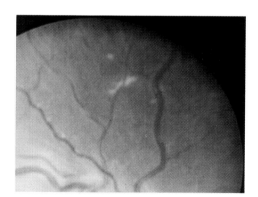

Fig. C. Roth spots. The hemorrhage is flame-shaped owing to its location in the nerve fiber layer, and it has a small, white center of malignant or inflammatory cells.

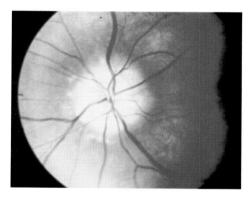

Fig. D. Drusen. These excrescences can be seen as isolated refractile bodies in the substance of the disc.

PLATE 2–II

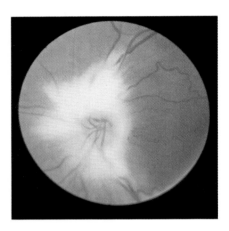

Fig. A. Medullated nerve fibers. The appearance is one of uniform whiteness, with an irregular, feathery, sharp border.

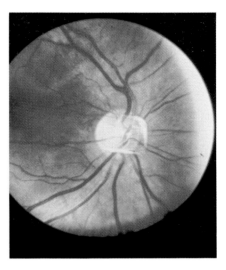

Fig. B. Epipapillary membrane. A normal variant of the resorption of the hyaloid artery complex.

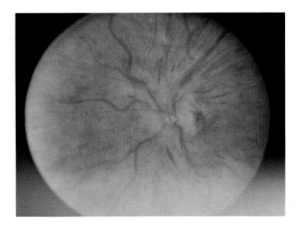

Fig. C. Hypertensive retinopathy. Attenuated arteries and papilledema are more prominent than hemorrhages, whereas the reverse is seen in central retinal vein occlusion.

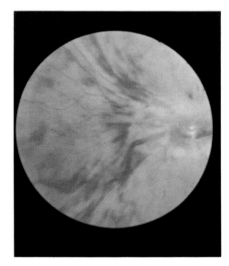

Fig. D. Central retinal vein occlusions. Hemorrhage is the most prominent feature, with papilledema only a secondary aspect.

maneuver, the headache becomes worse. Vascular headaches are frequently improved by Valsalva maneuver, and tension headaches are not affected at all.

PSEUDOPAPILLEDEMA

Drusen

These excrescences (Plate 2-ID) are a frequent cause of blurred disc, particularly in children. The drusen may cause enlarged blind spots, as well as other field defects, most commonly, inferonasally. Drusen may be buried deep in the disc and not easily seen in children, especially when the ophthalmoscope light is shined directly on the disc. Shining the light at the edge of the disc causes retro-illumination of the disc structures and frequently makes the yellow crystalline body more visible. Diagnosis is made more difficult when hemorrhages occur with the drusen.

Drusen tend to be less of a diagnostic problem in patients in their late teens and older, perhaps because with the patient's age the drusen increase in number or migrate forward in the disc and become more visible. Examining the pediatric patient's parents or older siblings for evidence of drusen may be helpful in identifying a familial tendency.

Kamin reported two children with decreased vision secondary to optic nerve drusen. This loss of vision is extremely rare in children since most of us see this problem in that age group as part of the differential diagnosis of a blurred disc rather than as loss of vision. Drusen have always been regarded as a curiosity of ophthalmoscopy for the most part. Our understanding of the pathology of drusen has been radically changed by the work of Spencer and Tso. Their work on the role of axoplasmic transport in the production of papilledema and drusen has radically changed our thinking. Although drusen uncommonly cause symptomatic defects, they are not all that benign. Of 38 eyes studied by Newman, using red free fundus

photography, 75% had abnormal fields and 97.2% had an abnormal appearance to the nerve fiber layer. The most interesting finding was an abnormal VEP response in 97.2% of the study.

When losses of vision and field occur, drusen may be even more difficult to accept as the only cause of disc blurring. If only one eye is involved, other causes must be evaluated to rule out the possibility that a retrobulbar tumor is compressing the nerve and causing loss of vision and field. If both eyes have loss of vision and field, the diagnosis is easier since field loss in both eyes does not fit into a recognized neurologic picture. However, a suprachiasmatic mass should be considered and evaluated with special studies, such as roentgenograms of the sella turcica, and computerized tomography (CT).

The computerized scan has essentially replaced the air study. This is even more true today with the use of contrast material and thinner computer scan slices.

Hemorrhages associated with drusen are occasionally seen by ophthalmologists. They may occur more frequently than we suspect because they usually produce no symptoms recognizable to the patient and, therefore, are not seen by a physician at the time they occur. Drusen as the cause of a hemorrhage on or near the disc has been reported many times and is a well-recognized entity. Sanders, Gay, and Newman divided hemorrhages associated with drusen into three classes because they felt that each had a different significance in regard to sequelae. The hemorrhages in the first group occur in the superficial nerve fiber layer. They rarely cause symptoms but can cause field defects that resolve. Vitreous hemorrhages cause a more dramatic loss of vision, particularly if they occur anterior to the fovea. These usually also resolve unless vitreous complications occur. The hemorrhages in the last group occur in association with optic nerve drusen and choroidal neovascularization. Patients with this type of hemorrhage have acute visual symptoms and seek consultation. Henkind and Wise felt that this group with neovascularization would develop permanent visual loss and require vigorous treatment. Harris, however, recently reported on 4 patients (7 eyes) with drusen, hemorrhage, and subpigment epithelial neovascularization. All but 1 of these 7 patients did well with no treatment. The follow-up evaluation ranged from 1 to 10 years. It would seem that this group of hemorrhages associated with drusen and a choroidal neovascular membrane should be looked at more seriously even though they also appear to have an excellent prognosis.

It is still true that over all, drusen of the optic disc is a benign ophthalmoscopic finding; however, in view of the new reports on changes in the nerve fiber layer, VEP, and complications associated with neovascular membranes, more cautious observation is indicated in anyone with optic nerve drusen.

Myelination of Nerve Fibers

For the ophthalmologist, who sees myelination of the nerve fibers from time to time, the anomaly is not usually a problem in the differential diagnosis of papilledema. The condition is caused by myelination that has continued past the lamina cribrosa on to the retina itself, but usually does not cover the entire disc (Plate 2-IIA). The appearance of the myelin is white and solid, with an irregular feathery border, as opposed to the appearance of an edematous disc, which blends into the surrounding retina.

The myelin may extend along the arcuate fibers to a lesser degree, giving the appearance of edema in the fibers. The only field defect that may occur is enlargement of the blind spot. Myelination does not cause the other signs of papilledema. If they are present, another process must also be considered.

Since the presence of myelin is presumed to depend on the integrity of a healthy axon, the reverse should also be true. The disappearance of myelin would be expected to occur if optic atrophy of these axons occurs. This combination of events is rare and it is even rarer to have the before and after pictures to document such an event. Schachat and Miller recently reported such a case in a man with anterior ischemic optic neuropathy. Therefore, patients with myelinated fibers should have them photographically documented. If they return with visual complaints, the appearance of early disc atrophy may be masked by the white appearance of the disc owing to the myelin. The reduction in the extent of the myelinated fibers may be the only early diagnostic sign. Myelinated fibers otherwise cause no clinical signs or symptoms, such as optic nerve drusen can.

Glial Veil

This sign is frequently seen in any ophthalmologic practice, and is rarely mistaken for papilledema. However, if the atrophy of the hyaloid artery system is incomplete and the epipapillary membrane in front of the disc is dense enough, it may obscure the disc structures and be misinterpreted as disc edema (Plate 2–IIB).

Papilledema of Hyperopia

This condition is usually seen in children who have moderate hyperopia—in the range of 3 diopters or more. No enlargement of the blind spot occurs; and none of the other signs of true papilledema, such as enlargement of veins, are present. It must be remembered that the presence of pseudopapilledema does not eliminate the possibility that the patient has true papilledema from other causes.

CAUSES OF PAPILLEDEMA AND DISC EDEMA

Hypertension

The disc edema caused by group 4 hypertension and that caused by increasing intracranial pressure appear essentially the same. The problem arises in trying to differentiate increased intracranial pressure with secondary hypertension from group 4 hypertension with papilledema and hypertensive encephalopathy. The papilledema secondary to increased intracranial pressure is limited to the posterior pole, whereas that caused by hypertension is accompanied by marked hypertensive changes that extend to the peripheral retina (Plate 2–IIC).

Subarachnoid Hemorrhage

A small group of patients with papilledema have preretinal hemorrhages that may be located in front of the disc or the macula (Fig. 2–1). This type of hemorrhage in adults almost always indicates subarachnoid hemorrhage. In infants, it suggests subdural hemorrhage. If the hemorrhage is located in front of the macula, it causes a severe decrease in vision. Unless it breaks into the vitreous humor, however, it will be absorbed and previous vision will return.

Intraocular hemorrhages secondary to subarachnoid hemorrhage occur in about 20% of patients. The presence of these hemorrhages is highly significant in predicting the mortality rate from ruptured aneurysms. The mortality rate is about 60% when fundus hemorrhages are present versus 27% when they are absent, as reviewed by Manschot, Richardson and Hyland, and Fahmy.

Mechanisms for the production of fundus and optic nerve sheath hemorrhages have been put forward by Ballantyne, Walsh and Hedges, and Muller and Deck. Some authors, like Ballantyne, felt the hemorrhages were caused by venous obstruction owing to increased intracranial pressure on intracranial venous structures, draining the eye and orbit. Walsh and Hedges felt that the cause was intracranial pressure transmitted to orbital structures. Muller evaluated 46 eyes, their orbits and optic canals, in patients with increased intracranial pressure; 87% had optic nerve sheath hemorrhage and 37% had intraocu-

lar hemorrhages. In this study, Muller and Deck concluded that orbital hemorrhages came from optic nerve sheath vessels. These hemorrhages probably do not result from increased intracranial pressure being transmitted to the orbital venous structures. Also, any increased orbital venous pressure can be dissipated by alternate venous drainage into the facial and pterygoid vessels. These two facts militate against optic nerve sheath hemorrhages resulting from intracranial subarachnoid blood being pushed into the optic nerve sheath. Hemorrhages can be found on the optic nerve sheath in cases of increased intracranial hemorrhage without subarachnoid hemorrhage. These hemorrhages in the nerve sheath occur predominantly in the subdural rather than the subarachnoid space. Muller and Deck believed that the hemorrhages in the sheath may be caused by the rupture of pial vessels when the sheath is rapidly expanded during a sudden severe rise of intracranial pressure.

Muller and Deck stated that intraocular hemorrhages have a different mechanism. These hemorrhages result from sudden increases in venous ocular pressure at a level in the nerve that precludes its dissipation by alternate drainage into the facial and pterygoid vessel systems.

Vitreous hemorrhages in subarachnoid hemorrhage were first described by Terson. Vitreous hemorrhages in this clinical setting are rare. They may occur initially as large hemorrhages breaking out into the vitreous or secondarily from a subhyaloid hemorrhage that subsequently breaks the posterior vitreous face and invades the vitreous body. Hemorrhages of this magnitude represent even more serious consequences from the intracranial disease than just preretinal hemorrhages. If the patient survives, the vitreous hemorrhage will clear, which may take up to a year.

Subhyaloid hemorrhage may occur from neovascularization of the retina, such as in diabetes, or from the neovascularization following a central retinal vein occlusion.

The retinal diagnostic clues in diabetes, such as the exudates, are readily seen. In an old central retinal vein occlusion, the vein looks white, with vessels sprouting from the site of the obstruction.

Central Retinal Vein Occlusion

The predominant picture in central retinal vein occlusion (Plate 2-IID) is one of blood, not edema or exudate. The branch retinal vein occlusions are more readily diagnosed by those unfamiliar with the fundus picture because the hemorrhages are limited to one quadrant of the retina.

The decrease in visual acuity associated with central retinal vein occlusion is usually marked and rapid in onset. This decrease in acuity is not seen with increased intracranial pressure, except over a long period of time and with a gradual onset. The disc in central retinal vein occlusion is plethoric. The disc in papilledema with vision loss shows a gliotic grayish appearance with white sheathing of the vessels. Papillophlebitis as initially described by Lyle and Wybar and subsequently by Lonn and Hoyt should not be confused with papilledema secondary to increased intracranial pressure. Papillophlebitis occurs unilaterally in young healthy adults. The fundus picture is usually much worse than the patient's complaints of minimal blurriness. The edema and hemorrhages on the disc and in the retina are more consistent with a vein occlusion than with papilledema. Unlike vein occlusions in adults, this entity has a good prognosis. Like vein occlusion in adults, however, there is no effective treatment unless some systemic cause is revealed.

The diseases to be considered in determining the cause of central retinal vein occlusion are glaucoma, diabetes, dysproteinemias, multiple myeloma, and polycythemia vera. The evaluation of diabetes requires a formal glucose tolerance test rather than a postprandial blood glucose determination. The dysproteinemias, such as Waldenström's macroglobulinemia, are best diagnosed by an electrophoresis of the patient's blood serum.

Leukemia and Septic Chorioretinitis

These disorders are discussed together because of the sign they have in common— Roth's spots (hemorrhages with white centers) (Plate 2-IC). In leukemia the white centers are tumor cells, whereas in septic chorioretinitis they are inflammatory white cells. Both diseases may cause disc edema. Many hemorrhages are present but usually only a few Roth's spots. When Roth's spots are present, they are located at the posterior pole and need not be looked for at the equator or beyond. The white centers in Roth's spots frequently are transient, and when they are looked for the next day, they may be filled in with blood and look like an ordinary retinal hemorrhage. Roth's spots are seen in other diseases, such as subacute bacterial endocarditis, pernicious anemia, scurvy, lupus erythematosus, and sickle cell anemia. Usually, these conditions do not cause disc edema.

Optic Neuritis

As a rule, disc edema with a decrease in visual acuity suggests optic neuritis. The appearance of the papillitis is not diagnostic; some patients with optic neuritis have good visual acuity. In these, the field defect may be so subtle that the patient is not aware of it; it must be looked for carefully.

A useful diagnostic test for evaluating papillitis with good visual acuity is the afferent pupillary defect, which indicates unilateral optic nerve disease. This phenomenon may be seen when damage to the nerve occurs for any reason, causing a conduction defect, even in cases of neuritis with good visual acuity. The test is performed in the following way. The physician shines a light in the affected eye, and the pupil in that eye responds, as expected, by constricting. A consensual response also occurs. The light is then moved quickly from the affected eye to the other eye— and the degree of pupillary constriction in both eyes comes down more. The light is then moved quickly back to the affected eye, whereupon the pupil of the affected eye dilates significantly, as does the pupil in the fellow eye. The light must be moved rapidly from one eye to the other in order not to lose the constrictor effect from the normal eye. The test should be done several times in order to differentiate the condition from a dilatation of the pupil owing to hippus.

Cells in the vitreous humor in front of the disc are an inconstant sign of papillitis or a retrobulbar optic neuritis. They can be seen only with the fundus contact lens, and they are not seen grossly with the ophthalmoscope. Cells in the vitreous humor can be seen in a variety of conditions—pars planitis, chorioretinitis, and cyclitis. In all these disorders, the cells cause a visible haze or debris in the vitreous humor and are not localized to the disc area.

The Hardy, Rand, Ritter (HRR) color plates are a useful screening device. Even in optic neuritis with good visual acuity, the ability to recognize the plates may be markedly different in each eye. This finding can be carried over into the field examination, in which a field defect may be more easily detected with colored test objects than with small white ones.

Infiltration of Nerve

Infiltration of the nerve head may give the appearance of papilledema on casual inspection. Fortunately, infiltration of the disc is rare and usually occurs unilaterally, which should alert one to an alternative diagnosis to true papilledema. Infiltration or masses on the nerve head can be seen with several disorders, such as tuberous sclerosis, sarcoid, and lymphoma, to name a few.

The eye and orbit are affected in about 25% of cases of systemic sarcoid. The perivenous candle wax dripping appearance of the retinal vasculitis is well known.

The four different manifestations of optic nerve involvement in sarcoid are optic atrophy, optic neuritis, optic nerve granuloma invasion of the nerve, and papilledema.

The papilledema may occur secondary to infiltration of the perioptic meninges or as papillitis. It may also occur secondary to true increased intracranial pressure from a mass effect or, more rarely, from direct infiltration of the disc. A case reported by Jampol and seen by us is one in which a patient responded dramatically to systemic steroids (Fig. 13–8 A,B).

Intracranial involvement occurs in about 5% of cases of systemic sarcoid. These cases may present as cranial nerve involvement, of which seventh nerve paresis is the most common, or with hypothalamic involvement and symptoms of diabetes insipidus. We have reported a case of a suprasellar tumor causing a mass effect. This mass produced diabetes insipidus, bitemporal hemianopia, and papilledema. The mass was biopsied and showed a typical noncaseating granuloma. The mass responded to steroids and all of the symptoms and signs were relieved or markedly improved.

A firm diagnosis without a biopsy is difficult to establish. A computerized tomogram is said to show a characteristic appearance. This has not held up in a series of cases reviewed by Powers and Miller. An increase in the serum angiotensin-converting enzyme has also shown promise as a laboratory aid in the diagnosis, but it is not universally elevated in all cases of sarcoid.

Other infiltrations of the optic nerve can be seen, such as in lymphoid reticulum cell sarcoma. We have seen lymphoma produce this ocular presentation on several occasions; however, these patients were well known to us as patients with lymphoma and did not have optic infiltration as their initial systemic complaint. The optic nerve masses resolved under therapy but left an infarcted nerve from the infiltration.

Reticulum sarcoma usually presents as a uveitis associated with subretinal and choroidal infiltrates and, occasionally, with disc hyperemia mimicking early papilledema.

Tumors

Orbital and optic nerve tumors can cause disc edema through obstruction of ocular venous drainage. They may also cause decrease in visual acuity, field defects, decrease in motility, and proptosis. The exophthalmos may be subtle, and exophthalmometer measurements should be part of the evaluation of unilateral papilledema or loss of acuity.

Digital exploration of the periorbital area may reveal a mass accessible to biopsy. Tumors that are truly retro-orbital or are in the muscle cone are the most difficult to diagnose, but they can be diagnosed by the ultrasound technique or the computerized tomogram. Roentgenograms of the optic canal are a necessity, and basal tomograms should be ordered as indicated.

Thyroid disease may cause unilateral loss of vision, exophthalmos, disc edema, and horizontal striae in the macular area. Although these conditions also suggest orbital tumor, a positive forced duction test and lid retraction point toward thyroid disease as the primary cause.

Intracranial tumors, particularly those along the sphenoid ridge, can cause changes that are more marked in one eye than in the other. In disc edema caused by venous compression in the superior orbital fissure, the veins appear to be disproportionately larger than in papilledema caused by increased intracranial pressure. This venous stasis may also be seen as a caput medusa (dilated veins) on the globe. As the tumor enlarges and the intracranial pressure increases, the relationship of papilledema and venous engorgement is more typical of true papilledema. A variation of this condition is the Foster Kennedy syndrome, in which the tumor, usually a frontal lobe glioma or an olfactory groove meningioma, compresses the optic nerve, causing optic atrophy. The atrophy occurs before the tumor takes up a significant amount of intracranial space. Then as the tumor grows, increased intracranial pressure develops and the other nerve shows papilledema while the atrophic side does not. When the Foster Kennedy syndrome occurs in persons 65 years of age or older, however, it is commonly caused by vascular disease.

Long-standing increased intracranial pressure from any cause and tumor of the chiasm both bring about a bilateral decrease in acuity. Bilateral papilledema with a decrease in acuity can be confused with bilateral optic neuritis, a mistake that is likely to occur when the plain roentgenograms of the sphenoid ridge and sella turcica are reported as normal. Slow progressive loss of acuity is not caused by optic neuritis, however, so a compressive lesion must be considered. Suprasellar masses, such as meningioma, craniopharyngioma, or aneurysm, may cause compression of the nerves without evidence of bony changes, even with adequate tomograms of the sella turcica. A computed tomographic (CT) examination with a contrast medium should be used to rule out a suprasellar mass. Careful inspection of the plain roentgenograms may reveal subtle calcification in some cases of meningioma and aneurysm. Suprasellar calcification can be seen in more than 85% of childhood craniopharyngiomas, but it is uncommon in the adult variety. If the Foster Kennedy syndrome is caused by an olfactory groove meningioma, anosmia ipsilateral with the optic atrophy also occurs.

The association of a spinal cord tumor and increased intracranial pressure is well known but occurs uncommonly. The mechanism is also poorly understood. When no intracranial reason for the papilledema can be found and before pseudotumor cerebri is accepted as the diagnosis, investigation for a spinal cord tumor should be considered. The usual lower extremity symptoms should dismiss serious consideration of pseudotumor cerebri. Plain roentgenograms of the lumbar sacral region may show atrophy and widening of the interpedicular distance. This, then, suggests a more definitive evaluation by myelography or CT. The cause of the papilledema is not necessarily mechanical obstruction of cerebrospinal fluid flow as has been shown by myelography. Since increased cerebrospinal fluid protein is a constant finding in these cases, the protein may obstruct the turnover of cerebrospinal fluid as occurs in the Guillain-Barré syndrome.

Brain Abscess

Such an abscess usually causes focal neurologic deficit, but occasionally it produces papilledema.

Juxtapapillary Choroiditis

The focal chorioretinitis next to the disc may be hard to see because of overlying inflammatory exudates. The focal nature of the changes suggests the diagnosis since the rest of the nerve looks normal. Since juxtapapillary choroiditis most fequently occurs on the temporal side of the disc, it is unlikely to be papilledema, which occurs first on the nasal side.

Posterior Scleritis

This disorder is usually referred to as brawny scleritis. It causes retinal edema with horizontal striae in the macula as well as low-grade disc edema. The best way to see the thickened choroid is with the fundus contact lens. Brawny scleritis is usually idiopathic, but it can be associated with thyroid disease.

Ocular Hypotension Secondary to Intraocular Operation

Cataract operation, even when it is uncomplicated and when the depth of the anterior chamber is normal, may be associated with a low intraocular pressure—in the range of 2 to 4 mm. The low pressure causes mild swelling of the disc and macula, with chronic loss of vision caused by macular disease. A dilated fundus examination using the indirect ophthalmoscope is necessary. A detailed view of the ciliary body may reveal ciliary body detachment, with secondary decrease in aqueous production. Seidel's test with fluorescein should be done, and the physician should look for a leak of the wound if an obvious filtering bleb is not present.

Ischemic Optic Neuropathy

Temporal Arteritis. This condition is usually thought of as occurring in older people who show signs of headache and a temporal artery that is prominent, very tender, and noncompressible. The usual history is one of sudden loss of vision without warning or associated symptoms. If asked about any previous signs and symptoms, the patient may admit to them but dismiss them as "just old age" or "wearing out." Frequently, temporal arteritis causes disc edema, but it is of the pale and ischemic variety, with small vessels, rather than the plethoric type seen with increased intracranial pressure. The diagnosis of temporal arteritis should be considered in a patient over 55 years of age, particularly one over 65 years of age, when sudden loss of vision occurs in one or both eyes. Temporal arteritis has been reported and confirmed by biopsy in much younger people, but only rarely. The condition usually attacks one eye at a time, but since the other eye may be affected within days, a diagnosis should be made promptly and therapy begun immediately. Temporal arteritis is a true ophthalmic emergency.

The physician should strongly suspect temporal arteritis whenever the blood sedimentation rate is elevated. The usual elevation is 45 mm or more, but even minimal elevations (in the range of 30 mm) warrant a temporal artery biopsy. In a positive biopsy, the typical multinucleated giant cells are present (see Figs. 14–1, 14–2). If the condition is strongly suspected because of an elevated sedimentation rate, systemic steroid therapy should be started immediately, even if the biopsy cannot be done for as long as 48 hours. Such a brief course of steroid therapy does not affect the biopsy, and it may protect the other eye. Since temporal arteritis is a segmental disease, it is imperative to get serial sections done on the specimen because the pathologic area may be missed. It is important to get a positive biopsy early so that patients who do not require steroid therapy will not continue to receive it. Since they are in the age group that tolerates steroids poorly and is prone to such diseases as diabetes and hypertension, a positive biopsy also puts the treatment on a firmer basis. It has been suggested that doing a temporal artery arteriogram will show the occluded areas more precisely and thus increase chances of a positive biopsy. This has generally not worked out. When a sudden loss of vision with ischemic disc edema occurs, an important differential diagnosis is infarction of the nerve immediately behind the disc from emboli, particularly from an atheromatous condition of the carotid or aortic arch.

Small Vessel Optic Neuritis (Anterior Ischemic Optic Neuropathy). This condition is associated with ischemic disc edema more often than is temporal arteritis. The loss of vision in patients with small vessel optic neuritis is gradual rather than cataclysmic; it tends to be a piecemeal loss of vision. In persons with small vessel optic neuritis, the other eye tends to be affected more consistently, although usually not simultaneously. Small vessel optic neuritis is not associated with an increased sedimentation rate, and the temporal artery biopsy is negative. The cause is considered to be small vessel occlusive disease, and the condition is not favorably affected by anticoagulant or steroid therapy. Although no effective specific therapy exists, associated conditions that decrease the vascular profusion ratio of the eye should be evaluated. These conditions are increased ocular pressure, decreased blood pressure, such as occurs in too sudden and too severe treatment for hypertension, and decreased ca-

rotid pressure owing to silent carotid occlusive disease, as evidenced by a decrease in ophthalmodynamometry.

Acute Anemia. Acute blood loss, such as occurs in gastrointestinal and uterine hemorrhages, does not commonly cause loss of vision or disc edema. When it does, the edema is of the pale ischemic variety, with attenuated vessels. About 25% of those who develop disc edema do so immediately, and the remainder develop it in the next few days or weeks. The loss of vision is usually unilateral, and it may be complete or partial or even present as a field defect, such as an altitudinal hemianopsia. The visual loss may be made worse by antecedent carotid occlusive disease or small vessel disease in the optic nerve or in the retina, which has already decreased the perfusion of the eye.

Chronic Anemia. This condition is also an infrequent but established cause of visual loss and disc edema. In the United States, it usually occurs in women who have begun a pregnancy with a low hemoglobin level and then compounded the problem with no prenatal care, thus making the hemoglobin level drop even lower. The edema is low grade and closer to the ischemic variety than the edema in papilledema. The diagnosis is easily made by hemoglobin and hematocrit determinations. Whatever visual loss ensues can be made worse by an associated eclampsia or hypertension that causes further ischemia.

Pseudotumor Cerebri

This disorder produces all the signs of increased intracranial pressure, including papilledema. The results of the neurologic and neuroradiologic examinations, however, are all within normal limits. The papilledema of pseudotumor cerebri has no features that distinguish it from papilledema from other causes.

The pathogenesis of pseudotumor cerebri has eluded accurate definition, possibly because all cases may not be caused by the same or even a single factor. Donaldson's review makes a valiant attempt at categorizing the factors and how certain kinds of disease associated with pseudotumor cerebri may make use of these factors. The first factor is increased venous pressure. This occurs in cases of the superior vena cava syndrome and in bilateral or unilateral jugular vein obstruction. The second factor is increased arachnoidal resistance. This may result from metabolism changes at the arachnoidal level in cases related to vitamin A intoxication. It may also be seen in blockage of arachnoid villi from protein in Guillian-Barré syndrome or in metastatic seeding of the arachnoid space. The third factor is cerebrospinal fluid hypersecretion, which has been implicated in cases of choroid plexus papillomas. Lastly, there is increased elastance of the cerebrospinal fluid space, seen in spinal cord tumors, which are frequently associated with an increased spinal fluid protein which contributes to absorption problems.

Some cases of pseudotumor cerebri may have a cause that can be identified and eliminated. Pseudotumor cerebri is seen in association with an overdose of vitamin A. It is rarely seen as an unusual reaction to tetracycline and steroids. It has also been reported as a complication of Addison's disease or hypoparathyroid disease.

Vitamin A toxicity is particularly interesting because it is not usually seen in adults. I have seen it in one 19-year-old girl who chronically ingested an excess of vitamin A to treat her acne. Vitamin A toxicity can be acute or chronic. The acute variety occurs when the patient ingests food with a high vitamin A content such as polar bear meat or shark liver. The toxicity is manifested by headache, nausea and vomiting, a decreased sensorium, and irritability. Acute toxicity in children may be caused by an accidental overdose of vitamins that the infant had access to. Chronic intoxication is a more common presentation with the signs and symptoms of pseudotumor cerebri.

Hydrocephalus and increased intracranial pressure have also occurred in vitamin A-deficient babies in association with other neurologic signs such as increased reflexes and a bulging fontanel. Administration of vitamin A in these patients quickly reverses the process. It is important to consider this entity in infants who cannot speak and give a history.

Carotid Cavernous Sinus Fistula

Among younger patients, carotid cavernous sinus fistula is more often seen in men and after trauma. Among older patients, it is more often seen in women and secondary to arteriosclerotic rupture of an intracavernous aneurysm. The increased venous flow to the eye, as well as the increased venous pressure, may cause only edema of the disc and fullness of the retinal veins without dilated veins on the conjunctiva, sclera, and lids. If the fistula is present long enough, the edema may become bilateral. Rarely, disc edema may even begin in the contralateral eye if a superior ophthalmic vein thrombosis occurs ipsilateral with the fistula. The associated signs of ocular bruits and ophthalmoplegia should be evaluated.

Pulsations, unless marked, may be missed. They are best seen by looking at the eye from the side rather than straight ahead. The more subtle pulsations are diagnosed when the physician uses direct ophthalmoscopy, noting that the fundus is going in and out of focus synchronously with the pulse at the wrist. If the applanation technique is used, the tonometer sign may be missed. The variation of the tonometer reading may be interpreted as unsteadiness of the patient in the headrest of the slit lamp. With the Schiøtz tonometer, however, the arm has wide rhythmic swings in the range of six scale readings rather than the usual two to three scale readings.

Peripheral Ocular Disease

Peripheral uveitis or pars planitis may cause a vitreitis that, in turn, causes disc edema and macular edema. Examination of the far periphery of the fundus with the indirect ophthalmoscope is indispensable. Fundus contact lens examination of the vitreous humor reveals cells. The cellular reaction is more generalized than that seen in papillitis located just in front of the disc.

Unilateral Neck Dissection

In radical neck dissection, a procedure for extensive carcinoma, the possibility that a particular dissection is incomplete with later metastasis to the brain is of real concern. If the patient later has a mild disc edema and engorged veins, the question of cerebral metastasis with increased intracranial pressure is raised. The physician may not consider the possibility of decreased venous drainage from the head because he presumes that the other jugular system is able to drain the head adequately. The other system is not always competent, however, and disc edema may result. The usual studies—skull roentgenograms, brain scan, CT, neurologic examination, complete ophthalmologic examination, including field examination—must be performed. If the other signs of increased intracranial pressure are present, contrast studies must be considered.

Disc edema caused by severe pulmonary disease, such as emphysema, can also be seen. It may be caused by decreased venous drainage from the head into the chest, or it may be secondary to an increase in blood P_{CO_2}.

Chronic lung disease is a well-known cause of increased intracranial pressure. Despite large numbers of people whom we see with various grades of COPD, the occurrence of papilledema is rare. The cause is believed to be the increased CO_2 that results from the COPD. Kety showed that, by raising the level of CO_2 in the blood, secondary vascular dilatation occurs, resulting in increased intracranial pressure. The secondary anoxia these patients suffer over a long period rarely causes optic nerve ischemia and decreased vision. If another complicating factor occurs, such as a reduction in optic nerve perfusion pressure, then decrease in vision can occur. The chronic anoxia increases erythropoiesis, and a secondary type of polycythemia occurs. This hyperviscosity of the blood may cause sludging and vascular congestion at the nerve head, with the appearance of papilledema. The increased volume of the blood also causes an increase in the intravascular space in the cranial vault, further increasing the intracranial pressure.

FLUORESCEIN TEST

Fluorescein dye injections are useful for separating true disc edema from pseudopapilledema. Fluorescein testing does not, however, distinguish among the different causes of disc edema. Moreover, in many cases of mild papilledema, no true leakage of the dye from the disc occurs, although one would expect this result. The fluorescein test can be done without a photographic setup. The main requirements are a cobalt blue filter for the indirect ophthalmoscope and access to the fluorescein dye. Detailed study of the fluorescein photographs is desirable. Whenever possible, the test should be performed in conjunction with retinal photography rather than as a casual office procedure.

TREATMENT

The surgical treatment of increased intracranial pressure is the province of the neurosurgeon. The one form of intracranial pressure that requires continuous ophthalmologic observation is that related to pseudotumor cerebri. The ophthalmic problem in pseudotumor cerebri is that, if the increased intracranial pressure does not go into spontaneous remission, the optic nerve may suffer damage. The treatment generally has been cautious observation, but steroid therapy has been advocated and is of some value. Diamox reduces spinal fluid production in the same manner that it reduces aqueous production.

The surgical procedure of decompressing the optic nerve in chronic papilledema is relatively new. Its particular value is in unexplained chronic papilledema with beginning loss of vision owing to the chronic pressure.

Long-standing papilledema, such as can occur in pseudotumor cerebri, can cause loss of vision. Fortunately, a healthy optic nerve withstands this increased pressure well. The intracranial pressure usually returns to normal before direct surgical intervention is required to preserve vision. In the past, surgical relief of increased intracranial pressure was accomplished by bilateral subtemporal decompression or lumboperitoneal shunting. More recently, decompression of the perioptic meninges has been a much less formidable procedure. It is not a new procedure and was initially described by DeWecker in 1872. Different surgical approaches have been described but the medial orbital approach outlined by Galbraith and Sullivan is the one most commonly used and gives the best exposure.

The mechanism by which this procedure preserves vision is not completely understood. Hayreh and Davidson believe that it relieves pressure directly on the optic nerve and does not relieve intracranial pressure. Intracranial pressure was measured in the animal experiments by Hayreh and Hayreh who found that there was only a unilateral decrease in papilledema and no lowering of intracranial pressure with a unilateral incision of the optic nerve sheath. Some authors believe that the cerebral spinal fluid leaks out of the dural sheath window, thus reducing intracranial pressure, and reduces papilledema bilaterally. These authors are in the minority. Our clinical experience and Hayreh's experiments do not agree with that conclusion. In support of the theory that a unilateral dural sheath window only reduces the pressure effects on one nerve and does not influence the intracranial pressure is supported by the case reported by Kaye, Galbraith, and King. In a case of pseudotumor cerebri with deteriorating vision, optic nerve sheath decompression was performed. The intracranial pressure was measured by a subarachnoid pressure transducer for 24 hours before and 48 hours after each optic nerve decompression. After each operation, the papilledema subsided rapidly with no change in intracranial pressure despite constant 24-hour monitoring of that pressure. This would seem to be strong evidence in support of a local effect on the optic nerve rather than a general lowering of intracranial pressure.

The treatment of several nonsurgical causes of chronic papilledema is the province of the ophthalmologist. Hydroxycobalamine in place of the usual vitamin B_{12} preparations is useful and specific in treatment of optic neuritis associated with pernicious anemia. Several British authors consider it useful also in tobacco-alcohol amblyopia, but I have found it to be of little value, and the latter disease does not cause papilledema.

The treatment for temporal arteritis consists of large doses of systemic steroids for a considerable period of time. Using the sedimentation rate as the only indicator for lowering the steroid dosage—or for discontinuing it—can frequently be misleading because the sedimentation rate does not always drop to normal. The usual duration of a course of steroid therapy is a matter of months rather than weeks.

BIBLIOGRAPHY

Arseni, C., and Maretsis, M.: Tumor of the lower spinal cord associated with increased intracranial pressure. J. Neurosurg. 27:105, 1967.

Bagdasar, D., and Marinescu, G.: Tumors of the lower spinal cord associated with increased intracranial pressure and papilledema. J. Neurosurg. 27:105, 1967.

Ballantyne, A.J.: The ocular manifestations of spontaneous subarachnoid hemorrhage. Br.J. Ophthalmol. 27:383, 1943.

Bass, M.H., and Caplan, J.: Vitamin A deficiency in infancy. J. Pediatr. 47:690, 1955.

Behrman, S.: Pathology of papilledema. Brain 89:1, 1966.

Bhowmick, B.K.: Benign intracranial hypertension after antibiotic therapy. Br. Med. J. 3:30, 1972.

Bray, P.F., Carter, S., and Taveras, J.M.: Brainstem tumors in children. Neurology 8:1, 1958.

Brodrick, J.D.: Drusen of the disc and retinal hemorrhages. Br.J. Ophthalmol. 57:299, 1973.

Buchheit, W.A., et al.: Papilledema and idiopathic intracranial hypertension—report of a familial occurrence. N. Engl. J. Med. 280:938, 1969.

Chambers, J.W., and Walsh, F.B.: Hyaline bodies in the optic discs: report of ten cases exemplifying importance in neurological diagnosis. Brain 74:95, 1951.

Chamlin, M., and Davidoff, L.M.: Drusen of optic nerve simulating papilledema. J. Neurosurg. 7:70, 1950.

Chamlin, M., and Davidoff, L.: Divergence paralysis with increased intracranial pressure. J. Neurosurg. 7:539, 1950.

Chisholm, I.A.: Optic neuropathy of recurrent blood loss. Br. J. Ophthalmol. 53:289, 1969.

Cohen, D.: Drusen of the optic disc and development of field defects. Arch. Ophthalmol. 85:224, 1971.

Collins, E.T.: Intraocular tension. The sequelae of hypotony. Trans. Ophthalmol. Soc. U.K. 21:100, 1901.

Cornfield, D., and Cooke, R.D.: Vitamin A deficiency: case report. Pediatrics 10:33, 1952.

Daroff, R.B., and Smith, J.L.: Intraocular optic neuritis with normal visual acuity. Neurology 15:409,1965.

Davidson, S.I.: A surgical approach to plesocephalic disc oedema. Trans. Ophthalmol. Soc. U.K. 89:669, 1969.

Dees, S.C., and McKay, H.W.: Occurrence of pseudotumor cerebri (benign intracranial hypertension) during treatment of children with asthma by adrenal steroids. Report of three cases. Pediatrics 23:1143, 1959.

DeWecker, L.: An incision of the optic nerve in cases of neuroretinitis. Int. Ophthalmol. Congr. Rep. 4:11, 1872.

Donaldson, J.O.: Pathogenesis of pseudotumor cerebri syndromes. Neurology 31:877, 1981.

Duffy, G.P.: Lumbar puncture in the presence of raised intracranial pressure. Br. Med. J. 1:407, 1969.

Ecker, A.: Irregular fluctuation of elevated cerebrospinal fluid pressure. Arch. Neurol. Psychiatry 74:641, 1955.

Ellenberger, J.C., and Messner, K.H.: Papillophlebitis: benign retinopathy resembling papilledema or papillitis. Ann. Neurol. 3:438, 1978.

Erkkila, H.: The central vascular pattern of the eyeground in children with drusen of the optic disc. Albrecht on Graffes Arch–Klin. Exp. Ophthalmol. 199:1, 1976.

Fahmy, J.A.: Fundal hemorrhages in ruptured intracranial aneurysm. I. Material, frequency and morphology. Acta Ophthalmologica 51:289, 1973.

Fahmy, J.A.: Fundal hemorrhages in ruptured intracranial aneurysm. II. Correlation with clinical course. Acta Ophthalmologica 51:299, 1973.

Feldman, M.H., and Schlezinger, N.S.: Benign intracranial hypertension associated with hypervitaminosis A. Arch. Neurol. 22:1, 1970.

Fields, J.P.: Bulging fontanel: a complication of tetracycline therapy in infants. J. Pediatr. 58:74, 1961.

Ford, F.R., and Walsh, F.B.: Guillain-Barré syndrome with increased intracranial pressure and papilledema. Report of two cases. Bull. Johns Hopkins Hosp. 73:391, 1943.

Francois, J., et al.: Pseudo-papillitis vasculaires. Ann. d'Oculist. (Paris) 195:830, 1962.

Freedman, B.J.: Papilledema, optic atrophy and blindness due to emphysema and chronic bronchitis. Br. J. Ophthalmol. 47:290, 1963.

Friedman, A., et al.: Drusen of the optic disc. Surv. Ophthalmol. 21:375, 1977.

Frisen, L., Hoyt, W.F., and Tengroth, B.M.: Optociliary veins, disc pallor and visual loss. Acta Ophthalmol. 51:241, 1973.

Galbraith, J.E.K., and Sullivan, J.H.: Decompression of perioptic meninges for relief of papilledema. Am. J. Ophthalmol. 76:687, 1973.

Goldstein, J.E., and Cogan, D.G.: Exercise and the optic neuropathy of multiple sclerosis. Arch. Ophthalmol. 72:168, 1964.

Greer, M.: Benign intracranial hypertension. II. Following corticosteroid therapy. Neurology 13:439, 1963.

Greer, M.: Benign intracranial hypertension. III. Pregnancy. Neurology 13:670, 1963.

Greer, M.: Benign intracranial hypertension. IV. Menarche. Neurology 14:569, 1964.

Gudeman, J., Selhorst, B., and Susac, J.O.: Sarcoid optic neuropathy. Neurology 32:597, 1982.

Halpern, L., Feldman, M.D., and Peyser, E.: Subarachnoid hemorrhage with papilledema due to spinal neurofibroma. Arch. Neurol. 79:138, 1958.

Harris, M.J., Fine, S.L., and Owens, S.L.: Hemorrhagic complications of optic nerve drusen. Am. J. Ophthalmol. 92:70, 1981.

Hayreh, S.S.: Pathogenesis of edema of the optic disc. Br. J. Ophthalmol. 48:522, 1964.

Hayreh, S.S.: Optic disc vasculitis. Br. J. Ophthalmol. 56:652, 1972.

Hayreh, S.S., and Hayreh, M.S.: Optic disc and raised intracranial pressure. Arch. Ophthalmol. 95:1245, 1977.

Henkind, P.: Sarcoidoses: an expanding ophthalmic horizon. J. Roy. Soc. Med. 75:153, 1982.

Henkind, P., Atterman, M., and Wise, G.: Drusen of the optic disc and subretinal and subpigment epithelial hemorrhage. In The Optic Nerve. Edited by J. Gant. London, Henry Kimpton, 1972.

Henkind, P., and Benjamin, J.V.: Vascular anomalies and neoplasms of the optic nerve head. Trans. Ophthalmol. Soc. U.K. 96:418, 1976.

Hollenhorst, R.W., Hollenhorst, R.W., Jr., and McCarty, C.S.: Visual prognosis of optic nerve sheath meningiomas producing shunt vessels on the optic disc. Mayo Clin. Proc. 53:84, 1978.

Jampol, L.M., Woodfin, W., and McLean, E.: Optic nerve sarcoidosis. Arch. Ophthalmol. 87:355, 1972.

Jampolsky, A.: Ocular divergence mechanisms. Trans. Am. Ophthalmol. Soc. 68:825, 1970.

Joynt, R.J.: Mechanism of production of papilledema in the Guillain-Barré syndrome. Neurology 8:8, 1958.

Kahn, E.A., and Cherry, G.R.: The clinical importance of spontaneous retinal venous pulsation. Univ. Mich. Med. Bull. *16*:305, 1950.

Kamin, D.F., Helper, R.S., and Foo, R.Y.: Optic nerve drusen. Arch. Ophthalmol. *89*:359, 1973.

Kane, E.K.: Arctic explorations in the years 1853, 1854, 1855. Vol. 1. Philadelphia, Childs and Peterson Pub., 1856.

Kaye, A.H., Galbraith, J.E.K., and King, J.: Intracranial pressure following optic nerve decompression for benign intracranial hypertension. J. Neurosurg. *55*:453, 1981.

Kearns, T.J., and Wagner, H.P.: Ophthalmologic diagnosis of meningiomas of the sphenoidal ridge. Am. J. Med. Sci. *226*:221, 1953.

Kilburn, K.H.: Neurologic manifestations of respiratory failure. Arch. Intern. Med. *116*:409, 1965.

Kirkham, T.H., Bird, A.C., and Sanders, M.D.: Divergence paralysis with raised intracranial pressure. Br. J. Ophthalmol. *56*:776, 1972.

Lascari, A.D., and Bell, W.E.: Pseudotumor cerebri due to hypervitaminosis A. Clin. Pediatr. *9*:627, 1970.

Levatin, P.: Pupillary escape in disease of the retina or optic nerve. Arch. Ophthalmol. *62*:768, 1959.

Levin, B.E.: The clinical significance of spontaneous pulsations of the retinal vein. Arch. Neurol. *35*:37, 1978.

Lillie, W.I.: The clinical significance of choked discs produced by abscess of the brain. Surg. Gynecol. Obstet. *47*:405, 1928.

Lonn, L.I., and Hoyt, W.F.: Papillophlebitis. Eye, Ear, Nose, Thr. Monthly *45*:62, 1966.

Love, J.G., Wagener, H.P., and Woltman, H.W.: Tumors of the spinal cord associated with choking of the optic discs. A.M.A. Arch. Neurol. Psychiatry *66*:171, 1951.

Lowenstein, O.: Clinical pupillary symptoms in lesions of the optic nerve, optic chiasm and optic tract. Arch. Ophthalmol. *52*:385, 1954.

Lowenstein, O., and Givner, I.: Pupillary reflex to darkness. Arch. Ophthalmol. *30*:603, 1943.

Lyle, T.K., and Wybar, K.: Retinal Vasculitis. Br. J. Ophthalmol. *45*:778, 1961.

Manschot, W.A.: The fundus oculi in subarachnoid hemorrage. Acta Ophthalmol. *22*:281, 1944.

Marr, W.G., and Chambers, R.T.: Pseudotumor cerebri syndrome following unilateral radical neck dissection. Am. J. Ophthalmol. *51*:605, 1961.

Michelson, J.B., and Michelson, P.E.: Ocular reticulum cell sarcoma. Arch. Ophthalmol. *99*:1409, 1981.

Miller, A.J., and Cuttino, J.T.: On the mechanism of production of massive preretinal hemorrhage following rupture of a congenital medial defect intracranial aneurysm. Am. J. Ophthalmol. *31*:15, 1948.

Miller, G.R., and Smith, J.L.: Ischemic optic neuropathy. Am. J. Ophthalmol. *62*:103, 1966.

Moore, L.A., and Sykes, J.F.: Cerebrospinal fluid pressure and vitamin A deficiency. Am. J. Physiol. *130*:684, 1940.

Muller, P.J., and Deck, J.H.N.: Intraocular and optic nerve sheath hemorrhage in cases of sudden intracranial hypertension. J. Neurosurg. *41*:160, 1974.

Otradovec, J., and Vladykova, J: Zur Frage der Blutungen und der Venosen Stauung bei der Drusen-Papille. Ophthalmologica *161*:21, 1970.

Palmer, R.F., Searles, H.H., and Boldrey, E.B.: Papilledema and hypoparathyroidism simulating brain tumor. J. Neurosurg. *16*:378, 1959.

Paton, L.: VII Diseases of the nervous system. 1. Ocular symptoms in subarachnoid hemorrhage. Trans. Ophthalmol. Soc. U.K. *44*:110, 1924.

Paunoff, F.: Glaskorperblutungen bei Subarachnoidalblutung (Terson-Syndrome). Klin. Mbl. Augenheilk. *141*:625, 1962.

Phelps, C.D.: The association of pale centered retinal hemorrhages with intracranial bleeding in infancy. Am. J. Ophthalmol. *72*:348, 1971.

Porsaa, K.: Papilledema in iridocyclitis. Acta Ophthalmol. (KbH.)*21*:316, 1944.

Powers, W.J., and Miller, E.M.: Sarcoidosis mimicking glioma: case report and review of intracranial sarcoid mass lesions. Neurology *31*:907, 1981.

Primrose, J.: Mechanism of production of papilledema. Br. J. Ophthalmol. *48*:19, 1964.

Richardson, J.C., and Hyland, H.H.: Intracranial aneurysms. A clinical and pathological study of subarachnoid and intracerebral hemorrhage caused by berry aneurysms. Medicine (Balt.) *20*:1, 1941.

Rose, A., and Matson, D.D.: Benign intracranial hypertension in children. Pediatrics *39*:227, 1967.

Rosenbaum, T.J., MacCarty, C.S., and Buetnner, H.: Uveitis and cerebral reticulum-cell sarcoma. J. Neurosurg. *50*:660, 1979.

Rosenberg, M., Savino, P., and Glaser, J.: A clinical analysis of psuedopapilledema. 1. Population, laterality, acuity, refractive error, ophthalmoscopic characteristics and coincident disease. Arch. Ophthalmol. *97*:65, 1979.

Sanders, T.E., Gay, A.J., and Newman, N.: Hemorrhagic complications of drusen of the optic disc. Am. J. Ophthalmol. *71*:204, 1971.

Schachat, A.P., and Miller, N.R.: Atrophy of myelinated retinal nerve fibers after acute optic neuropathy. Am. J. Ophthalmol. *92*:854, 1981.

Schatz, N.J., and Smith, J.L.: Non-tumor causes of the Foster Kennedy syndrome. J. Neurosurg. *27*:37, 1967.

Simmons, R.J., and Cogan, D.G.: Occult temporal arteritis. Arch. Ophthalmol. *68*:8, 1962.

Spalter, H.F., and Bruce, G.M.: Ocular changes in pulmonary insufficiency. Trans. Am. Acad. Ophthalmol. *68*:661, 1964.

Spencer, W.H.: primary neoplasms of the optic nerve and its sheaths. Clinical features and current concepts of pathogenetic mechanisms. Trans. Am. Ophthalmol. Soc. *70*:490, 1972.

Spencer, W.H.: Drusen of the optic disc and aberrant axoplasmic transport. The XXXIV Edward Jackson Memorial Lecture. Am. J. Ophthalmol. *85*:1, 1978.

Spencer, W.H., and Hoyt, W.F.: Chronic disc edema from neoplastic involvement of perioptic meninges. *In* Ocular Pathology. Edited by M.E. Smith. Boston, Little, Brown and Co. 1971.

Stanley, J.A.: The swinging flashlight test to detect minimal optic neuropathy. Arch. Ophthalmol. *80*:769, 1968.

Stevens, R.A., and Newman, N.M.: Abnormal visual evoked potentials from eyes with optic nerve head drusen. Am. J. Ophthalmol. *92*:857, 1981.

Sutphin, A., Albright, F., and McCune, D.J.: Five cases of idiopathic hypoparathyroidism associated with moniliasis. J. Clin. Endocrinol. *3*:625, 1943.

Terson, A. Hémorragie dans le corps vitré au cours d'une hémorragie cérébrale. Ann. Oculist *147*:410, 1912.

Thompson, S.H.: Afferent pupillary defects. Am. J. Ophthalmol. *62*:860, 1966.

Timberlake, W.H., and Kubik, C.S.: Follow up report with clinical and anatomical notes on 280 patients with subarachnoid hemorrhage. Trans. Am. Neurol. Assoc. *77*:26, 1952.

Tso, M.O.: Pathology and pathogenesis of drusen of the optic nerve head. Ophthalmology *88*:1066, 1981.

Vanderlinden, R.G., and Chisholm, L.D.: Vitreous hemorrhages and sudden increased intracranial pressure. J. Neurosurg. *41*:167, 1974.

Van Uitert, R.L., and Eisenstadt, M.L.: Venous pulsations not always indicative of normal intracranial pressure. (Letter) Arch. Neurol. *35*:550, 1978.

Walker, A.E., and Adamkiewicz, J.J.: Pseudotumor cerebri associated with prolonged corticosteroid therapy. Reports of four cases. JAMA *188*:779, 1964.

Walsh, F.B., and Hedges, T.R.: Optic nerve sheath hemorrhage. The Jackson Memorial Lecture. Am. J. Ophthalmol. *34*:509, 1951.

Walsh, T.J., and Smith, J.L.: Sarcoidosis and suprasellar mass. Neuro-ophthalmology, Symposium of Univ. of Miami and Bascom Palmer Eye Institute. Edited by J.L. Smith. 1968, p. 167.

Weaver, R.G., and Davis, C.H.: Subhyaloid hemorrhage. Am. J. Ophthalmol. *52*:257, 1961.

Weisberg, L.A.: Benign intracranial hypertension. Medicine (Balt.) *54*:197, 1975.

Williamson-Noble, F.A.: Venous pulse. Trans. Ophthalmol. Soc. U.K. *72*:317, 1952.

Wise, G., Henkind, P., and Alterman, M.: Optic disc drusen and subretinal hemorrhage. Trans. Am. Acad. Ophthalmol. Otolaryngol. *78*:212, 1974.

Chapter 3

Pupillary Abnormalities

THOMAS J. WALSH

FUNCTION AND ANATOMY OF THE PUPIL

The pupil performs many functions. It regulates the amount of light entering the eye. By not dilating to its fullest extent, it reduces the spheric and chromatic aberration induced by the peripheral lens. By becoming small, it increases the depth of focus. All these pupillary phenomena can be observed by the physician who puts a miotic and a mydriatic in his own eye.

The sphincter muscle is innervated by parasympathetic fibers that come to the eye with the third cranial nerve. Pupillary dilatation is occasionally the earliest sign of third cranial nerve paralysis. The dilator muscle innervation comes in mainly by way of the ophthalmic nerve trunk through the superior orbital fissure.

Rare cases of congenital mydriasis exist. Pupils with this disorder respond to light but not to convergence or accommodation. They constrict to 4% pilocarpine, confirming that a sphincter is present. These pupils also react to 10% phenylephrine hydrochloride, confirming a functioning dilator muscle. There is no reaction to potent cholinesterase inhibitors, suggesting an abnormality in the activity of acetylcholine.

PUPILLARY SIZE

Sometime during the first 6 months of life, the pupils begin to increase in size, reaching their maximum size during early adulthood. An occasional complaint of adolescent patients is that their pupils are too large. Largeness of pupils is not significant if the pupils are equal in size and if they contract equally well. In older people the pupils become small.

It appears that, just as Hering's law applies to yoke muscles serving motility and levator function, it also applies to accommodation. For example, if one paralyzes the pupil and accommodation in one eye with a cycloplegic drug, and the person then tries to fix his vision up close with the cycloplegic eye, there is excessive miosis and accommodative response in the eye without cycloplegia. In a second experiment, a mydriatic drug is instilled in one eye. If a patient now fixes with this eye, the accommodative response is normal in that eye and the fellow eye does not show the excessive responses of the previous experiment when a cycloplegic drug was used. This appears to support the application of Hering's law to accommodation and that the accommodative function of the near reflex can be separate from the miotic component.

NORMAL PUPILLARY REFLEXES

Three normal pupillary reflexes deserve discussion.

Physiologic Pupillary Unrest. This normal pupillary movement goes on constantly, even when the stimulation of the pupil does not vary. The degree of movement varies from very active to barely perceptible. Both extremes may be (and usually are) normal. Abnormally active pupillary movement is said to represent a pathologic state. I have not found the separation of pupillary motion into physiologic movement and hippus valuable or valid.

Ciliospinal Skin Reflex. This phenomenon is frequently tested, but its mechanism is often misunderstood. Pinching the skin at the neck should dilate the pupils. In the unconscious patient the test is useful for determining the depth of coma. The reflex is mediated by the pain fibers of the descending branch of the fifth cranial nerve, and is not (as was once thought) initiated by squeezing the sympathetic chain in the neck.

Pupillary Light Reflex. The degree of pupillary contraction does not always indicate the state of vision. It is not unusual, for instance, for a patient to have finger-counting vision caused by central chorioretinitis and still maintain not only a good pupillary light reflex but also one that is equal to the reflex pupillary contraction to light of the uninvolved eye. If, however, one pupil is sluggish to light (compared with its fellow eye) but better to accommodation, a defect in the afferent arc of the light reflex is indicated. If the loss of vision is severe enough, an afferent defect or pupillary escape phenomenon may be present.

Tournay Phenomenon. The Tournay phenomenon refers to the dilatation of the pupil in the abducting eye on sustained lateral gaze. There is also a lesser contraction of the pupil in the abducting eye. This reaction does not occur immediately, but after a few seconds of sustained gaze. Sharpe and Glaser studied 30 patients, using infrared photography, and found no instances of the Tournay phenomenon. Loewenfeld, Friedlander, and McKennon, in studying 150 patients, found the phenomenon occasionally and suggested that it may occur in up to 10% of people. No matter how often it occurs, it has always been thought to be benign in nature and this is the only reason for recognizing the phenomenon at all.

IRREGULARITY OF THE PUPIL

This condition, another consideration in pupillary function, may be due to an old inflammation that has caused posterior adhesions (synechiae) to the lens. The condition may prevent adequate dilatation in the dark or adequate contraction in the light in one or more quadrants, depending on the extensiveness of the synechiae. Colobomas of the iris are always in the area of the fetal cleft, which is to the temporal side of the six o'clock position. Surgery, iris tumors, and blunt trauma can also distort the iris. If the blunt trauma tears the sphincter, the pupil is peaked. If the trauma tears the base of the iris, the tear may not be seen without a gonioscopic examination. A tipoff that the condition exists, however, is that a segment of the iris is displaced centrally and the pupil is flattened in the same area. Gonioscopic examination shows the tear at the base of the peripheral iris. A history of significant blunt trauma to the eye, such as a hyphema or a blow-out fracture of the orbital floor, would indicate enough force to cause such a tear.

GENERAL EXAMINATION TECHNIQUES

The first step in the examination is to notice the anisocoria, a step that may not be as easy as it sounds.

Anisocoria Identification

If you are unsure of the anisocoria in bright illumination, test for it in semidarkness, observing the other conditions for correct pupil testing. A carefully taken history may explain the pupil abnormality. Eye drops, trauma, or neck operation that has injured the sympathetic chain may produce anisocoria.

The mechanics of testing are not difficult, but they must be scrupulously employed. Do not stand in front of the patient and do not shine the light directly at him. Stand with the light off to one side, and have the patient look off at a distance to eliminate factors that might stimulate accommodation and invalidate the testing. Be sure that the beam of light is small enough that only one eye at a time is stimulated. Check the light reflex several times to be sure that the pupillary contraction is the result of the light and not of physiologic pupillary unrest.

The second step in the examination is to compare the reaction of the pupil to light and accommodation so that you can decide whether it is the larger or the smaller pupil—or whether both pupils are abnormal. Signs of fatigue may be a more subtle indication of a pupillary defect. Fatigue may not be apparent with one testing of the light reflex, and multiple retesting may be of value.

Traumatic mydriasis and iridoplegia can be complete, incomplete, or segmental. The causes of these findings after blunt eye trauma can be multiple. The sphincter can be torn or mechanically stunned. If the trauma is severe enough to cause recession of the angle, branches of the short ciliary nerve may be injured at the iris root. Lastly, retrobulbar hemorrhages may damage the ciliary ganglion or the short ciliary nerves.

The final step, particularly if function is intact and only anisocoria is present, is to check for associated signs, such as ptosis, muscle imbalance, or heterochromia.

Differentiating Miosis from Mydriasis

Tables 3–1 and 3–2 outline the causes of miosis and mydriasis and give the examiner information in a compact form that will help him in the differential diagnosis.

TONIC PUPIL

A tonic pupil (Adie's pupil) is of interest because of the diseases that may be confused with it. When a tonic pupil appears to be nonreactive, it may be confused with a third cranial nerve paralysis that is secondary to an aneurysm—a mistake that results in unnecessary hospitalization and, usually in an arteriogram. When a tonic pupil shows light-near dissociation, the patient may be labeled syphilitic. The tonic pupil has several clinical features that easily distinguish it from third cranial nerve

TABLE 3–1. Types and Causes of Miosis

Type	Causes
True Argyll Robertson	Syphilis
Pseudo Argyll Robertson	Pseudotabes pituitaria; pseudotabes diabetica; third cranial nerve misdirection; periaqueductal syndrome
Horner syndrome	Congenital; cluster headache; Raeder paratrigeminal syndrome; migraine headache; carotidynia
Drug-induced (topical medication)	Glaucoma medication
Drug-induced (systemic medication)	Narcotics; barbiturates
Posterior synechia	Iritis; hyphema
Pontine (coma)	

TABLE 3–2. Types and Causes of Mydriasis

Types	Causes
Oculomotor paralysis	Aneurysm; diabetes; trauma; tumor; syphilis
Tonic pupil	
Drug-induced (topical medication)	Mydriatics
Drug-induced (systemic medication)	Doriden
Traumatic	
Essential iris atrophy	
Absent sphincter muscle	

paralysis and from syphilis. It is usually unilateral, and it occurs predominantly in women between 20 and 40 years of age. It occurs uncommonly in males. Bilateral in only about 10% of the cases, involvement of the second pupil usually occurs at a later time rather than simultaneously.

There are two groups of tonic pupils. The first group is related to orbital disease that affects the ciliary ganglion. The cause for the majority of these cases is unknown (true Adie's pupil) and carries with it no long-term bad prognosis for life or vision. A small number of orbital cases can be secondary to severe orbital trauma or orbital infections. The second group is neuropathic in their cause and can be seen in association with diabetes, autonomic neuropathies (e.g., Ross syndrome) and Guillian-Barré syndrome.

Light-Near Dissociation

The initial complaint in a patient with a tonic pupil is usually that one pupil is larger than the other. The patient may or may not experience blurring, but she will have some visual complaints owing to the large pupil. On casual examination, the pupil does not appear to react to light or near. In addition, the patient may have a tension-related headache. The combination of internal ophthalmoplegia or partial third cranial nerve paralysis and headache immediately suggests an aneurysm. The diagnosis may be difficult if the pupil is truly unresponsive, and it may be unresponsive very early in the course of the disorder. A tonic pupil initially may be frozen to any light or to accommodation, no matter how prolonged the stimulus. Within days or several weeks, however, the more typical light-near dissociation phenomenon appears. The light-near dissociation pupil differs from the true Argyll Robertson pupil in that the true Argyll Robertson pupil does not have the tonic light and near response that an Adie's pupil has.

When initially evaluated, many patients demonstrate light-near dissociation, a fac-

tor that simplifies the problem. Some persons who have tonic pupil also have cycloplegia, which adds to the confusion that the defect is a third cranial nerve paralysis. The cycloplegia is transient, and near-normal accommodation returns. In examining for pupillary reactions, use a prolonged stimulation by a bright light, such as that from an indirect ophthalmoscope. An excellent approach is to seat the patient in front of the slit lamp and to use that light to examine her. The slit lamp is a bright-light source, and the magnification aids in the observation of pupillary narrowing.

The keys to diagnosing the tonic pupil are for the physician to have an index of suspicion, particularly when the patient is a young female, and to look for the typical clinical signs. A partial third cranial nerve paralysis should not show any light-near dissociation and thus be ruled out. Lack of ptosis or of any vertical muscle imbalance in any field of gaze, although not absolute proof, is strong evidence against third cranial nerve paralysis.

Tonic Movement

Movement to light or accommodation is also typical in tonic pupil. Observe the patient at the slit lamp or with some magnification, such as a loupe or hand magnifier, and stimulate the pupil reflex steadily. The pupil contracts, but it does so slowly, appearing to the observer like a light reflex in slow motion. If the condition were a partial third cranial nerve paralysis, the remaining pupillary reflex, although diminished in amplitude, would be brisk. In tonic pupil, the movements of the sphincter are not only slow but also irregular. The pupil contracts in segments, rather than simultaneously, for 360 degrees, giving the appearance of a bag of worms moving. This phenomenon is not seen in third cranial nerve paralysis or syphilis unless as a manifestation of third cranial nerve misdirection. This irregular contraction is due to segmental paresis of the iris sphincter. This seems to imply that one sector of the iris is innervated by one nerve with no lateral spread of innervation. This distribution may also be true in the Edinger-Westphal nucleus as suggested in the case report of Selhorst, Hoyt, and Feinsod on midbrain correctopia.

In the area of the cornea corresponding to the sector of iris paresis, there may be associated decreased corneal sensation.

Initially accommodative paresis is common, with gradual improvement over time. Just as there is tonicity of pupillary function, there is also tonicity of accommodation. This can cause asymmetric accommodation, giving rise to complaints of blurred vision, depending on which is the fixing eye. The contraction of the ciliary muscle may be somewhat segmental just as iris contraction is segmental owing to segmental paresis. There is clinical evidence in support of this phenomenon. In one third of the patients, astigmatism is induced when accommodation is stimulated.

Size

A tonic pupil is usually larger initially than its fellow pupil. When reinnervation of the tonic pupil occurs, the pupil becomes somewhat smaller, but anisocoria remains. Occasionally, the tonic pupil is smaller when examined than its fellow pupil. The tonic nature of the pupil is also seen when it is redilating, as well as when it is contracting. Thus, if a patient to be examined has been reading in the physician's waiting room for a period of time, both her pupils will have contracted. The physician examining the patient observes that the unaffected eye quickly redilates but the tonic pupil remains small for awhile—a phenomenon that may persist throughout the examination. Such a pupil is likely to be confused with a luetic pupil because it is small.

Mecholyl Test

The more peripheral the lesion is in a nerve, the more likely it is to develop supersensitivity to the motor end-plate excitor substance. The lesion in the tonic pupil is just behind the globe, in the ciliary ganglion. A patient with a tonic pupil develops supersensitivity to a 2.5% mecholyl solution, whereas the normal pupil does not contract with even a 15% solution. The supersensitivity is often not present initially, and if the test results are negative, the test should be repeated at a later date. To perform the test, measure both pupils at distance fixation and then instill one drop of a 2.5% mecholyl solution in each eye. Dismiss the patient for 45 minutes, telling her not to read or do any other close work. When she returns, measure the pupils again at distance fixation under the same lighting conditions. The tonic pupil will be smaller than before and frequently smaller than the pupil of the normal eye. If both pupils are tonic, both react; thus the physician cannot be sure that the patient is not one of those rare people who react to a 2.5% mecholyl solution. (Mecholyl sensitivity can also be seen in the Riley-Day, Goldenhar and cri-du-chat syndromes, all of which are easily differentiated from the tonic pupil.)

If mecholyl is not available, a 0.125% pilocarpine solution can be used. The normal pupil will react with less miosis to a 0.125% pilocarpine solution, than the tonic pupil. It is not important if the normal pupil also constricts to 0.125% pilocarpine; the tonic pupil will constrict proportionately more.

Tonic Pupil Syndrome

Some patients with a tonic pupil also have loss of knee and ankle reflexes. Other reflexes, such as those in the arms, can be absent or depressed also. This condition is known as the tonic pupil syndrome. The loss of the reflex may be unilateral or bilateral, and it is not necessarily ipsilateral with the abnormal pupil. Since the patient is asymptomatic, loss of the reflex is not brought out in the history; however, the reflexes can be tested easily. The reason for the association of tonic pupil and loss of reflexes is not understood. The reflex loss does support the tonic pupil diagnosis if the pupil is in the early phase of no reaction to light or accommodation.

Significance

The important feature of the tonic pupil syndrome and of the isolated tonic pupil is that neither condition is related to any ocular or nervous system disease that needs to be evaluated and treated. It is important, however, to inform the patient about the condition so that she in turn may inform any future physician of her eye and reflex changes and thus prevent his trying to fit them into another diagnosis. The patient should also carry some medical identification so that, should she ever become unconscious, the tonic pupil will not be thought of as a sign of a subdural hematoma and hence lead to a craniotomy.

ARGYLL ROBERTSON PUPIL

Classic Signs

The pupillary phenomenon of Argyll Robertson or light-near dissociation has been known since 1869, but its chief cause—syphilis—is as old as man. A light-sensitive retina and miosis are the essential features; an amaurotic eye also has a pupil that is rigid to direct light stimulation and that contracts to an imaginary target at near. The true Argyll Robertson pupil does contract to near but usually not normally. It is also a smaller pupil as compared to a tonic pupil. Long-standing Adie's may also become small but not as small as an Argyll Robertson pupil. The Argyll Robertson pupil is usually bilateral, but if it is initially unilateral, it is the smaller of the two pupils. Before and after pupil photographs under the same lighting and distance fixation circumstances are important to accurately document the results of the test. Argyll Roberston pupil is usually bilateral, but if initially it is unilateral, it is the smaller of the two pupils. Irregularity of the pupil,

a phenomenon frequently noted, is not one of the basic criteria. Argyll Robertson pupils become irregular because iritis occurs and posterior synechiae or iris atrophy from chronic inflammation develops. Argyll Robertson pupils also dilate poorly with atropine; however, this sign is difficult to evaluate and is not useful clinically.

Light-Near Dissociation

The classic signs of Argyll Robertson pupil, therefore, are rigidity to light and contraction to accommodation. If one used these criteria, the phenomenon represented tertiary syphilis 99% of the time. Since the advent of antibiotics, however, syphilis is less prevalent. The light-near dissociation is now more commonly a sign of Adie's pupil or tonic pupils caused by diabetic or alcoholic neuropathies.

In the 1800s, the bright lights of the indirect ophthalmoscope or the slit lamp were not available. Many of the then light-rigid pupils perhaps would not be considered rigid today. Therefore, I prefer to use the criterion of light-near dissociation. The small amount that the pupil reacts to light is normal and not slow as in the tonic pupil.

Causes

The fact that Argyll Robertson pupil represents *tertiary* syphilis means that the usual blood tests may be negative. If they are, an FTA-ABS test should be done. Argyll Robertson pupil may be (and often is) present without other signs of tertiary syphilis. Once syphilis is suspected, the physician should look for other ocular signs of the disease, such as peripheral chorioretinitis. If congenital syphilis is a possibility, the physician should look for salt-and-pepper retinopathy, as well as the ghost vessels of interstitial keratitis. (The ghost vessels should be looked for at the superior cornea beneath the upper lid since they may be subtle and missed unless the lid is elevated when the slit-lamp examination is performed.)

Herpes zoster, encephalitis, and

syringobulbia rarely cause Argyll Robertson pupils. Still, the possibility that a patient with one of these diseases may also have had syphilis with a negative blood test (not unusual in tertiary syphilis) cannot be ruled out.

Mass lesions in and around the aqueduct of Sylvius, between the third and fourth ventricle, can cause Argyll Robertson pupils. The lesions frequently cause other signs, such as paralysis of up gaze and retraction nystagmus. If retraction nystagmus is not obvious, it can be elicited by bringing optokinetic targets from above down. In this way, the quick component of the nystagmus is up and reinforces the retraction nystagmus, which is brought out in up gaze or attempted up gaze. The patient under consideration is obviously not a syphilitic patient.

Pseudo Argyll Robertson Pupil

This disorder is seen in pseudotabes pituitaria, pseudotabes diabetica, and third cranial nerve misdirection. In *pseudotabes pituitaria*, the light reaction is poor because of the underlying disease, in which the optic nerves are affected at the chiasm. In *pseudotabes diabetica*, the poor light reaction is secondary either to poor vision or to neuropathy of the short ciliary nerves.

Third cranial nerve misdirection is not common, but it can be mistaken for unilateral Argyll Robertson pupil. It is the unilateral nature of the pseudo Argyll Robertson pupil that should bring third cranial nerve misdirection to mind. The pupillary reaction to near occurs not because the pupil contracts on near gaze but because the medial rectus muscle is stimulated on near gaze. The stimulation is due to a misdirection after recovery from third cranial nerve paralysis, in which some relationship develops between the medial rectus muscle and the pupillary fibers. The pupillary reaction can also be demonstrated by observing the pupil when the patient is looking at a distant point and turning his gaze to the right or left so as to stimulate the

appropriate medial rectus muscle. This procedure causes contraction of the pupil, just as in accommodation, and differentiates the condition from a true Argyll Robertson pupil. The significance of the sign is that it occurs more commonly after a traumatic third cranial nerve paralysis or because of an aneurysm and rarely with tumors or syphilis, and it has never been reported after diabetic third cranial nerve paralysis. Therefore, if a patient has third cranial nerve misdirection *and* diabetes, the previous third cranial nerve paralysis was caused not by the diabetes but by something else—in the absence of a history of severe trauma, most likely it is an aneurysm.

It should be mentioned that some clinicians describe a pupil that is large and does not react to light but does contract to near (and that is associated with a positive blood test) as an Argyll Robertson pupil.

FIXED PUPIL

Amaurotic Pupil

The diagnosis of an amaurotic pupil is often made incorrectly because all four of the criteria for the condition are not evaluated. The observer frequently relies only on the fact that the pupil does not react to light. The criteria are that (1) the blind eye has no direct reaction to light but (2) it does react consensually, and (3) the normal eye has a good direct reaction to light but (4) it does not react consensually from a light shined in the amaurotic eye. If one were to use the lack of direct reaction to light as the only criterion, the Argyll Robertson and tonic pupils would be considered blind—and obviously they are not. If the affected eye has not only no direct reaction but also no consensual reaction, both limbs of the pupillary arc are involved. This involvement suggests an orbital apex syndrome since the third cranial nerve, as well as the optic nerve, is affected.

A more difficult situation arises when the patient complains of blurred vision and has a large nonreactive pupil. The initial impression may suggest optic nerve involvement also; however, the distance vision may be blurred because of an uncorrected refractive error, and the near vision may be blurred because of the loss of accommodation that becomes manifest with cycloplegia. In addition, a good consensual reaction exists in the normal eye.

Drug-Induced Cycloplegia

The possibility that the patient has either accidentally or intentionally put a cycloplegic drug in his eye should be considered. Accidental dilatation and cycloplegia can come about through the use of unlabeled eye drops that were prescribed for other eye diseases. Rubbing the sap of certain plants and flowers can also result in cycloplegia. (Most of the night-blooming flowers contain scopolamine.) The physician who is confronted either with background or with a negative neurologic examination should put one drop of a 0.5% pilocarpine solution in the affected eye. If no reaction occurs in either eye, then the test is inconclusive concerning pharmacologic blockade. In these cases and particularly in brown eyes, 1% pilocarpine may be needed. If the patient's mydriasis is drug induced, the motor end-plates will not react to such a dilute pilocarpine solution. If the condition represents a partial third cranial nerve paralysis, however, the motor end-plates are intact and will respond with the appropriate miosis.

AFFERENT PUPILLARY DEFECT

One of the functions of the pupil is regulation of the amount of light falling on the retina. Too much or too little light prevents the retina from working at peak efficiency.

Swinging Flashlight Test

If the amount of light shining into a pupil is reduced, both pupils dilate in order to gather in more light. If the intensity of the light is not reduced and the optic nerve has developed a conduction defect, less light is transmitted, a phenomenon that the brain interprets as less light getting onto the retina. The response to this light "reduction" is the same as in the first instance—both pupils dilate to an appropriate amount.

The afferent pupillary defect (Marcus Gunn pupillary escape phenomenon) is dependent on the light-reduction response that occurs in the presence of a conduction defect in the optic nerve. In attempting to elicit the afferent pupillary defect in a patient, the physician shines the light into each eye separately. Both pupils respond, even though one optic nerve has a conduction defect. A difference may exist in the quality of the response of each pupil to direct light, but the difference cannot usually be appreciated clinically unless the optic nerve is severely affected. However, when the light is brought quickly from the normal pupil to the side with the conduction defect, both pupils dilate. The brain interprets the decrease in signals from the nerve with the conduction defect as it would if the intensity of the light were reduced.

The afferent pupillary defect is more easily seen in dim illumination with distance fixation. The observer must be careful not to stimulate accommodation by standing in front of the patient or by putting a light directly in front of the pupil.

A conduction defect in one optic nerve causes the afferent pupillary defect, but it does not account for unequal pupils, which is a separate entity that requires additional explanation if it occurs.

The afferent pupillary defect is seen only in unilateral optic nerve disease; it is not generally a useful sign when the chiasm is involved. It can occasionally be seen in chiasmal disease if one nerve is more involved. It can also occur on a retinal basis, but only when extensive destruction has occurred. Such lesions as those in macular degeneration or the large macular lesions in toxoplasmosis can cause it. A lesion such as diffuse diabetic retinopathy, with proliferation and loss of most of the retinal architecture, or a complete retinal detachment can cause it. Therefore, if the patient has some minor retinal disease and exhibits the afferent pupillary defect, he has two diseases, one in the retina and one in the optic nerve.

The main use of the afferent pupillary defect is in evaluating the patient who complains about the vision in one eye but who has a normal ophthalmoscopic examination. The afferent pupillary defect is valuable in retrobulbar neuritis, particularly in patients with relatively good vision. It can be elicited even in cases of optic neuritis with only one Snellen line difference in acuity between the two eyes.

The afferent pupillary defect attests to the presence of the conduction defect, not to its time of onset. This defect lasts as long as there is a conduction difference between the two eyes.

THIRD CRANIAL NERVE PARALYSIS

An early sign of third cranial nerve disease may be simply mydriasis; however, careful evaluation may show that other functions of the third cranial nerve are affected. Look for a small vertical muscle imbalance that may be seen only on up gaze, for a slight ptosis, or for an ipsilateral decrease in accommodation. Repeated testing of the pupil with light may show pupillary fatigue in the abnormal eye, whereas the fellow eye continues to constrict normally, even when repeatedly tested.

Partial internal ophthalmoplegia has the same differential diagnosis and serious implications as described for total third cranial nerve paralysis. The most serious and urgent implication is an aneurysm.

Kerr and Hollowell confirmed Sunderland's work on the location of the pupil fibers in the third nerve. They are located dorsomedially and medially in the nerve. This has particular significance in predicting the ability to produce mydriasis with pressure on the third nerve. It takes pressure of a lesser magnitude on the medial aspect of the nerve than on the dorsal or lateral aspect to cause mydriasis. For instance, displacement of the brain with compression of the third nerve against the tentorial edge readily causes mydriasis whereas increased intracranial pressure with pseudotumor cerebri does not.

It is important, therefore, to identify other causes that can produce internal ophthalmoplegia. Infections, such as varicella and botulism, on occasion have been reported to cause internal ophthalmoplegia. Internal ophthalmoplegia has also been reported after panretinal photocoagulation. The probable mechanism created by the photocoagulation is damage to the short ciliary nerves traveling anteriorly in the sclera.

Accommodation problems have been reported to occur during the regulation of diabetes. This is besides the usual refractive error so commonly encountered. These findings are not associated with pupillary or motility signs. The accommodative changes are usually mild and often missed; however, they can be severe on occasion and their possible association with diabetes should be remembered. The cause is unknown, but it is suggested that a similar mechanism that affects the resiliency of the lens during changes in blood sugar accounts for changes also in accommodation.

Aberrant regeneration of the third cranial nerve can also affect only pupillary fibers. The aberrant association of pupillary contraction with innervation of the medial rectus has been well described by Ford, Walsh, and King.

Czarnecki and Thompson described three other pupillary signs of misdirection: (1) contraction of the iris sphincter to eye movements similar to that described by Ford, Walsh, and King but only in certain sectors of the iris, suggesting not only aberrant but partial regeneration of the third cranial nerve; (2) also similar sector contractions to light stimulation; (3) in the dark and in the absence of light stimulation and with pupils that had no light reaction, there was hippus but asynchronous with the normal eye. Since there is no efferent arc to stimulate the pupil, one explanation is that fibers intended for the third cranial nerve muscle group now innervate the pupil.

HORNER SYNDROME

This condition of the eye and eyelids is caused by paralysis of the cervical sympathetic nerves.

Anatomic Considerations

The long course of the sympathetic chain and the many syndromes encountered along it make essential at least a cursory knowledge of the anatomy involved (Fig. 3–1, Table 3–3). The first neuron of the sympathetic fibers begins in the posterior hypothalamus, traverses the midbrain and reticular substance of the pons, and ends in the anterior lateral gray substance of the spinal cord. It synapses somewhere between C-8 and T-2, in what is referred to as the ciliospinal center (Budge's center). The second neuron begins when the fibers leave the spinal cord via the white rami communicantes of C-8 to T-2, traveling through the stellate ganglion and vertical sympathetic trunk to synapse at the superior cervical ganglion, where the second

neuron is completed. Palumbo's work suggests that the preganglionic neurons controlling the pupil enter the upper one half of the stellate ganglion by a separate paravertebral root. The stellate ganglion contains the fibers from the lower cervical and first thoracic ganglia. He noted that, unlike taking the entire stellate ganglion, when he resected the preganglionic root and only the lower one half of the ganglion, he did not produce a Horner's pupil in 93% of the cases. He concluded that the pupillary fibers must travel by a separate root to only the upper half of the ganglion.

The third neuron is composed of fibers that form a plexus around the carotid artery. As the carotid artery bifurcates, the fibers subserving sweating follow the external carotid artery, a fact that is important in the localization of the lesion producing Horner syndrome. The main fibers go with the internal carotid artery into the carotid canal, in which a thin-walled structure separates the carotid artery from the tympanic cavity. The sympathetic fibers penetrate the carotid tympanic wall and form the caroticotympanic nerve, which runs submucosally in the middle ear. They then pass through the cranial vault near the pterygoid canal and enter the cavernous sinus. Passing over the gasserian ganglion,

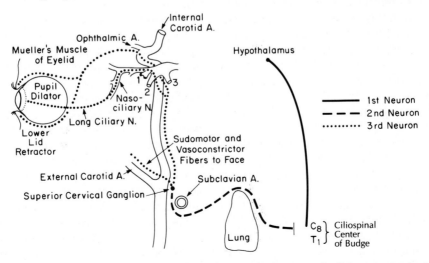

Fig. 3–1.   Course of sympathetic nerves from hypothalamus to the eye and adjacent anatomic structures.

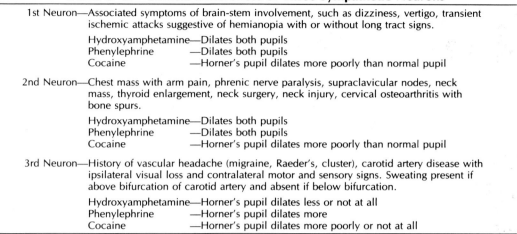

TABLE 3–3.   Clinical Differences of Three Sympathetic Neurons

1st Neuron—Associated symptoms of brain-stem involvement, such as dizziness, vertigo, transient ischemic attacks suggestive of hemianopia with or without long tract signs.

Hydroxyamphetamine	—Dilates both pupils
Phenylephrine	—Dilates both pupils
Cocaine	—Horner's pupil dilates more poorly than normal pupil

2nd Neuron—Chest mass with arm pain, phrenic nerve paralysis, supraclavicular nodes, neck mass, thyroid enlargement, neck surgery, neck injury, cervical osteoarthritis with bone spurs.

Hydroxyamphetamine	—Dilates both pupils
Phenylephrine	—Dilates both pupils
Cocaine	—Horner's pupil dilates more poorly than normal pupil

3rd Neuron—History of vascular headache (migraine, Raeder's, cluster), carotid artery disease with ipsilateral visual loss and contralateral motor and sensory signs. Sweating present if above bifurcation of carotid artery and absent if below bifurcation.

Hydroxyamphetamine	—Horner's pupil dilates less or not at all
Phenylephrine	—Horner's pupil dilates more
Cocaine	—Horner's pupil dilates more poorly or not at all

they enter the orbit via the superior orbital fissure. They travel with the nasociliary nerve to the long ciliary nerves, penetrate the sclera, and then pass forward to innervate the dilator muscle. Before the fibers enter the globe, a branch goes to the smooth muscles of the lids.

Signs

Ptosis. This condition is never severe in Horner syndrome since the levator portion of the third cranial nerve does most of the lid elevation. The ptosis varies, depending on how tired or alert the patient is. It is not uncommon to observe a ptosis when the patient is evaluated after admission in the evening (when he is tired) and to find it has improved in the morning. This improvement is not real since the levator and frontalis muscles and uninjured sympathetic fibers act to overcome the ptosis. Occasionally, no ptosis exists in the presence of sympathetic fiber damage, namely when the fiber to Müller's muscle has already branched off in the orbit proximal to the site of injury. Müller's muscle may also be spared in cases of slight damage to the sympathetic fibers. (I feel that this sparing is rare.) The lack of ptosis makes the diagnosis of Horner syndrome more difficult, but its absence or presence does not

usually help much in determining the anatomic location since the other factors just mentioned influence the degree of ptosis.

An additional problem in diagnosing the ptosis of Horner syndrome occurs in the elderly patient who may also have pseudoptosis secondary to blepharochalasis. In such a case, attention should be directed to the lower lid, which also has sympathetic innervation. I prefer to call the reaction Kearns' lower lid sign since it was Kearns who pointed out to me the significance of sympathetic innervation of the smooth muscle of the lower lid. This innervation normally holds the lower lid down and against the globe. When the muscle is paralyzed, the lid rides up slightly (Fig. 3–2A,B). The test for the lower lid sign is performed by having the patient fixate on a hand light and then moving the light up until the side with the suspected Horner syndrome has the six o'clock position of the cornea barely touching the lower lid. Then the other eye is observed. Instead of its being in the same position, some white sclera shows between the lower cornea and the lower lid. Thus in Horner syndrome there is upper lid ptosis and often lower lid elevation as well.

Apparent Enophthalmos. The position of the upper and lower lids makes the pal-

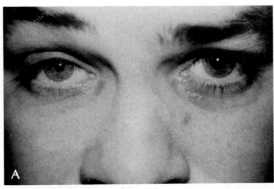

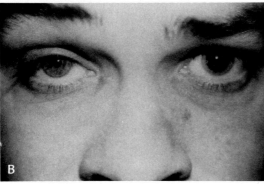

Fig. 3–2. Paredrine test on third neuron Horner syndrome. **A.** Right pupil is smaller. **B.** Thirty minutes after topical hydroxyamphetamine. Right pupil does not change and left pupil dilates. Notice that more sclera is seen between the lower lid and six o'clock position of limbus in the left eye than in the right. This raising up of the lower lid is seen on the side of any neuron Horner syndrome.

pebral fissure narrower in Horner syndrome; thus less of the eye is seen. Unlike man, some animals have functional smooth muscle in the orbit, and paralysis of this muscle results in enophthalmos. In man, the position of the lids gives the impression of enophthalmos; however, the enophthalmos cannot be documented by exophthalmometer readings. It is apparent rather than real.

Miosis. This condition may seem to vary in Horner syndrome. The brightness of the background light in which the patient is examined may make the anisocoria difficult to detect. The same can be said of the physician's standing in front of the patient during the examination and thereby stim-

ulating the patient's accommodation and reducing the size of both pupils. To overcome these two problems, the patient should be examined in a semidark room with his gaze at a distant point and the observer off to one side. Because of the slowness of the affected pupil to dilate in the dark, the anisocoria is greater during the first 5 seconds of dark adaptation than at 15 seconds.

The miosis may vary also according to the extent of the defect, patient alertness, extent of reinnervation, and degree of denervation sensitivity. As a result of denervation supersensitivity, a patient may complain of an occasionally larger pupil on the side on which the physician observes a smaller pupil. This situation rarely occurs, but it probably represents the patient's supersensitivity to his own circulating epinephrine, a phenomenon that can be elicited by the instillation of one drop of a 1:1000 aqueous epinephrine solution topically onto both corneas. In the patient with Horner syndrome, the pupil that has developed supersensitivity dilates, whereas the other pupil shows no reaction.

Systemic drugs such as the barbiturates and narcotics can also cause miosis but without ptosis. A notable exception to the rule is glutethimide (Doriden) which tends to enlarge the pupils, particularly when taken in toxic doses. Topical medications (including most of the antiglaucoma drugs) also cause miosis.

Miosis is greater in postganglionic lesions than in preganglionic ones.

Ocular Hypotony. The intraocular pressure on the side of a Horner syndrome is at least 5 mm less than the pressure in the fellow eye.

Heterochromia. The human iris is blue or slate-gray at birth. Those irises that become brown do so by the end of the first year of life, a change that involves sympathetic innervation. Therefore, the iris of a patient with congenital or neonatal Horner syndrome usually remains lighter, since no sympathetic stimulation occurs to make it darker blue or brown than the iris of its fellow eye. This phenomenon is obvious if the other eye is brown and the eye with the Horner syndrome is blue. It is not as apparent in blue-eyed patients, in whom the difference may be more subtle and can easily be overlooked. The difference is more easily seen in daylight than in artificial indoor light. In acquired adult Horner syndrome, depigmentation is said to occur, but for all practical purposes it can be considered a rare phenomenon. Therefore Horner syndrome with heterochromia has a congenital or neonatal onset—a fact that may be of value in medicolegal testimony.

Increase in Accommodation. Cogan demonstrated that an increased amplitude of accommodation occurs on the side with Horner syndrome. He also proved that the increase is caused not by the miosis but by change in the ciliary muscle that amounts to 0.5 to 1.5 diopters. It is difficult to use the phenomenon as a test in patients under 35 years of age. Young people can read almost up to their nose; thus any variations in accommodation are difficult to detect clinically. In examining a patient who needs glasses, be sure that he is wearing the correct distance prescription, with an equal reading prescription over it. With the use of the near reading card, you will find that the patient reads signficantly closer on the side with Horner syndrome.

Anhidrosis. Lesions from the posterior hypothalamus to the bifurcation of the carotid artery result in ipsilateral loss of sweating ability on the face. If Horner syndrome occurs above the carotid artery bifurcation, the sweating mechanism is intact, a good localizing sign. Nonetheless, demonstrating the loss of sweating ability or eliciting a history of it from the patient is not easy.

Chemical Tests

The clinical usefulness of cocaine and epinephrine was outlined by Foerster and Gagel. These authors believed that using either a 4% cocaine solution or a 1:1000 aqueous epinephrine solution can differentiate the neurons anatomically. Cocaine prevents the re-uptake of norepinephrine at the motor end-plate, and thus prolongs its action on the effector cell. If the sympathetic pathways are interrupted, norepinephrine should not be released, and therefore, a mydriatic effect should not occur. Epinephrine, on the other hand, works directly as a stimulator of the motor end-plate. A 1:1000 aqueous epinephrine solution should not dilate a normal pupil; however, if supersensitivity exists (as can occur in postganglionic [third-neuron] lesions), the pupil will dilate. Therefore, Foerster and Gagel believed that the scheme shown in Table 3–4 was a good one for localizing a Horner syndrome to one of 3 neurons; however, the scheme usually does not work. Third-neuron Horner syndrome rarely shows supersensitivity to 1:1000 aqueous epinephrine. It is better to use 1 or 2% phenylephrine. This drug may dilate both pupils but will have a greater effect on the supersensitive pupil. It is important to document both pupil signs before and after the test to evaluate the relative effectiveness of the drug on both pupils. In theory, cocaine should not dilate any Horner syndrome pupil, no matter what neuron is involved, since no impulse comes to the motor end-plate to release norepinephrine in the first place. If the Horner syndrome pupil does dilate, it is probably because the Horner syndrome is incomplete or because a small amount of norepinephrine has been released at the end-plate constantly without direct central nervous system stimulation. Thompson and Mensher have modified Foerster and Gagel's scheme by the use of hydroxyamphetamine, which works differently from the other two agents by releasing endogenous norepinephrine from an intact motor end-plate. If the condition is a third-neuron Horner syndrome and the nerve and end-plate have degenerated, epinephrine is not present and thus no mydriasis

TABLE 3–4.   Effects of Cocaine and Epinephrine on the Pupils in Horner Syndrome (Foerster and Gagel schema)

Agent	Effect on Pupil When Lesion Is Central (First-Neuron)	Effect on Pupil When Lesion is Preganglionic (Second-Neuron)	Effect on Pupil When Lesion is Postganglionic (Third-Neuron)
Cocaine	Normal mydriasis	None or slight dilatation	No dilatation
Epinephrine	No dilatation	No dilatation	Dilatation

occurs with hydroxyamphetamine (Fig. 3–2A, B).

If the condition involves a first or second neuron, the third neuron is left intact, with the norepinephrine stores present. Even though no central nervous system innervation exists, hydroxyamphetamine releases the norepinephrine and the pupil should dilate. My experience with the hydroxyamphetamine test makes it seem valuable. I think that is has good theoretic points to recommend it and that it should be tried. Maloney, Younge, and Moyer evaluated the hydroxyamphetamine test and found it 84% accurate in predicting and 96% accurate in confirming a third-neuron Horner syndrome. Grimson and Thompson agreed that the test may be inconclusive in 15 to 20% of cases and this number rises unless photographs are taken. The test is particularly unreliable in cases of congenital Horner syndrome. My experience with the test has been more limited than that of these authors, but I find it more useful than cocaine and 1:1000 aqueous epinephrine.

The cocaine test should be discussed further. The cocaine should be in a 4% solution and not a 10% solution as some advocate. A 10% solution adds nothing to the test and copious use may do some transient damage to the epithelium. Changing the corneal tear film or epithelium by drops or corneal sensitivity testing only alters the topical pharmacologic sensitivity tests such as epinephrine and mecholyl.

Causes and Significance

A usual question is, Why bother about Horner syndrome since the majority of patients are not symptomatic or, at the worst,

have only a slight ptosis? The reason for bothering is that Horner syndrome may be the tip of an iceberg, indicating a more serious condition.

In determining the cause of Horner syndrome, the usual approach is to try to localize it to a specific neuron. In older patients, one of the most common causes of Horner syndrome is a vascular infarct of the sympathetic chain. The syndrome may occur along the first neuron in the brain stem owing to the obstruction of the small penetrating vessels from the basilar artery. It occurs also along the distribution of the third neuron sympathetic chain associated with the carotid artery. The latter has been shown by Sears, Kier, and Chavis to occur experimentally.

The congenital variety of Horner syndrome is considered by most to be caused by neck injury from manipulation during a difficult forceps or breech delivery. Trauma is the most frequently found cause in those beyond infancy and under the age of 21. Patients older than 20 years of age, and particularly those over 50 years of age, with a second-neuron Horner's, should be investigated for the presence of tumor (usually malignant) when the onset of an isolated Horner syndrome occurs. The most common tumors are metastatic and bronchogenic carcinoma, particularly apical, or Pancoast tumors. Benign tumors, such as neurofibromas and thyroid adenomas, are less common.

The causes of isolated Horner syndrome have changed somewhat since the report of Giles and Henderson. Third-neuron Horner syndrome carries a high incidence of nontumor disease as the cause. Third-neuron Horner syndrome is more likely caused by a headache syndrome (e.g., Raeder's, cluster), trauma (e.g., basal skull fracture), or inflammations (e.g., Tolosa Hunt, otitis media, herpes zoster).

The second-neuron Horner syndrome still carries a high incidence of tumors as the cause as was pointed out by Giles and Henderson and confirmed in the recent reviews by Grimson and Thompson and by Maloney, Younge, and Moyer. Grimson and Thompson stated that the incidence is as high as 50%, and Maloney, Younge, and Moyer found that 72% of the tumors causing a Horner syndrome were along the second-neuron distribution. Younge makes an additional observation: Most of the tumors in their series were Pancoast-type, and Horner syndrome was rarely the presenting sign. Their patients also had arm pain, which should serve as a clue to the real cause of the Horner Syndrome.

Workup

How does the physician evaluate Horner syndrome once he has made the diagnosis? The time of onset may be difficult to establish. The time the patient says it started may be only the time that he noticed it. One of the best ways to establish the time of onset is by examining old photographs of the patient, particularly job, army, or passport identification photographs. Such photographs are usually unretouched, and often the pupils can be seen with a magnifying glass or the large indirect ophthalmoscope lens. If these types of photographs are not available, ask the patient to supply some pictures from his high school or college yearbook or some wedding pictures. The fact that a Horner syndrome has been present for 10 years or more points to a benign cause even when the exact reason for the condition remains obscure.

Ask the patient about any neck operation (such as thyroid surgical procedure) that may have injured the sympathetic chain. Scars from such operations can easily be overlooked. Ask also about a chest or heart operation, which could also account for

Horner syndrome. In the past, when more carotid arteriograms were done using the direct carotid artery injection route, both permanent and transient Horner syndromes were sometimes seen.

Question the patient carefully about any neck trauma as a youth. If he played sports, ask whether he wore a neck collar for several months because of an athletic injury. Photographs showing the patient's pupils around that time, when any miosis would have been more evident before reinnervation, may document the time of onset. Horner syndrome can also be seen in severe whiplash injuires, such as those occurring in automobile accidents.

The examination should include palpation of the neck for masses, thyroid nodules, or supraclavicular nodes. Apical views of the lung to visualize a Pancoast tumor, as well as skull and cervical roentgenograms, should be ordered. Hematologic evaluation to rule out lymphomas or Hodgkin's disease is also indicated.

Types

First-Neuron Horner Syndrome. The most common cause of first-neuron Horner syndrome is vertebral-basilar insufficiency as in Wallenberg syndrome. A Horner syndrome may be the only residual sign of a transient ischemic episode. Severe osteoarthritis of the neck, with obvious bony spurs visualized on roentgenographic examination, is known to have caused compression of the sympathetic fibers as they leave the cervical canal. I have also seen Horner syndrome occur with severe whiplash injury without other obvious neurologic deficits. Horner syndrome can be transient or permanent, and it may be the only evidence of the severity of the injury, particularly when the patient has multiple post-traumatic complaints.

Second-Neuron Horner Syndrome. Among the most common causes of second-neuron Horner syndrome is apical lung cancer (such as Pancoast tumor), which is best demonstrated by apical views of the lung. Mediastinal tumor is also a cause, but it is not as easily detected.

Third-Neuron Horner Syndrome—Group One. This type of Horner syndrome can be broken down into two groups. The first group includes patients with Raeder paratrigeminal syndrome, cluster headaches, and migraine. These three conditions may be aspects of the one disease, but each condition is worthy of comment because of its individual characteristics.

Raeder Paratrigeminal Syndrome. Essentially a painful Horner syndrome, the major complaint is pain over the first and second divisions of the trigeminal nerve. The patient shows all the signs of a Horner syndrome, except that the sweating mechanism is intact because the lesion is located above the bifurcation of the carotid artery. There may be a small area of anhidrosis on the ipsilateral forehead. This area is supplied by terminal frontal branches coming in with the carotid artery. This is a variable sign. Raeder syndrome occurs overwhelmingly in men, and usually in those in their forties. The major consideration is that the condition is benign. The pain subsides, but frequently the Horner syndrome remains. The first reported case of Raeder syndrome involved a meningioma of the gasserian ganglion, but most subsequent reported cases have been benign. Davis, Daroff, and Hoyt reported one case associated with an extracranial aneurysm. Law and Nelson also had one case of a supraclinoid aneurysm and Cohen, Zakov, and Solanga reported two cases associated with fibrous dysplasia.

Raeder syndrome can be broken down into 2 groups. Group 1 has a Horner syndrome, trigeminal pain, and other parasellar cranial nerve involvement and is not benign. Group 2 is the same without parasellar nerve involvement. Group 2 is usually caused by a vascular or inflammatory mechanism affecting the sympathetic chain and sensory fibers that run in the carotid artery sheath and is benign. If the pain is atypical or persists more than 3 months, these patients should be investigated even in the absence of other cranial nerve involvement. No specific treatment exists.

Cluster Headaches. Patients with third-neuron Horner syndrome may have headache as a primary finding. These patients are also usually in their forties. The headache is not steady, and it is predictable as to time of day and duration (usually several hours). These patients also have tearing and ocular hyperemia, as well as ipsilateral nasal stuffiness. The associated Horner syndrome may be transient. The condition is benign. At one time it was treated with histamine desensitization, but this treatment has fallen out of favor. In any case, it is usually a self-limited process, although episodes do recur (hence the name cluster headaches).

Migraine. In any form, even with a typical homonymous scotoma, migraine may affect the carotid artery and result in Horner syndrome. The condition is usually self-limited.

Third-Neuron Horner Syndrome—Group Two. The second group of third-neuron Horner syndrome involves the facial sweating mechanism. The syndromes are (1) idiopathic hemifacial hyperhidrosis, (2) postsympathectomy facial hyperhidrosis, and (3) hemifacial anhidrosis.

Idiopathic Hemifacial Hyperhidrosis. The patient with idiopathic hemifacial hyperhidrosis syndrome complains only of increased sweating on one side of the face, particularly on the forehead. Usually, the condition is aggravated by the eating of spicy foods. No other signs of Horner syndrome are present. The increased sweating is caused by the overactivity of the sympathetic fibers that subserve sweating, and it disappears with sympathetic nerve blockade. This is probably aberrant regeneration of the sudomotor fibers along the external carotid.

Postsympathectomy Facial Hyperhidrosis. After a complete cervical sympathectomy, anhidrosis is present in the ipsilateral affected area. Then after a long time, adjacent autonomic fibers from the vagus nerve sprout to innervate the sympathetic nerves. Thereafter, patients sweat and tingle when they eat. Since sweating is cholinergic and tingling is caused by pilomotion, which is adrenergic, the vagus nerve must make preganglionic connections where all fibers are of the cholinergic variety. No associated pupillary or palpebral signs are present.

Hemifacial Anhidrosis. Sweating over the ipsilateral face is lost with sympathetic interruption below the bifurcation of the carotid artery, where the facial sweat fibers leave the artery. Occasionally, however, sweating may be preserved on the forehead because some sympathetic fibers have gone with the orbital division, innervating the forehead directly. Therefore, anhidrosis of the face below the eye and above the upper lip has the same significance even if the sweating mechanism remains intact in regard to the forehead.

Phrenic Nerve Syndrome. A new triad involving a Horner syndrome has been reported: Horner syndrome, a hoarse voice, and paralysis of the hemidiaphragm. This triad involves the second neuron of the sympathetic chain, the phrenic nerve, and paralysis of the recurrent laryngeal nerve. The only place these three nerves are in close apposition is at the level of the sixth cervical vertebra. This syndrome occurs with local or recurrent tumors to this area. The three cases reported by Rowland and Payne involved recurrences of breast carcinoma.

HETEROCHROMIA

If heterochromia exists, one iris is different in color from its fellow iris. All patients with congenital Horner syndrome do not have one brown eye and one blue eye, or the detection of Horner's would be simple. Some blue-eyed patients show a much more subtle difference in color between their irises. Check the color difference in daylight (by the office window) rather than

in fluorescent light. The difference thus revealed is often striking.

Larger-sector pigmented areas are nevi and do not represent true heterochromia.

Darker-Eye Heterochromia

This heterochromia is not seen as frequently as is lighter-eye heterochromia. A diffuse iris *melanoma* is best evaluated with the slit lamp, since the darker brown area will appear as a mass rather than simply as pigmented iris stroma. In *neurofibromatosis,* associated signs help identify the disorder. A thorough physical examination is called for, with the physician looking for other neurofibromas and, particularly, for café-au-lait spots. If the physician finds 5 café-au-lait spots that are more than 2 cm in diameter each, the diagnosis of neurofibromatosis is almost a certainty, even if the patient lacks other signs and symptoms. A single café-au-lait spot may point to neurofibromatosis, but it is not conclusive evidence.

If *hemosiderosis* is present, a carefully taken history of trauma or ocular penetration, as well as slit-lamp, indirect ophthalmoscopic, and gonioscopic examinations, is mandatory.

Hemochromatosis of the iris is associated with a history of repeated bleeding in the anterior chamber.

Lighter-Eye Heterochromia

This heterochromia is seen more frequently than darker-eye heterochromia because the iris does not become pigmented until late in the first year of life. Iris pigmentation requires sympathetic stimulation. Congenital or neonatal sympathetic paralysis is a leading cause of heterochromia. The lack of pigmentation is not universally present.

Waardenburg syndrome is a variation of congenital Horner syndrome. In addition to lighter-eye heterochromia, the patient has a prominent white forelock, lateral displacement of the medial canthus, deafness, hypertrichosis, a broad nasal root, and lighter pigmentation of the ipsilateral fundus.

Fuchs' heterochromic cyclitis is worthy of comment because of its resistance to therapy. Most prolonged cases of iritis cause atrophy of the iris stroma and result in secondary heterochromia. Fuchs' iritis has specific corneal endothelial deposits that are stellate in shape. It has a low level of activity and is resistant to therapy of any kind. Secondary glaucoma and cataract also may develop, but they can be treated as the need arises.

Essential iris atrophy is a rare but interesting problem that occurs predominantly in young women. It is progressive. Since secondary glaucoma is the main complication, patients should be examined for glaucoma periodically.

BIBLIOGRAPHY

Adie, W.J.: Argyll Robertson pupils true and false. Br. Med. J. 2:136. 1931.

Adie, W.J.: Tonic pupils and absent tendon reflexes. Brain 55:98, 1932.

Bell, R.A., and Thompson, H.S.: Relative afferent pupillary defect in optic tract hemianopsia. Am. J. Ophthalmol. 85:538, 1978.

Bell, R.A., and Thompson, H.S.: Ciliary muscle dysfunction in Adie's syndrome. Arch. Ophthalmol. 96:638, 1978.

Bloor, K.: Gustatory, sweating and other responses after cervico-thoracic sympathectomy. Brain 92:137, 1969.

Boniuk, M. and Schlezinger, N.S.: Raeder's paratrigeminal syndrome. Am. J. Ophthalmol. 54:1074, 1962.

Bourgon, P., Pilley, S.F., and Thompson, H.S.: Cholinergic supersensitivity of the iris sphincter in Adie's tonic pupil. Am. J. Ophthalmol. 83:373, 1978.

Burde, R.M., The pupil. Int. Ophthalmol. Clin. 7:849, 1967.

Caccamise, W.C.: Bilateral congenital mydriasis. Am. J. Ophthalmol. 81:515, 1976.

Cannon, W.B.: A law of denervation. Am. J. Med. Sci. 198:737, 1939.

Clarke, A.M., and Behrendt, T.: Solar retinitis and pupillary reaction. Am. J. Ophthalmol. 73:700, 1972.

Cobb, S., and Scarlett, H.W.: A report of eleven cases of cervical sympathetic nerve injury causing the oculopupillary syndrome. Arch. Neurol. Psychol. 3:626, 1920.

Cogan, D.G.: Accommodation and the autonomic nervous system. Arch. Ophthalmol. 18:739, 1937.

Cohen, D.N., and Zakov, Z.N.: The diagnosis of Adie's pupil using 0.0625% pilocarpine solution. Am. J. Ophthalmol. 79:883, 1975.

Cohen, D.N., Zakov, N., and Salanga, V.: Raeder's paratrigeminal syndrome. Am. J. Ophthalmol. 79:1045, 1975.

Collin, J.R., Beard, C., and Wood, I.: Terminal course of nerve supply to Müller's muscle in the rhesus monkey and its clinical significance. Am. J. Ophthalmol. 87:234, 1979.

Czarnecki, J.S.C., and Thompson, H.S.: The iris sphincter in aberrant regeneration of the third nerve. Arch. Ophthalmol. 96:1606, 1978.

Davis, R.H., Daroff, R.B., and Hoyt, W.F.: Hemicrania, oculosympathetic paresis and subcranial carotid aneurysm. Raeder's paratrigeminal syndrome (Group 2), case report. J. Neurosurg. 29:94, 1968.

Ford, F.R., Walsh, F.B., and King, A.: Clinical observations on the pupillary phenomena resulting from regeneration of the third nerve with especial reference to the Argyll Robertson pupil. Bull. Johns Hopkins Hosp. 68:309, 1941.

Foerster, O., and Gagel, O.: Die Vorderseitenstrangdurchschneidung beim Menschen. Zschr. Neurol. Psychiatr. 138:1, 1932.

Geltzer, A.I.: Autonomic innervation of the cat iris. Arch. Ophthalmol. 81:70, 1969.

Giles, C.L., and Henderson, J.W.: Horner's syndrome: an analysis of 216 cases. Am. J. Ophthalmol. 46:289, 1958.

Glaser, J.S.: The nasal visual field. Arch. Ophthalmol. 77:358, 1967.

Grimson, B.S., and Thompson, H.S.: Horner's Syndrome: Overall View of 120 Cases. *In* Topics in Neurophthalmology. Edited by H.S. Thompson. Baltimore, Williams & Wilkins, 1979.

Gunn, M.R.: Retro-ocular neuritis. Lancet 3:412, 1904.

Harriman, D.G.F., and Garland, H.: The pathology of Adie's syndrome. Brain 91:401, 1968.

Hedges, T.: The tonic pupil: familial incidence, recognition and progression. Arch. Ophthalmol. 80:21, 1968.

Hedges, T.R., and Gerner, E.W.: Ross' syndrome. Br. J. Ophthalmol. 59:387, 1974.

Holmes, G.: Partial iridoplegia associated with symptoms of other disease of the nervous system. Trans. Ophthalmol. Soc. U.K. 51:209, 1931.

Hurwitz, B.S., et al.: The effects of the sympathetic nervous system on accommodation. 1. Beta sympathetic nervous system. Arch. Ophthalmol. 87:668, 1972.

Hurwitz, B.S., et al.: The effects of the sympathetic nervous system in accommodation. 2. Alpha sympathetic nervous system. Arch. Ophthalmol. 87:675, 1972.

Jagerman, L.S.: Hering's law applied to the near reflex. Am. J. Ophthalmol. 70:579, 1970.

Keane, J.R.: Tonic pupils with acute ophthalmoplegic polyneuritis. Ann. Neurol. 2:393, 1977.

Kerr, F.W., and Hollowell, O.W.: Location of pupillomotor and accommodation fibers in the oculomotor nerve. Experimental observations on paralytic mydriasis. J. Neurol. Neurosurg. Psychiat. 27:473, 1964.

Khurana, K.M., and Hunter, P.J.: Horner's syndrome produced by hypertrophic spurs from the cervical spine. Br. J. Ophthalmol. 48:227, 1964.

Kupfer, C., Chumbley, L., Downes, J.: Quantitative histology of optic nerve, optic tract and lateral geniculate nucleus of mass. J. Anat., 101:393, 1967.

Laties, A.M., and Scheie, H.G.: Adie's syndrome: duration of methacholine sensitivity. Arch. Ophthalmol. 74:458, 1965.

Law, W.R., and Nelson, E.R.: Internal carotid aneurysm as a cause of Raeder's paratrigeminal syndrome. Neurol. 18:431, 1968.

Levatin, P.: Pupillary escape in disease of the retina or optic nerve. Arch. Ophthalmol. 62:768, 1959.

Loewenfeld, I.E.: "Simple central" anisocoria: a common condition, seldom recognized. Trans. Am. Acad. Ophthalmol. Otolaryngol. 83:OP832, 1977.

Loewenfeld, I.E., Friedlaender, R.P., and McKennon, P.F.: Pupillary inequality associated with lateral gaze (Tournay's phenomenon). Am. J. Opthalmol. 78:449, 1974.

Loewenfeld, I.E., and Thompson, H.S.: The tonic pupil: a re-evaluation. Am. J. Ophthalmol. 63:46, 1967.

Lowenstein, O.: Clinical pupillary symptoms in lesions of the optic nerve chiasm and optic tract. Arch. Ophthalmol. 52:385, 1954.

Lowenstein, O., and Givner, I.: Pupillary reflex to darkness. Arch. Ophthalmol. 30:603, 1943.

Lowenstein, O., and Loewenfeld, I.E.: Pupillotonic pseudotabes. Surv. Ophthalmol. 10:129, 1965.

Maloney, W.F., Younge, B.R., and Moyer, N.J.: Evaluation of the causes and accuracy of pharmacologic localization in Horner's syndrome. Am. J. Ophthalmol. 90:394, 1980.

Marmor, M.F.: Transient accommodative paralysis and hyperopia in diabetes. Arch. Ophthalmol. 89:419, 1973.

McCrary, J.A., and Webb, N.R.: Anisocoria from scopolamine patches. JAMA 248:353, 1982.

Moore, R.F.: The non-luetic Argyll-Robertson pupil. Trans. Ophthalmol. Soc. U.K. 51:203, 1931.

Neidle, E.A.: Pilocarpine sensitization in the parasympathetically denervated pupil of the cat. Am. J. Phsysiol. 160:467, 1950.

Newsome, D.A.: Tonic pupil following retinal detachment surgery. Am. J. Ophthalmol. 86:233, 1971.

Okajima, T., Imamura, S., and Kawasaki, S.: Fisher's syndrome: a pharmacological study of the pupils. Ann. Neurol. 2:63, 1977.

Palumbo, L.T.: A new concept of the sympathetic pathways to the eye. Ann. Ophthalmol. 8:947, 1976.

Purcell, J.J., Krachmer, J.H., and Thompson, H.S.: Corneal sensation in Adie's syndrome. Am. J. Ophthalmol. 84:496, 1977.

Raeder, J.G.: Paratrigeminal paralysis of oculopupillary sympathetic. Brain 47:149, 1924.

Rogell, G.D.: Internal ophthalmoplegia after argon laser panretinal photocoagulation. Arch. Ophthalmol. 97:904, 1979.

Rowland Payne, C.M.E.: Newly recognized syndrome in the neck: Horner's syndrome with ipsilateral vocal cord and phrenic nerve palsies. J. Roy. Soc. Med. 74:814, 1981.

Russell, G.F.M.: Accommodation in the Holmes–Adie's syndrome. J. Neurol. Neurosurg. Psychiatry 21:290, 1958.

Schatz, N.J., Savino, P.J., and Corbett, J.J.: Primary aberrant oculomotor regeneration: a sign of intracavernous meningioma. Arch. Neurol. 34:29, 1977.

Sears, M.L.: The cause of the Argyll Robertson pupil. Am. J. Ophthalmol. 72:488, 1971.

Sears, M.L., Kier, L., and Chavis, R.M.: Horner's syndrome caused by occlusion of the vascular supply to sympathetic ganglia. Am. J. Ophthalmol. 77:717, 1974.

Selhorst, J.B., Hoyt, W.F., and Feinsod, M.: Midbrain correctopia. Arch Neurol. 33:193, 1976.

Sharpe, J.A., and Glaser, J.S.: Tournay's phenomenon. Am. J. Ophthalmol. 77:250, 1974.

Smith, T.L.: Raeder's paratrigeminal syndrome. Am. J. Ophthalmol. 46:194, 1958.

Stanley, J.A., and Baise, G.R.: The swinging flashlight test to detect minimal optic neuropathy. Arch. Ophthalmol. 80:769, 1968.

Sunderland, S.: Mechanism responsible for changes in the pupil unaccompanied by disturbances of extraocular muscle function. Br. J. Ophthalmol. 36:638, 1952.

Symonds, C.: A particular variety of headache. Brain 79:217, 1956.

Thompson, H.S.: Afferent pupillary defects. Am. J. Ophthalmol. 62:860, 1966.

Thompson, H.S.,: Pupillary signs in the diagnosis of optic nerve disease. Trans. Ophthalmol. Soc. U.K. 96:377, 1976.

Thompson, H.S.: Adie's syndrome. Some new observations. Trans. Am. Ophthalmol. Soc. 75:587, 1977.

Thompson, H.S.: Segmental palsy of the iris sphincter in Adie's syndrome. Arch. Ophthalmol. 96:1615, 1978.

Thompson, H.S.: Pharmacologic localization in Horner's syndrome. Am. J. Ophthalmol. 91:416, 1981.

Thompson, H.S., and Mensher, J.H.: Adrenergic mydriasis in Horner's syndrome. Am. J. Ophthalmol. 72:472, 1971.

Thompson, H.S., Montague, P., and Cox, T.A.: The relationship between visual acuity, pupillary defect and visual field loss. Am. J. Ophthalmol. 93:681, 1982.

Thompson, H.S., Newsome, D.A., and Loewenfeld, I.E.: The fixed dilated pupil. Arch. Ophthalmol. 86:21, 1971.

Thompson, H.S., and Pilley, S.F.: Unequal pupils. A Flow chart for sorting out the anisocorias. Surv. Ophthalmol. 21:45, 1976.

Walsh, J.C., Low, P.A., and Allsop, J.L.: Localized sympathetic overactivity: an uncommon compli-

cation of lung cancer. J. Neurol. Neurosurg. Psychiatry 39:93, 1976.

Weinstein, J.M., Zweifil, T.J., and Thompson, H.S.: The clinical diagnosis of pupil disorders. J. Contin. Ed. Ophthalmol. May, p. 15, 1979.

Williams, D., Brust, J., and Abrams, G.: Landry-Guillain-Barré Syndrome with abnormal pupils and normal eye movements. Neurology 29:1033, 1979.

Zee, D.S., Griffin, J., and Price, D.L.: Unilateral pupillary dilatation during adversive seizures. Arch. Neurol. 30:403, 1974.

Chapter 4

Exophthalmos

THOMAS J. WALSH

The term exophthalmos refers to abnormal protrusion of one or both eyes. Some forms are occasionally associated with pulsations of the globe. Determination of the cause of exophthalmos can be challenging because it involves many skills in ocular and orbital physical diagnosis. The discussion at hand includes a general review of these skills, with particular reference to specific diseases when they seem appropriate to the topic or have special diagnostic features. Because tumors are frequently encountered, some of the most common ones are discussed; however, a detailed description of the signs and symptoms of every possible tumor has not been attempted because many tumors are not distinguishable from one another without a biopsy. Neither has a detailed discussion of the various modes of surgical treatment been undertaken, because to do so would go beyond the purpose of this chapter, which is to introduce the reader to the diagnosis of the conditions of which exophthalmos is a sign. I refer those readers who desire a more detailed discussion of individual tumors, treatment, or surgical techniques to the works on orbital tumors by Henderson and by Reese.

Exophthalmos is only one sign of orbital disease. Moreover, it is not limited exclusively to orbital tumors; other conditions, such as thyroid disease, orbital varix, arteriovenous fistula, collagen vascular disease, infections, pseudotumor, prolapse of cranial contents into the orbit, and congenital cranial-orbital defects, may also cause exophthalmos. In addition, exophthalmos may sometimes be a remote or indirect effect of orbital passive congestion from carotid cavernous sinus fistula or orbital encephalocele. On the other hand, although exophthalmos occurs over 75% of the time, it should not be assumed that the absence of exophthalmos rules out a primary or secondary orbital tumor, since optic nerve gliomas and meningiomas may cause loss of vision or papilledema before exophthalmos is obvious.

Listed in order of relative frequency, the groups of orbital disorders causing exophthalmos are as follows:

1. Thyroid diseases
2. Tumors
3. Inflammations
4. Vascular disorders
5. Orbital anomalies
6. Miscellaneous disorders

This chapter discusses the characteristics

of these disorders. First, however, it reviews the various manifestations of exophthalmos, as well as some of the techniques used in diagnosis of the condition.

MEASURING EXOPHTHALMOS

If an orbital neoplasm or thyroid disease is suspected, reliance on simple observation can be grossly misleading and may result in an erroneous diagnosis of exophthalmos. At best, with any of the instruments available, it is difficult to duplicate exactly the readings of another observer or even the readings from one examination to another. I prefer the Krahn exophthalmometer, an instrument that measures the relationship between the anterior corneal surface and the lateral rim of the orbit. The advantage of the Krahn exophthalmometer is its reflecting mirror with two vertical lines that must be lined up before a reading on the scale is taken. This feature helps to ensure that the observer's head is in approximately the same position during each examination.

In evaluating exophthalmometer findings, it should be noted that the upper limits of normal vary somewhat. Ninety-five percent of the population measures 19 mm or less, and most people have readings that are in the 16 to 17 mm range. The observer should also keep in mind that some people either measure or look more exophthalmic because of family or racial characteristics. In his appraisals, the observer must evaluate not only the difference between both eyes but also the absolute results of exophthalmometry, since thyroid disease may affect both eyes simultaneously. A difference of up to 2 mm is usually considered normal; however, even a small discrepancy should be recorded on the patient's chart, because subsequent measurements may show progressive increases in exophthalmos that will make a presumably normal difference found on the first examination more significant. A slight degree of exophthalmos (about 1 to 2 mm) may result from a total third cranial nerve paralysis with relaxation of the extraocular muscles, or it may be brought about by venous congestion during a Valsalva maneuver.

TYPES OF OCULAR DISPLACEMENT

Vertical displacement of the eye may be a sign of tumor in a position opposite to the displacement, but it should not be confused with the different levels of the pupils when third cranial nerve paralysis or some other strabismus problem is present. Vertical displacement of the eye should be assessed from the standpoint of the change in position of the eye in relation to its bony orbit.

Since most orbital tumors (particularly benign tumors and cysts) occur in the upper two quadrants, the eye is usually displaced downward. If the tumor is upper temporal, the eye displacement will be downward and nasal; if the tumor is upper nasal, the eye displacement will be downward and temporal. If the eye is displaced upward, more commonly occurring inferior masses, such as lymphomas or carcinomas extending from the maxillary sinus, should be considered. Lateral displacement of the eye is frequently caused by extension of mucoceles or malignant tumors from the ethmoid sinuses. Medial displacement of the globe is least commonly seen because tumors giving rise to this condition extrude anteriorly from the orbit much earlier than do nasal tumors, and are thus palpable and available for biopsy. Henderson (1973) astutely pointed out that more displacement than exophthalmos occurs with anterior lesions (Figs. 4–1 and 4–2), whereas posterior lesions cause more exophthalmos. Tumors in the muscle cone area also cause more exophthalmos than displacement. An exception is the hemangioma of infancy, in which tumors push themselves out around the eye more than they displace it. Henderson believed that, if despite increasing exophthalmos the two eyes can maintain binocularity, the condition is more likely to be caused by expansion of a benign lesion

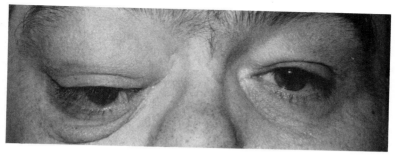

Fig. 4–1. In this patient, a meningioma has infiltrated the orbit and there is more displacement than exophthalmos. In thyroid disease, there is usually more exophthalmos.

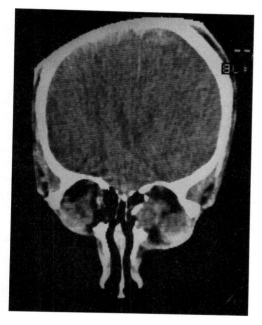

Fig. 4–2. CT examination of ethmoid sinus mass causing displacement of the globe rather than exophthalmos.

rectly behind the eye in the orbit or of an encephalocele. The pulsation, which is frequently hard to detect, is best seen by observing the eye laterally. If this technique fails, examination of the fundus with the direct ophthalmoscope will reveal that the pulsations of the eye are causing the disc to go in and out of focus synchronously with the pulse. Pulsating exophthalmos may be accompanied by bruits, which should be listened for directly over the eye, over the orbit, or in the temporal fossa. If Schiøtz's tonometer is placed on the cornea, the pulsations cause a much greater than usual rhythmic movement of the tonometer arm. Although an applanation tonometer may also be used, it gives a reading that may be less obvious.

In an adult, pulsating exophthalmos is most commonly caused by an arteriovenous fistula; in children, by neurofibromatosis with dehiscence in the orbital roof and extension of pulsations from the brain cavity.

EVALUATION TECHNIQUES

History and Patient Complaints

Although exophthalmos occurs in 30% of the patients suffering from orbital tumor, pain, diplopia, swelling, tearing, and blurred vision are much more common presenting complaints. Since most gliomas occur in the first few decades of life, loss of vision in children, with or without optic atrophy, suggests optic nerve glioma, par-

than by a malignant growth invading adjacent muscle tissue. Although this observation is generally valid, notable exceptions do exist. For example, thyroid disease, which is a benign lesion, can cause marked ophthalmoplegia and loss of binocularity with minimal exophthalmos.

PULSATING EXOPHTHALMOS

Pulsating exophthalmos is symptomatic either of an arteriovenous malformation di-

ticularly if some degree of exophthalmos exists. In a child, the presence of a retro-bulbar mass with ecchymosis of the lids and subconjunctival hemorrhage associated with exophthalmos suggests a malignant tumor, particularly medulloblastoma. Bluish masses on the lid or globe that change size with crying suggest hemangioma. Rapid onset of swelling and pain accompanied by inflammation most likely signals an orbital infection, particularly one from a paranasal sinus, or, in adults, pseudotumor of the orbit.

Ask the patient whether he hears a swishing sound. Such a sign suggests a carotid cavernous sinus fistula and may also be associated with pulsations of the globe. With the use of a bell stethoscope, the bruit may be heard above the eyebrow or eye itself.

A history of thyroid disease that has been successfully treated surgically or with radioisotopes suggests endocrine exophthalmos, which may come on later and in an even more virulent form than when the thyroid was hyperactive. Since the thyroid disease seems to the patient remote and not related to his present difficulty, he may not volunteer information about the earlier condition.

Mucormycosis should be considered in a diabetic patient suffering from rapidly advancing exophthalmos with loss of vision and impaired motility. Examination for the presence of mucormycosis is discussed later in this chapter. Exophthalmos in a patient with a history of nasal or sinus operation for polyps may indicate that an undiagnosed tumor has spread to the orbit. Sometimes, inspection with a nasal speculum reveals masses that were not previously suspected but are readily accessible for biopsy.

Examination should not be restricted to the eyes and orbits alone. It is important to look for adenopathy elsewhere or for café-au-lait spots or angiomas, which, although remote signs, may lead to a correct diagnosis of orbital disease.

Simple Inspection

As in other medical disciplines, simple external inspection is the basic tool for diagnosis of diseases of the eye. Such examination should include the lids, lacrimal apparatus, fornices, and external surfaces of the globe (Fig. 4–3), and it may require rotation of the globe or eversion of the lid over a retractor to check all recesses.

Inspection of the Eyelids

Generally speaking, the most common cause of localized lid swelling is probably a chalazion. If swelling is limited to one lid (or part of the lid), a tumor in that area may be suspected. With exophthalmos, swelling of the lids, particularly in the absence of other signs of infection (redness and elevated temperature), may indicate an anteriorly placed tumor. Lateral swelling of the upper lid points to a lacrimal gland tumor; nasal swelling of the upper lid, to mucoceles. Lower lid swelling suggests lymphoma, which may be visible or palpable in the inferior fornix. Edema of both lids, with proportionately greater swelling of the lower lid, may be symptomatic of meningioma.

The most intense rubor associated with lid edema and infection of the globe occurs in orbital cellulitis. I have also seen an equally high degree of rubor in some cases of pseudotumor of the orbit. Orbital and lid inflammation and minimal exophthalmos may also occur after trauma to a dermoid tumor that has resulted in extrusion of its contents into the orbit. Inflammation can also accompany rapidly growing tumors, such as rhabdomyosarcoma in children and metastatic carcinoma in adults.

Lid retraction can occur without exophthalmos (Fig. 4–4); however, Henderson has made an interesting distinction between exophthalmos owing to endocrine disease and that owing to orbital tumor. The distance between the lid margin and the superior palpebral fissure is a constant 3 mm. According to Henderson, lid retraction owing to endocrine disease shortens

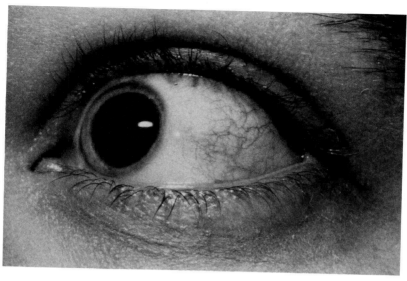

Fig. 4–3. Increase in conjunctival veins over lateral rectus muscle but not extending to limbus is a common sign of thyroid disease.

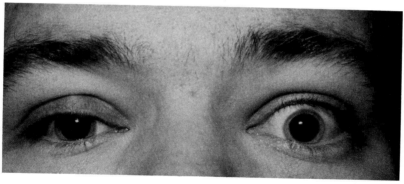

Fig. 4–4. This patient appears more exophthalmic than he really measures because of upper lid retraction. Notice how far left lid is retracted above superior limbus as compared with the right eye. Notice shortening of distance from lid margin to palpebral fissure in the left eye.

the distance; whereas in orbital tumor, the distance remains the same.

Similarly, lid lag (failure of the lid to follow the globe in down gaze) may also be indicative of endocrine disease. In endocrine exophthalmos, the lid-to-limbus distance increases in down gaze; in other forms of exophthalmos with lid retraction above the upper limbus, the ratio of the lid margin to its upper limit remains relatively constant.

Vascular dilatation and congestion can vary in degree with the rapidity of the development of exophthalmos and in relation to its underlying cause. Some forms of epibulbar vascular dilatation are diagnostic of specific disease entities. Dilatation of the vessels over the lateral rectus muscles that does not extend to the limbus is highly suggestive of endocrine exophthalmos (Fig. 4–3). In this condition, the remaining epibulbar vessels are of normal color and caliber, whereas those over the lateral rectus muscle are purple and tortuous and associated with chemosis of the adjacent conjunctiva.

If the vessels are dilated, violaceous, and tortuous, and if they extend to the limbus in many quadrants, but the conjunctiva between the vessels is not red and chemotic, a vascular anomaly is suggested (perhaps carotid cavernous sinus fistula, orbital arteriovenous fistula, or orbital hemangioma).

Palpation

A frequently overlooked but valuable technique is palpation (use of the tip of the little finger to probe around the eye). At the Mayo Clinic, this procedure has been used in diagnosing 70% of all orbital tumors and 85% of the more common tumors, such as lacrimal gland tumors, malignant lymphomas, dermoid tumors, and hemangiomas, many of which are anteriorly placed in the orbit.

Since most tumors occur in the upper orbital quadrants, palpation in these areas can be most productive. Childhood hemangioma and adult mucocele are two of the most commonly occurring upper nasal masses. On light touch, a hemangioma is smooth, but, as is characteristic of vascular masses, appears to collapse on firm palpation, as if the mass were emptying. A mucocele, on the other hand, does not collapse, but feels doughy on firm pressure.

The upper temporal quadrants are frequently the site of dermoid tumors as well as of lacrimal gland tumors. Dermoid tumors can not only be felt but frequently also seen when the upper lid is doubly everted over a Desmarres retractor and the eye is rotated downward and toward the nose. The same procedure may make lacrimal gland tumors more accessible for palpation. It is difficult, however, to differentiate between a benign and a malignant tumor by palpation. A common error is to mistake a lobule of the lacrimal gland for a tumor. Sometimes the tumor is behind the protruding lobule of the lacrimal gland, in which case a negative biopsy of the lobule may be misleading. In some races (among blacks, for example), the anterior lobe of the lacrimal gland usually protrudes into the upper fornix. One feature of adenocarcinoma of the lacrimal gland that may help in selecting a site for biopsy is a firmness relative to a normal gland, with fixation to the periorbita as the tumor breaks out of the gland capsule. The fact that adenocystic tumors tend to be more tender on palpation than other tumors is also helpful in arriving at a diagnosis. The fat hypertrophy of endocrine disease and inflammatory changes owing to a pseudotumor may also be mistaken for a real tumor. The associated signs should help differentiate these entities from a real tumor.

Malignant lymphomas are most frequently found in the inferior quadrants and may also be seen in the area of the lacrimal gland. These tumors are easily palpated, and their nodular-like surface makes them easily identifiable. Through the conjunctiva they appear to be salmon colored. On the roentgenogram, secondary malignant neoplasms, particularly from the sinuses or from the anterior cranial fossa via the sphenoid ridge or superior orbital fissure, show changes suggestive of the diagnosis. When the superior orbital fissure is involved, ocular motility is also impaired.

Loss of Visual Acuity

This loss can occur with exophthalmos from any cause; however, a retrobulbar tumor, particularly in the muscle cone, is the first consideration in the case of slowly progressive exophthalmos and loss of acuity. If the acuity can be restored by plus lenses and if increasing hyperopia is suggested, a retrobulbar tumor that is causing a flattening of the posterior surface of the eye should be considered. This is not pathognomonic of a retrobulbar tumor, since it can be seen also in posterior scleritis or with mild subretinal edema from other causes that displace the retina anteriorly.

In endocrine exophthalmos, loss of vision is usually minimal and it frequently varies, suggesting some problem with the corneal epithelium secondary to exposure or to disturbance in the tear film owing to dryness or decreased blinking. In some cases, when exophthalmos is rapid and accompanied by considerable chemosis and inflammation, the loss of vision can be profound and may be caused by optic nerve involvement.

In some cases of thyroid disease, there is more pronounced swelling of the muscles in the posterior orbit with minimal signs of exophthalmos. A loss of vision then becomes hard to ascribe to thyroid disease until one sees a CT Scan of the posterior orbit. In Figure-4–5, it is easy to imagine compression of the nerve and its blood supply by a large medial rectus muscle.

Ophthalmoscopy

Tumors that indent the posterior part of the globe, particularly in the muscle cone, can cause horizontal striae in the macula that are similar in appearance to the vertical lines on the temporal side of the disc seen in papilledema. Folds are seen not only with retrobulbar tumors; they may also be seen in association with ocular hypotony, intraocular tumors, scleritis, uveitis, after scleral surgery, and occasionally in thyroid disease. Norton, in his histologic study of these folds, concluded that they represented folds in Bruch's membrane. He postulated three contributory factors: shortening of the posterior sclera, papilledema, and congestion of the choroid. By the time most tumors cause striae, however, at least some degree of exophthalmos is present

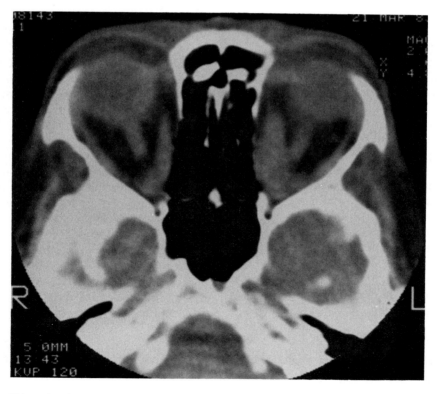

Fig. 4–5. This patient has minimal exophthalmos owing to thyroid disease, but has progressive loss of vision. On CT examination in the left eye, the posterior portion of the medial rectus muscle is markedly enlarged and is seen as compressing the optic nerve and causing ischemia. This anatomic fact would not be appreciated on external examination alone without a CT evaluation of the posterior orbit.

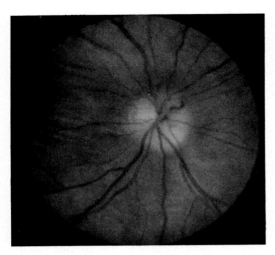

Fig. 4–6. Horizontal striae can cause a decrease in vision and can be due to a tumor in the muscle cone, thyroid disease, or posterior scleritis.

(Fig. 4–6). Tumors in the muscle cone may also cause optic atrophy or papilledema because of their proximity to the optic nerve and to major venous channels.

Dilatation and tortuosity of vessels, particularly of the veins, suggest some arteriovenous connection in the orbit or cavernous sinus. This condition may be grossly evident in the fundus even when no vascular changes appear in the orbital adnexa. As mentioned, pulsation synchronous with the radial pulse, confirming the vascular nature of the problem, may be observed with the ophthalmoscope as the disc goes in and out of focus.

Leukemic infiltrates in the orbit may also affect the fundus. The presence of Roth's spots would confirm this diagnosis, because Roth's spots arising from other conditions do not cause exophthalmos or ophthalmoplegia.

Evaluation of Motility

Orbital tumors and some endocrine disorders can cause exophthalmos without impairment of motility. Benign orbital masses frequently cause only minor limitation of local rotation, usually in the field of action where the mass is located. Although the two conditions usually occur together, in some cases of endocrine disease ophthalmoplegia may occur before frank exophthalmos appears. Forced duction tests are usually positive in endocrine disease; however, some limitation may be experienced—and the test is less than specific—if considerable orbital edema or inflammation from other causes exists. Endocrine ophthalmoplegia usually occurs in up gaze, owing to restriction of the inferior rectus and inferior oblique muscles. The unilateral nature of the paralysis should not induce the observer to reject endocrine disease as the causative factor, particularly if lid retraction and enlarged vessels over the lateral rectus muscle are present.

Other orbital entities may affect motility more than cause exophthalmos. The effect that may be limited to one muscle or movement of the glove in one direction may even result in a slight enophthalmos, which may be a subtle clue to the diagnosis. This includes abnormal muscle innervation such as is seen in third nerve misdirection and Duane syndrome. It can occur after excessive or complicated surgery on the extraocular muscles with secondary scarring or myositis limited to one muscle or to tumor invasion of one muscle.

Metastatic carcinomas that have invaded muscle tissue, acute orbital infections from adjacent sinuses (particularly the ethmoid sinuses), and acute pseudotumor are the diseases that cause severe ophthalmoplegia. Of all tumors, scirrhous adenocarcinomas from the breast seem to cause the worst ophthalmoplegia and, because of their nature, also cause contraction of orbital tissue and enophthalmos rather than exophthalmos.

Tonometry

Elevated intraocular pressure does not always signify the presence of glaucoma. It may point to the pseudoglaucoma of thyroid disease, a condition that can be seen best with Schiøtz's tonometer, with the patient lying down. As the patient looks farther toward his brow, the restricted inferior muscle compresses the globe and raises the pressure artificially. Pseudoglaucoma on progressive up gaze can be looked for specifically when it is uncertain whether thyroid disease is the cause of the exophthalmos. If the patient's head position is adjusted and his lids are elevated, the phenomenon can be demonstrated with the applanation tonometer, but not as readily as with Schiøtz's tonometer because with the applanation technique the patient is sitting up and looking ahead.

Glaucoma, probably of the ischemic variety, may be a factor in advanced cases of carotid cavernous sinus fistula. By the time this symptom appears, however, all the other signs of the disease are so evident as to make the diagnosis certain.

Laboratory Studies

Such studies are usually of little value. If leukemia or multiple myeloma is suspected, a complete blood count is revealing. In cases of lymphoma, an evaluation of the bone marrow is helpful. Thyroid studies are often disappointing because thyroid exophthalmos and ophthalmopathy may occur when the thyroid appears to be functioning normally. In a certain percentage of such cases, however, results of the Werner suppression test are positive, thus providing valuable evidence that the problem is endocrine-dependent even though results of other tests are normal.

Roentgenographic Studies

These studies as they apply to the orbit are covered in detail in Chapter 8; however, a few general comments are appropriate here. It is always good diagnostic medicine to start with a simple examination and then select more sophisticated studies as indicated. In the case of roentgenography, the best orbital roentgenograms should include (1) a Caldwell view for comparing the size of the two orbits, (2) a Water's view, (3) a lateral view, and (4) good views of the optic canal. Since small differences in the size of the optic canal are important, imperfections in technique (such as poor positioning of the head) must be avoided if the roentgenogram is to be reliable.

Only a moderate percentage of orbital tumors are revealed in roentgenographic studies, except in CT examination—and the studies are diagnostic in an even smaller percentage of cases. The combination of palpation (to evaluate the tactile quality and location of the lesions) and roentgenographic studies (to reveal bony or sinus changes) may give significant clues to the diagnosis, along with a CT examination with contrast material.

Tomography has the advantage of filming sections at measured intervals; thus a bony defect can be well localized. Basal tomograms, rather than the usual frontal views, are particularly useful in evaluating enlargement of the optic canal. The technique allows the viewer to see the entire optic canal in each film section.

With the institution of femoral catheterization and selected arteriography, angiography has reached a high degree of accuracy. Orbital angiography has not been as useful as intracranial angiography, and it is used primarily to demonstrate an arteriovenous connection in the orbit. I have not found the technique as useful in detecting hemangiomas.

I consider venography a difficult technique and one that has rarely added to information obtained by the use of other techniques. Venograms have outlined orbital varices and hemangiomas, but these conditions were equally well delineated by the ultrasound technique. Although orbital contrast studies using Renografin have been advocated for intraorbital injection and outlining masses, I have not employed these studies in some time.

Computerized tomography has revolutionized the technique for examination of the retrobulbar space. It is the best single test currently available, and it is being improved all the time. Some instruments have achieved such a high degree of sophistication that they reveal minute details of ocular structures and other anatomic aspects of the orbit.

Digital venous arteriography has also been a great step forward in the evaluation of transient ischemic attacks. This test, when properly done, is as good as regular arteriography, but far safer. The quality of this digital examination is extremely good up to the carotid siphon. This covers the surgically treatable areas (see Fig. 13–2A, B).

Ultrasonography

Using ultrasonography with the B-scan technique has proved most valuable in locating and evaluating the size of orbital tumors. It has been particularly useful in evaluating masses in the retrobulbar space, where palpation is of little use. For some time, B-scan ultrasonography with Polaroid picture documentation has been the best way to judge the size, location, and quality (cystic or solid) of masses behind the eye; and it remains a useful test even with the institution of computerized tomography. It gives a certain dynamic quality to the examination that a CT scan does not possess and complements the CT examination in preoperative evaluations of orbital masses.

Biopsy

Although considered a definitive test, biopsy too has its problems. Sometimes, the inflamed tissue surrounding the tumor is the first part seen and chosen for biopsy, thus resulting in an inconclusive or false diagnosis. If one takes only a portion of tissue for biopsy (deferring definitive treatment until diagnosis), the result may be spread of the tumor, with widespread and devastating recurrence. Inadequate preoperative evaluation of a mass may cause problems at biopsy, such as taking a biopsy of an arteriovenous malformation or hemangioma. Inappropriate or poorly performed biopsies may cause more problems than they resolve. In cases of pseudotumor or thyroid disease, it is not uncommon to see increased inflammation after biopsy. A partially excised dermoid tumor may leak its contents into the orbit and cause a severe inflammatory reaction. Finally, it is most important that a pathologist experienced in ophthalmic tumors read the specimens so that no mistake is made as to the benign or malignant nature of the tumor. Some forms of pseudotumor can be mistaken for lymphoma, and some lymphomas may be called benign hyperplasia.

CAUSES

Thyroid Disease

Although thyroid eye disease is discussed fully in Chapter 6, a few comments are appropriate here.

The lid retraction of thyroid disease may give a normal eye the appearance of exophthalmos. Lid retraction is indicative of thyroid disease, not of orbital tumor. Difficulty in retropulsion may be caused by either condition, and forced ductions may be misleading if a tumor has directly involved muscles.

A few features of thyroid disease may help to establish it as the diagnosis. A careful inspection of the "normal" eye may reveal lid retraction or limitation of motility to a lesser degree than in the involved eye. The bilaterality certainly suggests thyroid disease. CT scan or ultrasonograms of the extraocular muscles can easily detect enlargement compatible with thyroid disease. This enlargement may be present before any disturbance in ocular motility (Fig. 4–7).

The patient with ocular thyroid disease has multiple and constant complaints, not the least of which is the cosmetic appearance. Lateral tarsorraphy for mild cases of exophthalmos is useful and simple to perform, but if the exophthalmos is severe, a tarsorraphy may actually accentuate the poor appearance of the patient. Procedures to drop the upper or raise the lower lid

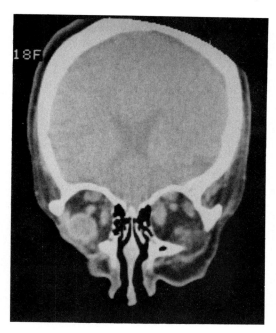

Fig. 4–7. A coronal CT examination demonstrating that all extraocular muscles are enlarged in this case, despite a predominantly vertical limitation to ocular movement.

constitute another approach. This can be done by inserting banked sclera into the tarsus and thus lengthening it. Extreme cases, in which there is progressive loss of vision, are treated more aggressively with an orbital decompression as seen in Figure 4–8A,B. This patient not only stopped losing vision but improved her vision and field and also markedly improved her appearance.

Tumors

Most tumors cannot be diagnosed on the basis of their appearance alone; however, a knowledge of some features of the more common tumors is helpful in making a preliminary diagnosis.

Lymphoma. By the time a patient suffering from lymphoma complains of swelling and exophthalmos, there is usually a palpable mass that, in my experience, originates most commonly in the inferior and anterior orbit. (Authors do not universally agree on this location.) Depending on the

location of the mass, the globe may be more displaced than it is exophthalmic, a phenomenon that is more common with masses in the anterior orbit.

The orbital condition may progress more rapidly in children than in adults, since it is only one aspect of a systemic disease and the true nature of the disease may not be suspected. Chloroma is an important differential diagnosis, particularly in children. Chloroma occurs most often in conjunction with myelogenous leukemia, but it may be present also in lymphatic leukemia. Chloroma appears as a green-colored mass, and is fairly easy to diagnose. It has a predilection for the bones of the skull and, particularly, the orbit, and it is usually bilateral. Hemorrhage into the lids and the orbits is a common associated sign.

Malignant Melanoma. Primary malignant melanoma is rare. Recurrence after enucleation for malignant melanoma of the globe should be suspected with the appearance of a brownish mass or with extrusion of the implant or with sudden poor retention or fitting of the prosthesis.

Rhabdomyosarcoma. The onset of exophthalmos with rapid progression in an infant or child should suggest rhabdomyosarcoma. The differential diagnoses are leukemia, neuroblastoma, and histiocytosis. In cases of neuroblastoma, the child may have a spontaneous retrobulbar hemorrhage, with ecchymosis of the upper lid limited by the orbital septum. If the rhabdomyosarcoma is located anteriorly, the chemosis, redness, and lid swelling may suggest cellulitis and thus confuse the issue initially. Other signs of infection are not present, however: the ethmoidal roentgenograms are normal, and the white blood cell count does not show the typical inflammatory neutrophilic response.

Retinoblastoma. Almost exclusively a disease of children, the average age of patients with retinoblastoma is 13 months. Approximately 25% of the cases are bilateral, involving separate sites of origin rather than the spread of a primary tumor.

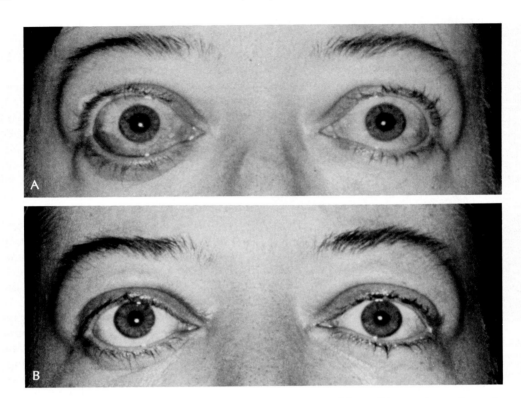

Fig. 4–8. **A.** Severe bilateral exophthalmos, with marked upper and lower lid retraction and vascular engorgement, particularly on the temporal aspect of both globes. **B.** Marked improvement in all cosmetic aspects after orbital decompression.

The tumor begins intraocularly and then escapes along the optic nerve to grow intracranially or through the sclera to form an orbital mass. The endophytum type of tumor begins in the inner retinal layers and grows into the vitreous cavity. Its pink-cream color, caused by the newly formed blood vessels over its surface, makes it easy to see. The exophytum type of tumor grows in the outer layers of the retina, causing a detachment of the overlying retina. It is not as easy to see as the endophytum type, but transillumination as well as ultrasonography help to evaluate it. Many retinoblastomas undergo some necrosis and calcification. The calcification can be seen as a granular shadow in the orbit on roentgenograms.

The child with retinoblastoma may come to the clinic with esotropia, but frequently he is brought for treatment when someone notices that he has leukocoria. In the child with a white pupil, a number of different conditions should be considered as the cause. Thus a digression at this point to discuss the differential diagnosis of leukocoria seems warranted.

LEUKOCORIA—DIFFERENTIAL DIAGNOSIS

The differential diagnoses to be considered when leukocoria is present include the following:
1. Retinoblastoma
2. Retrolental fibroplasia
3. Persistent hyperplastic vitreous
4. Retinal dysplasia
5. Metastatic retinitis
6. Massive retinal fibrosis
7. Nematode endophthalmitis
8. Glioma
9. Coats' disease

Retrolental Fibroplasia

This condition manifests itself as leukocoria in its cicatricial stages in infants about 3 to 5 months of age.

The disease occurs primarily in premature infants. Some degree of microphthalmos and associated shallow anterior chamber with grayish opaque vascularized tissue in the vitreous humor behind the lens is present. The microphthalmos and shallow chamber militate against a diagnosis of retinoblastoma. The ciliary processes are seen in the periphery of the tissues—a phenomenon that does not occur in retinoblastoma. (In retrolental fibroplasia, the ciliary processes are seen because they are abnormal and long; they are also seen in persistent hyperplastic vitreous but because they are pulled into the vitreous.) The roentgenograms do not show calcium.

Persistent Hyperplastic Vitreous

This condition occurs in full-term infants. The leukocoria is frequently seen at birth, and it is unilateral. The white mass, which tends to be on the posterior surface of the lens, is densest at the center and thins out toward the periphery of the lens. The vessels in it may radiate from the central area and around the lens. The ciliary processes are seen, and they are smaller and longer than normal. Usually, a small degree of microphthalmos is present. The capsule of the lens may show a dehiscence at the posterior pole, with, characteristically, a local cataract at the same time. If the dehiscence is large, the patient may go on to develop a total cataract. The iris stroma shows prominent iris vessels, a phenomenon that is as suggestive of this disease as the shallow chamber is of retrolental fibroplasia.

Retinal Dysplasia

This condition is associated with diffuse anomalies of the central nervous and other body systems. Retinal dysplasia is always bilateral, and a certain familial tendency exists. Some of the other associated anomalies are mental retardation, obstructive hydrocephalus, numerous cardiovascular defects, polydactylism, cleft palate, and cleft lip. A view of the fundus shows the presence of an opaque tissue somewhat adherent to the posterior surface of the lens and, behind this mass, a grayish-white tissue in the vitreous humor that represents the elevated and malformed retina.

Metastatic Retinitis

This condition can cause the retina to organize and contract and lead to retinal detachment and leukocoria.

Massive Retinal Fibrosis

This condition shows protrusion from the retina of a grayish-white mass owing to organization of massive retinal hemorrhages that may have occurred at birth. Studies have shown that the number of at least small hemorrhages into the retina is quite high, even in normal deliveries. These hemorrhages would have to be massive, however, to cause the secondary contraction and organization.

Nematode Endophthalmitis

This disorder is characterized by massive focal inflammatory changes that are localized to one side in the vitreous humor and retina. The usual cause, Toxocara canis, can now be identified by serologic tests.

Coats' Disease

This disease occurs primarily in young men, usually those in their late twenties. It is usually unilateral. The whitish pupillary reflex is caused by a massive exudative retinitis in the macular area, with some glistening cholesterol deposits and hemorrhages. If the condition goes untreated, it leads to massive organization of the retina and to retinal detachment.

Neurofibroma. Like optic nerve gliomas, neurofibromas tend to occur in the first decade of life. They commonly occur in the superior orbit. Ptosis, a frequent sign, is caused by infiltration of the lid by a plexiform neuroma that on palpation feels like a bag of worms. Patients with neurofibromas frequently have other stigmata of neurofibromatosis. Ipsilateral glaucoma may be present.

In addition to optic nerve glioma, other causes of exophthalmos in this disease are other orbital tumors, including nerve sheath meningiomas; defects in the sphenoid bone, causing orbital encephalocele and pulsating exophthalmos; and a large deformed buphthalmic eye from congenital glaucoma.

Glioma. These slow-growing tumors most frequently appear during the first decade of life; 80% of gliomas occur in persons under 20 years of age. I have not found pain to be a prominent feature. Most children with gliomas are referred to the ophthalmologist because strabismus, particularly esotropia, has developed. These patients are found to have poor vision and some pallor or edema of the disc. Other children with gliomas often are referred to the specialist because during a school vision-screening test they were found to have poor vision in one eye. On further examination, these children are frequently found to have some degree of exophthalmos, but not so obviously as do persons with rhabdomyosarcoma or neuroblastoma.

Roentgenograms of the optic canal may demonstrate enlargement, a finding that suggests intracranial extension. If the field in the other eye shows no upper temporal cut, the tumor has not extended into the chiasm. Computerized tomography and ultrasonography demonstrate optic nerve enlargement, thus suggesting the presence of a glioma rather than other types of orbital masses. When enlargement of the optic nerve is questionable, the other optic nerve should be used for comparison. The physician should always look for other signs of neurofibromatosis even though only about 25% of optic nerve gliomas are associated with it.

Some authors feel that these tumors are hamartomas and that they should be observed rather than operated on or even subjected to a biopsy. There is evidence that optic nerve gliomas associated with neurofibromatosis are more benign than those not associated with neurofibromatosis. I feel that since meningiomas of the optic nerve sheath do occur, a biopsy should be done in order to obtain a positive tissue diagnosis. The management of the meningioma is by operation, and to leave the tumor to observation could be disastrous. It is true that glioma of the optic nerve is more common than meningioma of the optic nerve sheath, but this type of meningioma is not as rare as was once thought.

Meningioma. Usually occurring in the fourth and fifth decades of life, meningiomas appear more frequently in women than in men. Exophthalmos and loss of vision are the predominant signs. Plain roentgenograms of the optic canal and sphenoid ridge that show bony hyperostosis often establish the diagnosis. The exophthalmos may be secondary to the tumor in the orbit, or it may be a result of hyperostosis of the orbital bones that has caused displacement of the globe. Diplopia is not a common initial complaint; swelling of the upper lid is.

Dermoid Tumors. These tumors are rarely a presenting complaint in infants or in persons over 50 years of age. The most common ages for recognition are from 3 to 10 years. Dermoid tumors are usually superior and anterior in location and, in my experience, upper temporal more often than upper nasal. They grow at an irregular rate, and they rarely cause exophthalmos or displacement. No treatment is indicated, unless for cosmetic reasons. Occasionally, a dermoid tumor is traumatized and its contents leak into the orbit, causing an inflammatory reaction; however, this action is not common.

Lacrimal Gland Tumors. The presentation of lacrimal gland tumors depends on their location. If they are superior and posterior in location, the eye is displaced downward and forward, and no mass can be felt. If they are superior and anterior in location, there is less exophthalmos and more displacement of the globe downward. The differential diagnoses include pseudotumor of the orbit, lymphoma, dermoid tumor, and adenocystic carcinoma. (Adenocystic carcinoma differs from lacrimal gland tumors in that palpation of adenocystic carcinoma causes the patient to have pain.)

Since increases in the size of the lacrimal gland fossa and in bone density are subtle and may be missed on routine roentgenography, lateral tomograms should be done of all masses located in the upper temporal quadrant of the orbit.

Carcinoma. Although adenocystic carcinoma tends to have more characteristic signs, the most common form of carcinoma is squamous carcinoma. Frequently the adenocystic variety is located in the upper temporal orbit and shows exophthalmos and downward displacement of the globe. As the tumor grows, it spreads to the periorbita and along adjacent nerves and becomes painful.

Mucocele. These tumors arise from obstruction of sinus drainage with secondary buildup in sinus pressure and erosion of the bone. Frontal mucoceles are the most common ones. As they invade the orbit, they push the eye downward and forward. The mass frequently feels firm, is not compressible, and does not transilluminate. Since roentgenograms do not always show a bony defect, the physician must have a high index of suspicion. Occasionally, the roentgenogram shows a fluid level.

Ethmoid and maxillary sinus mucoceles are much less common than are frontal mucoceles. Malignancies of the maxillary sinus extending into the orbit are more common than mucoceles, and they should be so considered in making a diagnosis. Since mucoceles in the sphenoid sinus may cause pain and ophthalmoplegia, they are often mistaken for ophthalmoplegic migraine.

Inflammations

Pseudotumor. This disease is always a consideration in unexplained exophthalmos with or without inflammatory signs. The diagnosis is arrived at by careful exclusion of other disease entities.

Two of the main differential diagnoses of orbital pseudotumor are Wegener's granulomatosis and lymphoma. Wegener's granulomatosis classically involves the respiratory and genitourinary system in a necrotizing granulomatous vasculitis. The incidence of eye involvement in Wegener's granulomatosis is about 42%, including other ocular manifestations than pseudotumor of the orbit, such as corneal and scleral ulcerations and keratitis. Biopsy of pseudotumor associated with Wegener's granulomatosis reveals a necrotizing granulomatous vasculitis; however, the pathologic findings are not unlike those of periarteritis nodosa, which can also cause proptosis and is a major differential diagnosis of Wegener's granulomatosis. Also included in the differential diagnosis of necrotizing angiitis are Boeck's sarcoidosis, allergic granulomas, and allergic angiitis. There are limited forms of Wegener's granulomatosis without renal involvement, and orbital forms that initially are limited only to the orbit. In prolonged orbital pseudotumor cases, Wegener's should be kept in mind. Wegener's granulomatosis in gen-

eral does not respond as well to steroids as does the non-Wegener's form of pseudotumor, which may be a clue to the cause of the inflammatory proptosis. Lymphoma, on the other hand, may respond to steroids and should still be considered in the absence of an adequate biopsy.

Some cases of pseudotumor are chronic in onset, with lid edema and chemosis occurring months before frank exophthalmos and diplopia. Other cases of pseudotumor come on quickly. Pain, a variable sign, is said not to be severe, but my patients have found it quite severe. The results of forced duction tests may be positive. The inflammation may be diffuse, or a solitary nodule (Fig. 4–9) may be palpable—and should be looked for. The age of onset ranges from the third to the sixth decade, and the condition affects both sexes about equally. According to Reese, up to one third of the cases show some degree of bilaterality, if not simultaneously, then at least within several months. I have not found the incidence of bilaterality to be nearly that high. In treating pa-

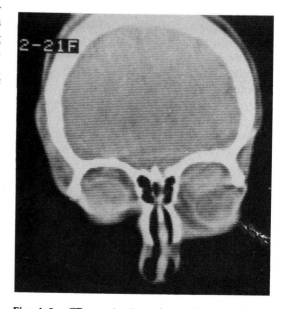

Fig. 4–9. CT examination of pseudotumor of the orbit. It presents in this case as a solitary mass and displaces the eye down and laterally.

tients with pseudotumor, it is important to remember that the disease may go on for months and that it may be difficult to discontinue steroid therapy without recurrence of the disease.

Myositis. This rare condition may be difficult to distinguish from pseudotumor. If pain on motion and ophthalmoplegia are significant features and if the external inflammatory signs are minimal, myositis is a more likely diagnosis. Fortunately, both myositis and pseudotumor respond to steroid therapy.

Infections

Orbital cellulitis occurs most commonly as an extension of contiguous sinus disease. The most common site is the ethmoid sinus, with its paper-thin separation from the orbit. In children under 12 years of age, the maxillary sinus may also be the site, whereas after age 12 the frontal sinus is the second most common site. Delay in diagnosis or treatment of cellulitis may cause severe orbital disease and life-threatening complications. One of the possible complications is an anesthetic cornea, with increased chance of severe keratitis along with the exposure problems that come with exophthalmos. Papillitis and compression of arteries and veins can lead to loss of retinal function as well as to direct abscess formation into the nerve or the eye itself. The most serious complication, however, is a phlebitis that spreads from the orbital veins to the cavernous sinus. The signs that warn of this complication are a rapid worsening of the patient's general condition, engorgement of the veins in the forehead, rapid pulse, involvement of all the other extraocular muscles, and, perhaps, signs of meningitis.

If roentgenograms show gas in the orbit, the possibility of gas gangrene should be considered. The background for the development of gas gangrene may be a penetrating injury rather than a spreading from the paranasal sinus.

If an orbital abscess occurs in children

between 3 and 30 months of age, osteoperiostitis should be considered. The most common cause of osteoperiostitis is a staphylococcal osteomyelitis in the superior maxilla resulting from an infection of a tooth bud, particularly of an unerupted first molar. The illness is usually ushered in by high fever, loss of appetite, bowel disturbances, swelling of the lower lid, and redness of an eye. This infection can lead to the same problems found in other orbital cellulitis disorders, and it requires swift and specific therapy. As osteoperiostitis develops, edema is characteristically seen in the nasal part of the lower lid, in the region of the lacrimal sac. Occasionally, the condition may be mistaken for a dacryocystitis; however, dacryocystitis is not seen in children under 1 year of age.

Occasionally, the physician sees a limited form of orbital infection in which the infection is localized under the periosteum, causing severe pain (because of the stretching of the periosteum) but few signs of orbital inflammation. Such cases are more difficult to diagnose unless a tender mass can be palpated.

Mucormycosis. This rarely seen disease occurs in conjunction with acidotic diabetes or debilitating disease or in patients on long-term antibiotic or steroid therapy. The infection usually begins rapidly, with edema and hemorrhages and subsequent involvement of the ophthalmic and other orbital arteries caused by invasion of the blood vessels by the mucormycosis. Making the diagnosis in time requires a high index of suspicion. The physician should examine one of the nasal turbinates, particularly the middle turbinate, for a small black crust that would ordinarily be passed off as dried blood. If the crust is removed and examined under a microscope with potassium chloride stain, the picture typical of mucormycosis can be identified and appropriate treatment with amphotericin B can be instituted. The differential diagnoses are cavernous sinus thrombosis and lethal midline granuloma.

Vascular Disorders

Orbital varix is a major cause of intermittent exophthalmos. In infants, the typical history is that the eye bulges forward when the child cries or performs the Valsalva maneuver. The exophthalmos may occur also when the head is bent over, with the eye in a dependent position, allowing the varix to fill. For diagnosis, compression of the jugular veins may bring out the exophthalmos. During the exophthalmos and depending on its severity, ophthalmoplegia, pupillary abnormalities, and decreased vision may occur. Orbital varix is the one disease in which orbital venography may be of particular help in establishing the diagnosis. Treatment of it is difficult and should always be evaluated with a neurosurgeon. The condition is usually limited to the orbit, but any association with an intracranial arteriovenous malformation should be carefully ruled out. Occasionally, spontaneous orbital hemorrhage may occur. When it does, neuroblastoma, hemophilia, and scurvy should be considered.

Cavernous Sinus Thrombosis. As mentioned, cavernous sinus thrombosis secondary to orbital infection may occur. It can also occur spontaneously in debilitated patients with dehydration and decreased blood pressure, resulting in increased blood coagulability. The thrombosis may give rise to signs involving the third, fourth, and sixth cranial nerves as they traverse the cavernous sinus. Usually ipsilateral exophthalmos is present unless a thrombosis of the ipsilateral superior ophthalmic vein prevents the buildup of venous pressure in the orbit.

Orbital Anomalies (Craniostenosis)

The most common forms of craniostenosis are oxycephaly and craniofacial dysostosis (Crouzon's disease). These conditions are caused by abnormal closure of the cranial suture lines. In normal children, at age 7, the orbits are as large as those of adults, but the cranium continues to grow. First the coronal sutures close, then the sagittal sutures, and, last, the lambdoidal sutures.

Oxycephaly. Tower skull, or oxycephaly, is associated with shallow orbits. The orbits are so shallow that spontaneous dislocation of the globe may occur during crying. Syndactyly, prognathism, high palate, and, frequently, loss of vision at about 7 years of age (from increased intracranial pressure) are associated conditions. Roentgenograms show convolutional atrophy secondary to intracranial pressure. Intracranial pressure accounts also for the digital impressions, which are the most prominent features the roentgenograms show.

Craniofacial Dysostosis. Often called Crouzon's disease, craniofacial dysostosis is caused by premature closure of all the cranial sutures. Persons with this condition have exophthalmos, with occasional subluxation of the globe. They also have an antimongoloid slanting of the palpebral fissure. Loss of vision may result from increased intracranial pressure. Atrophy of the maxilla, enlargement of nasal bones, and prognathism are also present.

Other Disorders

Occasionally, exophthalmos has been reported to be associated with acromegaly, multiple myeloma, myxedema, Paget's disease, or periarteritis nodosa. Normally, exophthalmos is not associated with migraine, but Hedges has reported a case of intermittent exophthalmos owing to migraine that probably represents some vascular alteration in the orbit.

With the notable exception of sphenoid ridge meningioma, intracranial tumors do not generally cause exophthalmos. Pituitary adenoma, however, occasionally produces a mild degree of exophthalmos, presumably because of a pressure effect on the cavernous sinus, with secondary filling of the orbital veins and subsequent displacement of the globe. I have seen such a condition only once.

The periorbital edema induced by high-

TABLE 4–1.   Differential Diagnoses in the Evaluation of Exophthalmos

Type of Exophthalmos	Differential Diagnoses
Intermittent exophthalmos	Orbital varix, vascular neoplasm, angioneurotic edema, recurrent orbital hemorrhage, voluntary nervous system stimulation, sympathetic nervous system stimulation (Claude Bernard syndrome)
Pulsating exophthalmos	Vascular disorders (venous varix, vascular tumor, cavernous sinus thrombosis, carotid artery aneurysm in cavernous sinus), cerebral disorders (congenital absence of roof in neurofibromatosis, trauma)
Bilateral exophthalmos	Edema, systemic disease in histiocytosis and Wegener's granulomatosis, inflammation from ethmoid sinus, developmental craniofacial dysostosis (infantile cortical hyperostosis, fibrous dysplasia, osteitis deformans, yaws, osteopetrosis, rickets, acromegaly), chloroma

dosage steroid therapy is common. Edema fluid may also be present in the orbit, which causes mild exophthalmos, but this condition is much less common than the periorbital edema.

Table 4-1 is a list of conditions that would help to establish the differential diagnosis of exophthalmos.

ENOPHTHALMOS

This condition rarely occurs. When it does, the normal eye is mistakenly reported as exophthalmic, and it appears so because it seems more prominent than the affected eye—the enophthalmic eye.

The many causes of enophthalmos include ocular and orbital diseases. The enophthalmos may be owing to either an acquired or a congenital small globe. The acquired small globe, called phthisis bulbi, is caused by disorganization of the globe secondary to end-stage disease such as glaucoma or to trauma.

The eye may only appear to be smaller because less of the globe is seen, such as with ptosis from any cause, but particularly minimal ptosis (for example, that in Horner syndrome).

Orbital disease, such as floor fractures that cause a prolapse of orbital contents into the maxillary antrum, with a secondary sinking into the orbit of the globe, can cause enophthalmos. Severe orbital trauma with hemorrhage or prolonged infections (such as cellulitis) or inflammations (such as pseudotumor of the orbit) can cause secondary absorption of orbital fat and en-

ophthalmos. Muscle contractions can occur secondary to orbital infections, myositis, pseudotumor, or muscle operation and can result in enophthalmos in general or in one field of gaze.

PSEUDOEXOPHTHALMOS

This disorder is caused by some extraocular factor that makes the globe appear prominent. The most common cause is lid retraction (Fig. 4–4). Contractions or sagging of the lower lid from contracted scar expose the eye abnormally.

The second most common cause of pseudoexophthalmos is a globe that is abnormally large even though it is located correctly in the orbit. This type of globe is seen in buphthalmos secondary to congenital glaucoma, high axial myopia, and staphyloma.

BIBLIOGRAPHY

Albert, D.M., Rubenstein, R.A., and Scheie, H.G.: Tumor metastasis to the eye. I. Incidence in 213 adult patients with generalized malignancy. II. Clinical study in infants and children. Am. J. Ophthalmol. 63:723, 1967.

Albright, F., et al.: Syndrome characterized by osteitis fibrosa disseminata, areas of pigmentation and endocrine dysfunction, with precocious puberty in females: report of five cases. N. Engl. J. Med. 216:727, 1937.

Alfano, J.E.: Ophthalmological aspects of neuroblastoma: a study of 53 cases. Trans. Am. Acad. Ophthalmol. Otolaryngol. 72:830, 1968.

Anderson, R.L., and Linberg, J.V.: Transorbital decompression in Graves' disease. Arch. Ophthalmol. 99:120, 1981.

Bard, L.A., and Schulze, R.R.: Unilateral proptosis as the presenting sign of metastatic carcinoma of the prostate. Am. J. Ophthalmol. 58:107, 1964.

Berge, H.L.: Meningiomas: an ophthalmic problem;

diagnosis and results of treatment. Am. J. Ophthalmol. *39*:828, 1955.

Billson, F.A., and Hudson, R.L.: Surgical treatment of chronic papilledema in children. Br. J. Ophthalmol. *59*:92, 1975.

Blodi, F.C., and Gass, J.D.M.: Inflammatory pseudotumor of the orbit. Trans. Am. Acad. Ophthalmol. Otolaryngol. *71*:303, 1967.

Blue, P.W., and LaPiana, F.G.: Superficial vertical corneal striations: a new eye sign of Graves' disease. Ann. Ophthalmol. *12*:635, 1980.

Brenner, E.H., and Shock, J.P.: Proptosis secondary to systemic lupus erythematosus. Arch. Ophthalmol. *91*:81, 1974.

Brown, D.H.: The urinary excretion of vanilmandelic acid (VMA) and homovanillic acid (HVA) in children with retinoblastoma. Am. J. Ophthalmol. *62*:239, 1966.

Brownstein, M.H., Elliott, R., and Helwig, E.R.: Ophthalmologic aspects of amyloidosis. Am. J. Ophthalmol. *69*:423, 1970.

Bruwer, A.J., and Keirland, R.R.: Neurofibromatosis and congenital unilateral pulsating and non-pulsating exophthalmos. Arch. Ophthalmol. *53*:2, 1955.

Bullock, J.D., and Egbert, P.R.: Experimental choroidal folds. Am. J. Ophthalmol. *78*:618, 1974.

Bullock, L.J., and Reeves, R.J.: Unilateral exophthalmos: roentgenographic aspects. Am. J. Roentgenol. Radium Ther. Nucl. Med. *82*:290, 1959.

Burch, F.E.: Orbital metastasis from malignant tumor of the suprarenal gland. Arch. Ophthalmol. *7*:418, 1932.

Burton, C.V., and Goldberg, M.F.: Exophthalmos from ruptured intracavernous carotid aneurysm without pulsation, bruit or murmur. Am. J. Ophthalmol. *70*:830, 1970.

Calhoun, F.P., Jr., and Reese, A.B.: Rhabdomyosarcoma of the orbit. Arch. Ophthalmol. *27*:558, 1942.

Cassady, R., Jr., et al.: Radiation therapy for rhabdomyosarcoma. Radiology *91*:116, 1968.

Cassan, S.M., et al.: Pseudotumor of the orbit and limited Wegener's granulomatosis. Ann. Intern. Med. *72*:687, 1970.

Chutorian, A.M., et al.: Optic gliomas in children. Neurology (Minneap.) *14*:83, 1964.

Coop, M.E.: Pseudotumor of the orbit. A clinical and pathological study of 47 cases. Br. J. Ophthalmol. *45*:513, 1961.

Cushing, H.: The meningiomas (dural endotheliomas): their source and favoured seats of origin. Brain *45*:282, 1922.

Day, R.M.: Ocular manifestations of thyroid disease: current concepts. Trans. Am. Ophthalmol. Soc. *57*:572, 1959.

Dayton, G.O., Jr., Langden, E., and Rochlin, D.: Management of orbital rhabdomyosarcoma. Am. J. Ophthalmol. *68*:906, 1969.

Dixon, R.: The surgical management of thyroid-related upper eyelid retraction. Ophthalmology *89*:52, 1982.

Donaldson, S.S., Bagshaw, M.A., and Kriss, J.P.: Supervoltage orbital radiotherapy for Graves'

ophthalmopathy. J. Clin. Endocrinol. Metab. *37*:276, 1973.

Doughman, D.J.: Ocular amyloidosis. Surv. Ophthalmol. *13*:133, 1968.

Doxanas, M.T., and Dryden, R.M.: The use of sclera in the treatment of dysthyroid eyelid retraction. Ophthalmology *88*:887, 1981.

Fauci, A.S., and Wolf, S.M.: Wegener's granulomatosis: studies in eighteen patients and a review of the literature. Medicine *52*:535, 1973.

Faulds, J.W., and Wear, A.R.: Pseudotumor of the orbit and Wegener's granuloma. Lancet: *2*:955, 1960.

Ferry, A.P., and Naghdi, R.N.: Bronchogenic carcinoma metastatic to the orbit. Arch. Ophthalmol. *77*:214, 1967.

Font, R.L., Yanoff, M. and Zimmerman, L.E.: Benign lymphoepithelial lesion of the lacrimal gland and its relationship to Sjögren's syndrome. Am. J. Clin. Pathol. *48*:365, 1967.

Forrest, A.W.: Epithelial lacrimal gland tumors: pathology as guide to prognosis. Trans. Am. Acad. Ophthalmol. Otolaryngol. *38*:848, 1954.

Gaynes, P.M., and Cohen, G.S.: Juvenile xanthogranuloma of the orbit. Am. J. Ophthalmol. *63*:755, 1967.

Greer, C.H.: Choroidal carcinoma metastatic from the male breast. Br. J. Ophthalmol. *38*:312, 1954.

Harper, J.M., and Hunter, W.A.: Unilateral exophthalmos secondary to metastatic carcinoma of the prostrate: case report and review of the literature. J. Urol. *89*:75, 1963.

Hayreh, S.S.: Pathogenesis of oedema of the optic disc. Doc. Ophthalmol. *24*:289, 1968.

Hedges, T.R.: Alternating exophthalmos with painful ophthalmoplegia. Arch. Ophthalmol. *74*:625, 1965.

Henderson, J.W.: Orbital Tumors. Philadelphia, W. B. Saunders Co., 1973.

Henderson, J.W., and Antine, B.E.: Brain scanning in neuro-ophthalmologic diagnosis. Trans. Am. Ophthalmol. Soc. *64*:274, 1966.

Henderson, J.W., and Schneider, R.C.: The ocular findings in carotid-cavernous fistula in a series of 17 cases. Trans. Am. Ophthalmol. Soc. *56*:123, 1958.

Hoyt, W.F., and Baghdassarian, S.A.: Optic glioma of childhood: natural history and rationale for conservative management. Br. J. Ophthalmol. *53*:793, 1969.

Huber, A.: Arteriography and phlebography in the diagnosis of orbital affections. Bull. N.Y. Acad. Med. *44*:409, 1968.

Jensen, V.J.: Sarcoidosis of the orbit. Acta Ophthalmol. (Kbh) *35*:416, 1957.

Jones, I.S., and Pfeiffer, R.L.: Lacrimal gland tumors: roentgenographic diagnosis. Trans. Am. Acad. Ophthalmol. Otolaryngol. *58*:841, 1954.

Jones, I.S., Reese, A.B., and Kraut, J.: Orbital rhabdomyosarcoma: an analysis of 62 cases. Am. J. Ophthalmol. *61*:721, 1966.

Kearns, T.P., Wagner, H.P.: Ophthalmologic diagnosis of meningiomas of the sphenoidal ridge. Am. J. Med. Sci. *226*:221, 1953.

Keltner, J.E., Albert, D.M., and Lubow, M.: Optic

nerve decompression. Arch. Ophthalmol. *96*:97, 1977.

Kennerdall, J.S., Rosenbaum, A.E., and El-Hosky, M.H.: Apical optic nerve compression of dysthyroid optic neuropathy on computed tomography. Arch. Ophthalmol. *99*:807, 1981.

Kramar, P.: Management of eye changes in Graves' disease. Surv. Ophthalmol. *18*:369, 1974.

Leeds, N., and Seaman, W.B.: Fibrous dysplasia of the skull and its differential diagnoses: a clinical and roentgenographic study of 46 cases. Radiology *78*:570, 1962.

LeWald, L.T.: Congenital absence of the superior orbital wall associated with pulsating exophthalmos: report of four cases, Am. J. Roentgenol. Radium Ther. Nucl. Med. *30*:756, 1933.

Linberg, J.V., and Anderson, R.L.: Transorbital decompression. Arch. Ophthalmol. *99*:113, 1981.

Marshall, D.: Glioma of the optic nerve as a manifestation of von Recklinghausen's disease. Am. J. Ophthalmol. *37*:15, 1954.

McGavic, J.S.: Lymphomatoid diseases involving the eye and its adnexa. Arch. Ophthalmol. *30*:179, 1943.

McGavic, J.S.: Lymphomatous tumors of the eye. Arch. Ophthalmol. *53*:236, 1955.

Melmon, K.L., and Goldberg, J.S.: Sarcoidosis with bilateral exophthalmos as the initial symptom. Am. J. Med. *33*:158, 1962.

Meyer, D., Yanoff, M., and Hanno, H.: Differential diagnosis in Mikulicz's syndrome. Mikulicz's disease and similar disease entities. Am. J. Ophthalmol. *71*:516, 1971.

Norton, E.W.D.: A characteristic fluorescein angiographic pattern in choroidal folds. Proc. R. Soc. Med. *62*:119, 1969.

Osher, R.H., Schatz, N.J., and Duane, T.D.: Acquired orbital retraction syndrome. Arch. Ophthalmol. *98*:1798, 1980.

Putterman, A.M., and Vrist, M.: Surgical treatment of upper eyelid retraction. Am. J. Ophthalmol. *87*:401, 1972.

Ravin, J.G., Sisson, J.C., and Knapp, W.T.: Orbital radiation for the ocular changes of Graves' disease. Am. J. Ophthalmol. *79*:285, 1975.

Reese, A.B.: The treatment of expanding lesions of the orbit with particular regard to those arising in the lacrimal gland. Am. J. Ophthalmol. *41*:3, 1956.

Reese, A.B.: Tumors of the Eye, 2nd Ed. New York, Harper & Row, Haber Medical Division, 1963.

Reese, A.B., and Ellsworth, R.M.: The evaluation and current concept of retinoblastoma therapy. Trans. Am. Acad. Ophthalmol. Otolaryngol. *67*:164, 1963.

Rucker, C.W., and Kearns, T.P.: Mistaken diagnoses in some cases of meningioma: clinics in perimetry. Am. J. Ophthalmol. *51*:15, 1961.

Sanders, T.E.: Infantile xanthogranuloma of the orbit: a report of three cases. Am. J. Ophthalmol. *61*:1299, 1966.

Skalka, H.W.: Perineural optic nerve changes in endocrine orbitopathy. Arch. Ophthalmol. *96*:468, 1978.

Trokel, S.L., and Potter, G.D.: Hypocycloidal tomography of the optic canal. Arch. Ophthalmol. *81*:797, 1969.

Walsh, F.B., and Dandy, W.E.: Pathogenesis of intermittent exophthalmos. Arch. Ophthalmol. *32*:1, 1944.

Weiter, J., Farkas, T.G.: Pseudotumor of the orbit as a presenting sign in Wegener's granulomatosis. Surv. Ophthalmol. *17*:106, 1972.

Wheeler, J.M.: Exophthalmos associated with diabetes insipidus and large defects in the bones of the skull. Arch. Ophthalmol. *5*:161, 1931.

Wheeler, J.M.: Exophthalmos caused by eosinophilic granuloma of bone. Am. J. Ophthalmol. *29*:980, 1946.

Wolfe, S.A.: Surgical treatment of exophthalmos and enophthalmos. Ann. Ophthalmol. *13*:995, 1981.

Wolter, J.R.: Parallel horizontal choroidal folds secondary to an orbital tumor. Am. J. Ophthalmol. *77*:669, 1974.

Yanoff, M., and Scheie, H.G.: Malignant lymphoma of the orbit: difficulties in diagnosis. Surv. Ophthalmol. *12*:134, 1967.

Chapter **5**

Ptosis

THOMAS J. WALSH

Blepharoptosis, usually referred to as ptosis, can be described as the condition in which the upper lid is at a lower position over the cornea than normal. The question arises, What is the normal position? The usual adult position, with the eyes straight ahead, is for the lid to be about 1.5 mm below the upper limbus of the cornea. It is usually not this low in infants, and it is frequently lower in older persons. It may be lower in some people as a familial trait. If the ptosis is unilateral or asymmetric, the diagnosis is usually made more easily. In some diseases, however, both bilateral and symmetric ptosis occurs, making the diagnosis of ptosis more difficult. (A normal form of bilateral and symmetric ptosis is the condition referred to colloquially as bedroom eyes.)

Two groups of muscles and nerves elevate the upper lid. The major contributor is the levator muscle, which is innervated by the third cranial nerve. This muscle extends as a broad band and inserts into the anterior surface of the cartilaginous tarsal plate. A secondary system inserts into the upper border of the tarsus; it is called Müller's muscle, and it has an associated pupillary sign. Müller's muscle is innervated by the sympathetic nervous system. A pe-

culiar feature of anatomy, which requires understanding, is the intimate relationship between the superior rectus muscle, which elevates the eye, and the levator muscle. Both muscles come from the same anlage, at Zinn's ligament. Not infrequently, both are affected, particularly when trauma is involved.

EXAMINATION TECHNIQUES

Measure the distance between the two lid margins by measuring the lid fissures with a millimeter ruler and with the patient's eyes looking straight ahead. This method is more accurate than measuring how much of the lid is below the theoretically normal lid position, which, as mentioned, can vary. In planning any surgical correction, it is also important to know where the other normal lid sits in relation to the cornea.

Another feature to consider is the function of the levator muscle. Using the millimeter ruler again, observe the excursion of the lid from eyes in the full down-gaze position to the full up-gaze position. Normal excursion is about 15 mm. A major error in evaluating the amount of ptosis can occur when a patient overcomes his ptosis by employing the frontalis muscle. If you observe a wrinkling over one eye and not over the other, suspect a slight ptosis that is being overcome by the use of the frontalis muscle, giving some lift to the ipsilateral lid. Have the patient close his lid, and press your thumb over the center of his eyebrow. Do not push up—and thus do the same thing the patient's frontalis muscle does—or push down, thereby depressing the lid and causing a ptosis. Press in toward the bone so as to prevent the frontalis muscle action on the skin overlying the lid. This maneuver should also be done when measuring excursions of the lid.

True ptosis is due to a neuropathic process either in the third cranial nerve innervation to the levator muscle or in the sympathetic innervation to Müller's muscle or to one of several myopathic processes.

PSEUDOPTOSIS—TYPES AND CAUSES

Protective Ptosis

Pseudoptosis has many manifestations, the most common one being protective ptosis associated with an irritated eye. The irritation may be an internal inflammation, such as iritis. Photophobia is an early sign of iritis, and frequently it is present before any external inflammatory sign, such as redness. Photophobia may also be seen with inflammation in the posterior segment of the eye, but not as consistently as in iritis. The possibility of a corneal foreign body, abrasion, or retained foreign body under the upper lid should be considered. Careful inspection of the upper lid when everted, particularly when doubly everted over a Desmarres retractor, is a necessity.

Hysterical Ptosis

This condition is usually unilateral, and the wrinkling of the orbicularis muscle can be seen as the cause. Cases of flaccid hysteric ptosis do occur, but they are rare.

Enophthalmos

The lid may be ptotic because of lack of support from the globe, a condition that occurs with enophthalmos secondary to a loss of orbital fat. The loss of fat occurs most often after blunt trauma with orbital hemorrhage or after trauma causing a blowout of the orbital floor with damage to the orbital contents.

Microphthalmia and Phthisis Bulbi

In congenital microphthalmia, the lid is not supported properly. A more common variety of microphthalmia is phthisis bulbi, a shrinking of a normal eye after total blindness occurs and internal disruption of all functions such as in end-stage glaucoma or severe disorganization after trauma.

Blepharochalasis

A common finding, and one that may mask an associated subtle but true ptosis, such as exists in Horner syndrome, is the blepharochalasis of the elderly. This condition results from loss of fascial attachments of the overlying skin to the levator muscle, causing the skin to fall down and cover the lid margin. Usually the skin can be gently lifted by pushing up on the brow; and the lid margin may then be found to be in a normal position.

Ptosis after Operation

Minimal ptosis may occur after cataract or retinal detachment operation, with traction sutures under the superior rectus muscle, or after temporary removal of that muscle.

Vertical Muscle Imbalance

The most subtle type of ptosis, and one that is frequently overlooked, is that caused by vertical muscle imbalance. If the patient fixes with the lower eye, the action causes the other eye to move up and places the lid lower on the cornea, thereby giving the appearance of ptosis. To detect this condition, alternately cover one eye and then the other. Two observations can be made. The apparently ptotic side will have that eye come down to fix when the cover is moved to the other eye. When each eye

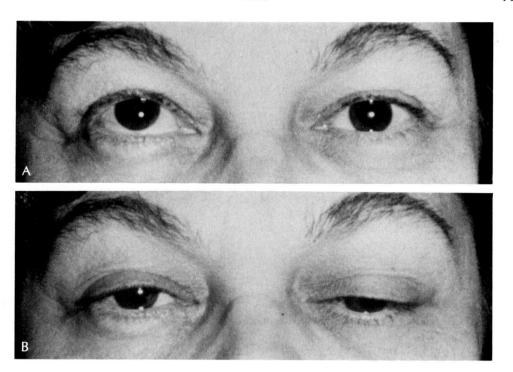

Fig. 5–1. This patient has a right hypertropia. **A.** She is fixing with the hypotropic eye, and no difference in the lids is noticed. **B.** She is fixing with the hypertropic eye, causing the left eye to look down and the left lid to also be down, giving the impression of a ptosis.

The relative position of the pupil as a result of a tropia will influence which eye appears to have a pseudoptosis.

fixes, each lid will be in the same position in reference to the pupil and the cornea. The measurement of the fissures will also be found equal (Fig. 5–1A, B).

Apraxia of Lid Opening

This condition is not true ptosis. A patient with this disorder has difficulty in opening the lids after forced closure. The condition is not related to blepharospasm, and the patient shows no contraction of the orbicularis muscle. Characteristically, to initiate movement, the patient may thrust his head back, as if to break some neuronal connection inhibiting lid opening. No ptosis occurs between attacks, which are associated with a variety of supranuclear lesions, including Huntington's chorea.

TRUE PTOSIS

Congenital Ptosis

Most kinds of congenital ptosis are not hereditary, with one notable exception. The ptosis associated with epicanthus inversus and blepharophimosis, which is usually bilateral, is frequently familial and may be a dominant characteristic. The other kinds of congenital ptosis have no familial association (and the ptosis is unilateral in 70% of the cases).

Superior Rectus Muscle Weakness

A feature often overlooked in congenital ptosis—and sometimes in acquired ptosis—is an associated weakness of the superior rectus muscle (found in about 10% of the cases). This feature is an essential one to consider in evaluating a patient for correction of ptosis. It is also important to evaluate the patient's Bell's phenomenon. Failure to know about a superior rectus muscle weakness or an inadequate Bell's phenomenon may result in a corneal exposure problem that may be more serious than the original ptosis. Once a corrective surgical procedure has been performed on the lid, the superior rectus muscle weakness may be more of a cosmetic problem than the ptosis ever was. The patient may complain that the now obvious vertical displacement of the eye was caused by the operation. Improper selection of operative procedure may make the vertical problem worse.

Horner Syndrome

This disorder has ptosis as one of its prime signs. Just as the ptosis may be overlooked because of associated frontalis muscle assistance, incompleteness of Horner syndrome or degree of alertness of the patient may cause the miosis to be overlooked if all the pupil-influencing factors are not considered. A detailed description of these factors is given in Chapter 3. The presence of heterochromia on the side of the ptosis should alert one to look even harder for a smaller pupil on that side since it goes along with a congenital Horner syndrome (Fig. 5–2). Heterochromia is seen only in a ptosis caused by sympathetic paralysis with a congenital or neonatal onset.

Cyclic Third Cranial Nerve Paralysis

This paralysis is a rare entity. It usually begins in childhood, remains throughout life, and is benign. Cyclic paralysis of the third cranial nerve may be complete or incomplete. It is gradual in onset until a certain point, and then it gradually recovers without any deficit. An entire episode lasts only a few minutes. After pupillary involvement, ptosis is one of the most constant features of this syndrome. The inclusion of other parts of the third cranial nerve varies from patient to patient. Lid twitching occurring prior to the onset of each new phase is a characteristic sign. The extra-ocular muscles are infrequently involved and then only the medial rectus muscle. The onset in childhood, repetitiveness of course, and lack of residual deficit essentially differentiate it from those cases of third cranial nerve paralysis associated with diabetes or aneurysm, which come on later in life. The cause is unknown, as is the treatment.

Acquired Ptosis

Hereditary ptosis coming on later in life is not common. The main example that I see is that associated with chronic progressive external ophthalmoplegia. The leading initial sign of the condition is ptosis, and it may be the only sign for many years. Observing other members of the patient's family, either in person or from photographs, is important. Many patients either suppress a family history or are truly unaware of it; since all members look alike, nobody thinks to comment about it. The Tensilon test is negative and excludes myasthenia gravis. The normal pupil and normal accommodation absolve the third cranial nerve.

Myasthenia Gravis

Ptosis is usually the first sign of this condition in young people, just as it is in chronic progressive external ophthalmoplegia. The ptosis caused by myasthenia gravis, however, is responsive to a Tensilon injection. In addition, no pupillary or accommodative abnormalities exist, and the ophthalmoplegia that usually comes on later is similar to other myopathies, with the elevation of the eye being primarily affected. Keeping the eyes in sustained up gaze for 1 to 2 minutes causes the ptosis to get worse. This factor is almost pathognomonic of myasthenia gravis and is not seen in Horner syndrome or third cranial nerve disease.

In cases in which the question of the cause of the ptosis is still in doubt, the lid peek sign may be useful. Just as the levator is weakened to hold the upper lid in its

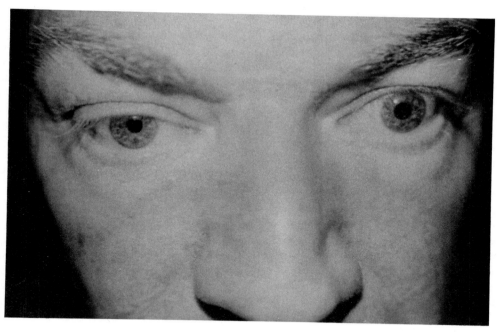

Fig. 5–2. A typical Horner syndrome with right ptosis and miosis of right pupil. Even in a black and white photograph, the light color of the right iris can be appreciated, which is in keeping with a congenital Horner syndrome.

proper position, the orbicularis is also weak in keeping the fissure closed for a prolonged period. When a patient is asked to close his eyes and keep them closed, the fissure opens up in a few seconds because of the orbicularis weakness. This phenomenon needs to be differentiated from motor inpersistence, which is part of the syndrome of the nondominant hemisphere or which occasionally can be seen in bilateral hemisphere lesions. The associated hemisphere signs and symptoms should easily differentiate it from the lid peek sign of myasthenia gravis.

Lid retraction in myasthenia gravis is uncommon as compared with ptosis. When it occurs, three different types are categorized by the duration of the lid retraction. The most common form is the lid retraction associated with weakness of the contralateral levator muscle. This may be a prolonged lid retraction. This form of the lid retraction is an example of Hering's law of equal innervation to yoke muscles at work.

Hering's law can be temporarily altered toward the more normal side during the Tensilon test. During this test, less effect is required of the myasthenic lid and no lid retraction develops in the other lid. The second form of lid retraction is Cogan's lid twitch sign. The upper lid overshoots when the eyes are moved rapidly from down gaze to a position straight ahead. There is no sustained lid retraction in these instances. The third type of lid retraction was reported by Puklin, Sacks, and Boshes in a small series of myasthenic patients. This type of lid retraction is over a few seconds and is caused by post-tetanic facilitation of the levator, seen particularly after prolonged up gaze. A similar mechanism was postulated for a comparable phenomenon in the small muscles of the hand of myasthenic patients.

Third Cranial Nerve Paralysis

One of the major causes of ptosis is third cranial nerve paralysis owing to an aneurysm. If the ptosis is associated with diplopia or, more significantly, with a pupillary abnormality, aneurysm as the cause must be the first consideration. The condition is one that requires prompt evaluation and treatment because of its catastrophic characteristics. Not all third cranial nerve paralyses come on with marked involvement of all parts of the third cranial nerve. In the overwhelming majority of patients with aneurysms causing third cranial nerve paralysis, however, the pupil is affected to some degree. Subtle changes in pupil size in dim illumination with distance fixation should be scrupulously evaluated. The extraocular muscle weakness may not be apparent or considered since the patient does not complain of diplopia. When the patient is examined with his eyes in the extremes of gaze, particularly with the affected eye turned up and out in the field of action of the superior rectus muscle, a small hypotropia may be seen that is not present in the opposite field of gaze.

The other prime cause of third cranial nerve paralysis, diabetes, does not always spare the pupil and accommodation. In about 20% of the cases of diabetic third cranial nerve paralysis, the pupil is involved; and these cases cannot be differentiated clinically from those caused by aneurysm even when the urine gives a 4 plus reaction for sugar. A third cranial nerve paralysis with the pupil involved must be considered as being caused by an aneurysm until that is adequately ruled out. Some degree of ptosis is almost always present in third cranial nerve paralysis from any cause.

Adults with acquired Horner syndrome do not have the heterochromia associated with congenital Horner syndrome (Chapter 3). In any case of ptosis, examination of the pupils for size abnormalities is essential. When in doubt as to the equality of pupils, observe the pupils in dim light with the patient's gaze directed at a distance. The other test is to measure the near point of accommodation or the point at which the patient begins to notice blurring. The side with Horner syndrome will read considerably closer. Measure with the patient's glasses on for his full distance correction and an equal amount of bifocal correction if needed. The procedure is most effective with patients over 40 years of age who require reading glasses. The high degree of residual accommodation in the young person makes the measurement difficult in those under the age of 35.

Trauma

Any injury often causes either direct damage to the levator muscle or damage to its oculomotor innervation. Since the superior rectus muscle has a common origin with the levator muscle, it is also frequently injured, with a resultant muscle imbalance. The damage may not be immediately apparent if the ptosis is severe enough to cover the pupil and prevent diplopia. The recovery from ptosis may take many months, and no corrective surgery should be considered until at least 6 months have elapsed with no improvement. Resorption of edema of the lids should not be interpreted as improvement of ptosis. Be conservative and do not overestimate the final outcome to the patient.

External Tumors of the Lid

Any such tumors sufficiently large to pull the lid down are readily visible. Those that are in the superior orbit or in the upper fornix between the lids and the globe may not be appreciated on simple inspection. Diagnosis may require digital palpation of the area beneath the superior bony orbital rim, as well as double eversion of the upper lid and observation beneath it. Plexiform neuromas of the lid feel like a bag of worms rather than a single mass, and they frequently extend laterally beneath the skin of the cheek and into the temporal fossa. These neuromas are associated with generalized neurofibromatosis and have other signs, such as café-au-lait spots and epilepsy.

Strabismus Operation

When such an operation shortens the superior rectus muscle, it may also pull the levator muscle down, causing ptosis. Superior rectus muscle operation, if carried too far posteriorly, may cause damage to the nerve going to the levator muscle (because the nerve passes through the superior rectus muscle on its way to the levator muscle). Ptosis thus caused would come on at the time of the surgical procedure, of course, and not months or years later.

Myotonic Dystrophy

This disorder does not start with ptosis and therefore is not usually a problem in diagnosis. The other muscular signs of myotonia, as well as the age of the patient at onset, make the diagnosis rather easy. Cataracts of all types are seen in association with myotonic dystrophy, but the Christmas tree cataract is pathognomonic. It is seen only with the slit lamp, and it appears as multiple scattered red and green crystalline dots throughout the lens.

SYNKINETIC PTOSIS

In synkinetic ptosis, the change in degree of ptosis is related to some other facial movement, such as that of the nostril, ear, or jaw. Those cases of synkinetic ptosis associated with jaw movement (referred to as the Marcus Gunn, or jaw-winking, phenomenon) are the only ones of clinical significance.

The patient exhibiting the Marcus Gunn phenomenon moves the lid up and down by opening and closing the mouth, with associated contraction of the masseter muscle. The same lid action can be achieved by contracting the masseter muscle when the jaw is moved from side to side. The lid movement can be brought out by having the patient chew gum or suck on a hard candy. As long as the masseter muscle is contracted, the ptosis is improved. A feature that has been observed is that the jaw-winking component seems to disappear with age in many patients but the ptosis does not. The reason for this difference is not known.

Third Cranial Nerve Misdirection

Synkinetic retractions may be seen in third cranial nerve misdirection between the levator muscle and the inferior rectus muscle; they are referred to as the pseudo von Graefe's sign. After third cranial nerve paralysis owing to trauma or aneurysm, a misdirection phenomenon may occur between the levator muscle and the inferior rectus or medial rectus muscle. When the eye is moved in the direction of either of these muscles, the lid may be innervated, causing lid retraction.

LID RETRACTION

A consideration of lid retraction should be included in any discussion of lid abnormalities.

When looking at a patient with ptosis, the physician must decide whether one lid is ptotic or the other lid is retracted, regardless of which lid the patient thinks is abnormal. The patient interprets his condition according to what is more cosmetically disturbing to him. If retraction is present, a small white area of sclera appears between the lid and the upper cornea, a phenomenon that is always abnormal.

Thyroid Disease

Although the causes of lid retraction are numerous, over 90% of the time the condition represents thyroid disease. As pointed out by McLean and Norton, the sign may be unilateral, and it may occur prior to the onset of systemic and chemical signs of thyroid disease. A discussion of the chemical tests that are most valuable currently for the diagnosis of thyroid disease are discussed more fully in Chapter 6, Diplopia.

Collier's Lid Retraction

The next most common cause of lid retraction is Collier's sign in midbrain disease occurring particularly at the posterior commissure. Usually, no problem exists in differentiating patients with this condition from those with thyroid disease.

Hydrocephalus

The setting-sun sign of hydrocephalus in children is not well explained; possibly it is a variant of Collier's sign and is caused by transmitted pressure.

Third Cranial Nerve Misdirection

Third cranial nerve misdirection may produce a combination of ptosis and lid retraction. It occurs predominantly after trauma or aneurysm—and never results from diabetes, which fact is the reason for observing this sign. If a patient has developed third cranial nerve misdirection after a third cranial nerve paralysis, it must be concluded that, even if the patient has diabetes, the cause of the misdirection was either trauma or an aneurysm that was unsuspected. Diabetes causes third cranial nerve paralysis but never misdirection. When the third cranial nerve recovers, there may be a slight ptosis or none at all. As the eye is adducted, the lid retracts because of a new relationship established between the innervation of the medial rectus muscle on adduction and the lid. This sign is best seen in examining the horizontal excursion of the eye in question on down gaze rather than in the straight-ahead position. A similar relationship may occur between the levator muscle and the inferior rectus muscle on down gaze.

Adversive Seizures

Frontal lobe or adversive seizures have associated ocular signs that are of interest. When one frontal lobe is stimulated, the head and eyes are driven toward the other side and the upper lids retract. Between seizures, the lids and the gaze mechanisms are normal.

Lid Retraction after Operation

Previous operation for ptosis with secondary overcorrection or a surgical procedure for laceration of the lid with contraction of the scar in a vertical direction may result in retraction of the lid. These causes of lid retraction may be identified readily from the history or from simple inspection.

Claude Bernard Syndrome

This rare syndrome is the opposite of Horner syndrome. In Claude Bernard syndrome, lesions stimulate the sympathetic chain, causing ipsilateral lid retraction. The lesions that cause Horner syndrome also cause Claude Bernard syndrome. Occasionally, a patient voices complaints typical of those made in Claude Bernard syndrome but on examination will be found to have a slight Horner syndrome rather than lid retraction and enlarged pupils. Such a patient may have a peripheral Horner syndrome in which a supersensitivity to his own circulating epinephrine has developed. This possibility is confirmed by placing a 1:1000 aqueous solution of epinephrine in both eyes and observing them 30 minutes later. The side the patient has complained about will show a larger pupil and a variable amount of upper lid retraction.

Myasthenia Gravis

In cases of myasthenia gravis, one always thinks of ptosis, not of lid retraction. Occasionally, the degree of the myasthenic process affecting each lid is different and does not affect the frontalis muscle at all. As a result, the patient uses his frontalis muscle to improve the side with the ptosis. In accordance with Hering's law of equal innervation, the same effort is transmitted to the other side (the normal one), causing the lid to retract. The clue is frontalis muscle wrinkling on the side of the lid retraction.

Voluntary Subluxation of the Globe

In this frightening spectacle, the patient is able to markedly retract the upper and lower lids to near the equator of the globes. At the same time, he subluxates the globes enough to get the lids behind the equatorial plane. He then squeezes the orbicularis muscle and closes the lids, thus pushing the globes further out. The patient can usually reverse the process unless the lids go into spasm or secondary swelling occurs. At this point, the patient may require a partial facial nerve block to release the lid spasm and replace the globes.

Myotonic Lid Lag

There are cases of myotonic lid lag in both hypo- and hyperkalemic periodic paralysis that initially look like lid retraction. Myotonic lid lag is more common in the hyperkalemic form, but can occur in the hypokalemic form, making the institution of potassium therapy sometimes puzzling.

TESTS

Tensilon Test

Any ptosis that is not of obvious origin deserves a Tensilon test, which is given as a 1 ml intravenous injection. Traditionally, it has been advised that an adequate dose of atropine be given to the patient prior to injection. A problem involved in giving the atropine dose is that the medication lasts much longer than is required for the test and becomes uncomfortable to the patient. Another problem in giving the atropine is that most patients are given it intramuscularly and then almost immediately—before the atropine has a chance to work—are given the Tensilon test. Many physicians feel that the use of atropine is unnecessary, but that is should be available.

To do the Tensilon test, give the patient 0.1 ml of Tensilon as a screening dose while looking for any overreactions to the drug. If none occur within 1 minute, then give the rest of the dose fairly rapidly intravenously. An improvement in the ptosis should be seen within 30 seconds; the entire effect will pass within 3 minutes. The important part of the test is to find the area of maximum ocular deficit, either in extraocular muscle imbalance or as ptosis, before giving the test. Then examine that entity or position during the test period. A positive response reflects significant improvement in these areas and pinpoints the cause as myasthenia gravis. Ptosis is more easily evaluated with the Tensilon test than is diplopia.

Quinine Challenge

Before the Tensilon test came into use, an opposite approach was in vogue, namely, seeing whether one could make the myasthenia worse. The physician gave the patient quinine, which reduced the sensitivity of the motor end-plate and thus aggravated the myasthenia. This approach is no longer taken, but the reaction to quinine may still be seen in two other situations: (1) a patient who drinks tonic water may ingest enough quinine to cause a worsening of any myasthenia and (2) quinine given to many older people as a treatment for night leg cramps may at the same time aggravate a myasthenic process.

Electromyography

In my experience, electromyograms for ocular myasthenia gravis are not useful. The electrical pattern obtained may be typical of myasthenia gravis but not entirely diagnostic. Furthermore, the technique is inadequate because the recording needle is frequently inserted in the levator aponeurosis rather than in the muscle, which is farther back in the orbit. Testing other muscles, such as the biceps muscle, may give false-negative results if the patient has only the ocular form of myasthenia gravis.

Biopsy

This procedure is also of limited value because, first, one has to get some muscle and not the aponeurosis, and second, the specific features that are diagnostic of myasthenia gravis are not commonly seen in biospy specimens. The basic defect is not in the muscle anatomy; it is a biochemical defect in the number of packets of acetylcholine in the motor end-plate. The biochemical defect is evaluated by the Tensilon test. The pathologic changes are indirect evidence of the disease. None of the other myopathic processes involve significant enough differential pathologic changes to warrant a biopsy. Drachman points out that one cannot differentiate a neuropathic process from a myopathic one by a biopsy. In addition, good experimental evidence now exists that an antigen-antibody reaction at the motor end-plate also interferes with the motor end-plate function.

TREATMENT

Treatment depends on the problems involved. If the ptosis causes skeletal deformity owing to head position or if the lid covers the pupil in a child in whom amblyopia may develop, repair must be undertaken early.

If the ptosis is caused by recent trauma, delay and careful observation for many months are indicated before embarking on a surgical procedure. If the condition is a myopathy and up gaze is affected—or may be affected in the future—surgical caution is the word because severe corneal exposure (owing to inadequate Bell's phenomenon and the associated orbicularis muscle weakness during sleep) becomes a problem. Cautious neglect may be the treatment of choice in these cases.

Surgical Treatment

The type of operation varies according to the degree of ptosis, the amount of levator muscle function, and the judgment of the surgeon. In-depth discussion of the possibilities is best left to surgical texts. The two approaches I recommend are the tarsal-conjunctival approach of Iliff for a small ptosis (3 mm or less) and the skin approach of Berke for a larger one. For ptosis associated with the Gunn lid phenomenon, the frontalis sling, along with the cutting of the innervation to the lid so as to prevent the

recurrence of jaw-winking, is recommended. Crutch glasses can be used, but they seldom are tolerated by the patient.

Corticosteroid Therapy

Oral corticosteroids have been used in the treatment of ocular myasthenia gravis for several years. Despite the lack of universal agreement as to the efficacy of this treatment in purely ocular cases, certainly it may be worthwhile in a number of cases, particularly when the patient does not have an adequate response to anticholinesterase drugs. In addition, some evidence suggests that long-term anticholinesterase therapy may destroy some of the smaller nerve terminals and therefore may not be the best treatment over long periods of time.

Treatment of Lid Retraction

The treatment of lid retraction is the treatment of the underlying process. In the case of thyroid disease, the lid retraction usually does not go away completely with control of the hyperthyroidism, but it can be further improved by lateral and, if necessary, a small medial tarsorrhaphy. In extreme cases, a reverse ptosis procedure can be performed, in which part or all of the tarsal attachments of the smooth and striate muscles are detached.

Guanethidine Therapy

The use of topical guanethidine to create a chemical Horner syndrome was first reported by Gay and his associates and subsequently popularized in the British literature. It has not been useful in my hands and has a history of ocular irritation. Recent studies with topical 0.5% thymoxamine have been more promising but also have the same irritating effects when applied topically. The thymoxamine is an alpha-adrenergic blocker and, therefore, ideal to effect abnormal stimulation of Müller's muscle. Thymoxamine does relieve about 2 to 3 mm of lid retraction even if thickened muscles are demonstrable on computerized tomography. It does not work on stable, long-standing thyroid eye disease. It also does not affect normal persons, nor does it work in a variety of other neuromuscular diseases. It is in this latter category, as a diagnostic agent to confirm thyroid disease and rule out other neuromuscular diseases that thymoxamine may find its greatest use.

BIBLIOGRAPHY

Aita, J.F., and Wanamaker, W.: Body computerized tomography and the thymus. Arch. Neurol. 36:20, 1979.

Almon, R.R., and Appel, S.H.: Serum acetylcholine receptor antibodies in myasthenia gravis. Ann. N.Y. Acad. Sci. 274:235, 1975.

Armaly, M.F.: Effect of corticosteroids on intraocular pressure and fluid dynamics. Part III. Changes in visual function and pupil size during topical dexamethasone application. Arch. Ophthalmol. 71:636, 1964.

Beard, C.: A new treatment for severe unilateral congenital ptosis and for ptosis with jaw-winking. Am. J. Ophthalmol. 59:353, 1965.

Becker, B.: The side effects of corticosteroids. Invest. Ophthalmol. 3:492, 1964.

Berke, R.N.: An operation for ptosis utilizing the superior rectus muscle. Arch. Ophthalmol. 42:685, 1949.

Berke, R.N.: Results of resection of the levator muscle through a skin incision in congenital ptosis. Arch. Ophthalmol. 61:177, 1959.

Berke, R.N., and Wadsworth, J.A.C.: Histology of levator muscle in congenital and acquired ptosis. Arch. Ophthalmol. 53:413, 1955.

Boruchoff, S.A., and Goldberg, B.: Tensilon in diagnosis of ocular myasthenia gravis. Arch. Ophthalmol. 53:718, 1955.

Bradley, W.G., and Toome, B.K.: Synkinetic movements of the eyelid: a case with some unusual mechanisms of paradoxical lid retraction. J. Neurol. Neurosurg. Psychiatry 30:578, 1967.

Burian, H.M., and Burns, C.A.: Ocular changes in myotonic dystrophy. Am. J. Ophthalmol. 63:22, 1967.

Caplan, L.R.: Ptosis. J. Neurol. Neurosurg. Psychiatry 37:1, 1974.

Cogan, D.G.: Myasthenia gravis. A review of the disease and description of lid twitch as a characteristic sign. Arch. Ophthalmol. 74:217, 1965.

Cole, M.: Eyelid tone: a sign of facial paresis. Neurol. 18:413, 1968.

Collier, J.: Nuclear ophthalmoplegia with special reference to retraction of the lids and ptosis and to lesions of the posterior commissure. Brain 50:488, 1927.

Cuénoud, S., Feltkamp, T.E.W., and Fulpuis, B.W.: Antibodies to acetylcholine receptor in patients with thymoma but without myasthenia gravis. Neurology 30:201, 1980.

Dixon, R.S., Anderson, R.L., and Hatt, M.U.: The use of thymoxamine in eyelid retraction. Arch. Ophthalmol. 97:2147, 1979.

Drachman, D.B.: Myopathic changes in chronically denervated muscle. Arch. Neurol. 16:14, 1967.

Fischer, K.C., and Schwartzman, R.J.: Oral corticosteroids in the treatment of ocular myasthenia gravis. Neurology 24:795, 1974.

Frankel, M.: Myasthenia gravis: current trends. Am. J. Ophthalmol. 61:522, 1966.

Gay, A.J., Salmon, M.L., and Windsor, C.E.: Hering's law, the levators and their relationship in disease states. Arch. Ophthalmol. 77:157, 1967.

Goldstein, J.E., and Cogan, D.G.: Apraxia of lid opening. Arch. Ophthalmol. 73:155, 1965.

Henderson, J.W.: Relief of eyelid retraction. Arch. Ophthalmol. 74:204, 1965.

Iliff, C.E.: A simplified ptosis operation. Am. J. Ophthalmol. 37:529, 1954.

Johnson, C.C.: Blepharoptosis. Arch. Ophthalmol. 66:793, 1961.

Johnson, C.C.: Blepharoptosis. Arch. Ophthalmol. 67:18, 1962.

Keesey, J., Bein, M., and Mink, J.: Detection of thymoma in myasthenia gravis. Neurology 30:233, 1980.

Kennard, D.W., and Glaser, G.H.: An analysis of eyelid movements. J. Nerv. Ment. Dis. 139:31, 1964.

Kennard, D.W., and Smith, G.L.: Reflex regulations of the upper eyelids. With observations on the onset of sleep. J. Physiol. (Lond.) 166:168, 1964.

Lindstrom, J.: An assay for antibodies to human acetylcholine receptor in serum from patients with myasthenia gravis. Clin. Immunol. Immunopathol. 7:36, 1977.

Loewenfeld, I.E., and Thompson, H.S.: Oculomotor paresis with cyclic spasms. A critical review of the literature and a new case. Surv. Ophthalmol. 20:81, 1975.

McLean, J.M., and Norton, E.W.D.: Unilateral lid retraction without exophthalmos. Arch. Ophthalmol. 61:681, 1959.

Mink, J., et al.: Computed tomography of the anterior mediastinum in patients with myasthenia gravis and suspected thymoma. Am. J. Roentgenol. 130:239, 1978.

Newsome, D.A., Wong, V.G., and Cameron, T.P.: "Steroid-induced" mydriasis and ptosis. Invest. Ophthalmol. 10:424, 1971.

Nichols, J.P.: Topical corticosteroids and aqueous humor dynamics. Arch. Ophthalmol. 72:189, 1964.

Osher, R.H., and Griggs, R.C.: Obicularis fatigue. Arch. Ophthalmol. 97:677, 1979.

Penfield, W., and Rasmussen, T.: The Cerebral Cortex of Man. New York, Macmillan, 1950.

Pochin, E.E.: The mechanism of lid retraction in Graves' disease. Clin. Sci. 4:91, 1939.

Pochin, E.E.: Unilateral retraction of the upper lid in Graves' disease. Clin. Sci. 3:197, 1938.

Puklin, J.E., Sacks, J.G., and Boshes, B.: Transient eyelid retraction in myasthenia gravis. J. Neurol. Neurosurg. Psychiatry 39:44, 1976.

Resnick, J.S., and Engel, W.K.: Myotonic lid lag in

hypokalemic periodic paralysis. J. Neurol. Neurosurg. Psychiatry *30:*47, 1967.

Simpson, D.G.: Marcus Gunn phenomenon following squint and ptosis surgery. Arch. Ophthalmol. *56:*743, 1956.

Smith, J.L.: Therapy for ocular myasthenia gravis. Trans. Am. Acad. Ophthalmol. Otolaryngol. *78:*795, 1974.

Summerskill, W.H., and Molnar, G.D.: Eye signs in hepatic cirrhosis. N. Engl. J. Med. *266:*1244, 1962.

Susac, J.O., and Smith, J.L.: Cyclic oculomotor paralysis. Neurology *24:*24, 1974.

Van der Ged, H., et al.: Multiple antibody production in myasthenia gravis. Lancet *2:*373, 1963.

Walsh, F., and Ford, F.: Clinical observations on the pupillary phenomenon resulting from regeneration of the third nerve with especial reference to the Argyll Roberston pupil. Bull. Johns Hopkins Hosp. *68:*309, 1941.

Walsh, F.B., and Hoyt, W.F.: Clinical Neuro-ophthalmology, 3rd Ed. Vol. 1. Baltimore, William & Wilkins, 1969.

Walsh, T.J., and Gilman, M.: Voluntary propulsion of the eyes. Am. J. Ophthalmol. *67:*583, 1969.

Chapter 6

Diplopia

THOMAS J. WALSH

DEFINITION OF TERMS

Patients frequently complain of "double vision," a term they often use to describe a condition other than diplopia. Many patients use the term double vision to describe a decrease in visual acuity such as occurs with polyopia caused by a cataract. In examining a patient who complains of diplopia, it is important to discover which symptom he really has—diplopia or blurred vision.

Diplopia is synonymous with double vision. Since this medical term is relatively unknown to the public, the patient complains of seeing double rather than of having diplopia. Double vision in neuro-ophthalmology is that which disappears on the closure of either eye—which means that the patient sees a duplication of one particular object or two images of the same object, which are related to the physical position of each eye. This discussion does not concern so-called "monocular diplopia," in which the patient sees double even when one eye is closed. This condition is usually caused by physical interference between the object and the photoreceptor of the particular eye. This chapter does not refer to the double vision reported with receptor problems, in which the image in one eye is blurred as compared with that in the other and appears as a halo over the clear image in binocular vision.

This can be caused by irregular astigmatism of the cornea secondary to keratoconus or from some external pressure such as a chalazion. Intraocular causes include early cataract changes, partially dislocated lenses, and vitreous opacities. Intracranial causes are rare. Receptor problems have occasionally been reported with pituitary tumors that bisect fixation and with hemorrhages in the occipital cortex that spread the receptor elements of the visual cortex.

True binocular diplopia has two components. The motor aspect deals with the position of each eye as controlled by the oculomotor mechanism; the sensorial part is a response to the visual direction of each eye, which is acquired during the development of the binocular reflexes in childhood, assuming that no interruption occurs during the period of time needed for the reflexes to become permanently fixed.

The egocentric development of the visual directions begins shortly after birth when the developing macula assumes the straight-ahead directional position in each eye. At the same time each eye is divided sensorially into halves, temporal and nasal, in such a manner that any object imaged in these areas appears egocentrically localized in the opposite direction. By the same token, owing to the decussation of the optic nerve, the macula in each eye achieves the same direction, and the whole visual field in one eye is physiologically superimposed over that of the other in such a manner that every part of the visual field in one eye has an exact counterpart in the other eye. In this manner, the temporal retina corresponds to the nasal retina and vice versa. Thus, in order for one object to be seen singly in space, it must stimulate corresponding points in each retina. If it stimulates non-corresponding points, that is, nasal in one eye and temporal in the other or macula in one eye and another part of the retina that is not the macula in the other, diplopia is present. The relationship between the motor and sensorial development is very close. The eye muscles serve two main purposes:

1. When the image of an object that is attractive to the organism is imaged in the periphery of the retina, the eye muscles move the eye so that the object is imaged in the macula where it can be seen better. At the same time, the other eye moves in the same manner.
2. Once the image of this object is centrally placed, the eye muscles in both eyes try to keep it there in all positions of gaze, whether in versions or in vergences.

During the first 3 or 4 months of life, fixation, versions, and vergences are developed; at the same time, the macula is developing anatomically and physiologically as the center of the visual system and the seat of the best visual acuity. If a muscle imbalance is present and a turn in an eye affects either a version or a vergence movement before the age of visual maturity (7 years), a fleeting type of diplopia occurs, the image in the turning eye is suppressed, and the patient does not report diplopia. Once visual maturity has occurred, any motor defect in the system is accompanied by double vision.

When an eye is turned, each macula receives an image that corresponds to objects in the direction in which each eye is facing; this situation causes "confusion," which is very unpleasant. Therefore, the person, through mental processes that are not understood, selects one of the objects as the object of regard and suppresses the image hitting the macula of the other eye. Now the object of regard is imaged in the macula looking at it and in a non-corresponding point in the other eye, giving rise to two images of the same object. One of the images is straight ahead, and the other corresponds to the directional value of the retina on which it is imaged. As an example, in esotropia the false image hits the nasal retina and is directed to the same side as the turned eye so the diplopia is uncrossed or homonymous. In exotropia the image hits the temporal retina and is directed to the side opposite the turned eye, so the condition is crossed or heteronymous diplopia. If an eye is turned down, the image of that eye is seen higher than the image of the straight eye, because it is hitting the lower retina, which has an upward direction.

Monocular diplopia is caused by a defect in the refractive medium that divides the image. A patient with this condition speaks of a second shadow (like a TV ghost image) rather than of two separate images. The most common cause of this symptom is a nuclear sclerotic cataract. Other opacities, such as corneal scars or vitreous opacities, may cause a similar problem, as can dislocation of the lens that is caused by trauma or occurs spontaneously in homocystinuria and Marfan syndrome. Dislocation, which may be subtle if the lens is only partially dislocated, can be detected by asking the patient to look up and then quickly look you in the eye. Tremulousness of the iris (iridodonesis), which is most easily seen in patients who have undergone a cataract operation, indicates a dislocated or partially dislocated lens. Polyopia may be caused by excessive secretion of the meibomian glands. The onset of oblique or irregular astigmatism as seen with keratoconus can cause diplopia. Although an early complaint, this condition is not immediately obvious on slit lamp examination.

Intermittent diplopia and variable diplopia are more frequently seen in persons with ophthalmoplegias, such as myasthenia gravis, than in those with paralysis of the third, fourth, or sixth cranial nerves. If caused by a partial involvement of these nerves, the diplopia is intermittent because it occurs only when the patient turns his eye into the maximum field of action of the affected muscle. Thus paralysis of the left lateral rectus muscle may produce diplopia only when the patient looks into moderate or extreme left gaze. This phenomenon differs from the variability related to fatigue and prolonged use of the offending muscles that occurs in myasthenia. Occasionally, vascular disease can affect cranial nerves intermittently, as in vertebral basilar insufficiency.

Intermittent diplopia or variable diplopia can be extremely difficult to diagnose, and careful history taking and repeated examination are necessary to evaluate the significance of this symptom.

IDENTIFICATION OF MUSCLES INVOLVED

When it is determined that true diplopia is present, the offending muscle(s) must be identified. To do this, examine each eye separately, instructing the patient to follow a hand light into all the cardinal fields of gaze (duction) while one eye is covered. If a muscle is severely affected, some limitation of movement will occur in one or more fields, which will facilitate identification of the offending muscle. If limitation is not obvious, the muscle is weak only in

regard to maintaining fusion with the other eye (version). Since, as a rule, ductions are stronger than versions, muscular weakness affecting fusion usually occurs first.

Limitation of movement can be caused by structural changes in the muscles that prevent their stretching or to tumor masses or hemorrhage. Tumor or hemorrhage may cause diplopia for several reasons, including neuropathic or myopathic changes and displacement of the globe. Blow-out fractures of the orbital floor with entrapment of the muscle tendons also produce diplopia.

The forced duction test is a simple, easily performed, and useful diagnostic technique for evaluating limitation of ocular rotation and determining whether lack of innervation or some other condition is responsible. The test involves anesthetizing the eye with a 0.5% solution of tetracaine or of proparacaine HCl. If further anesthesia is required, as is frequently the case in the limbal area, a cotton-tip applicator dipped in a 4% solution of cocaine may be employed. Then, using a small-tooth forceps, grab the conjunctiva at the limbus where it joins the cornea in the area opposite to the direction in which the eye is to be moved. If a paralysis of the right lateral rectus muscle has been discerned, apply the forceps at the three o'clock position (on the nasal side of the cornea); and as the patient attempts to look to his right, move his eye in the same direction. If it moves freely, it may be assumed that the muscle is not restricted but merely lacks innervation. Sometimes a patient resists the forced movement of his eye, and a false-positive result occurs. In this event, observation of the other eye is important. If the patient moves his eyes to the right on command but the right eye resists movement with the forceps, the presumption is that a restriction of the right eye occurs owing to inelasticity of the medial rectus muscle. If neither eye moves, no assumption of entrapment can be made since the patient made no effort to move the normal eye to the right. In fact, he may be actively resisting the test, thus giving the false impression of entrapment. This test is just as valuable in the vertical as in the horizontal plane.

Horizontal Diplopia

Horizontal movement of the eye is accomplished by means of the medial rectus muscle, which is innervated by the third cranial nerve, and by means of the lateral rectus muscle, which is innervated by the sixth cranial nerve. The medial rectus muscle moves the eye toward the nose; the lateral rectus muscle turns the eye out. Diplopia involving these muscles is purely horizontal. When the medial rectus muscle is involved, the images are crossed; that is, the left image disappears when the right eye is covered. Diplopia involving the lateral rectus muscle produces homonymous, or uncrossed images, and may be evident only when an attempt is made to look into the field of action of that muscle. Therefore, examination should include right and left as well as straight ahead gaze.

With right lateral rectus muscle weakness, diplopia may not occur in left gaze; however, an uncrossed diplopia will occur in the right gaze, and the right image will disappear when the right eye is covered.

Vertical Diplopia

Four muscles produce vertical diplopia (Table 6–1). Three of these, the superior rectus and the inferior oblique muscles, which move the eye up, and the inferior rectus muscle, which moves it down, are controlled by the third cranial nerve. The fourth muscle, the superior oblique muscle, which moves the eye down, is innervated by the fourth cranial nerve. Unlike

the medial and lateral rectus muscles, which have a single function, these muscles cause the eye to intort or extort and, in addition, assist the medial and lateral rectus muscles to move the eye medially or laterally. Because of these secondary functions, vertical diplopia is rarely just vertical; the images are usually obliquely located, at least to some degree.

The terms intorsion and extorsion refer to the rotation of the eye around an imaginary axis running from the posterior orbital apex through the center of the globe and out through the cornea when the head is tilted toward either shoulder. This movement keeps the visual axis parallel to the ground.

The principal function of these muscles is elevation or depression of the eye, primarily in one position. The superior oblique muscle, for instance, is a depressor only when the eye is adducted. When it is abducted, this muscle acts as an intorter, rotating the eye toward the nose. The primary vertical function of the superior and inferior rectus muscles takes place when the eye is abducted. The primary vertical action of the inferior oblique muscle occurs when the eye is adducted.

Vertical Diplopia Testing

Evaluation of vertical diplopia involves three steps.

Step I. Since four muscles in each eye may be implicated, it must first be determined in which eye the visual axis is deviated upward. The answer is easily ascertained by the cover-uncover test while the patient fixes on a light. If it is determined that the condition is a true tropia and not a phoria, one can use the alternate cover test, which is easier and quicker to perform. As each eye is covered alternately, one will come up and the other come down to fix. The one that comes down is the higher, or hypertropic, eye. Even if the other eye is suspected of being the affected eye, the eye that comes down to fix should be selected for this evaluation. From the

TABLE 6–1. Actions of Cyclovertical Muscles

Muscle	Vertical Actions	Torsions
Superior rectus	Elevation	Intorsion
Inferior rectus	Depression	Extorsion
Inferior oblique	Elevation	Extorsion
Superior oblique	Depression	Intorsion

eight muscles that could cause vertical diplopia, all the combinations of muscles that could cause the test results should be considered. In the higher eye, weak depressor muscles, such as the inferior rectus and superior oblique muscles, may be responsible. On the other hand, the elevator muscles in that eye can be eliminated, since only overactions secondary to weak antagonists—not primary muscle overactions—should be considered. Another possibility is that there are weak elevators in the hypotropic eye, which suggests the superior rectus and inferior oblique muscles. Thus, possible involvement has been reduced from eight to four muscles, two in each eye and all different.

Step 2. In this step, the degree of diplopia in right and left gaze is examined. Since the vertical muscles function most strongly in one field of gaze, when they are weakened the greatest vertical separation will be in that field. The vertical action of the superior and inferior oblique muscles occurs primarily in adduction; in abduction, the superior and inferior rectus muscles come into play. If the diplopia is worse in right, as opposed to left, gaze, from the muscles isolated in step 1, the one in each eye that would have the greatest vertical effect in right gaze should be selected.

At this point, it should be determined whether the muscles chosen are intorters or extorters. If one is an extorter and one an intorter, the error is in selection, and the diagnostic steps must be checked.

Step 3. The Bielschowsky head tilt test is now used to determine torsional malfunction of the vertical muscles (Table 6–2). Because of the partial or complete paresis of one muscle, extra innervation is given to it in order to help the muscle perform its torsional function. Following Herings' law of equal innervation to yoke muscles, an equal amount of innervation is given to the yoke muscle in the other eye. This causes an excessive response in the unaffected muscle, creating an increased deviation. When the head is tilted to the left, the left eye intorts and the right eye extorts, and when the head is tilted to the right, the right eye intorts and the left eye extorts. If the diplopia worsens in left tilt, either a weak intorter in the left eye or a weak extorter in the right eye is responsible. The fact that both mucles chosen in step 2 were either intorters or extorters facilitates selection of the muscles to be considered in step 3. If both intorters were selected in step 2 and the diplopia is worse on left head tilt, the only intorters involved are those in the left eye. Since the two intorters selected in step 2 were in different eyes, the intorter in the left eye is the offending muscle.

In order to compensate for the double vision, we adjust the position of our head, face, and chin and place all three in a position where fusion may be restored. Depressing or elevating the chin compensates for vertical movement. Turning the face to the right or left compensates for a lack of abduction or adduction. Head tilting compensates for the tortional component. In the case of the medial and lateral rectus muscles, only the face turn is necessary, since there is no vertical or tortional component to be compensated. In theory, the head positioning should be universally adapted. It is not. In fact, it is most commonly seen with paresis of the lateral rectus, superior rectus, and superior oblique muscles. Even then, patients may not adopt a compensatory head position, or may even assume a reverse head position. This latter type head positioning lets the eyes drift farther apart since it may be easier to suppress widely separated images than to fuse images in an uncomfortable

TABLE 6–2. Bielschowsky Head Tilt Test

Muscle	Hypertropic Eye	Direction of Head Tilt to Increase Diplopia
Right superior rectus	Left	Right
Right superior oblique	Right	Right
Left superior rectus	Right	Left
Left superior oblique	Left	Left

position. Knowing the three functions of the vertically acting muscles of elevation or depression, adduction or abduction, and incycloversion and excycloversion is enough to decide the correct head position. A summary of compensatory head, face, and chin positions is listed in Table 6–3.

In order to bring this diagnostic method into focus, let us consider two hypothetic cases in which this type of testing would be standard procedure.

Case 1—Paralysis of the Superior Oblique Muscle. In step 1, a patient complaining of diplopia is found to have the left eye higher on the alternate cover test (Table 6–4). Possibly involved are the weak depressor muscles (the superior oblique and the inferior rectus muscles) in the left eye, or the weak elevators (the superior rectus and the inferior oblique muscles) in the right eye.

In Step 2, the diplopia is determined to be worse in right gaze. Of the four muscles selected in step 1, the only ones having maximum vertical action in right gaze are the left superior oblique and the right superior rectus muscles. Both are intorters.

In step 3, the diplopia is found to be worse on left head tilt, which brings into play the left eye intorters and the right eye extorters. Since only intorters were selected in step 2, malfunction of the left superior oblique muscle is indicated, because the other intorter in that eye (the superior rectus muscle) was eliminated in step I.

Case 2—Paralysis of the Superior Rectus Muscle. In step 1, a patient with a vertical diplopia is found on alternate cover testing to have the left eye higher (Table 6–5). The muscles involved must be either the weak elevators of the right eye (right superior rectus and right inferior oblique muscles) or the weak depressors of the left eye (the left superior oblique and left inferior rectus muscles).

In step 2, the diplopia is determined to be worse in right gaze. Of the muscles selected in step 1, the only purely vertical muscles in right gaze are the left superior oblique and the right superior rectus, both of which are intorters.

In step 3, the diplopia is found to be worse on right head tilt, which involves the right eye intorters and the left eye extorters. Since only intorters were selected in step 2, the intorter of the right eye, the right superior rectus, must be the muscle at fault.

The foregoing cases illustrate the most common forms of isolated paralysis to which the three-step evaluation method is applicable. A similar program can be worked out for the inferior rectus and inferior oblique muscles. However, these

TABLE 6–3. Compensatory Head Positioning

Paretic Muscle	Face Turn	Chin	Head Tilt
Left medial rectus	Right	—	—
Left lateral rectus	Left	—	—
Left superior rectus	Right	Up	Right
Left superior oblique	Left	Down	Right
Left inferior rectus	Right	Down	Left
Left inferior oblique	Left	Up	Left

TABLE 6–4. Three-Step Test for Paralysis of the Left Superior Oblique Muscle

Muscles Possibly Involved	Muscles Selected—Step 1	Muscles Selected—Step 2	Muscles Selected—Step 3
Right superior rectus		Right superior rectus	
Right superior oblique	Right superior rectus		
Right inferior oblique	Right inferior oblique		
Right inferior rectus			Left superior oblique
Left superior rectus			
Left superior oblique	Left superior oblique	Left superior oblique	
Left inferior oblique			
Left inferior rectus	Left inferior rectus		

TABLE 6–5. Three-Step Test for Paralysis of the Right Superior Rectus Muscle

Muscles Possibly Involved	Muscles Selected—Step 1	Muscles Selected—Step 2	Muscles Selected—Step 3
Right superior rectus	Right superior rectus		
Right superior oblique		Right superior rectus	
Right inferior rectus	Right inferior oblique		
Right inferior oblique			Right superior rectus
Left superior rectus	Left superior oblique	Left superior oblique	
Left superior oblique	Left inferior rectus		
Left inferior rectus			
Left inferior oblique			

muscles are more usually involved in cases of local disorders of the orbit, such as inflammation, tumors, and blow-out fractures of the floor; only rarely are they causative factors in isolated paralysis owing to neuropathic processes.

It should be noted that diagnosis of vertical diplopia is not always easy. Not infrequently, more than one muscle may be involved, as in a partial third cranial nerve paralysis. Where diplopia is minimal, failure to make sure that the patient's head is in the correct erect straight-ahead position is a common error. A mild degree of vertical and oblique diplopia can be compensated for by unconscious head tilting on the part of the patient, which may obscure results. On the other hand, head tilting is much more common in superior oblique than in superior rectus muscle paralysis, and observation of abnormal head posture prior to formal testing may facilitate diagnosis.

The oblique character of diplopia tends to confuse the diagnostic program, and it will be totally misleading if it is simultaneously considered in the course of the evaluation. When both vertical and oblique separation of images occurs, only the vertical component should be considered. If so much horizontal separation exists that it is difficult or impossible to determine whether the vertical component is greater in left or right gaze or to evaluate the significance of the torsional component in step 3, the horizontal displacement should be removed by prism correction. The extent of this correction should be such that, on testing, the vertical movement of the eyes is more apparent to the patient and

to the observer. Such a correction is more easily done with loose prisms than with the prism bar, which is cumbersome to move correctly when testing in the various cardinal fields of gaze.

If the vertical diplopia is not of recent onset, step 1 and step 2 of the testing procedure will fall in line, but step 3 will usually be inconclusive, because the head tilt test may not separate out the last two malfunctioning muscles. Smoothing out or development of comitancy is common, and may come on soon after the onset of the initial paralysis. In such an event, an indication of what muscle is involved may be derived from the patient's history, which may reveal local trauma to one eye, associated ptosis with a superior rectus muscle weakness, or a previous third cranial nerve paralysis on one side.

With vertical diplopia testing, it is difficult to follow the three-step diagnostic procedure while keeping the correct muscles in mind. Thus it is recommended that the three primary observations be made and noted, but that the muscle selection for each step be deferred until the testing is completed. At that time, results based on primary observations can be checked and rechecked more simply and efficiently.

During the alternate cover test, some cases of diplopia are not grossly obvious because the diplopia may be caused by minimal paralysis of the muscle or fusion may overcome or obscure the problem. In these cases, the red lens test can sometimes be of great help. When a red lens is put over one eye as the patient looks at the hand light in the extremes of gaze, he sees two images, because the red lens helps to break up fusion. The image as the patient sees it will be in a position opposite to that of the position of the eye. Thus, if the red lens is over the right eye and the patient sees the red image as the lower of the two images, the right eye is the higher eye in terms of the straight-ahead position.

If the patient maintains fusion even with the red lens in position, the Maddox rod, which changes a beam of light into a line by multiple prisms, should be used. With the Maddox rod, the patient sees a bar of light in one eye and a pinpoint of light in the other and obviously cannot fuse these two dissimilar images. If the rod is red, this feature further helps the patient to discriminate between the two objects. The Maddox rod can be rotated so that the line of light is vertical in one situation, thus allowing the patient to experience horizontal separation of images. The Maddox rod can then be rotated 90° to measure the vertical separation.

NEUROPATHIC CAUSES

Third Cranial Nerve Paralysis

General Testing Signs

The third cranial nerve (oculomotor nerve) has many functions. It supplies innervation (1) to the levator muscle, which lifts the lid, (2) to the superior rectus and inferior oblique muscles, which elevate the eye, and (3) to the inferior rectus muscle, which depresses the eye. Accommodation and pupillary constrictions are also dependent on the third cranial nerve.

When a patient is being examined for possible third cranial nerve paralysis, all the areas innervated by the third cranial nerve must be tested. If ptosis is present, the diplopia may not be evident to either the patient or physician when the patient is tested in the straight-ahead position; however, when the patient is instructed to look up and laterally in the field of vertical action of the superior rectus muscle, the imbalance may be obvious to both the pa-

tient and the observer. This subtle finding may also be true of the other muscles as well as the pupillary and accommodation reactions. Owing to their common origin at the annulus of Zinn, a combination of ptosis and superior rectus muscle weakness is the most frequently occurring of all possible associations within the third cranial nerve. Isolated ptosis and isolated superior rectus muscle weakness are usually of traumatic or congenital origin.

Third Cranial Nerve Misdirection. Although the physician does not often look for this sign, it is of real significance because it occurs after recovery from a third cranial nerve paralysis; however, it may not be obvious for 6 months to a year after the onset of and recovery from the paralysis. Several signs of this condition must be looked for, any one of which may occur alone and be as significant as multiple signs of misdirection. The most common form of misdirection is the pseudo von Graefe's sign. When the patient looks down, his upper lid retracts and the superior sclera is exposed (as in thyroid disease). In another form of misdirection, lid gaze dyskinesis, the lid is elevated when the patient moves the eye medially and innervates the medial rectus muscle on pure horizontal gaze. When he looks laterally, the lid returns to normal position. Lid gaze dyskinesis may be missed when the affected eye is examined in the horizontal plane, and is best seen in horizontal movements of the eye in down gaze (Fig. 6–1 A,B,C,D). (In a normal eye, no elevation or depression of the lid should exist in pure horizontal gaze excursion.) If lid gaze dyskinesis is present, pupillary signs frequently are seen. The pupil becomes smaller in near gaze on innervation of the medial rectus muscle as well as in horizontal gaze, when the patient turns his eyes toward the nose, again innervating the medial rectus muscle. This reaction is termed a pseudo Argyll Robertson pupil, referring to a lack of pupillary response to light but a better reaction to accommodation-convergence. In

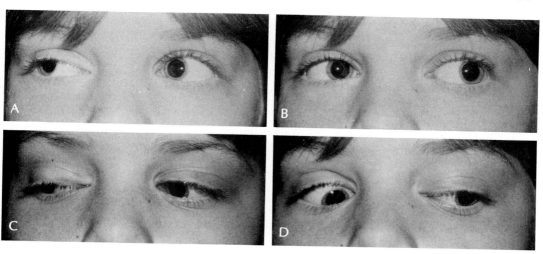

Fig. 6–1. This patient has a right third-nerve misdirection of the lid. In moving the eyes from right to left gaze (**A, B**), the lid elevates. This sign is more easily seen when the test is performed with the eyes in down gaze rather than straight ahead (**C, D**).

patients with the misdirection phenomenon, however, the pupil is contracted, not because of the accommodation reflex, but because of some crossover innervation between the medial rectus muscle and the pupil. This phenomenon can be demonstrated by making the medial rectus muscle work on distant horizontal gaze movement and show the same contraction of the pupil as would occur via the accommodation-convergence mechanism. (This phenomenon also differentiates the condition from one related to tertiary syphilis.)

Third cranial nerve misdirection (1) occurs more frequently after third cranial nerve paralysis owing to trauma or after an aneurysm, (2) is infrequently caused by tumor or syphilis, and (3) has not been reported after third cranial nerve paralysis owing to diabetes. Therefore, if a diabetic patient shows third cranial nerve misdirection, it is likely that a subtle aneurysm has been overlooked and should now be considered in the absence of a significant history of trauma.

Anatomic Types

Once diplopia has been diagnosed as being caused by dysfunction of the third cranial nerve, the next step is to determine what part of the nerve is affected and what disease is the cause. For the purpose of this discussion, disorders of the third cranial nerve have been grouped into six categories according to anatomic location.

Nuclear Lesions. Even though the two third cranial nerve nuclei are separate, they show some interaction. Most authors believe that the fibers of the superior rectus muscle are the ones that are interdependent; therefore, in identifying an isolated third cranial nerve paralysis as being nuclear in location, the following comment should be helpful. Total third cranial nerve paralysis affecting one eye but with no limitation of up gaze in the other eye rules out a nuclear lesion as the causative factor. In paralysis owing to a nuclear lesion, the contralateral superior rectus muscle would have to be limited because of interdependence. Vascular disease is the most frequent cause of this type of paralysis.

Fascicular Lesions. Disease in the fascicular fiber bundle, which is also intrinsic to the brain stem, involves two well-recognized syndromes. A disorder in the dorsal fascicular area produces the syndrome of Benedikt, with ipsilateral third cranial nerve paralysis and a contralateral hemi-tremor that is produced by proximity to the red nucleus. Disorder in the ventral fascicular area produces the syndrome of Weber, with ipsilateral third cranial nerve paralysis and contralateral hemiparesis. The degree of involvement of the third cranial nerve and the severity of the tremor or paralysis vary from mild to severe. Once again, vascular disease, particularly arteriosclerosis, is the main cause of these symptoms. The syndrome of Weber may also occur as an extrinsic brain stem phenomenon owing to lesions in the interpeduncular fossa, where the third cranial nerve exits from the brain stem, but it cannot be differentiated from the intrinsic variety on clinical grounds alone. In addition to vascular disease, venous malformation and tumors may also cause this condition in the interpeduncular fossa.

Subarachnoid Lesions. The subarachnoid space is the most common location for third cranial nerve paralysis, particularly if the pupil is involved, no matter how minimally. When the pupil is involved, the major cause to be considered is an aneurysm at the junction of the internal carotid and posterior communicating arteries. If aneurysm proves to be the cause, other signs of subarachnoid hemorrhage usually occur, such as pain, stiffness of the neck, photophobia, and a change in the level of consciousness. These additional symptoms are not always present, however, and their absence does not rule out an aneurysm if the pupil is involved. Pupillary involvement owing to an aneurysm is usually significant: the pupils usually are large and fixed; however, any change in size and function is equally significant. Absence of pupillary involvement used to be considered rare, occurring (according to Rucker) in about 3% of cases owing to aneurysm. More recent studies by Kissel, et al., and Nadeau and Trobe indicate that it is not all that rare. This is particularly true in partial third nerve paresis, in which pupillary response may initially be normal, but the pa-tient should be observed for subsequent development of pupillary signs.

Diabetes is the second most common cause of third cranial nerve paralysis in the subarachnoid space. In third cranial nerve paralysis secondary to diabetes, the pupillary function is usually unimpaired, owing, theoretically, to collateral circulation from the pial vessels in the peripheral part of the nerve, where the pupil fibers are located. On the other hand, studies by Cogan and Goldstein and by Rucker indicate that pupillary involvement may occur in as many as 20% of cases of diabetic ophthalmoplegia, and that pain indistinguishable from that associated with aneurysm can occur in as many as 50%. Therefore, it is incumbent on the physician to consider the possibility of aneurysm even if the patient is a known diabetic. Clearness of spinal fluid does not rule out an aneurysm since evidence of subarachnoid hemorrhage is not always present. The 2-hour postprandial serum glucose test is not sufficient for identifying diabetes as the underlying cause of third cranial nerve paralysis. In the majority of such cases, it will be found that the patient has occult diabetes that may be suggested only by a formal glucose tolerance test. Since the treatment for third cranial nerve paralysis secondary to diabetes is to do nothing, the physician may be tempted to wait the 6 or 8 weeks it takes almost all cases to clear up. By delaying, the physician can differentiate between a condition owing to diabetes and one owing to an aneurysm since the latter is unlikely to improve. Such an approach is still foolish and dangerous since the time of peak incidence for spontaneous rebleeding from an aneurysm is within 12 to 14 days, a period well short of the healing time for diabetic third cranial nerve paralysis. Moreover, some aneurysms do not progress and the third cranial nerve returns to normal—thus, a potential time bomb is left untreated. The best rule is to regard an isolated third cranial nerve paralysis with pupillary involvement as being caused by aneurysm until it is proven otherwise.

Infrequently, subarachnoid involvement of the third cranial nerve can be caused by cranial arteritis. I have rarely found this situation, but Meadows has found subarachnoid involvment of the third nerve in 12 to 15% of the cases of temporal arteritis he has seen.

In 40% of cases involving patients with third cranial nerve ophthalmoplegia owing to tumor, the tumor is metastatic. In 2 large series on ophthalmoplegia, nasopharyngeal carcinoma was found to be the most common metastatic tumor.

Infection accompanying third cranial nerve paralysis is not common; however, varicella and botulism have been reported as causing isolated internal ophthalmoplegia involving accommodation and pupillary function, and thus deserve special mention. At one time, diphtheria was a frequent cause of isolated pupillary paralysis, but today diphtheria is rarely reported.

Cavernous Sinus Involvement. Another form of paralysis can occur where the third cranial nerve runs through the cavernous sinus—the point at which it is associated with the fourth and sixth cranial nerves, the first and second divisions of the fifth cranial nerve, and the ocular sympathetic nerves. An isolated third cranial nerve paralysis in this location is rare, but it can occur; however, signs of cavernous sinus involvement soon become evident on repeated examination.

An intracavernous aneurysm underlying third cranial nerve paralysis is readily differentiated from other cerebral aneurysms. An important distinction is that, even if an intracavernous aneurysm ruptures, bleeding occurs into another vascular compartment rather than into the subarachnoid space; thus the signs and symptoms of a subarachnoid hemorrhage are absent. Pain is usually intermittent and not a prominent feature of an intracavernous aneurysm, which frequently develops a fibrous coat

as it enlarges and progressively compresses the cavernous sinus nerves. One of the earliest signs of third cranial nerve paralysis owing to a disorder in the cavernous sinus is depression of the ipsilateral corneal reflex. Presence of a cephalic murmur that can be altered by carotid compression may help in differential diagnosis. Symptoms of an intracavernous aneurysm occur, on the average, when the patient is over age 50; whereas aneurysms located on the internal carotid artery produce symptoms at least 10 years earlier. Exophthalmos is usually moderate, occurs later in life than aneurysms in other parts of the internal carotid artery, and frequently appears without chemosis, all of which symptoms differ from those of arteriovenous cavernous sinus fistula. Optic atrophy owing to enlargement of the aneurysm and compression of the optic nerve is of major concern.

Arteriovenous fistulas are of two varieties—those caused by trauma and those that are spontaneous and arteriosclerotic. In this era of the automobile and motorcycle, more than 75% of such cases are caused by trauma and are seen mostly in young men, as might be expected. The remainder are spontaneous and arteriosclerotic in origin, and occur primarily in elderly women.

Arteriovenous fistulas can affect the third cranial nerve as well as the other nerves of the cavernous sinus. Exophthalmos and chemosis may be much more prominent than in cavernous sinus aneurysm. Dilated veins around the cornea give the appearance of a caput medusa. Bruits are easily heard by both the physician and the patient, while the ability to change their character by carotid compression is variable and dependent on the degree of collateral circulation.

Schiøtz's tonometer can be a valuable tool in diagnosing arteriovenous cavernous sinus fistula. Normal pulsations in the eye cause the arm of this instrument to move 2 or 3 scale readings on the average, but the wider pulse swings of an arteriovenous cavernous sinus fistula may cause the arm to swing 10 scale readings or more. (This wide swing may occur without the physician's having noted any obvious pulsation on simple inspection.) Abnormal pulsation of the globe can be seen with applanation tonometry as well, although not as easily as with Schiøtz's tonometer.

Another subtle feature of pulsation may be seen during direct ophthalmoscopic examination of the fundus. As the fundus is observed, the disc and vessels go in and out of focus synchronously with the pulse at the wrist. This phenomenon is distinct from the variation in focus that occurs with variation in accommodation. The pulsations just described are more easily perceived with the direct than the indirect ophthalmoscope. Both types of ocular pulsation may be seen when gross movement of the globe is not apparent.

Both secondary glaucoma and ischemic optic atrophy are of major concern and are the usual reasons for a decision to operate on patients suffering from arteriovenous fistula. The results of an operation can be disastrous, however, and the desirability of surgical intervention is presently being widely debated. The more conservative view is expressed by Hoyt (Spencer, Thompson, and Hoyt; and Sanders and Hoyt), who believes that present surgical techniques tend only to increase the ischemia in many cases and thus make matters worse.

Not all fistulas have the signs described. Some may only have the dilated episcleral and conjunctival vessels. This type of fistula is small and is usually a dural-cavernous sinus fistula rather than a larger one between the internal carotid artery and cavernous sinus. The most common complication of the smaller fistulas is open-angle glaucoma. This is most likely caused by the increase in episcleral venous pressure.

A third variety of tumor invasion of the cavernous sinus occurs in two different ways: (1) by intracavernous growth of a metastatic tumor and (2) by lateral extension of a pituitary tumor into the cavernous sinus with or without the bitemporal field loss usually associated with this condition. In the latter disorder, which is termed pituitary apoplexy, the onset is usually sudden and the patient appears quite ill. The third cranial nerve is rarely solely involved, and the optic nerve on the same side may also be involved owing to extension of the tumor forward into the optic nerve sheath. The fact that most persons exhibiting this syndrome have not had a known pituitary tumor prior to the onset of the apoplexy may delay a proper diagnosis.

Superior Orbital Fissure Involvement. Tumors impinging on the superior orbital fissure can also cause third cranial nerve paralysis. Because the nerves involved are the same as those involved in disorders located in the cavernous sinus, differentiation usually cannot be made on clinical grounds alone; however, indications of bony changes owing to tumor provide a clue to diagnosis. The most common tumor in this area is a sphenoid ridge meningioma that frequently causes prominent changes readily discernible on the plain roentgenogram.

Tolosa-Hunt syndrome is a condition entirely unrelated to other disorders causing ophthalmoplegia. Pain usually precedes the ophthalmoplegia, and is usually steady rather than throbbing or episodic. The ophthalmoplegia may involve the third, fourth, and sixth cranial nerves separately or in combination. Symptoms may last for several weeks or longer, and then usually remit spontaneously, although some residual ophthalmoplegia may continue. It is not unusual to have a remission of the syndrome involving the third cranial nerve, and then a quick relapse with involvement of the sixth or fourth cranial nerve. Bilateral involvement is rare but not unheard of.

In diagnosing this condition, all other possible causes of this symptom complex must be ruled out. This procedure usually includes roentgenograms of the sinuses (to exclude infection) and the sphenoid ridge, ultrasonograms, or computerized tomograms of the retro-orbital structures, and perhaps cerebral arteriograms. Diagnosis of Tolosa-Hunt syndrome is by exclusion, and should therefore be made only after exhaustive evaluation.

Orbital Lesions. Ophthalmoplegia affecting the third cranial nerve in the orbit involves not only the same nerves as in superior orbitalfissure and cavernous sinus but also the optic nerve. As a consequence, the patient may experience loss of vision and perhaps exhibit exophthalmos. In the orbit, the third cranial nerve separates into two divisions, so a partial third cranial nerve paralysis of one or the other division is possible. The upper division innervates the lid and the superior rectus muscles; all the other third cranial nerve functions are in the inferior division.

A decrease in vision or merely an afferent pupillary defect on the affected side may be enough of a clue to lead to a diagnosis of third cranial nerve paralysis in the orbit. Among possible causative factors, orbital tumor and contiguous sinus disease, such as mucocele, tumor, or infection, should receive major consideration. Infection may not be immediately obvious if the patient has no sinus symptoms and does not appear toxic; however, progressive pain and exophthalmos should suggest this possibility, and appropriate roentgenographic evaluation is indicated. Since roentgenograms of the sinus area are frequently difficult to read, expert opinion should be sought (1) as to the views to be taken and (2) in the interpretation of the roentgenograms.

Other Causes

Ophthalmoplegic migraine is a well-established, although hard-to-prove, cause of third cranial nerve paralysis.This condition may be accompanied by all the oculomotor nerve signs of an aneurysm; however, a distinguishing feature is that its onset is commonly in the first and second decades of life, far earlier than the emergence of symptoms of aneurysm. In addition, the condition usually (but not always) clears. In some instances, diagnosis is facilitated by a history of classic migraine, the patient even having ophthalmoplegia during a classic migraine attack.

Experience indicates that migraine patients have a significantly higher rate of complications from arteriography than do other types of patients. It must be said, however, that most of the pertinent studies were done in the days of direct carotid arteriography; present techniques using the femoral catheter route may have changed the statistics significantly. Nevertheless, whether an arteriogram should be done on a patient who presents with a third cranial nerve paralysis, questionably migraine in origin, with pupillary involvement, even though it clears, remains a problem for the physician.

The main diagnostic features of migrainous third cranial nerve paralysis are the transient nature of the ophthalmoplegia, recurrence, rapid clearing of the paralysis, and, frequently, a personal or family history of migraine.

The Kernohan notch syndrome is a variation of a frequently occurring condition. Ordinarily, supratentorial pressure from a tumor or subdural hematoma compresses the third cranial nerve as it crosses the tentorial edge. Since the pupillary fibers are in the peripheral superior medial part of the nerve, these fibers are frequently affected first, without significant involvement of other parts of the third cranial nerve. The ipsilateral cerebral peduncle is compressed at the same time, and signs of ipsilateral pupillary enlargement and contralateral hemiparesis can be observed.

In the Kernohan notch variation, compression of the ipsilateral third cranial nerve is associated with cross-compression of the contralateral cerebral peduncle, resulting in ipsilateral third cranial nerve paralysis and ipsilateral hemiplegia. This situation leads to confusion as to which side of the head the expanding lesion is on, since these two signs are normally crossed. In determining the location of the lesion, a rule of thumb is to rely on the pupillary sign rather than on the hemiparesis.

Orbital bone fractures can trap muscles and result in diplopia. The most common fracture is one that occurs in the orbital floor, trapping the inferior oblique and inferior rectus muscles as they form into Lockwood's ligament. Rare cases also exist of simulated superior oblique tendon sheath syndrome with a floor fracture. Medial wall fractures can trap the medial rectus muscle and may look like a lateral rectus palsy; however, the globe retracts with attempts at lateral gaze. This entrapment and pseudo lateral rectus palsy can be diagnosed by a forced duction test and by saccadic velocity testing.

Orbital roof fractures are less common but have their own set of complications. These complications may be insidious and delayed in onset and, therefore, often missed. The most serious of these complications are meningitis and brain abscess secondary to a connection between the intracranial space and the frontal sinuses.

Herpes zoster ophthalmoplegia occurs when the skin lesions over the first division of the fifth cranial nerve are almost healed. The diagnosis is obvious since all the symptoms of the herpetic disease are present. The ophthalmoplegia will clear slowly without therapy.

Congenital third nerve palsies are generally considered to be traumatic in origin because of the high incidence of misdirection that occurs in the peripheral nerve. They tend to be an isolated neurologic event without other brain stem signs.

Third cranial nerve paralysis occurs infrequently in connection with lupus erythematosus, encephalitis, amyloidosis, Hodgkin's disease, temporal arteritis, tetanus, sarcoidosis, and rarely, after dental anesthesia. The mechanism in dental anesthesia may be retrograde flow of the an-esthetic. More rarely, fat emboli can cause blindness owing to arterial obstruction. Multiple sclerosis rarely causes ophthalmoplegia, and when it does, it is usually in the form of a sixth cranial nerve paralysis.

Fourth Cranial Nerve Paralysis

Unlike the third cranial nerve, the fourth cranial nerve (trochlear nerve) innervates only one muscle, the superior oblique, which causes the eye to intort and turn down. Minimal weakness in this muscle may result in symptoms, since the eye is much less able to overcome vertical than horizontal imbalance. In paralysis of the oblique muscle, the versions are mostly affected; the ductions are frequently full.

A frequent error in testing for a minimal defect in motility is permitting the patient's head to be tilted during testing, which masks the defect. Testing should be done with the patient's head erect, even if it has to be supported manually.

Head Tilt

In the three-step test outlined earlier, step 3 is the critical point for identifying the superior oblique muscle as the cause of the muscle imbalance. The Bielschowsky head tilt test is positive if further separation of the images occurs when the head is tilted to the side of the affected superior oblique muscle. For instance, in paralysis of the left superior oblique muscle that causes a left hypertropia, the diplopia increases with left head tilt.

In general, the head tilt test is useful in distinguishing paralysis of the superior oblique muscle in one eye from paralysis of the superior rectus muscle in the other, since, for all practical purposes, the possibility of isolated paralysis of the inferior oblique and inferior rectus muscles is uncommon.

An outline of the procedure for practical head tilt testing is given in Table 6–2. In recording a head position, it is always important to describe three facets of the position rather than the shoulder toward which the head is tilted. The first facet to record is whether the chin is elevated or is depressed in an attempt to overcome the vertical aspect of the imbalance. The second facet to record is whether the face is turned to the right or whether it is turned to the left in order to overcome weakness in adduction or abduction. Finally, it should be noted whether the head is tilted toward the left shoulder or toward the right shoulder to overcome tortional weakness. A description of these three head positions represents the attempt to compensate for the three functions of the vertically acting muscles. As an example, in paralysis of the left superior oblique muscle, the chin is tilted down to overcome the weak depression effect of the left superior oblique muscle; the face is turned to the right to overcome the weak abductions; and, last but not least, a right head tilt causes the left eye to extort, thereby overcoming the weak intorsion effect of the paralysis of the left superior oblique muscle (Table 6–4).

Head tilt tests for the other vertically acting muscles can be similarly worked out by reference to the three primary functions outlined in Table 6–1.

Exceptions to the foregoing rules are rare, but they do occur. For instance, a patient chooses a head position presumably in order to maintain fusion. On rare occasions, however, he may elect the reverse position in order to further separate the images, thus making it easier to suppress the more distant image (Owens and Owens). Actual testing by the three-step method will show that the head tilt assumed makes the images move farther away rather than nearer. Thus the head position initially seen should not be considered absolutely indicative of the muscle involved.

Sandifer syndrome, an unusual form of head tilting, is seen in children with a short esophagus. In such cases, the head can be easily lifted manually (suggesting no contraction of neck muscles), but the tilt to one shoulder will be resumed as soon as the supporting hand is removed. No muscle imbalance is found on repeated motility testing, which rules out the two common causes of head tilting. If the child is old enough, it may be possible to elicit from him a history of gastrointestinal disturbances that are relieved when the head is tilted and depressed, thus shortening the esophagus. Patients with this condition are best referred to a pediatric surgeon, who can readily diagnose hiatus hernia using a barium swallow and treat it.

Testing of Fourth Cranial Nerve Paralysis in Presence of Third Cranial Nerve Paralysis

In evaluating any third cranial nerve paralysis, it is important to detect any associated defects in the fourth and sixth cranial nerves, which may place the lesions in the cavernous sinus or superior orbital fissure. Since third cranial nerve paralysis prevents the eye from being adducted in order to test the vertical action of the superior oblique muscle, another form of testing must be chosen. The patient should be instructed to attempt to look down and in with the paretic eye while the examiner confirms the effort by observing the fellow eye, which should move down and out. A small intorting maneuver of the affected eye, not vertical depression, is an indication of good fourth cranial nerve function in an eye that cannot be adducted because of third cranial nerve paralysis. The intorsion, which reflects the action of the superior oblique muscle when it is not in the abducted position, is small, and it must be looked for specifically. Watching the movement of a horizontally located conjunctival vessel makes the intorsion easier to see.

Congenital Paralysis

This fairly common defect frequently goes undetected. Many patients' features are cosmetically acceptable and congenital paralysis of the fourth cranial nerve does not usually involve amblyopia; thus, they usually remain undiscovered until they have a routine eye examination. Types of congenital paralysis diagnosed in children of preschool age are either cosmetically obvious or accompanied by a head tilt that suggests a muscle imbalance requiring evaluation.

Brown's syndrome, which involves restriction of the muscle and sheath as it slides through the trochlea, is not innervational but mechanical, and it is therefore an entirely different problem. In a typical case, as the eye is adducted in up gaze, it turns down and in as if an inferior oblique muscle paralysis existed. The forced duction test easily differentiates this movement from that occurring in inferior oblique muscle paralysis; it is positive when the examiner attempts to move the eye up and in.

Trauma is the leading cause of acquired superior oblique muscle paralysis. The trauma can be local, with damage to the trochlea, or more severe, with intracranial damage. A form of trauma that does not appear to be severe at first glance occurs as the result of a rear-end automobile collision.

The history has been similar in the cases I have seen. The stopped car in which the patient was seated was hit from behind, causing a typical whiplash movement, with sudden hyperextension of the head and neck. In some instances, the head struck the steering wheel or dashboard. Usually, the patient was not rendered unconscious nor did he sustain more than a bump on the head. Onset of diplopia was immediate. On examination, the eye was neither red nor swollen, indicating little if any local injury to the trochlea or to the superior oblique muscle in the orbit. The muscle imbalance was minimal and usually cleared over a period of 3 to 6 months.

Acquired Paralysis

In cases of acquired paralysis of the fourth cranial nerve, the exact location of the injury to the nerve is uncertain; how-

ever, a clue may be gleaned from three bilateral cases that I have seen in which the head injury was slightly more serious. Two of these patients had experienced a period of unconsciousness, but in all three, superior oblique muscle paralysis was the only sign of intracranial trauma despite the severity of the head blow. Since both fourth cranial nerves come together only in the anterior medullary velum where they cross, it seems likely that the injury occurred in this area. Of further note, the bilateral cases that I have seen have not cleared spontaneously but have required a surgical procedure to resolve the problem. The sign that suggests that there is bilateral fourth nerve involvement is the alternating hypertropia. There is a left hypertropia in right gaze and a right hypertropia in left gaze. The Bielschowsky head tilt test also changes from side to side if one looks to the right or to the left when performing the test.

In certain surgical approaches to frontal sinus disease, the trochlea is moved and may be damaged; however, these procedures are now rarely used. Other causes of superior oblique muscle paralysis, such as vascular disease and diabetes, have been diagnosed, but trauma is by far the most frequent cause. Although isolated fourth cranial nerve paralysis owing to diabetes is uncommon, a glucose tolerance test is indicated in certain patients.

A form of intermittent Brown's tendon sheath syndrome occurs in adults. The usual complaint is intermittent diplopia immediately preceded by what is described as a popping sensation in the area of the trochlea, sometimes accompanied by mild pain and tenderness. The diplopia may last from minutes to days or weeks. The same forced duction findings seen in a true Brown's syndrome are found while the patient is symptomatic. Although the cause of this disorder is unknown, systemic steroids seemed to help in two cases that I have treated. I have not tried local injection of steroids.

Sixth Cranial Nerve Paralysis

Like the fourth cranial nerve, the sixth cranial nerve (abducens nerve) innervates only one muscle, the lateral rectus, which moves the eye laterally. Unlike the superior oblique muscle, the lateral rectus muscle has no secondary or tertiary function. It comes into play primarily when the eye is fixed on a distant object. Many a case of minimal sixth cranial nerve paralysis has been missed because the patient was asked to look at a light 3 feet distant rather than 20 feet distant during the alternate cover test.

Just as head positioning can mask a fourth cranial nerve paralysis, so a head turn can mask a minimal sixth cranial nerve paralysis if the patient is examined only in the straight ahead or near position. The diplopia that occurs with lateral rectus muscle paralysis is homonymous owing to the esotropia that is created; that is, when two images are seen, the ipsilateral image disappears when the ipsilateral eye is covered.

The measurement of horizontal vergences reveals the ability of a muscle to overcome stress. Some people can overcome 30 prism diopters of muscle imbalance, which permits certain muscle weaknesses to be overcome before diplopia is experienced. This compensation is different from that of muscles innervated by the fourth cranial nerve, which work primarily in a vertical direction and may overcome only 1 or 2 prism diopters of imbalance. If a patient has a progressive weakening of the lateral rectus muscle, as may occur with increasing intracranial pressure, it will show up in the distance muscle balance. In successive examinations (either days or weeks apart) of the distance phoria, the measurements increase significantly toward the esophoric side. The first readings may be an esophoria of 2 diopters, indicating a small degree of esophoria at distance that will become moderate as the intracranial pressure increases. The increase

in measurement will take place before the occurrence of frank diplopia, owing to the vergence reserve of the horizontal fusional mechanism. This testing technique is particularly useful in deciding whether a blurred disc is true papilledema. While the disc problem is being evaluated, over several days, the change in the measurements of the distance phoria may be significant. By the time a frank sixth cranial nerve paralysis has developed or both sixth cranial nerves are shown to be involved, the diagnosis of increased intracranial pressure is obvious.

Although isolated sixth cranial nerve paralysis is not uncommon, it is almost impossible to make an adequate identification of its cause or specific anatomic location. Therefore, it is important that the physician be familiar with the syndromes and associated signs, both major and minor, that may help to identify either the location or the cause of this disorder.

Congenital Paralysis

Möbius syndrome involves complete bilateral paralysis of the sixth and seventh cranial nerves. Its cause is unknown, but a carefully taken drug history may be revealing. I had two patients whose mothers had taken thalidomide during pregnancy. In most cases, however, the cause is unexplainable.

Duane syndrome is one form of congenital sixth cranial nerve paralysis. Since most patients with this condition are not esotropic in the primary straight-ahead position, the condition is frequently not discovered early in life. When it is finally diagnosed, whether the sixth cranial nerve paralysis is old or of recent origin becomes a serious question. Bilateral paralysis of recent onset may be caused by increased intracranial pressure or brain stem glioma. Bilateral Duane syndrome is rare.

Examination for the additional signs of Duane syndrome assists the observer in differentiating between this condition and an acquired sixth cranial nerve paralysis.

Patients with Duane syndrome are not usually esotropic in the primary position, and they do not develop amblyopia as a rule. If they look into the field of the paretic muscle, no diplopia results, because this movement brings into play a mechanism called facultative amblyopia rather than the amblyopia ex anopsia usually seen with esotropia. The key sign, however, is a narrowing of the lid fissure on adduction and return of the fissure to normal when the eye reverts to the straight-ahead position. In at least some cases, lid narrowing is caused by simultaneous innervation of the lateral and medial rectus muscles. This has been confirmed by electromyographic studies and autopsy material reported by Hoyt and Nachtigaller and again by Hotchkiss, Miller, Clark, and Green. Auditory evoked material by Jay and Hoyt further suggests a primary brain stem malfunction rather then a peripheral cause. On adduction, therefore, the medial and lateral rectus muscles co-contract, causing enophthalmos and narrowing of the lid fissure. Once lid narrowing is observed, the malfunction can be diagnosed as congenital, and further diagnostic procedures are unnecessary. In rare circumstances Duane syndrome can be acquired. I have seen one case caused by trauma and at least one case has been reported in a patient with rheumatoid arthritis. The electromyographic studies are much different in these cases then in the congenital form, which shows co-contraction of the lateral and medial rectus muscles. In addition, superior or inferior oblique muscles may overact.

Acquired Paralysis

Vascular Occlusion. Vascular accidents involving the brain stem occur frequently. The two syndromes that usually accompany such accidents are (1) Foville syndrome, which combines sixth and peripheral seventh cranial nerve paralysis with homolateral gaze paralysis, and (2) the Millard-Gubler syndrome, which consists of sixth and peripheral seventh cranial nerve paralysis and contralateral hemiplegia.

In elderly patients, spontaneous isolated sixth cranial nerve paralysis can occur and frequently disappears within several months. One explanation of this malfunction, proposed as far back as Cushing's time, holds that it is caused by compression of the sixth cranial nerve on the anterior surface of the pons by the lateral branches of the basilar artery, particularly the anterior inferior cerebellar artery.

Gradenigo Syndrome. This syndrome is seen in this age of antibiotics, but rarely. The inflammation often involves severe otitis media and mastoiditis with secondary petrositis, in the course of which the area of the petrous bone called Dorello's canal is affected and the sixth cranial nerve becomes paretic. In more extensive cases, the gasserian ganglion is affected, causing severe pain in the temporoparietal area. Further extension of the infection may also involve the seventh and eighth cranial nerves. The most serious complications of unchecked infection are meningitis, epidural abscess, or dural sinus thrombosis with secondary pseudotumor cerebri.

Lateral Sinus Thrombosis. This thrombosis is frequently idiopathic. The resulting inflammation extends to the inferior petrosal sinus, which is adjacent to the sixth cranial nerve, thus causing malfunction of this nerve. Thrombosis may occur postpartum, or from distant emboli, as, for example, in venous stasis of the legs.

Superior Orbital Fissure Syndrome. Also called Tolosa-Hunt syndrome, this condition may begin as an isolated sixth cranial nerve paralysis. The course, diagnosis, and treatment of this syndrome were discussed earlier in the chapter.

In treating patients having symptoms located at the superior orbital fissure, the physician must be careful not to err by failing to rule out all the diseases possible in the cavernous sinus, superior orbital fissure, and posterior orbit. In addition to carotid arteriography, testing procedures should include plain roentgenograms, tomograms of the superior orbital ridge and orbit, and ultrasonograms and computerized tomograms of the orbit. The same rule applies to suspected lesions in the cavernous sinus, such as arteriovenous fistulas and tumors. It is unusual to see only an isolated sixth cranial nerve paralysis without symptoms relating to the other cavernous sinus nerves; however the literature includes several cases of a sixth cranial nerve paralysis in the cavernous sinus, with further signs developing only 6 months after onset of the paralysis.

Cerebellopontine Angle Tumors. Although these tumors cause paralysis of the sixth cranial nerve, other prominent signs frequently precede their onset. The seventh and eighth cranial nerves are affected, and frequently anesthesia of the cornea is present. All three nerves should be tested when an obscure sixth cranial nerve paralysis is seen. Sixth cranial nerve paralysis is not the presenting sign of an angle tumor, but it may be the complaint that leads the patient to seek medical attention. Appropriate roentgenograms, selective audiograms, and an air study outlining the cerebellopontine angle will demonstrate an acoustic neuroma, the type of tumor most commonly found in that area. Of cerebellopontine angle tumors, 90% are acoustic neuromas. The most common causes of the remaining 10% are meningioma and cholesteatoma. In the case of meningiomas, radiographic studies may show osteoblastic changes in adjacent bones. In the case of cholesteatomas, contrast studies demonstrate a scalloped edge to the tumor unlike the smooth surface of an acoustic neuroma. A facial tic is also more common with cholesteatoma. Although not 100% accurate, spinal fluid protein tends to be normal rather then markedly elevated as it is in other tumors located in that area of the angle, which obstruct the flow of cerebrospinal fluid as do acoustic neuromas.

Spinal Anesthesia. Transient sixth cranial nerve paralysis following spinal anesthesia is a rare but definite occurrence. In a review of 10,400 cases involving spinal anesthesia, Phillips found that transient sixth cranial nerve paralysis had occurred in 8 patients. Thorsen felt it was more common, with an incidence of 1 in 400 procedures. This condition is much less common in my experience. I agree that it is more common with the injection of contrast material than with a simple spinal tap. The incidence is too small to be sure of this fact, however.

One explanation for the cause is a toxic response to the injected material. This is unlikely since there is a delay of 1 or 2 weeks before the symptoms develop.

The second explanation is more plausible. The patients that have experienced lateral rectus paresis have other post-spinal-tap symptoms, such as headache in the erect position. This has generally been considered to be caused by chronic leakage of spinal fluid from the tap site with displacement of the brain and traction on pain-sensitive structures. It is not hard to extrapolate this theory to include traction on the sixth nerve with compression over firm structures such as the petrous bone.

Spinal fluid examinations to determine the presence of a cellular reaction indicative of arachnoiditis are not usually performed. Paralysis owing to spinal anesthesia clears rapidly (within days or a week or two), and requires no further investigation if the rest of the neurologic examination is normal. In summary, the cause of this type of nerve malfunction is obscure, and the treatment is to do nothing.

Wernicke-Korsakoff Syndrome. This syndrome, when associated with chronic alcoholism, includes several eye signs, among which are nystagmus of a nonspecific character, horizontal gaze paralysis, sixth cranial nerve paralysis, and, rarely, vertical gaze paralysis. If a patient with sixth cranial nerve paralysis has a history of alcoholism, Wernicke-Korsakoff syndrome is frequently the diagnosis; however, the physician should not fail to rule out the possibility that an alcoholic patient may have sustained some intracranial trauma, and that the sixth cranial nerve paralysis could be the result of increasing intracranial pressure from a subdural hematoma. In addition, the patient may suffer from ataxia of gait and from somnolence, the other two symptoms in the triad described originally be Wernicke. The confabulation symptom of the Korsakoff syndrome was added later, and although it is frequently seen, it is not an essential feature of the Wernicke syndrome.

Toxic Drug Reactions. Such reactions should always be considered in cases of sixth cranial nerve paralysis, and the taking of a careful drug history is essential. Lateral rectus muscle paralysis has been reported in connection with such drugs as furaltadone and iodochlorhydroxyquin. Optic neuritis is a much more common problem with iodochlorhydroxyquin, but sixth cranial nerve paralysis has also been reported.

Increased Intracranial Pressure. Sixth cranial nerve paralysis secondary to increased intracranial pressure is well known. What produces paralysis (stretching of the nerve with bony impingement owing to downward displacement of the brain stem? compression by branches of the basilar artery?) is not completely understood. The early sign of this condition, increasing esophoria, has been discussed earlier in this chapter.

An unusual but dramatic form of sixth cranial nerve paralysis is one that is transient but occurs suddenly and repeatedly. Patients with this disorder develop sudden headaches that are accompanied by paralysis of one or both lateral rectus muscles. All symptoms disappear within minutes or hours. While the signs are present, the patient is usually active rather than lethargic, and he frequently shakes or hits his head as if to push out whatever is causing the symptoms. This maneuver suggests that some ball valve mechanism may be causing sudden changes in intracranial pressure. A colloid cyst of the third ventricle which is intermittently closing off the aqueduct can do this.

Compared with tumor, pseudotumor cerebri is a relatively infrequent cause of increased intracranial pressure. If this condition is to be ruled out as a causative factor, however, (1) diagnostic tests should reveal signs of increased intracranial pressure; (2) the results of a spinal fluid examination should be negative except for increased opening pressure; (3) the neurologic examination should be totally negative, except for the possible presence of a sixth cranial nerve paralysis if the intracranial pressure is high enough; and (4) a CT examination should reveal a normal size ventricular system. If there were a small lesion near to and compressing the aqueduct then the ventricles would be enlarged, suggesting a noncommunicating hydrocephalus. In the past an air study was required.

Most cases of pseudotumor cerebri are idiopathic. Some are related to specific causes (such as chronic vitamin A intoxication, tetracycline overdose, postpartum dural sinus thrombosis, the institution or withdrawal of steroids in treating nephrosis) or are a complication of Addison's or hypoparathyroid disease. Treatment varies, but it usually consists of steroid therapy over a period of several weeks.

Pseudotumor cerebri is self-limited, but it may persist for months. The real danger of a prolonged course is secondary atrophy of the optic nerve. Thus, vision and fields should be checked frequently, and the disc should be observed for beginning gliosis—all of which indicate optic nerve decompensation and suggest the need for more vigorous treatment of the intracranial pressure.

Nasopharyngeal Malignancy. This malignancy (Godtfredsen syndrome) is an uncommon disease that usually affects the sixth cranial nerve. (In a series of 53 cases reviewed by Smith and Wheliss, sixth cranial nerve paralysis was present in 29.) A significant feature of this type of sixth cranial nerve paralysis is associated pain or paresthesia over the second division of the fifth cranial nerve. This combination of signs should impel the physician to look for other signs that suggest nasopharyngeal malignancy.

The main presenting complaints usually include cervical lymphadenopathy, pain in the ear, pain in the face, and symptoms of nasal obstruction. Most patients have also experienced unexplained weight loss prior to seeking medical attention, at which time a mild or frank sixth cranial nerve paralysis may be present. The third and fourth cranial nerves may also be affected initially, but not as frequently as is the sixth cranial nerve. Usually, by the time multiple orbital nerves are involved, exophthalmos is also present. Mention of serous otitis media, another significant symptom of this disorder, may be omitted by the patient as of minor importance compared with the diplopia and pain he is experiencing. Intermittent blockage of the eustachian tube, causing a popping sensation or a blocked ear, is another and more subtle symptom of this disease.

Even when a nasopharyngeal malignancy is suspected, it may be difficult to establish. Examination is frequently misleading, since the tumor initially arises submucosally in the nasopharynx. It then grows intracranially but extradurally, affecting one cranial nerve after another before becoming a significant space-occupying lesion. Therefore, a biopsy is indicated even if the nasopharyngeal mucosa looks normal. A good location for biopsy is in the area called Rosenmüller's fossa, which is a common site for this type of tumor.

Special roentgenographic views may reveal another feature of a nasopharyngeal malignancy. A nasopharyngeal tumor usually gains entrance to the cranium by way of the basilar foramina. The usual skull series does not include these openings; therefore roentgenographic views of the basilar foramina should be ordered specifically since they may reveal significant erosion of one or more foramina.

On the basis of cell type, lymphoepithelioma is the most common form of tumor found in the nasopharyngeal area. Such tumors are relatively radiosensitive, and radiotherapy may result in a temporary amelioration of symptoms; however, the 5-year survival rate for patients with this type of malignancy is only about 25%. Although malignant nasopharyngeal tumors are rarely seen in the United States, this condition is the leading cause of cancer among males in mainland China. It is not common among people of Chinese descent living in enclaves in Hawaii and San Francisco.

Sixth Cranial Nerve Paralysis in Children. When sixth cranial nerve paralysis develops suddenly in an otherwise normal child, it is certainly cause for concern as to the possible presence of a serious disorder. Such disorders as increased intracranial pressure or a pontine glioma are always a possibility.

In 1967, Knox Clark, and Shuster reported on a series of children with spontaneous sixth cranial nerve paralysis that occurred about 7 to 21 days after a nonspecific illness. Spinal fluid tests were usually negative, and no attempt was made to establish that the paralysis was infectious in origin. The patients developed no other symptoms, and the paralysis cleared within several weeks. I have seen 2 such cases in my practice, and I believe that it is proper to wait if no other signs of increased intracranial pressure exist and the remainder of the neurologic examination is normal. Some noninvasive studies such as CT may be performed, but the invasive studies (such as a posterior fossa air study) may be deferred a week or 2, provided that the foregoing criteria are met. A spontaneous sixth cranial nerve paralysis begins to clear in a week or 2, whereas a pontine glioma does not. Nevertheless, a week's delay probably does not affect the outcome of a pontine glioma.

Synkinetic phenomena of the third cranial nerve are well known and not rare. Synkinetic phenomena involving the sixth cranial nerve are rare. I have not seen a case, but Spaeth reported on a small series in 1950.

MYOPATHIC CAUSES

Thyroid Disease

Signs and Symptoms

Signs of a thyroid disorder can be seen in the eye at different stages of the disease. Symptoms may include some of the signs of hyperthyroidism, as are seen in Graves' disease, and thus the diagnosis is obvious. More frequently, the patient consults an ophthalmologist, complaining of lid retraction and mild exophthalmos before the onset of the systemic signs of hyperthyroidism or before results of laboratory tests are positive. The most frustrating form of eye involvement is that which sometimes occurs after ablation of the hyperactive thyroid gland, when all the systemic signs and laboratory tests have returned to normal.

Although exophthalmos is the best-known symptom of thyroid disease, it may not always be obvious. Even though the condition is present, some patients neither look nor measure particularly exophthalmic owing to the position of their eyes. In such cases, comparison of the patient's present appearance with that in old photographs may be of help. Conversely, some patients who appear exophthalmic may have appeared that way all their lives; or prominent or protruding eyes may be a family characteristic. More rarely, a patient may complain of unilateral exophthalmos, the condition most obvious to him, when in reality he may have enophthalmos on the other side owing to an old orbital cellulitis or he may have suffered trauma with orbital hemorrhage and perhaps a fracture of the orbital floor. All of these conditions can cause absorption of orbital fat and enophthalmos.

Exophthalmic measurements are not difficult, but practice with the instruments involved is required in order to get reliable results. I prefer the Krahn instrument because of the lining-up mechanism that is built into the system. The part of this instrument that brackets the eye includes mirrors with a millimeter scale. This device permits measurement of the anterior surface of the cornea. In addition, the presence in the mirror of 2 red lines that the observer must line up before he takes this reading ensures that the testing circumstances will be the same for every examination. A measurement of 19 mm represents the upper limit of normal for the anterior surface of the cornea: 95% of the population have measurements below this figure; however, as previously indicated, if a patient who normally measures 16 mm now measures 19 mm, he is becoming exophthalmic.

Ophthalmoplegia is a prominent feature, whereas diplopia is not a prominent feature of thyroid disease. If it is present, the patient will probably mention it; however, he will usually not compensate for it by putting a patch over one eye or closing an eye as does a patient who has experienced the sudden onset of a sixth cranial nerve paralysis. Limitation of ocular motion is usually in the upward direction and is caused by restriction of the globe by the inferior muscles rather than by weakness of the elevator muscles. This condition can be confirmed by finding restriction of the globe in the forced duction test, which is a particularly significant test when the extraocular muscles are affected before exophthalmos or lid retraction indicates the nature of the disease. Since the inferior muscles are primarily affected, an attempt at up gaze causes compression of the globe owing to restriction caused by these muscles. This compression in turn raises the intraocular pressure and creates a false impression of glaucoma. Measurement of the difference in intraocular pressure between the eye in down gaze as opposed to up gaze should demonstrate such a variation.

Lid retraction, as has been pointed out by McLean and Norton, may be unilateral and precede all other signs of hyperthyroidism by years. Moreover, lid retraction may occur even in the absence of exophthalmos. The lid is considered retracted when the sclera shows between the upper lid margin and the superior limbus. The fact that the sclera is showing above the limbus indicates that that eye is more likely to be the affected one rather than that the other eye has a ptosis. An exception to this rule occurs when one eye is hypotropic to the other eye, which is fixing. This condition may leave sclera showing above in the hypotropic eye (Fig. 5–1A,B).

Periorbital edema may be caused by several conditions in addition to thyroid disease. As the lid tissues become more relaxed with age, some patients, particularly women, may complain of swelling that is worse on arising in the morning. Periorbital edema also occurs in association with orbital infection, trichinosis, renal disease, and myxedema. In early thyroid disorders, the skin edema is usually pale and soft, rather than red and brawny, as it usually is in severe infection. In Graves' disease, which is marked by the rapid onset and progression of exophthalmos, the edema is firm and the eyes red and swollen. In fact it may be stated that the more severe the exophthalmos and the more acute its onset, the greater the chemosis, redness, and congestion of the globe.

Prominent conjunctival vessels over the lateral rectus muscles are often seen before significant chemosis and congestion of the rest of the ocular vessels occur (Fig. 4–3).

Foreign body sensation is a common complaint, particularly in patients with a combination of up-gaze defect, exophthalmos, and lid retraction—all of which lead to corneal exposure, which is most easily seen in the inferior cornea. Examination following application of fluorescein is best done with the slit lamp, because the punctate staining will be superficial and mild in contrast to the obvious staining usually seen in the case of an outright abrasion. Patients frequently complain of foreign body sensation early in the course of thyroid disease, even though no staining is evident. Photophobia is also a frequent complaint in thyroid disease, even with minimal corneal involvement.

Severe corneal exposure can lead to corneal ulcers, to infection, and, eventually, to scarring or perforation. Extreme exophthalmos requires constant observation and appropriate treatment to prevent such complications. On occasion, the treatment may even include operation to decompress the orbit.

Optic nerve involvement in the form of decreased visual acuity is seen in the most severe cases of exophthalmos, and it is most likely to develop when the exophthalmos is rapidly progressive and accompanied by numerous inflammatory signs. Optic neuropathy is certainly not caused by mechanical stretching of the optic nerve, since the intraorbital portion of the nerve measures about 30 mm—the distance from the posterior aspect of the globe to the beginning of the optic canal is 18 mm. Thus, there are 12 mm of play in this S-shaped nerve before mechanical stretch occurs—far in excess of the 7 to 10 mm of exophthalmos seen in the most severe cases. It may be caused by compression of the nerve and its vascular supply by enlarged muscles (Fig. 4–5). A decrease in acuity can also be ascribed to changes in the corneal epithelium owing to a lack of adequate precorneal tear film or to punctate epithelial changes.

Brawny scleritis, which causes a decrease in acuity owing to macular involvement, can also occur as a consequence of hyperthyroidism. Dilation of the pupil and examination with the fundus contact lens may reveal horizontal retinal macular striae and a thickened elevated choroid in the posterior pole (Fig. 4–6).

Unusual Complications

Myasthenia gravis develops in about 5% of patients with hyperthyroidism, usually late in the course of the disease. Myasthenia gravis should be suspected in a patient whose hyperthyroidism has been arrested but who suddenly begins to complain of diplopia and shows increased muscle imbalance. A resurgence of the signs and symptoms of hyperthyroidism is usually presumed, even though the patient is euthyroid by laboratory standards. Steroid therapy usually results in minimal improvement.

A Tensilon test is usually diagnostic of myasthenia gravis. Also helpful in diagnosing cases of secondary myasthenia after hyperthyroidism is a lessening of the previous lid retraction or the development of an outright ptosis. A Tensilon test may not only reduce the ptosis but also return the lid to its previously retracted position during the period when the Tensilon is effective.

In rare instances, resurgence of ocular symptoms in treated cases of hyperthyroidism is iatrogenic in origin. Many patients who have undergone thyroid ablation with ^{131}I are given thyroid replacement therapy. Since over a long period some normal thyroid function may return, the initial replacement dosage may require adjustment in order to avoid an iatrogenic recurrence of hyperthyroidism.

Thyroid Function Tests

Basal Metabolic Rate. Following Magnus Levy's observation (in 1896) that thyroid gland activity has a profound effect on total oxygen consumption and regulation of metabolic activity, determination of the basal metabolic rate became a classic method for evaluating thyroid function. Although its clinical imprecision has detracted from its acceptance, determination of the basal metabolic rate, when performed under research laboratory conditions, can still be useful in measuring the impact of thyroid hormone on end-organ responses (heat production and oxygen consumption).

Thyroid Hormone Analyses—Thyroxine.
The level of concentration of thyroid hormone in plasma or blood is usually a valuable index of thyroid activity. A number of early tests that measured iodine content, such as the protein-bound iodine test, are now only of historic interest. These tests do not accurately measure thyroxine concentration in serum probably contaminated with a number of compounds that contain organic or nonorganic iodine. Newer testing methods, such as the competitive protein-binding test and radioimmunoassay, identify the molecular configuration of thyroxine rather than its iodine content, and when combined with an estimate of thyroxine-binding globulin capacity, measure effective, or free, thyroxine concentration.

Free thyroxine concentration, which most accurately parallels the physiologic role of thyroxine, can be determined by measuring the total thyroxine concentration radioimmunoassay (RIA) and the triiodothyronine (T_3) resin uptake of the same sample. The T_3 resin uptake is a measurement of serum thyroxine-binding capacity only. It is not a direct thyroid function test, and it should not be confused with a new test of thyroid function, the serum T_3 concentration by RIA test.

New Concepts in Thyroid Physiology. Concepts of thyroid physiology have been changed recently by the rediscovery of the vital role of T_3 as the only form of thyroid hormone that can interact with specific hormone receptors in the cytoplasm and nucleus of cells influenced by thyroid hormone.

Iodide Physiology. Over the past 20 years, the amount of iodine consumed as part of the daily diet has increased almost 300%. When iodine is ingested by healthy people, it is reduced to iodide in the intestine (where it is absorbed almost completely) and is removed from the plasma by the kidneys and the thyroid gland. The thyroid cells extract iodide and concentrate it in the cell interior and in the follicle colloid.

In testing for hyperthyroidism, the uptake of radioactive iodide by the thyroid, as measured externally by a sodium iodide crystal probe detector, can be correlated with thyroid function if the total organic and inorganic iodide pools are normal (no reduction by operation or radioactive iodine therapy in the case of the organic pool; no increase in or reduction of dietary iodide in the case of the inorganic pool). Determination of the plasma thyroid-stimulating hormone (TSH) concentration is at present the most accurate method of testing for primary hyperthyroidism, and it should be used to confirm low-normal corrected or free thyroxine levels. The iodine that enters the thyroid is quickly organically bound to tyrosine in thyroglobulin, and coupled to form thyroxine and T_3 still connected to the large storage protein, thyroglobulin, in the colloid space. Follicular microvilli "pinch off" small bits of colloid and pull them into the follicle cells, where they are broken down into constituent thyroxine, T_3, iodide, and amino acids. The average daily secretion in a normal male is 94 to 110 g of thyroxine and 16 to 22 g of T_3. About 25% of this secreted thyroxine is converted to T_3 in hepatic, renal, and other tissues as yet unidentified. Thyroxine may be considered a prohormone since most of its activity comes from its conversion to T_3, which is three times more potent.

In hyperthyroidism, T_3 is not only secreted by the thyroid in increased amounts but also converted into increased amounts of secreted thyroxine. Generally, a parallel exists between the increased amounts of thyroxine and T_3, so measurement of the effective serum thyroxine can be used to diagnose the hyperthyroid state.

T_3 measurements are not as widely available as measurements of thyroxine-RIA, and they cost about three times as much. T_3 should be measured in any hyperthyroid-like clinical presentation in which effective or free, thyroxine measurements are not high. I have noted better correlation of symptoms with T_3 than with thyroxine

levels in hyperthyroid patients whose thyroxine levels were above normal.

T_3 toxicosis presents with signs and symptoms of hypermetabolism (congestive heart failure, arrhythmias, and myopathy are common), a normal serum thyroxine, free thyroxine, T_3 resin uptake and thyroid-binding globulin concentrations, and a high radioactive iodide uptake. In its pure form, this condition occurs primarily in elderly patients. A radioactive iodide scan reveals that a hyperfunctioning adenoma of the thyroid gland is suppressing normal thyroid tissue. At its onset, T_3 toxicosis is frequently confused with malignant disease, neuromuscular degenerative disease, and cardiac conditions.

Exophthalmos is rarely seen in cases of T_3 toxicosis, but may occur in cases of thyrotoxicosis associated with lymphocytic thyroiditis. According to Basterne, about 66% of patients suffering from Graves' disease with exophthalmos are affected with autoimmune thyroiditis. Most American thyroidologists would agree with this concept, but would question the rate of incidence, basing their objections on data from thyroid antibody studies.

Exophthalmos of thyroid origin is associated, although rarely, with thyroiditis with high microsomal and thyroglobulin antibody titers. It is also associated with evidence of lack of suppressibility of the thyroid-pituitary axis to feedback control: excessive production of thyroxine and failure of T_3 to shut off more hormone production by the overactive gland. The Werner suppression test (T_3 suppression test) to demonstrate this lack of response may now be replaced by the thyroxine-releasing hormone (TRH) stimulation test. The major disadvantage of the Werner test is the hazard involved in giving possibly toxic amounts of T_3 to a hyperthyroid patient with heart, hypertensive, or vascular problems.

Since it is now available for intravenous testing purposes, the TRH stimulation test will probably replace the Werner test in diagnosing lack of pituitary-thyroid responsiveness. The infusion of this hypothalamic tripeptide fails to elicit from the pituitary a rise in TRH in Graves' disease before hyperthyroid signs have become overt. Although the TRH stimulation test is expensive and occasionally causes nausea, it should be safer than the Werner test.

Measurement of the long-acting thyroid stimulator (LATS) has also been used in the early diagnosis of exophthalmos when thyroid dysfunction has not been clearly established as the underlying causative factor. Unfortunately this test involves bioassay in mice, and is not sensitive enough to ensure clear results in more than 40% of serum samples tested. If the thyroid membrane radioreceptor assay of Rees Smith, which has demonstrated thyroid-stimulating immunoglobulins (TSI) in 100% of patients with Graves' disease, can be developed for wide clinical use, measurement of TSI concentration may be the most sensitive of all tests for thyroid disease as the underlying cause of exophthalmos.

Treatment

In all forms of thyroid disease, restoration of a euthyroid state is the ultimate goal. In regard to ocular involvement, treatment falls into both the medical and surgical categories.

Medical Treatment. The aim of medical treatment is to minimize the patient discomfort that accompanies thyroid disease with ocular involvement. Severe periorbital swelling in the morning can be lessened somewhat if the patient sleeps with his head elevated. If corneal exposure owing to severe exophthalmos or paralysis of up gaze is a problem, taping the lid shut or filling the palpebral fissure with some bland ointment at night can be of value. Lid taping may not be totally successful, however, because the partially open palpebral fissure may allow the tape to scrape the cornea. Should this problem occur, creating a moisture chamber by taping the edges of a piece of plastic wrap (like Saran) to the skin at the orbital rim may afford some relief. The frequent use of some form of artificial tears can help to alleviate the foreign body sensation as well as the symptoms of mild superficial punctate keratitis. Occasionally, the physician must resort to rather thick artificial tears in the form of a 1% solution of methylcellulose. I usually reserve this type of medication for the most severe cases since it is rather sticky and esthetically repugnant to the patient.

Lid retraction is probably the sign most obvious to patients and the one that bothers them the most cosmetically. A method of treatment devised by Gay involves the use of topical guanethidine to create a chemical Horner syndrome with slight ptosis. Although this treatment aroused considerable interest in England, it is not standard accepted treatment in the United States. I have tried Gay's method on several patients, but found it of little value in facilitating normal lid function, particularly if the lid retraction was of long-standing, with fibrotic changes in the levator tendon. The use of systemic steroids should be reserved for cases of diplopia in which the onset is rapid and progressive, and for exophthalmos accompanied by significant inflammatory signs.

Surgical Treatment. In my opinion, surgical treatment should be restricted to cases in which the ocular involvement is severe.

In some patients, the eyes appear paralyzed with respect to up gaze, when in fact, changes in the inferior muscles are restricting the upward movement of the globe. Surgical correction of this defect primarily involves weakening the depressor muscles, which are really the main offenders.

Surgical procedure to improve the appearance of patients with exophthalmos and lid retraction should be considered only if these two signs are stable. If they are, a small lateral tarsorrhaphy may be performed to reduce the prominent appearance of the eye. (A too-aggressive lateral tarsorrhaphy may give the eyes a squashed appearance.) Most patients are grateful for an improvement in their appearance, even though the lids have not been brought down to a fully normal position.

Cases of severe progressive exophthalmos with loss of vision, severe recurrent corneal ulcers, and exposure keratitis require careful treatment to prevent permanent loss of vision. In the past a lateral Krönlein resection to decompress the orbit was the standard procedure. More recently there has been some interest in combining the lateral Krönlein procedure with the creation of a surgical blow-out fracture, thus, it is hoped, improving both the exophthalmos and the vision. On the other hand, many cases involving acutely progressive signs can be managed with systemic steroids, constant care of the corneal exposure problem, and a little patience.

Myasthenia Gravis

As Drachman et al. have so well pointed out, the pathologic differences between neuropathic and myopathic processes are not as clear-cut as was once believed. Myasthenia gravis is a chronic disease marked by weakness of the voluntary muscles, particularly the muscles involved in facial expression, mastication, swallowing, movement of the proximal limb girdle, and lid and ocular motility. Myasthenia gravis affecting ocular and lid motility can occur first as an isolated ptosis owing to a weak levator muscle. Biopsy of the affected muscle is rarely helpful in diagnosing myasthenia gravis, since it seldom reveals the specific changes that occur as a result of this disease. Moreover, because the biopsy is performed on the levator tendon rather than the muscle itself, the test is often inconclusive.

Signs and Symptoms

Although myasthenia gravis affects many muscle groups, the ocular signs, particularly ptosis, are frequently the earliest indication of the presence of this disease.

In fact, ocular symptoms are the only sign in at least 15% of patients. Ptosis without ophthalmoplegia may be present for some time before weakness of the extraocular muscles is detectable.

Some patients may mask or partially overcome a minimal ptosis (as in Horner syndrome) by contracting the frontalis muscle (furrowing the brow). A patient suffering from myasthenia gravis is usually unable to furrow his brow, since his frontalis muscle is just as weak as his levator muscle is. A rare exception occurs in cases of asymmetric myasthenia gravis. When patients with this condition attempt to contract the frontalis muscle, no correction for the ptosis occurs on the abnormal side. On the unaffected side, the contraction of the frontalis muscle causes the lid to retract. This action may lead to an erroneous diagnosis of thyroid myopathy.

The Tensilon test is helpful in the diagnosis of asymmetric myasthenia gravis, because after the injection of this drug the lid on the ptotic side retracts immediately. With the Tensilon test, lid retraction may occasionally be observed on the normal side also, even though the patient is not contracting his frontalis muscle. This retraction indicates some bilateral, although asymmetric, levator weakness.

Up gaze is the direction in which the patient initially develops symptoms of diplopia. Weakness of convergence, particularly during extensive reading, also causes symptoms to develop. These symptoms are frequently misinterpreted as signs that the patient needs stronger eyeglasses. Thus, many different strengths of eyeglasses, even some with prisms, are prescribed before myasthenia gravis is discovered as the true cause of the diplopia. In an attempt to strengthen weakening convergence the entire near reflex may be invoked, causing an increase in accommodation. This will cause a pseudomyopia.

Since weakness of up gaze may not be manifest on primary gaze, the patient should be instructed to rotate his eye well up and to sustain it in that position. Sustained up gaze tends to make the ptosis clearly evident, and may also reveal a diplopia that may not be obvious on simple inspection. Some physicians prefer to have the patient move his eyes up and down rapidly and to open and close his lids quickly in order to fatigue the muscles. I find the sustained up gaze maneuver to be equally successful. The patient may not be aware that he is suffering from weak ocular motility since the ptosis that has led him to seek treatment may cover the pupil in extremes of up gaze and therefore obscure the diplopia.

The worsening of the diplopia and ptosis seen on exercising those muscles in myasthenia gravis does not occur in patients with partial third cranial nerve paralysis, regardless of how long the patient sustains a gaze in the field of action of the weak muscles.

The key sign differentiating myasthenia gravis from third cranial nerve paralysis is the absence of pupillary signs in myasthenia gravis. If pupillary signs are present, either two disease conditions are present or the diagnosis of myasthenia gravis is incorrect.

In contrast to the good orbicularis muscle function but weak elevator muscle function typical of third cranial nerve paralysis, a patient with weak elevator muscles owing to myasthenia gravis may also have weak orbicularis muscles. Ignoring this fact, particularly in view of the possibility that the patient may have some difficulty with up gaze, may lead to a severe corneal exposure problem if a surgical procedure for ptosis is attempted. (The orbicularis muscle can be tested by forcing the lids open after the patient has been instructed to squeeze them shut.)

The myasthenic crisis is one of the most feared complications of myasthenia gravis. Overtreatment of myasthenia gravis with cholinergic drugs results in clinical findings similar to those in the myasthenic crisis. The most serious complication of both conditions is respiratory paralysis, with tracheotomy sometimes required.

Myasthenia gravis takes three forms in infancy and childhood. All of them respond to anticholinesterase medication. All three also show similar and appropriate EMG responses of a decrement in motor units in response to repetitive nerve stimulation. Other features of the disease serve to differentiate the causes of all three types.

The neonatal form is seen in infants born of myasthenic mothers and is probably secondary to the transfer of antibodies to the acetylcholine receptors. Symptoms occur during the first day of life and in over 78% of cases, which differs from the original description. The most common sign is a poor sucking reflex despite an alert infant eager to eat. Eye signs, such as ptosis and motility disturbances, which are so common in adult onset myasthenia, occur in only about 15% of neonatal myasthenia.

The second type is the congenital form, which probably results from a genetically transmitted disease rather than a circulating antibody. A prominent sign is extraocular muscle abnormalities with a minor amount of generalized weakness, which is the reverse of the neonatal form.

The third form is called juvenile; its onset is usually after 1 year of age, and the majority of cases occur after the age of 10. As in the adult form, ptosis and diplopia are the prominent initial features.

An autoimmune response is suggested as the mechanism in the juvenile and adult forms, and an antiacetylcholine receptor antibody can be identified in a high percentage of cases. No antibody to the acetylcholine receptor is found in the congenital form, which is genetically transferred.

Eaton-Lambert Syndrome. This syndrome is a myasthenia gravis-like condition that occurs as a consequence of carcinoma elsewhere in the body. Eye signs in connection with this disorder are rare but not unheard of. Isolated eye signs, however, have not been reported; therefore Eaton-Lambert syndrome need not be considered if the presenting symptom is isolated ophthalmoplegia or isolated ptosis. The significant features are absent or decreased deep tendon reflexes, proximal muscle weakness, and increasing (rather than decreasing) muscle strength after voluntary exercise. Electromyography serves to definitely distinguish the Eaton-Lambert syndrome from true myasthenia gravis. In the Eaton-Lambert syndrome a recruitment of motor units occurs with continual stimulation, rather than the dropout that occurs in myasthenia gravis.

The myasthenic syndrome of Eaton-Lambert affects many different muscle groups but, remarkably, spares the ocular muscles, unlike true myasthenia. There have been isolated reports of diplopia, but these are extremely rare. A remote effect of carcinoma has been the development of polyneuropathies that develop slowly over months and are predominantly distal, symmetric, and sensorimotor in type. These patients develop severe weakness and atrophy, ataxia, and sensory loss in the limbs. A mixed sensorimotor form of myasthenic syndrome is 5 times more common than a pure sensory form; usually, there is no remission and steady progression. This is seen in 2 to 5% of all patients with malignancy. Carcinoma of the lung accounts for 50% of the sensorimotor form and 75% of the pure sensory form. There is also a type that takes the form of polymyositis and this syndrome, secondary to carcinoma, is seen in about 15% of all patients with polymyositis; it typically appears after the age of 50. The proportion of these cases owing to bronchogenic carcinoma is higher than in other forms of carcinoma.

Myasthenic-like syndromes can occur secondary to medication. The cause of these myasthenic syndromes varies from drug group to drug group. With d-penicillamine, an antiacetylcholine receptor antibody develops. With antibiotics such as neomycin, streptomycin, kanamycin, polymyxin B sulfate, dihydrostreptomycin, viomycin sulfate, and colistin sulfate neuromuscular blocking effects occur for other reasons. These effects may not be related only to the use of these medications, they have been more frequently reported after general anesthesia. They also may not necessarily be related to the stress of surgery but rather to other factors influencing neuromuscular transmission, such as neuromuscular blocking agents (succinylcholine, for example), or to a decrease in serum and tissue calcium.

Tests for Myasthenia Gravis

When evaluating patients suspected of having myasthenia gravis, the major procedure is the Tensilon test, which is specific for myasthenia gravis. It should be noted, however, that results of the Tensilon test are not always positive, even in obvious cases. It is also true that the Tensilon test may not be positive at the onset of the disease, but may become positive as the condition progresses. For this reason, the test should be repeated at intervals if results are negative early in the course of the disease.

The Tensilon test should be administered in 3 stages: (1) the patient is usually given an injection of atropine to prevent undue vagal response, (2) a 0.1 ml dose of Tensilon is administered, following which the patient should be observed for any overreaction or drug sensitivity and (3) if after 1 minute no undue reaction occurs, a 0.9 ml dose of Tensilon is administered. Since a positive response to Tensilon usually occurs in about 30 seconds and is over within 1 to 3 minutes, the precise ocular function to be tested should be determined before the testing procedure is begun. A total ocular motility examination should not be attempted during the short period in which Tensilon is effective, since the key signs of a positive reaction may be missed. If ptosis is the most obvious sign of myasthenia gravis, improvement in this condition is the sign to look for during the first 2 or 3 minutes of the testing procedure. A positive response to Tensilon is definitely diagnostic of myasthenia gravis since only in the presence of this disease does such a reaction occur.

The Tensilon test is not positive nearly as often as we suspect the diagnosis of myasthenia gravis. For confirmation, Miller, Morris, and Maguire use intramuscular neostigmine with detailed orthoptic measurements before and during the test. This procedure in association with electromyographic studies is said to yield a higher number of positive results for myasthenia then Tensilon alone.

Before Tensilon became available, small doses of curare were used to test for myasthenia gravis. Patients with myasthenia gravis are supersensitive to curare, however, so this difficult and dangerous drug was all but abandoned with the advent of Tensilon.

Another once-popular test that has fallen by the wayside involved the use of quinine—a drug that made the myasthenic process worse. Although quinine is no longer used in the testing procedure, this drug may still subtly alter the results of other tests, because many patients drink quinine water or take quinine compounds—which aggravate the myasthenia gravis symptoms. Therefore, unless history taking includes a specific question as to the use of quinine in any form, the physician may remain unaware that such a practice is making the myasthenia gravis worse or at least making treatment more difficult. The theory behind quinine ingestion is that the drug lessens the sensitivity of the motor endplate and thus holds the firing of the muscle neurofibrils to a minimum. It is commonly given for night leg cramps.

The Tensilon test may also be done in conjunction with tonography. In fact, this modification is recommended for patients who have responded negatively to the Tensilon test alone. In the combination test, the patient is given an intravenous drip of normal saline solution. The tonometer is placed on his eye, and the normal slope of the tonography curve is followed. A small amount of saline solution is then injected into the tubing, following which, the slope of the curve is again observed. The saline injection should cause no change. Tensilon is now injected into the same tubing. If the muscles are normal, no reaction occurs. A positive reaction, which consists of a sudden increase in the pressure in the eye owing to co-contraction of the extraocular muscles, is diagnostic of myasthenia gravis.

Treatment

In the treatment of myasthenia gravis, anticholinesterase medications, such as prostigmine, are the drugs of choice. The main problem with this group of drugs is the possibility of an overdose and consequent cholinergic crisis. Moreover, the use of these drugs is particularly difficult when the myasthenia gravis is confined to the ocular muscles. As a result, a therapeutic dose for the ocular muscles may be too toxic for normal skeletal muscles.

Steroids are now being used to treat advanced cases of myasthenia gravis that are not responding well to anticholinesterase medication. Such patients are started on steroids in daily doses of up to 100 mg per day and maintained at that level until symptoms stabilize. The dosage is then reduced to a minimal amount on an alternate-day program until the medication can be discontinued, perhaps after many months.

Thymectomy in women or removal of solitary thymomas is still appropriate and efficacious therapy. In some clinics, thymectomies are being performed with good success even on men without thymomas.

In myasthenic patients, surgical procedure for ptosis should be approached with extreme caution. A perfect ptosis repair may leave the cornea exposed during the day because of a weak orbicularis muscle, and at night because of an inadequate Bell's phenomenon owing to ophthalmoplegia. If the ptosis is severe and the lid covers the pupil, a surgical procedure may be considered; however, the amount of ptosis should be stable, the degree of Bell's phenomenon reasonable, and the ptosis repair less than complete.

Progressive External Ophthalmoplegia

Once a myopathy with ptosis as the most prominent feature has been diagnosed, the differential diagnosis is essentially either myasthenia gravis or progressive external ophthalmoplegia (PEO).

The onset of PEO can be between infancy and 50 years of age, but PEO commonly begins in person over 20 years of age. Frequently, a family history of this condition exists. As in myasthenia gravis, a long interval may elapse between the development of ptosis and involvement of the extraocular muscles. The muscles controlling up gaze are the first group involved in both myasthenia gravis and PEO. The two principal points of difference between these conditions are the negative Tensilon test and the absence of diurnal variation or relation to fatigue, both of which are usually present in myasthenia gravis.

The four syndromes disussed in the following paragraphs are not simply other forms of PEO. They are discussed here because they not only all have PEO as part of the clinical picture, but also have abnormalities of the nervous, cardiac, and hematopoietic systems that differentiate them from PEO. When PEO is diagnosed, it is essential that these other diseases be ruled out because they are more serious than PEO and are, in fact, life threatening.

Oculopharyngeal Dystrophy of Victor

This condition, which may occur sporadically or be inherited as a dominant trait, involves external ophthalmoplegia and pharyngeal weakness. Facial and limb girdle weakness have also been reported in association with this condition.

Kearns-Sayre Syndrome

This syndrome is made up of PEO, retinitis pigmentosa, and heart block in young people. Therefore, in all cases of PEO, a good ophthalmoscopic examination and electrocardiogram should be performed; if the PEO is associated with the Kearns-Sayre syndrome, death from heart block is a possibility.

Bassen-Kornzweig Syndrome

This syndrome consists of a broad mixture of signs, one of which includes PEO. Diarrhea owing to poor absorption of lipids from the gastrointestinal tract may precede the onset of PEO by a few weeks to several years. Patients with this syndrome are also deficient in serum cholesterol and beta-lipoproteins. Pigmentary degeneration of the retina is seen in some cases. Some patients have a positive Babinski reflex, suffer from sensory loss, ataxia, and optic atrophy, and show an increase in cerebrospinal fluid protein. Acanthocytosis of the red blood cells is another laboratory sign that is of assistance in diagnosing the Bassen-Kornzweig syndrome.

Refsum Syndrome

This syndrome, which is rather uncommon should be suggested by a combination of PEO, retinitis pigmentosa, and polyneuropathy. Presence of these conditions should prompt a test for phytanic acid level, which is elevated in this disorder. Less significant diagnostic signs are cerebellar ataxia, hearing loss, anosmia, ichthyosis, and epiphyseal dysplasia.

Pseudotumor of the Orbit

In addition to chemosis, pain, and exophthalmos, pseudotumor of the orbit has an inflammatory sign similar to that which occurs in orbital cellulitis. The congestion of the vessels is usually not as prominent as in cellulitis, but the difference is difficult to evaluate. Pseudotumor of the orbit is usually unilateral, and the ophthalmoplegia is usually marked. Onset can occur at any age, but I usually see it in women between 30 and 50 years of age. Occasionally, the inflammatory signs are minimal, and diplopia is present, with involvement of only 1 muscle and pain on motion—a combination that makes diagnosis more difficult. In early cases of pain in the orbit, exophthalmometer readings on each visit may reveal a gradual development of exophthalmos. This changing pattern facilitates diagnosis of pseudotumor of the orbit before the frank signs of this condition become obvious. The usual differential diagnosis of cellulitis or an infiltrating lesion must be ruled out because no specific tests are available to establish the presence of these diseases. On the other hand, the possibility of a lymphoma of the orbit should be considered.

Patients with pseudotumor of the orbit respond very well to systemic steroids; however, discontinuance of steroid therapy without a recurrence of the disease rarely occurs. I have had to keep many of my patients on steroid medication for months, and in some cases up to a year. Even when steroid medication is apparently withdrawn successfully, the disease can recur months or years later.

Myositis

Myositis has the same signs and symptoms as pseudotumor of the orbit, and it is treated with steroids with the same degree of effectiveness.

Trichinosis

This condition is uncommon in the United States, and in the few cases that occur, a carefully taken history will reveal that the patient has recently eaten pork. In addition to the gastrointestinal problems and eosinophilia that are symptomatic of trichinosis, the main ocular symptoms are periorbital swelling, marked pain on movement, and occasionally, diplopia. Examination of the globe itself does not reveal the inflammatory signs usually associated with pseudotumor or myositis. Petechial hemorrhages of the conjunctiva are frequently seen.

Myotonic Dystrophy

Although diplopia is not a sign of myotonic dystrophy, this disease is discussed in this chapter because it is a myopathic process. Patients suffering from myotonic dystrophy frequently have ptosis, which is also an early sign of myasthenia gravis and PEO. Therefore, prior to the onset of diplopia, the possibility of myotonic dystrophy should be considered in the course of the differential diagnosis.

Ptosis is certainly not the earliest sign of myotonic dystrophy; however, in known cases, ptosis is part of this syndrome and should be so regarded in the absence of other signs of third cranial nerve paralysis, such as pupillary involvement. Restriction of gaze occurs less frequently, but is also a sign of myotonic dystrophy. Other associated eye signs are a positive Schirmer's test, keratitis sicca, ocular hypotony averaging 10 mm of mercury, decreased corneal sensitivity, decreased dark adaption as shown by the electroretinogram, and, in a small number of cases, a starlike retinal pigmentary degeneration.

The handclasp sign is easily elicited and dramatic. After a firm handshake, the patient is unable to release his grasp. Similarly, after forced closure of the lids, the patient may be unable to open his eyes on command (or at will).

BIBLIOGRAPHY

Aberfeld, D.C., and Namba, T.: Progressive ophthalmoplegia in Kugelberg-Welander disease. Arch. Neurol. 20:253, 1969.

Alexander, W.S.: Phytanic acid in Refsum's syndrome. J. Neurol. Neurosurg. Psychiatry 29:412, 1966.

Asbury, A.K.: Diabetic ophthalmoplegia: a clinicopathologic investigation. Trans. Am. Neurol. Assoc. 94:64, 1969.

Avanzini, G., et al.: Oculomotor disorders in Huntington's chorea. J. Neurol. Neurosurg. Psychiatry. 42:581, 1979.

Barr, H.W.K., Blackwood, W., and Meadows, S.P.: Intracavernous carotid aneurysms. Brain 94:607, 1971.

Barricks, M.E., Traviesa, D.B., Glaser, J.S., and Levy, I.S.: Ophthalmoplegia in cranial arteritis. Brain 100:209, 1977.

Bassen, F.A., and Kornzweig, A.L.: Malformation of

the erythrocytes in a case of atypical retinitis pigmentosa. Blood 5:381, 1950.

Basterne, P.A., and Ermans, A.M.: Thyroiditis and Thyroid Function. New York, Pergamon Press, 1972.

Bender, M.B.: The nerve supply to the orbicularis muscle and the physiology of movements of the upper eyelid. Arch. Ophthalmol. 15:21, 1936.

Bender, M.B., and Fulton, J.F.: Factors in functional recovery following section of the oculomotor nerve in monkeys. J. Neurol. Neurosurg. Psychiatry 2:285, 1939.

Bender, M. B.: Polyopia and monocular diplopia of cerebral origin. Neurol. Psych. 54:323, 1945.

Benjamin, J.W.: The nucleus of the oculomotor nerve with special reference to innervation of the pupil and fibers from the pretectal region. J. Nerv. Ment. Dis. 89:294, 1939.

Berman, B.: Voluntary propulsion of the eyeballs. Arch. Intern. Med. 117:648, 1966.

Bevin, C.T., et al.: Penicillamine induced myasthenia gravis. Effects of penicillamine on acetylcholine receptor. Neurology 32:1077, 1982.

Biglan, A.W., Ellis, F.D., and Wade, T.A.: Supranuclear third nerve palsy and exotropia after tetanus. Am. J. Ophthalmol. 86:666, 1978.

Blodi, F.C.: Ophthalmic zoster in malignant disease. Am. J. Ophthalmol. 65:686, 1968.

Blodi, F.C., Van Allen, M.W., and Yarbrough, J.C.: Duane's syndrome: a brain stem lesion. Arch. Ophthalmol. 72:171, 1964.

Boniuk, M., and Schlezenger, N.: Raeder's paratrigeminal syndrome. Am. J. Ophthalmol. 54:1072, 1962.

Brain, R., and Henson, R.A.: Neurological syndromes associated with carcinoma. Lancet 275:971, 1958.

Brauston, B.B., and Norton, E.W.D.: Intermittent exophthalmos. Am. J. Ophthalmol. 55:701, 1963.

Breinin, G.M.: New aspects of ophthalmoneurologic diagnosis. Arch. Ophthalmol. 58:375, 1957.

Brougham, M., Heusner, A.P., and Adams, R.D.: Acute degenerative changes in adenomas of the pituitary body with special reference to pituitary apoplexy. J. Neurosurg. 7:421, 1950.

Brown, H.W.: Congenital structural muscle anomalies. *Strabismus ophthalmic symposium.* St. Louis, C.V. Mosby, 1950, p. 205.

Brown, H.W.: True and simulated superior oblique tendon sheath syndromes. Acta Ophthalmol. 34:123, 1973.

Brown, P.: Septic cavernous sinus thrombosis. Bull. Johns Hopkins Hosp. 109:68, 1961.

Bruce, G.M.: Ocular divergence—its physiology and pathology. Arch. Ophthalmol. 13:639, 1935.

Bryce-Smith, R., and Macintosh, R.R.: Sixth nerve palsy after lumbar puncture and spinal analgesia. Br. Med. J. 1:275, 1951.

Burger, L.J., Kalvin, N.H., and Smith, J.L.: Acquired lesions of the fourth cranial nerve. Brain 93:567, 1970.

Burgess, D., Roper-Hall, G., and Burde, R.M.: Binocular diplopia associated with subretinal neovascular membranes. Arch. Ophthalmol. 98:311, 1980.

Burian, H.M., Rowan, P.J., and Sullivan, M.S.: Absence of spontaneous head tilt in superior oblique muscle palsy. Am. J. Ophthalmol. 79:972, 1975.

Burke, G.: The triiodothyronine suppression test. Am. J. Med. 42:600, 1967.

Burnet, F.M.: The immunological significance of the thymus. Aust. Ann. Med. 11:79, 1962.

Byers, R.K., and Hass, G.M.: Thrombosis of the dural venous sinuses in infancy and in childhood. Am. J. Dis. Child. 45:1161, 1933.

Cape, C.A.: Ocular response to corticotropin in myasthenia gravis. Arch. Ophthalmol. 90:292, 1973.

Casey, E.B., Jellife, A.M., LeQuesne, P.M., and Millett, Y.L.: Vincristine neuropathy. Brain 96:69, 1973.

Chambers, J.W., and Walsh, F.B.: Hyaline bodies in the optic discs: report of ten cases exemplifying importance in neurological diagnosis. Brain 74:95, 1951.

Chapman, L.I., et al.: Acquired bilateral superior oblique muscle palsy. Arch. Ophthalmol. 84:137, 1970.

Cogan, D.G., and Goldstein, J.E.: Diabetic ophthalmoplegia with special reference to the pupil. Arch. Ophthalmol. 64:592, 1960.

Cogan, D.M., and Victor, M.: Ocular signs of Wernicke's disease. Arch. Ophthalmol. 51:204, 1954.

Cohen, S.M., and Waxman, S.: Myasthenia gravis, chronic lymphocytic leukemia and autoimmune hemolytic anemia. Arch. Intern. Med. 120:717, 1967.

Coleman, D.J.: High resolution B-scan ultrasonography of the orbit. Arch. Ophthalmol. 88:465, 1972.

Collier, J.: Nuclear ophthalmoplegia with especial reference to retraction of the lids and ptosis and to lesions of the posterior commissure. Brain 50:488, 1927.

Cross, H.E., and Pfaffenbach, D.D.: Duane's retraction syndrome and associated congenital malformations. Am. J. Ophthalmol. 74:442, 1972.

Crouch, E.R., and Urist, M.J.: Lateral rectus muscle paralysis associated with closed head trauma. Am. J. Ophthalmol. 79:990, 1975.

Cushing, H.: Strangulation of the nerve abducens by lateral branches of the basilar artery in cases of brain tumor. Brain 33:204, 1910.

Dailey, E.J., et al.: Evaluation of ocular signs and symptoms in cerebral aneurysms. Arch. Ophthalmol. 71:463, 1964.

Danta, G., Hilton, R.C., and Lynch, P.G.: Chronic progressive external ophthalmoplegia. Brain 98:473, 1975.

Daroff, R.B.: Chronic progressive external ophthalmoplegia. Arch. Ophthalmol. 82:845, 1969.

Davidson, T.M., Alesen, R.M., and Nachum, A.M.: Medial orbital wall fracture with rectus entrapment. Arch. Otolaryngol. 101:33, 1975.

Davis, R.H., Daroff, R.B., and Hoyt, W.F.: Hemicrania, pupillosympathetic paresis and subcranial carotid aneurysm: Raeder's paratrigeminal syndrome (group 2). J. Neurosurg. 29:94, 1968.

Dawson, B.H.: Acute massive infarctions of pituitary adenomas: a study of five patients J. Neurosurg. 37:275, 1972.

DeSanto, L.W.: Surgical palliation of ophthalmopathy of Graves' disease. Mayo Clin. Proc. 47:989, 1972.

Dimant, J., Grob, D., and Brunner, N.G.: Ophthalmoplegia, ptosis and miosis in temporal arteritis. Neurology 30:1054, 1980.

Dimsdale, H., and Phillips, D.G.: Ocular palsies with nasal sinusitis. J. Neurol. Neurosurg. Psychiatry 13:225, 1959.

Dornan, T.L., et al.: Remittant painful ophthalmoplegia. The Tolosa-Hunt syndrome? J. Neurol. Neurosurg. Psychiatry 42:270, 1979.

Drachman, D.A.: Ophthalmoplegia plus. Arch. Neurol. 18:654, 1968.

Drachman, D.A., et al.: Experimental denervation of ocular muscles. Arch. Neurol. 21:170, 1969.

Drachman, D.A., et al.: Myopathic changes in chronically denervated muscle. Arch. Neurol. 16:14, 1967.

Drews, L.C.: Exophthalmometry. Am. J. Ophthalmol. 43:37, 1957.

Dunnington, J.H., and Berke, R.N.: Exophthalmos due to chronic orbital myositis. Arch. Ophthalmol. 30:446, 1943.

Duvoisin, R.C.: Part 2: the cluster headache. JAMA 22:1403, 1972.

Eareckson, V.O., and Miller, J.M.: Third nerve palsy with sparing of pupil in diabetes mellitus. Arch. Ophthalmol. 47:607, 1952.

Eaton, L.M., and Lambert, E.H.: Electromyography and electric stimulation of nerves in diseases of motor unit: observations on myasthenic syndrome associated with malignant tumor. JAMA 163:1117, 1957.

Edgerton, A.E.: Herpes zoster ophthalmicus. Arch. Ophthalmol. 34:40, 1945.

Elizan, T.S., Spere, J.P., and Andiman, R.M.: Syndrome of acute idiopathic ophthalmoplegia with ataxia and areflexia. Neurology 21:281, 1971.

Ellenbery, M.: Diabetic neuropathy presenting as the initial clinical manifestation of diabetes. Ann. Intern. Med. 49:620, 1958.

Elmquist, D., and Lambert, E.H.: Detailed analysis of neuromuscular transmission in a patient with the myasthenic syndrome sometimes associated with bronchogenic carcinoma. Mayo Clin. Proc. 43:689, 1968.

Elmquist, D., et ai.: An electrophysiological investigation of neuromuscular transmission in myasthenia gravis. J. Physiol. 174:417, 1964.

Fenichel, G.M.: Clinical syndromes of myasthenia in infancy and childhood. Child Neurology. 35:97, 1978.

Fenton, R.H.: Histopathologic findings in eyes with paralysis of the oculomotor (third) nerve. Arch. Ophthalmol. 73:224, 1965.

Fields, J.D.: Bulging fontanel: a complication of tetracycline therapy in infants. J. Pediatr. 58:74, 1961.

Fisher, M.: An unusual variant of acute idiopathic polyneuritis (syndrome of ophthalmoplegia, ataxia and areflexia). N. Engl. J. Med. 255:57, 1956.

Flanagan, J.C., McLachlan, D.L., and Shannon, G.M.: Orbital roof fractures: Neurologic and neurosurgical considerations. Ophthalmology 87:325, 1980.

Fleming, R.: Refsum's syndrome. Neurology 7:477, 1957.

Flynn, J.T., et al.: Ocular motility complications following intranasal surgery. Arch. Ophthalmol. 97:453, 1979.

Foley, J.: Benign form of intracranial hypertension: toxic and otitic hydrocephalus. Brain 78:1, 1955.

Ford, F.R., and Walsh, F.B.: Raeder's paratrigeminal syndrome, a benign disorder, possibly a complication of migraine. Bull. Johns Hopkins Hosp. 103:296, 1958.

Ford, F.R., Walsh, F.B., and King, A.: Clinical observations on the pupillary phenomena resulting from regeneration of the third nerve with especial reference to the Aryll Robertson pupil. Bull. Johns Hopkins Hosp. 68:309, 1941.

Forster, R.K., Schatz, N.J., and Smith J.L.: A subtle eyelid sign in aberrant regeneration of the third nerve. Am. J. Ophthalmol. 67:696, 1969.

Foster, R.S., Metz, H.S., and Jampolsky, A.: Strabismus and pseudostrabismus with retrolental fibroplasia. Am. J. Ophthalmol. 79:985, 1975.

Friedman, A.P., Harter, D.H., and Merritt, H.H.: Ophthalmoplegic migraine. Arch. Neurol. 7:320, 1962.

Friedman, G., and Harrison, S.: Mucocele of the sphenoidal sinus as a cause of recurrent oculomotor nerve palsy. J. Neurol. Neurosurg. Psychiatry 33:172, 1970.

Fryer, D.G., Winckleman, A.C., Ways, P.O., and Swanson, A.G.: Refsum's disease: a clinical pathological report. Neurology 21:162, 1971.

Gay, A.J.: Topical guanethidine therapy for endocrine lid retraction. Arch. Ophthalmol. 76:364, 1966.

Gay, A.J.: Topical sympatholytic therapy for pathologic lid retraction. Arch. Ophthalmol. 77:341, 1967.

Gibberd, F.B., Navab, F., and Smith, C.L.: Treatment of ocular myasthenia with corticotrophin. J. Neurol. Neurosurg. Psychiatry 34:11, 1971.

Giles, C.L., and Westerberg, M.R.: Clinical evaluation of local ocular anticholinesterase agents in myasthenia gravis. Am. J. Ophthalmol. 52:331, 1961.

Glaser, J.S.: Myasthenic pseudointernuclear ophthalmoplegia. Arch. Ophthalmol. 75:363, 1966.

Glaser, J.S.: The edrophonium tonogram test in myasthenia gravis. Arch. Ophthalmol. 76:368, 1966.

Glaser, J.S.: Tensilon tonography in the diagnosis of myasthenia gravis. Invest. Ophthalmol. 6:135, 1967.

Godtfredsen, E., and Lederman, M.: Diagnostic and prognostic roles of ophthalmoneurologic signs and symptoms in malignant nasopharyngeal tumors. Am. J. Ophthalmol. 59:1063, 1965.

Goldhammer, Y., and Smith, J.L.: Acquired intermittant Brown's syndrome. Neurology 24:666, 1974.

Goldsmith, M.O.: Herpes zoster ophthalmicus with sixth nerve palsy. Can. J. Ophthalmol. 3:279, 1968.

Goldstein, J.E.: paresis of superior rectus muscle associated with thyroid dysfunction. Arch. Ophthalmol. 72:5, 1964.

Goldstein, J.E., and Cogan, O.G.: Diabetic ophthalmoplegia with special reference to the pupil. Arch. Ophthalmol. 64:592, 1960.

Gorman, C.A.: Optic neuropathy of Graves' disease. N. Engl. J. Med. *290*:70, 1974.

Gradenigo, G.: A special syndrome of endocranial otitic complications (paralysis of the motor oculi externus of otitic origin). Ann. Otol. Rhinol. Laryngol. *13*:637, 1904.

Green, W.R., Hackett, E.R., and Schlezenger, N.S.: Neuro-ophthalmologic evaluation of oculomotor nerve paralysis. Arch. Ophthalmol. *72*:154, 1964.

Greer, M.: Benign intracranial hypertension. IV. Menarche. Neurology *14*:569, 1964.

Haddad, H.M.: Tonography and visual fields in endocrine exophthalmos. Am. J. Ophthalmol. *64*:63, 1967.

Haddad, H.M.: Experimental endocrine exophthalmos. Ann. Ophthalmol. *6*:721, 1974.

Hamburger, J.I., and Sugar, H.S.: What the internist should know about the ophthalmology of Graves' disease. Arch. Intern. Med. *29*:131, 1972.

Hedges, T.R.: Visual field defects in exophthalmos associated with thyroid disease. Arch. Ophthalmol. *54*:885, 1955.

Hedges, T.R.: Alternating exophthalmos with pain ophthalmoplegia. Arch. Ophthalmol. *74*:625, 1965.

Helveston, E.M.: A new two-step method for the diagnosis of isolated cyclovertical muscle palsies. Am. J. Ophthalmol. *64*:914, 1967.

Henderson, J.W.: Optic neuropathy of exophthalmos. Arch. Ophthalmol. *59*:471, 1958.

Henderson, J.W.: Relief of eyelid retraction. Arch. Ophthalmol. *74*:205, 1965.

Henderson, J.W., and Schneider, R.C.: The ocular findings in carotid cavernous fistula in a series of 17 cases. Am. J. Ophthalmol. *48*:585, 1959.

Herman, J.S.: Isolated abducens paresis complicating herpes zoster ophthalmicus. Am. J. Ophthalmol. *54*:298, 1962.

Hilel, N., Ouaknine, G., and Kosarv, I.: The abducens nerve, anatomical variations in its course. J. Neurosurg. *41*:561, 1974.

Hitselberger, W.E., and Gardner, G.: Other tumors of the cerebellopontine angle. Arch. Otolaryngol. *88*:712, 1968.

Hotchkiss, M.G., Miller, N.R., Clark, A.W., and Green, W.R.: Bilateral Duane's retraction syndrome. Arch. Ophthalmol. *98*:870, 1980.

Hoyt, W.F., and Keane, J.R.: Superior oblique myokymia. Arch. Ophthalmol. *84*:461, 1970.

Hoyt, W.F., and Nachtigalle, H.: Anomalies of oculomotor nerves, neuroanatomic correlates of paradoxical innervation in Duane's syndrome and related congenital oculomotor disorders. Am. J. Ophthalmol. *60*:443, 1965.

Hunt, W.E., et al.: Painful ophthalmoplegia. Neurology *11*:56, 1961.

Hyans, S.W.: Oculomotor palsy following dental anesthesia. Arch. Ophthalmol. *94*:1281, 1976.

Igersheimer, J.: Visual changes in progresive exophthalmos. Arch. Ophthalmol. *53*:94, 1955.

Isenberg, S., and Urist, M.J.: Clinical observations with Duane's retraction syndrome. Am. J. Ophthalmol. *84*:419, 1977.

Ivy, H.K.: Medical approach to ophthalmopathy of Graves' disease. Mayo Clin. Proc. *47*:980, 1972.

Jackson, W.D., Tolis, G., and Chertman, W.: The TRH test: Its value in the diagnosis of Graves' ophthalmopathy. Can. J. Ophthalmol. *13*:10, 1978.

Jain, N.S.: Interpretation of synkinetic oculopalpebral phenomena in acquired ophthalmoplegias. Am. J. Ophthalmol. *53*:115, 1962.

Jampel, R.S., and Fells, P.: Monocular elevation paresis caused by a CNS lesion. Arch. Ophthalmol. *80*:45, 1968.

Jay, W.M., and Hoyt, C.S.: Abnormal brain stem auditory-evoked potentials in Stilling-Turk-Duane retraction syndrome. Am. J. Ophthalmol. *89*:814, 1980.

Keane, J.R.: Ocular skew deviation. Arch. Neurol. *32*:185, 1975.

Keane, J.R.: Delayed trochlear nerve palsy in a case of zoster oticus. Arch. Ophthalmol. *93*:383, 1975.

Kearns, T.P., and Sayre, G.P.: Retinitis pigmentosa, external ophthalmoplegia and complete heart block. Arch. Ophthalmol. *60*:280, 1958.

Kearns, T.P., and Wagner, H.P.: Ophthalmologic diagnosis of meningiomas of the sphenoidal ridge. Am. J. Med. Sci. *226*:221, 1953.

Kerns, J.J., Smith, D.R., and Alper, M.G.: Third nerve regeneration after aneurysm surgery. Am. J. Ophthalmol. *87*:225, 1979.

Kiloh, L.G., and Nevin, S.: Progressive dystrophy of the external ocular muscles. Brain *74*:115, 1951.

Kissel, J.T., Burde, R.M., Klingele, T.G., and Zeigler, N.E.: Pupil-sparing oculomotor palsies with internal carotid-posterior communicating artery aneurysms. Ann. Neurol. *13*:149, 1983.

Knapp, P.: The surgical treatment of double elevator paralysis. Trans. Am. Ophthalmol. Soc. *67*:304, 1969.

Knauer, W.J.: Gradenigo's syndrome: Review of the literature. Trans. Laryngol. Soc. *50*:110, 1946.

Knox, D.L., Clark, D.B., and Schuster, F.F.: Benign sixth nerve palsies in children. Pediatrics *40*:560, 1967.

Koeppen, A.H.: Abducens palsy after lumbar puncture. Proc. Weekly Sem. Neurol. *17*:68, 1970.

Kornzweig, A.L., and Bassen, F.A.: Retinitis pigmentosa, acanthrocytosis, heredo-degenerative neuromuscular disease. Arch. Ophthalmol. *58*:183, 1957.

Kroll, A.J.: Dysthyroid exophthalmos: palliation by lateral orbital decompression. Arch. Ophthalmol. *76*:205, 1966.

Kuroiwa, Y., and Furukawa, T.: Hemispheric infarction after herpes zoster ophthalmicus: computed tomography and angiography. Neurology *31*:1030, 1981.

Laing, D.: Nasopharyngeal carcinoma in the Chinese in Hong Kong. Trans. Am. Acad. Ophthalmol. Otolaryngol. *71*:934, 1967.

Lakke, J.P.W.F.: Superior orbital fissure syndrome. Arch. Neurol. *7*:289, 1962.

Law, W.R., and Nelson, E.R.: Internal carotid aneurysm as a cause of Raeder's paratrigeminal syndrome. Neurology *18*:43, 1968.

Leopold, I.H.: Local administration of anticholinesterase in ocular myasthenia gravis. Arch. Ophthalmol. *63*:544, 1960.

Lepore, F.E., and Glaser, J.S.: Misdirection revisited. Arch. Ophthalmol. 98:2206, 1980.

Lissell, S.: Supranuclear paralysis of monocular elevation. Neurology 25:1134, 1975.

Lopez, R.I., and Collins, G.H.: Wernicke's encephalopathy: a complication of chronic hemodialysis. Arch. Neurol. 18:248, 1968.

Lowes, M.: Chronic progressive external ophthalmoplegia, pigmentary retinopathy and heart block (Kearns-Sayre syndrome). Acta Ophthalmologica 53:610,1975.

Lyle, D.J.: Experimental oculomotor nerve regeneration. Am. J. Ophthalmol. 61:1239, 1966.

Macoul, K.L., and Winter, F.C.: External ophthalmoplegia secondary to systemic amyloidosis. Arch. Ophthalmol. 79:182, 1968.

Magoun, H.W., and Ranson, S.W.: The central path of the light reflex. Arch. Ophthalmol. 13:791, 1935.

Mahto, R.S.: Ocular features of hypothyroidism. Br. J. Ophthalmol. 56:546, 1972.

Marie, W.G., and Chambers, J.W.: Occlusion of the cerebral dural sinuses. Am. J. Ophthalmol. 61:45, 1966.

Marie, W.G., and Chambers, J.W.: Pseudotumor cerebri syndrome following unilateral radical neck dissection. Am. J. Ophthalmol. 51:605, 1961.

Marit, J., and See, G.: Acute hypervitaminosis A of the infant. Am. J. Dis. Child. 87:731, 1954.

Martins, H.: Treatment of myasthenia gravis with immunosuppressives. Exp. Neurol. 2:321, 1969.

Max, M.B., Deck, M.D.F., and Rottenberg, D.A.: Pituitary metastasis: incidence in cancer patients and clinical differentiation from pituitary adenoma. Neurol. 31:998, 1981.

Mayfield, F.H., and Wilson, C.B.: The pathological basis for postural (intermittent) exophthalmos. J. Neurosurg. 26:619, 1967.

McCormick, W.F., and Rodnitzky, R.L.: Varicella-zoster encephalomyelitis. Arch. Neurol. 21:559, 1969.

McLean, J.M., and Norton, E.W.D.: Unilateral lid retraction without exophthalmos. Arch. Ophthalmol. 61:681, 1959.

McQuillin, M.P., and Johns, R.J.: The nature of the defect in the Eaton-Lambert syndrome. Neurology 17:527, 1967.

Meadows, S.P.: Aneurysms of the internal carotid artery. Trans. Ophthalmol. Soc. U. K. 69:137, 1949.

Meadows, S.P.: Intracavernous aneurysms of the internal carotid artery. Arch. Ophthalmol. 62:566, 1959.

Meadows, S.P.: Temporal or giant cell arteritis. Vol. 4. Neuro-ophthalmology Symposium of the University of Miami and Bascom Palmer Eye Institute. Edited by J.L. Smith. St. Louis, C.V. Mosby Co., 1968. p. 148

Merz, M., and Wojtowicz, S.: The Möbius syndrome. Report of electromyographic examination in two cases. Am. J. Ophthalmol. 63:837, 1967.

Miller, E.A., Savino, P.J., and Schatz, N.J.: Bilateral sixth nerve palsy. Arch. Ophthalmol. 100:603, 1982.

Miller, J.E.: Surgical correction of hypotropias associated with thyroid dysfunction. Arch. Ophthalmol. 74:509, 1965.

Miller, N.R.: Solitary oculomotor nerve palsy in childhood. Am. J. Ophthalmol. 83:106, 1977.

Miller, N.R., Morris, J.E., and Maguire, M.: Combined use of neostigmine and ocular motility measurements in the diagnosis of myasthenia gravis. Arch. Ophthalmol. 100:761, 1982.

Millikan, C.H., and Eaton, L.M.: Clinical evaluation of ACTH and cortisone in myasthenia gravis. Neurology 1:145, 1951.

Millikan, C.H., and Haines, S.F.: The thyroid gland in relation to neuromuscular disease. Arch. Intern. Med. 92:5, 1953.

Nadeau, S.E., and Trobe, J.D.: Pupil-sparing oculomotor palsy: A brief review. Ann. Neurol. 13:143, 1983.

Nemet, P., Ehrlich, D., and Zayar, M.: Benign abducens palsy in varicella. Am. J. Ophthalmol. 78:859, 1974.

O'Donnell, J.J., and Howard, R.D.: Torticollis associated with hiatus hernia. (Sandifer's syndrome). Am. J. Ophthalmol. 71:1134, 1971.

Ogura, J.H.: Transorbital decompression for progressive exophthalmos. Med. Clin. North Am. 52:399, 1968.

Owens, W.C., and Owens, E.U.: Cyclovertical motor anomalies. Am. J. Orthoptic. 5:87, 1955.

Palentine, A.G., Younge, B.R., and Piepgras, D.G.: Visual prognosis in carotid-cavernous fistula. Arch. Ophthalmol. 99:1600, 1981.

Parkinson, D.: Collateral circulation of cavernous carotid artery anatomy. Can. J. Surg. 7:251, 1964.

Parkinson, D.: Transcavernous repair of carotid cavernous fistula. J. Neurosurg. 26:420, 1967.

Parkinson, D., and Shields, C.B.: Persistent trigeminal artery: its relationship to the normal branches of the cavernous carotid. J. Neurosurg. 39:244, 1974.

Parks, M.D.: Isolated cyclovertical muscle palsy. Arch. Ophthalmol. 60:1027, 1958.

Parks, M.D., and Brown, M.: Superior oblique tendon sheath syndrome of Brown. Am. J. Ophthalmol. 79:82, 1975.

Pasik, T., Pasik, P., and Bender, M.B.: Superior colliculi and eye movements. Arch. Neurol. 15:420, 1966.

Pfaffenbach, D., Cross, H., and Kearns, T.P.: Congenital anomalies in Duane's retraction syndrome. Arch. Ophthalmol. 88:635, 1972.

Phelps, C.D., Thompson, H.S., and Ossoinig, K.C.: The diagnosis and prognosis of atypical carotid-cavernous fistula (red-eyed shunt syndrome). Am. J. Ophthalmol. 93:423, 1982.

Phillips, O.C., et al.: Neurologic complications following spinal anesthesia with lidocaine. Anesthesiology 30:284, 1969.

Piemme, E.: Myasthenia gravis and auto-immune disease. Ann. Intern. Med. 60:130, 1964.

Raflo, G.T., Farrell, T.A., and Sioussat, R.S.: Complete ophthalmoplegia secondary to amyloidosis associated with multiple myeloma. Am. J. Ophthalmol. 92:221, 1981.

Records, R.E.: Monocular diplopia. Survey Ophthalmol. 24:303, 1980.

Refsum, S.: Heredopathia atoctica polyneuritiformis, J. Nerv. Ment. Dis. *116*:1046, 1952.

Riley, F.C.: Orbital pathology in Graves' disease. Mayo Clin. Proc. *47*:975, 1972.

Riley, F.C.: Surgical management of ophthalmopathy. Mayo Clin. Proc. *47*:986, 1972.

Robertson, D.M., Hines, J.D., and Rucker, C.W.: Acquired sixth nerve paresis in children. Arch. Ophthalmol. *83*:574, 1970.

Robles, R.: Cranial nerve paralysis after spinal anesthesia. Northwest Med. *67*:845, 1968.

Romano, P.E., and Stark, W.J.: Pseudomyopia as a presenting sign in ocular myasthenia gravis. Am. J. Ophthalmol. *75*:872, 1973.

Rose, A., and Matson, D.D.: Benign intracranial hypertension. Pediatrics *39*:227, 1967.

Rovit, R.L., and Fein, J.M.: Pituitary apoplexy: a review and reappraisal. J. Neurosurg. *37*:280, 1972.

Rucker, C.W.: Paralysis of the fourth and sixth cranial nerves. Am. J. Ophthalmol. *46*:787, 1958.

Rucker, C.W.: The causes of paralysis of the third and fourth and sixth cranial nerves. Am. J. Ophthalmol. *61*:1293, 1966.

Rush, J.A., and Younge, B.R.: Paralysis of cranial nerves 3, 4, and 6. Arch. Ophthalmol. *99*:76, 1981.

Rutkowski, P.C., and Burian. H.M.: Divergence paralysis following head trauma. Am. J. Ophthalmol. *73*: 660, 1972.

Sahs, A.L., and Joynt, R.J.: Brain swelling of unknown cause. Neurology *6*:791, 1956.

Sanders, M.D., and Hoyt, W.F.: Hypoxic ocular sequelae of carotid cavernous fistula. Br. J. Ophthalmol. *53*:82, 1969.

Sandford-Smith, J.H.: Superior oblique tendon sheath syndrome and its relationship to stenosing tenosynovitis. Br. J. Ophthalmol. *57*:859, 1973.

Satoyoshi, E., et al.: Distal involvement of the extremities in ocular myopathy. Am. J. Ophthalmol. *59*:668, 1965.

Schatz, N.J., Savino, P.J., and Corbett, J.J.: Primary aberrant oculomotor regeneration. Arch. Neurol. *34*:29, 1977.

Schneider, R.C., and Johnson, F.D.: Bilateral traumatic abducens palsy. J. Neurosurg. *34*:33, 1971.

Scott, A.B., and Wong, G.Y.: Duane's syndrome. Arch. Ophthalmol. *87*:140, 1972.

Scott, W.E.: Isolated inferior oblique paresis. Arch. Ophthalmol. *95*:1586, 1977.

Sevel, D., and Kassar, B.: Bilateral Duane syndrome. Arch. Ophthalmol. *91*:492, 1974.

Seybold, M.E., and Lindstrom, J.M.: Myasthenia gravis in infancy. Neurology *31*:476, 1981.

Seyfert, S., and Mager, J.: Abducens palsy after lumbar myelography with water-soluble contrast media. J. Neurol. *219*(3):213, 1978.

Shaw, R.E.: Cavernous sinus thrombophlebitis; a review. Br. J. Surg. *40*:40, 1952.

Shin Joong, O.H.: The Eaton-Lambert syndrome. Arch. Neurol. *27*:91, 1972.

Shrader, E.C., and Schlezenger, N.S.: Neuroophthalmologic evaluation of abducens nerve paralysis. Arch. Ophthalmol. *63*:84, 1960.

Slavin, M.L., and Glaser, J.J.: Idiopathic orbital myositis; report of six cases. Arch. Ophthalmol. *100*:1261, 1982.

Smith, J.L.: Raeder's paratrigeminal syndrome. Am. J. Ophthalmol.*46*:194, 1958.

Smith, J.L. and Creighten, J.B.: Sixth nerve palsy due to furadantin. Arch. Ophthalmol. *65*:61, 1961.

Smith, J.L., David, N.J., and Klintworth, G.: Skew deviation. Neurology *14*:96, 1964.

Smith, J.L., and Taxdal, D.R.: Painful ophthalmoplegia: the Tolosa-Hunt syndrome. Am. J. Ophthalmol. *61*:1466, 1966.

Smith, J.L., and Walsh, F.B.: Syndrome of external ophthalmoplegia, ataxia and areflexia. Arch. Ophthalmol. *58*:109, 1957.

Smith, J.L., and Wheliss, J.A.: Ocular manifestations of nasospharyngeal tumors. Trans. Am. Acad. Ophthalmol. Otolaryngol. *66*:659, 1962.

Smith, M.E.: Differential diagnosis of exophthalmos. Int. Ophthalmol. Clin. *9*:918, 1967.

Solomon, O.D., Moses, L., and Volk, M.: Steroid therapy in cavernous sinus thrombosis. Am. J. Ophthalmol. *54*:1122, 1962.

Somers, J.E., Irwin, R.L., and Shy, G.M.: The use of lycoramine derivatives in myasthenia gravis. Neurology *13*:543, 1963.

Sondheimer, F.K., and Knapp, J.: Angiographic findings in the Tolosa-Hunt syndrome. Painful ophthalmoplegia. Radiology *106*:105, 1973.

Spaeth, C.B.: A congenital levator and external rectus muscle internuclear associated reflex. Am. J. Ophthalmol. *33*:751, 1950.

Spencer, W.H., Thompson, H.S., and Hoyt, W.F.: Ischaemic ocular necrosis from carotid-cavernous fistula. Br. J. Ophthalmol. *57*:145, 1973.

Spoor, T.C., Martinez, A.J., and Kennerdell, J.: Dysthyroid and myasthenic myopathy of the medial rectus. Neurology *30*:939, 1980.

Steele, J.C., Richardson, J.C., and Olszewski, J.: Progressive supranuclear palsy. Arch. Neurol. *10*:333, 1964.

Steinberg, D.: Refsum's disease. A recently characterized lipidosis involving the nervous system. Ann. Intern. Med. *66*:365, 1967.

Summerskill, H.J., and Molnar, G.D.: Eye signs in hepatic cirrhosis. N. Engl. J. Med. *266*:1244, 1962.

Sunderland, S.: Mechanism responsible for changes in the pupil unaccompanied by disturbances of extraocular muscle function. Br. J. Ophthalmol. *36*:638, 1952.

Susac, J.O., Garcia-Mullin R., and Glaser, J.J.: Ophthalmoplegia in dermatomyositis. Neurology *23*:305, 1973.

Sutphin, A., Albright, F., and McCune, D.J.: Five cases of idiopathic hypoparathyroidism associated with moniliasis. J. Clin. Endocrinol. *3*:625, 1943.

Tamler, E., and Jampolsky, A.: Is divergence active? An electromyographic study. Am. J. Ophthalmol. *63*:452, 1967.

Trobe, J.D., Glaser, J.S., and Post, J.D.: Meningiomas and aneurysm of cavernous sinus. Arch. Ophthalmol. *96*:457, 1978.

Van Allen, M.W.: Transient recurring paralysis of ocular abduction. Arch. Neurol. *17*:81, 1967.

Victor, D.I.: The diagnosis of congenital unilateral third nerve palsy. Brain *99*:711, 1976.

Victor, M., Hayes, R., and Adams, R.D.: Oculopharyngeal muscular dystrophy, N. Engl. J. Med. 267:1267, 1962.

Von Sallmann, L.: Primary amyloidosis. Ann. Intern. Med. 52:668, 1969.

Vukov, J.G.: Intracavernous aneurysm with isolated sixth nerve palsy. Ann. Ophthalmol. 7:1071, 1975.

Wahner, H.W.: T$_3$ hyperthyroidism. Mayo Clin. Proc. 47:938, 1972.

Walsh, F.B.: Papilledema associated with increased intracranial pressure in Addison's disease. Arch. Ophthalmol. 47:86, 1952.

Walsh, J.P., and O'Doherty, D.S.: A possible explanation of the mechanism of ophthalmoplegic migraine. Neurology 10:1079, 1960.

Warwick, R.: Representation of the extra-ocular muscles in the oculomotor nuclei of the monkey. J. Comparative Neurol. 98:449, 1953.

Warwick, R.: The so-called nucleus of convergence. Brain 78:92, 1955.

Weber, R.B., Daroff, R.B., and Mackey, E.A.: Pathology of oculomotor nerve palsy in diabetics. Neurology 20:835, 1970.

Werner, S.C.: Classification of eye changes of Graves' disease. Am. J. Ophthalmol. 68:646, 1969.

Werner, S.C.: Classification of the eye changes of Graves' disease. J. Clin. Endocrinol. Metab. 29:982, 1969.

Werner, S.C.: The eye changes of Graves' disease. Mayo Clin. Proc. 47:969, 1972.

Wilcox, L.M., and Gittinger, J.W.: Congenital adduction palsy and synergistic diplopia. Am. J. Ophthalmol. 91:1, 1981.

Winand, R.J.: Increased urinary excretions of acidic mucopolysaccharides in exophthalmos. J. Clin. Invest. 47:2563, 1968.

Wolter, J.R., and Clark, R.L.: Ocular involvement in acute intermittent porphyria. Am. J. Ophthalmol. 74:666, 1972.

Wolter, J.R., Hoy, J., and Schmidt, D.M.: Chronic orbital myositis. Am. J. Ophthalmol. 62:292, 1966.

Wybar, K.C.: The nature of endocrine exophthalmos. Bibl. Ophthalmol. 49:119, 1957.

Zakharia, H.S., Osdourian, K., and Matta, C.S.: Unilateral exophthalmos: aetiological study of 85 cases. Br. J. Ophthalmol. 56:678, 1972.

Zauberman, H., Magora, A., and Chaco, J.: An electromyographic evaluation of the retraction syndrome. Am. J. Ophthalmol. 63:1103, 1967.

Zipf, R.F., and Trokel, S.L.: Simulated superior oblique tendon sheath syndrome following orbital floor fracture. Am. J. Ophthalmol. 75:700, 1973.

Chapter *7*

Retinal Disease

The Ocular Fundus: Its Relation to Central Nervous System and Systemic Disease

ROBERT B. WELCH

The specialty of neuro-ophthalmology in its truest sense is based on the effect of disease on the function of intracranial and related intraorbital structures. The eye, which is an anterior extension of the brain, is truly unique, for not only do we see with it, but we can also look inside it. Thus, in the fundus, we may visualize the effect of a lesion of the brain that produces increased intracranial pressure as papilledema, or a lesion involving the cavernous sinus as venous engorgement. Because the eye is also our organ of sight, we may record visual field defects and localize lesions involving the visual pathways, as well as recognize extraocular muscle palsies and chart diplopia fields. A basic understanding of the anatomic relationships of the associated structures of the eye and brain is essential to the diagnostic correlation of the physical signs and symptoms that we as clinicians discover on ophthalmologic examination.

In its broadest sense, neuro-ophthalmology encompasses all the fields of ophthalmology, for even the "super-specialist" must be constantly alert to the fact that his area of interest may be affected by a disease with widespread and protean manifestations. This fact is well illustrated by the extensive coverage of disease entities and syndromes in *Clinical Neuro-ophthalmology* by Walsh and Hoyt and its update by Miller in the fourth edition.

The signs and symptoms of intracranial lesions with respect to ocular motility, visual pathways, the optic nerve, and retinal vasculature are covered elsewhere in this book. This chapter emphasizes a systemic approach to retinal evaluation, considers fundus abnormalities related to systemic disease, such as the phakomatoses, and also considers other abnormalities involved in the differential diagnosis. In addition, diseases involving the optic nerve and its vasculature with common interest

127

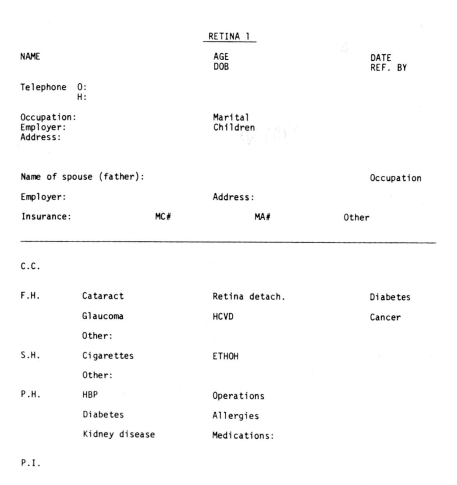

                                    <u>RETINA 1</u>

NAME   AGE   DATE
                                  DOB   REF. BY

Telephone   O:
            H:

Occupation: Marital
Employer: Children
Address:

Name of spouse (father):   Occupation

Employer: Address:

Insurance: MC#   MA#   Other

_____

C.C.

F.H.   Cataract   Retina detach.   Diabetes

          Glaucoma   HCVD   Cancer

          Other:

S.H.   Cigarettes   ETHOH

          Other:

P.H.   HBP   Operations

          Diabetes   Allergies

          Kidney disease   Medications:

P.I.

Fig. 7–1.   The retina flowsheet—a guide to a systematic review of systems and a means to record objective findings.

RETINA 2

NAME

EXAM

				c gl.		
Vision	RE		Reads			
c gl.	LE			s gl.		
s gl.						
Wearing	RE		Add			
	LE					
Ext.	RE		TN	RE	/5.5	/7.5
	LE			LE		
S.L.	RE					
	LE					

Fundus

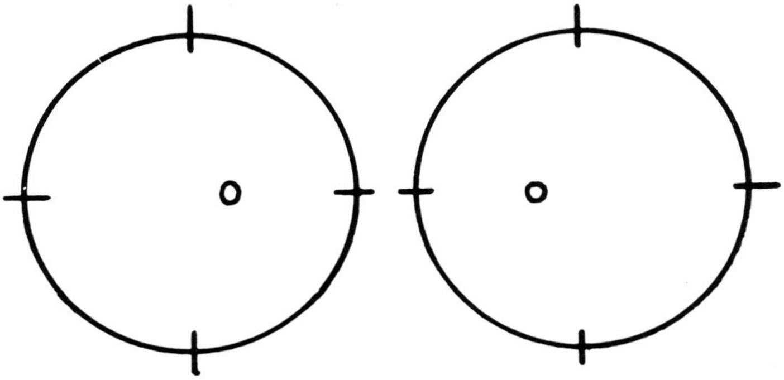

RE   LE

IMP

DISP

C.C.   Address:

Fig. 7–1 *Continued.*

to both neuro-ophthalmologists and retinal specialists are considered.

EVALUATION OF THE OCULAR FUNDUS

Evaluation of lesions of the fundus is often obtained by ophthalmoscopy alone. Although many lesions may be correctly diagnosed, it should be emphasized that this "morphologic approach" often leads to an erroneous diagnosis, whereas a systematic approach to examination might have permitted a correct analysis. The three most important aspects of ocular examination include (1) history taking, (2) examination techniques and instrumentation, and (3) interpretation. All three require expertise and the correlation of the three defines clinical acumen. A proper evaluation of the fundus should include a complete eye examination. A printed eye evaluation form or retina flow sheet (Fig. 7–1) is of value as a means to record data and as a guide to a thorough examination. The examination really begins as the patient enters the examining area, for we have a chance to evaluate his overall physical appearance, and abnormalities may be spotted before he ever sits down (e.g., abnormalities of gait and cutaneous lesions). In gathering preliminary data such as date of birth and occupation, we gain insight into the patient as a functioning individual and we are often alerted to alterations in affect or speech. Our introductory relationship provides us with a "feel for the patient" before beginning the examination.

One of the most important parts of the examination is taking the history. This aspect should include the chief complaint, family history (think genetics), social history (drugs, tobacco, and alcohol), past medical history (a careful systems review), and present illness. Often, at this point in the examination, we begin to formulate possible causes of the patient's problem, which primes our mental processes for what is yet to come.

The ocular examination now begins with visual acuity, refractive error, muscle balance, and external examination. Pupillary function is specifically noted, and the "swinging light" test for afferent pupillary defect is recorded. An undilated slit lamp examination is followed by tonometry and visual field testing (Goldmann perimetry) before dilating drops are instilled. The patient is requested to keep his eyes closed during dilatation, which prevents corneal clouding. When dilated, he is examined by the binocular indirect ophthalmoscope with scleral depression. The 30 D lens (American Bifocal Company, Cleveland, Ohio) is used for scanning the fundus and for examining patients with poorly dilated pupils, while the 20 D lens (Nikon) is used for more detail. Fundus pathology is drawn in the fundus circles on the retina flow sheet or on a standard retina sketch pad with a logical method for covering all aspects of the fundus, e.g., optic nerve, retinal vessels, and choroidal landmarks. The fellow eye should be carefully examined with the same thoroughness, as it often contains a valuable clue (Fig. 7–2). Following indirect examination, the fundus is observed with the direct ophthalmoscope. The dilated patient is now reexamined at the slit lamp where additional studies may be performed with the Hruby, contact, and three-mirror lens. Following this step, tests such as ophthalmodynamometry, transillumination, ultrasonography, and fluorescein funduscopy may be performed as well as fundus photography with or without fluorescein. Interpretation is formulated from a consideration of all the available data.

To summarize, we must learn the technique of indirect ophthalmoscopy and scleral depression to study the fundus adequately. However, it is the man behind the scope who really makes the difference in the long run. He uses history, examination techniques, and available instrumentation to interpret the cause of the problem. Instrumentation is only as advanced as the mind that applies it. We must

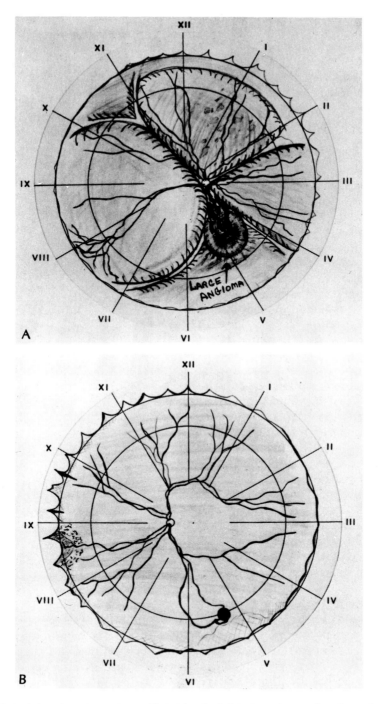

Fig. 7–2. **A.** Retinal drawing of a patient with total retinal detachment secondary to angiomatosis retinae previously undiagnosed. Angioma almost obscured by detachment and vitreous hemorrhage, but dilated vessels from the disc provided a clue, and examination of the fellow eye, **B,** which had been reported as normal, revealed an early angioma.

think when we look and look when we think.

PHAKOMATOSES

The importance of recognizing the phakomatoses is multifold. This term, proposed by van der Hoeve, is of value because of (1) its historical significance, (2) the concept of disease syndromes, (3) its approach to the classification of disease, and (4) its role as a prime example of the need for the cooperation of a variety of medical specialties in the full appreciation of a disease entity.

Van der Hoeve in 1932, in presenting the Doyne Memorial Lecture, correlated various aspects of Bourneville's, von Hippel-Lindau's, and von Recklinghausen's diseases, calling them the phakomatoses. He derived the name from the Greek word *phakos*, "a spot, congenital in orgin, often hereditary and familial in appearance, which can be found in different parts of the human body, either be present at birth or appear later on, which can vary in size, enlarge by proliferation of any part of the tissue, grow to real blastomas and even turn to malignancy, but does not contain nevus-cells." He closed his lecture by stating, "The phakomatoses are worthy of attention of neurologists, psychiatrists, neurosurgeons, surgeons, internists, pediatrists, pathologists, embryologists, teratologists, dermatologists and otologists—that means the whole medical profession—and we saw what a prominent role can be played in it by ophthalmology."

The phakomatoses may thus be regarded as diseases often of dominant autosomal inheritance with irregular penetrance and variable expressivity that affect the eye, brain, and peripheral organ systems. Although originally designated for the previously mentioned syndromes, van der Hoeve and Mahoney added Sturge-Weber disease in 1937. Since this time, various authors have added additional syndromes, so that today the designation, phakomatosis, represents a variable list.

I do not intend to present an in-depth treatment of all these various syndromes, but rather to stimulate an interest in this subject by emphasizing certain salient features.

Terminology of Classification

Van der Hoeve chose the stem word "phakos" carefully. With its use he could designate the individual tumor in its particular organ system as "phakomata," or the grouped anomalies as "phakomatoses." The name *phakomatosis* with its suffix, -osis, implies a syndrome with many symptoms. Since van der Hoeve's day, many authors have suggested other terminology for these syndromes, including heredofamilial neurocutaneous syndromes, neurocutaneous ocular syndromes, and hereditary hamartomatosis. The pathologic concept of hamartoma is important, yet I feel that the term phakomatosis merits retention in our system of classification of disease entities.

CLASSIC PHAKOMATOSES

Four syndromes comprise the classic phakomatoses of van der Hoeve:
1. Tuberous sclerosis (Bourneville's disease)
2. Neurofibromatosis (von Recklinghausen's disease)
3. Angiomatosis retinae and angiomatosis of the central nervous system (von Hippel-Lindau's disease)
4. Encephalotrigeminal or encephalofacial angiomatosis (Sturge-Weber syndrome)

All but Sturge-Weber's disease are of autosomal dominant inheritance with variation in penetrance and expressivity. All are system diseases affecting the brain, eye, and peripheral organs. Cutaneous manifestations are common to all, and a particular abnormality may be found in more than one syndrome, i.e., pheochromocytoma in von Recklinghausen's and von Hippel-Lindau's diseases.

Tuberous Sclerosis (Bourneville's Disease)

Tuberous sclerosis is a hereditary system disease classically manifest by mental deficiency and epilepsy, characteristic cutaneous lesions of the face (adenoma sebaceum), and retinal involvement by translucent mulberry tumors of the optic nerve and superficial retinal layers. Tumors of peripheral organs and other skin lesions may be recognized.

Historic Background

1. Recognized as a pathologic entity by Bourneville in 1880.
2. Triad of mental deficiency, epilepsy, and adenoma sebaceum elaborated by Vogt in 1908.
3. Referred to as epiloia by Sherlock in 1911.
4. Recognized as a familial disease by Berg in 1913.
5. Retinal lesions recognized by van der Hoeve in 1920 and classified as one of his phakomatoses in 1923 and 1932.

Basic Pathology

1. Astrocytic hamartomas (brain and eye).
2. Angiofibromas of the skin (adenoma sebaceum).
3. Hamartomas of peripheral organs

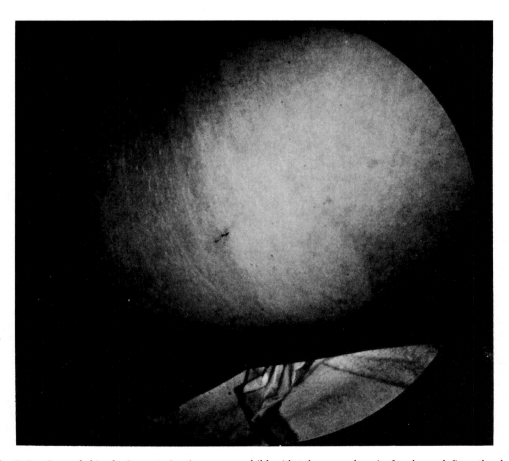

Fig. 7–3. Area of skin depigmentation in a young child with tuberous sclerosis. Its shape defines the designation, mountain ash leaf spot.

(rhabdomyomas, leiomyomas, angiomyolipomas).

Heredity

This autosomal dominant disorder has low penetrance and variable expressivity. Mutation is common enough to account for spontaneous cases, but because of low penetrance, familial cases may be overlooked.

Brain Involvement

Mental deficiency and epilepsy are the result of multiple astrocytic hamartomas of the brain with a predilection for cerebral cortex and periventricular tissue. Involvement of the basal ganglia is common, whereas cerebellar and spinal cord involvement is less frequent. The firm and rubbery consistency of the cortical tumors (potato-like masses) was the basis for Bourneville's designation of tuberous sclerosis. They often arise in the sulcus terminalis and project into the lateral ventricles. Calcification leads to the roentgenographic picture of "brain stones."

Eye Involvement

Astrocytic hamartomas of the optic nerve and retina are of two basic types. (1)

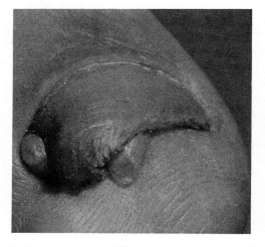

Fig. 7–4. A subungual fibroma in a patient with tuberous sclerosis.

Flat, soft, semitranslucent lesions lying superficial to the retinal vessels (Plate 7–I, Fig. 1) are slightly more frequent than the (2) elevated, solid, mulberry lesions containing calcium that are found at the disc and more rarely in the periphery (Plate 7–I, Fig. 2). The translucent lesions have been observed to change to the solid type with the passage of time, but either type may persist unchanged throughout the life of the individual. Intermediate lesions may be seen as well as areas of depigmentation, hyperpigmentation, and typical choroidal nevi. Patients may show papilledema from increased intracranial pressure. Vision is usually unaffected, but calcification of the hamartomas may cause macular traction, and portions of calcified hamartoma may break off and float in the vitreous to cause symptoms of a vitreous floater.

Skin Lesions

1. Adenoma sebaceum refers to the lesions that occur as symmetric tumors of the cheeks and nasolabial folds of the nose. They may be red and seed-like, or nodular and skin-colored. Rarely present at birth, they usually appear at 6 months of age or later.
2. Shagreen patches ar slightly raised, leathery tan plaques that are often found in the lumbosacral region.
3. Typical café-au-lait spots.
4. Areas of depigmentation—mountain ash leaf spots (Fig. 7–3).
5. Subungual fibromas (Fig. 7–4).

Bone Involvement

This aspect occurs in over 50% of patients and is manifest by cystic changes in the phalanges and cortical thickening of the metatarsal and metacarpal bones.

Peripheral Organ Involvement

Hamartomas of the kidney, heart, spleen, lungs, and uterus have been described. Angiomyolipoma of the kidney is the most frequent form of peripheral organ involvement.

PLATE 7–I

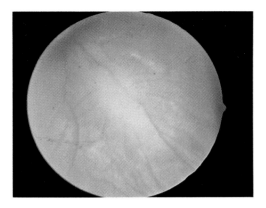

Fig. 1. The soft, translucent type of astrocytic hamartoma in a young child with tuberous sclerosis.

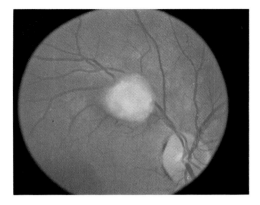

Fig. 2. The elevated, solid type of astrocytic hamartoma in a young female with tuberous sclerosis.

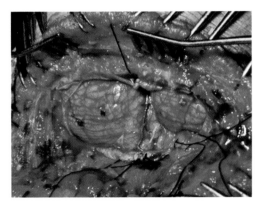

Fig. 3. A 47-year-old white female with a history of von Hippel-Lindau disease developed headaches and projectile vomiting. At surgery, the left cerebellar hemisphere is grossly distended.

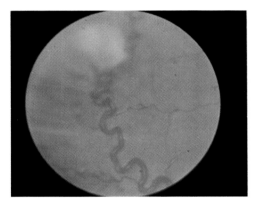

Fig. 4. A 19-year-old white male with a typical angioma of von Hippel-Lindau disease in the temporal periphery.

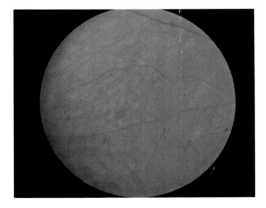

Fig. 5. A 21-year-old white male with early stage I angiomatosis retinae. This lesion did not demonstrate feeder vessels 21 months previously (see Fig. 7–12).

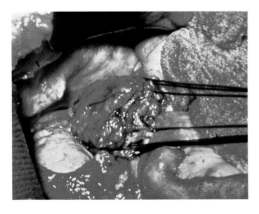

Fig. 6. The surgical removal of a pheochromocytoma from a 19-year-old white female with von Hippel-Lindau disease. This tumor is common in patients with this syndrome and should be considered in every case.

PLATE 7–II

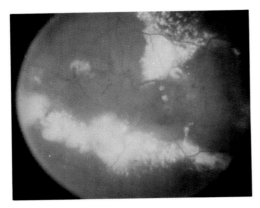

Fig. 1. A 19-year-old white male with Coats' disease of the left eye, with lipid deposition in the macula.

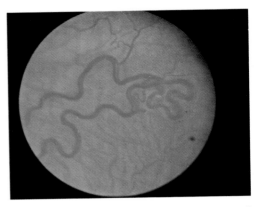

Fig. 2. A 15-year-old black female with a typical racemose aneurysm of the fundus.

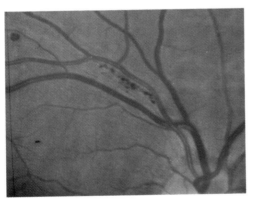

Fig. 3. A 22-year-old white male with a small cavernous hemangioma of the retina (see Figure 7–20).

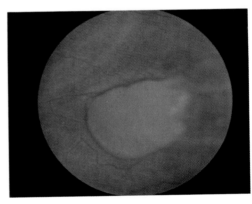

Fig. 4. A sub-internal limiting membrane hemorrhage in a young male with sickle cell hemoglobin C disease, producing a pseudoangioma.

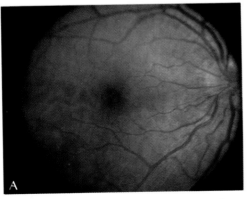

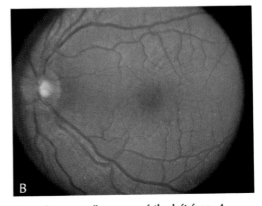

Fig. 5. A young woman with Sturge-Weber syndrome showed a nevus flammeus of the left face. *A.* The right fundus shows normal color and choroidal markings. *B.* The left fundus shows the red velvet appearance of diffuse hemangioma.

Plate 7–III

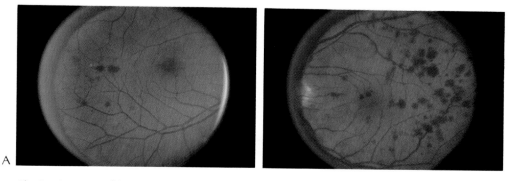

Fig. 1. A 53-year-old white male referred with bilateral hemorrhagic retinopathy. *A.* The right fundus. *B.* The left fundus. Slightest digital pressure blanched the central retinal arteries. The right carotid was 100% occluded, the left 99% occluded.

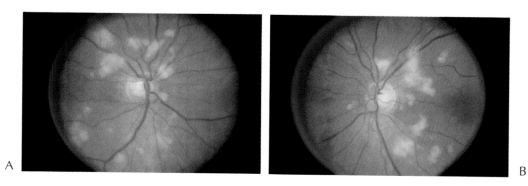

Fig. 2. A 67-year-old white female presented with blurred vision. *A.* The right fundus. *B.* The left fundus. In spite of classic symptoms of scalp tenderness, jaw claudication, and weight loss, 6 previous physicians had failed to make the diagnosis of giant cell arteritis.

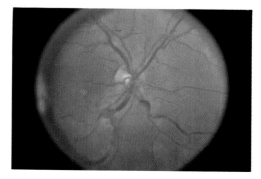

Fig. 3. A 28-year-old white female with papillophlebitis. This resolved in 3 months.

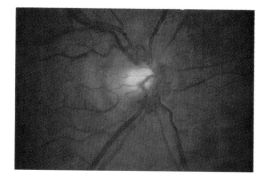

Fig. 4. A 70-year-old white female with shunt vessels of the optic nerve owing to chronic vascular obstruction.

Notable Points

1. This heredofamilial disease of auto-somal dominance has low penetrance an variable expressivity, character-ized by astrocytic hamartomas of the visceral organs.
2. The classic triad of mental deficiency, epilepsy, and adenoma sebaceum should be remembered, but almost 50% overall of patients are not re-tarded.
3. Some 50% of patients with tuberous sclerosis show retinal hamartomas.
4. Of patients with retinal involvement, a little over 50% show flat, semitrans-lucent lesions that may easily be over-looked. Indirect ophthalmoscopy is of benefit in finding these lesions.
5. Just under 50% of the patients with retinal involvement show the solid mulberry calcified lesion, which is usually at the disc margin, but may occur in the retinal periphery.
6. Bilaterality of retinal hamartomas occurs in approximately 50% of pa-tients with retinal involvment.
7. Skin lesions are prominent in this dis-ease. In addition to adenoma seba-ceum, which occurs on the face in the "butterfly area," shagreen patches and mountain ash leaf spots are com-mon.
8. In patients showing high expressivity of the disease, renal hamartomas are almost always found. They are mixed-tissue hamartomas commonly referred to as angiomyolipomas. They are locally destructive and may cause renal signs and symptoms, but do not metastasize.

Differential Diagnosis

1. *Retinoblastoma.* Small retinoblastomas may resemble the astrocytoma of tu-berous sclerosis. Fluorescein angiog-raphy is not of benefit since both le-sions contain capillaries. Careful clinical evaluation and other stigmata of tuberous sclerosis should permit diagnosis.

   Spontaneous regression of retino-blastoma has a cottage cheese ap-pearance and may be confused with the mulberry type of astrocytoma, but the surrounding degeneration in the retina and pigment epithelium seen in retinoblastoma should prevent confusion (Fig. 7–5).
2. *Neurofibromatosis (von Recklinghausen's disease).* Retinal hamartomas indistin-guishable from those in tuberous scle-rosis may be found, but associated stigmata of the two diseases should differentiate them.
3. *Astrocytomas.* The diagnosis of astro-cytomas without evidence of tuber-ous sclerosis is a matter of exclusion by system study and family study.
4. *Drusen of the optic nerves.* When su-perficial, drusen may be confused with the mulberry astrocytoma, but lack of other stigmata and careful evaluation should differentiate the two. No real evidence exists that this condition is a forme fruste of tuberous sclerosis (Fig. 7–6).
5. *Toxocara canis lesions.* Usually solid and smooth, the lesions show evi-dence of previous vitreous reaction and retinal traction folds (Fig. 7–7).
6. Epipapillary membranes and persist-ent hyaloid remnants are present.
7. Congenital hamartomas of the pos-terior pole occur in children and young adults (Fig. 7–8).

These lesions often overlie the disc, show pigment epithelial hyperplasia, and are often confused with toxocara canis le-sions.

Neurofibromatosis (von Recklinghausen's Disease)

This hereditary system disease is mani-fested by tumors of the sheath cells of nerves throughout the body, with associ-ated skeletal abnormalities, cutaneous le-

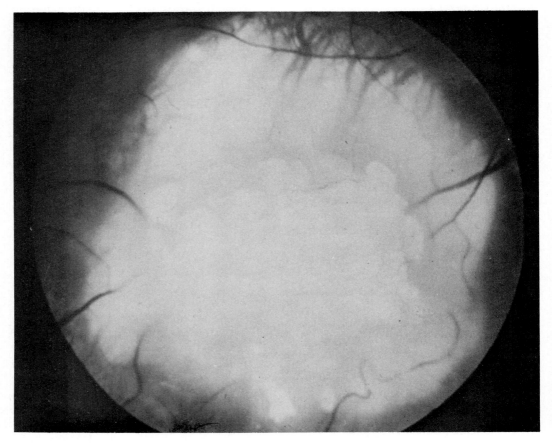

Fig. 7–5. Spontaneously regressed retinoblastoma in a 15-year-old white male. Note surrounding area of degeneration and atrophy as a differential point in distinguishing it from a solid mulberry astrocytoma.

sions, and visceral hamartomas. Multiple tumors of the brain, spinal cord, and meninges, as well as cranial, peripheral, and sympathetic nerve tumors may be encountered. Gliomas of the optic nerve and chiasm as well as meningiomas are associated with this syndrome. Cutaneous involvement is classically represented by café-au-lait spots, while the most characteristic visceral tumor is the pheochromocytoma. It is a disease of protean manifestation, with reference always leading to Schwannean and other neuronal hamartomas.

Historic Background

1. The disease was described by Robert William Smith of Dublin in his treatise on the *Pathology, Diagnosis and Treatment of Neuroma* in 1849, but was not appreciated as a disease syndrome until 1882.
2. In that year, von Recklinghausen presented his classic paper.
3. van der Hoeve included this disease as one of his phakomatoses in 1923 and 1932.

Basic Pathology

Neurofibromas with whorl-like proliferations of Schwann cells produce focal and diffuse thickenings as well as tortuosity of affected nerves. Neurolemmomas, fibromas, hemangiomas, psammomas, and pheochromocytomas occur. Central nerv-

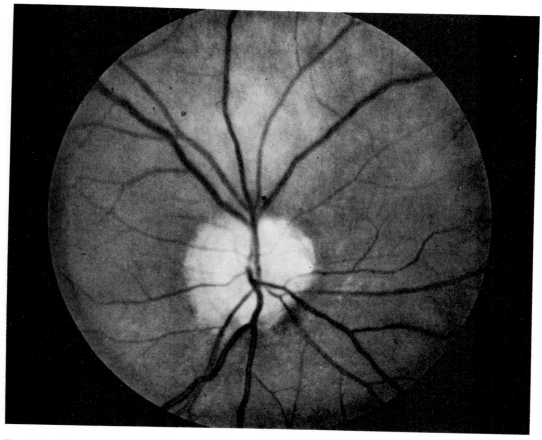

Fig. 7–6. Drusen of the optic nerve in an asymptomatic white female. Evidence does not point toward a forme fruste of tuberous sclerosis.

ous system gliomas, meningiomas, and developmental skeletal abnormalities are a part of the fundamental aspect of this pathologic process.

Heredity

Autosomal dominant inheritance shows high penetrance but variable expressivity. The gene mutation rate is high.

Brain Involvement

Central nervous system involvement is related to developmental anomalies of the bones of the skull and orbit, neuronal hamartomas of the cranial nerves and spinal cord, as well as gliomas and meningiomas. Manifestations show a wide range including exophthalmos or endophthalmos from

defects in orbital bones; optic atrophy and field defects from gliomas and meningiomas; auditory loss from acoustic neuroma; and the spinal cord compression syndrome. Increased intracranial pressure and epilepsy may be associated features.

Eye Involvement

Although fundus involvement in this phakomatosis is relatively rare, various other ocular structures may be involved.

1. Congenital glaucoma may be found, especially when a plexiform neuroma is present on the upper lid.
2. Corneal involvement manifested by thickened corneal nerves may occur alone or in association with other findings, such as the syndrome of

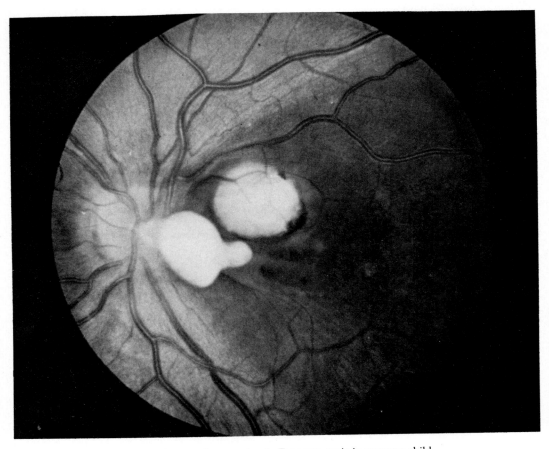

Fig. 7–7. Typical posterior pole granuloma owing to Toxocara canis in a young child.

medullary thyroid carcinoma, pheochromocytoma, and mucosal neuromata.

3. Iris lesions consisting of pigmented nodules may be found, but histologically, these are nevi rather than neurofibromata.

4. Choroidal involvement consists of hamartomas (ganglioneuromelanocytosis, which are usually plaque-like but have been reported to lead to retinal detachment in rare instances. Malignant melanomas have been found in patients with neurofibromatosis but the usual finding is only a typical choroidal nevus.

5. Lid lesions show cutaneous fibroma molluscum as well as plexiform neuromas. Thickening of the lid margins with rostral displacement of the lashes may be a feature.

6. Retinal lesions are manifest by optic atrophy in patients with glioma of the optic nerve as well as by astrocytic hamartomas that are indistinguishable from those seen in tuberous sclerosis. Medullated nerve fibers have been seen in patients with neurofibromatosis.

7. Orbital involvement may be manifest by pulsating enophthalmos or exophthalmos from defects in the bony orbit or proptosis from meningiomas or neurolemmomas within the orbit.

Skin Lesions

1. The café-au-lait spot is the classic lesion and may be the only sign of the

disease. Usually involving the trunk, these macular lesions show hyperpigmentation of the basal layers of the skin from melanocytes.

2. The fibroma molluscum may be found anywhere and is a pedunculated, pigmented nodule composed of cutaneous nerves with proliferation of Schwann cells.
3. The plexiform neuroma commonly seen in the lids is often referred to as a bag of worms. It consists of enlarged nerves with thickened perineural sheath (Fig. 7–9).
4. Elephantiasis neuromata refers to the hemihypertrophy of the face or extremity that is caused by proliferation of Schwannean elements in the dermis.

Bone Involvement

Osseous manifestations are varied and include defects in the bones of the skull and orbit, kyphoscoliosis, irregularity of long bones, and enlargement of the sella (box-like sella).

Peripheral Organ Involvement

Neural hamartomas may occur anywhere, but the classic involvement includes pheochromocytoma and medullary thyroid carcinoma. Cystic lung disease may occur, and endocrine abnormalities such as acromegaly are reported. Parathyroid adenomas and megacolon should be remembered as possible associated features.

Notable Points

1. This heredofamilial disease of autosomal dominance shows high penetrance but variable expressivity. Nerve sheath tumors are its hallmark, with involvement of cranial peripheral and sympathetic nerves.
2. Fundus involvement is unusual, although iris and choroidal nevi are common. Astrocytic hamartomas of the retina similar to those found in tuberous sclerosis are occasionally seen.
3. Gliomas of the optic nerve and chiasm as well as meningiomas may be associated with this syndrome.
4. Café-au-lait spots are the hallmark of cutaneous involvement, although fibroma molluscum and plexiform neuromas are commonly associated.
5. The pheochromocytoma is found in approximately 5% of patients with neurofibromatosis and may be associated with carcinoma of the thyroid in the medullary carcinoma syndrome.
6. Bony abnormalities may be widespread, but defects in orbital bones causing pulsating exophthalmos or enophthalmos are often recognized by the ophthalmologist.
7. Neurofibromatosis is a disease of protean manifestation. Whenever a lesion is thought to be related to neural elements, the syndrome should be suspected.

Differential Diagnosis

1. For neurofibromatosis, the differential diagnosis is the same as that for tuberous sclerosis for fundus involvement, since both may show astrocytic hamartomas of the retina.
2. Pheochromocytomas may be found in both neurofibromatosis and von Hippel-Lindau disease.
3. When seeing patients with malignant melanoma, choroidal nevi, or medullated nerve fibers, remember that all three may be seen in patients with this syndrome.

Angiomatosis of the Retina and Central Nervous System (von Hippel-Lindau Disease)

The third syndrome to be included in the phakomatoses by van der Hoeve is a hereditary system disease involving the retina, cerebellum, and peripheral organs. The classic picture includes hemangioblas-

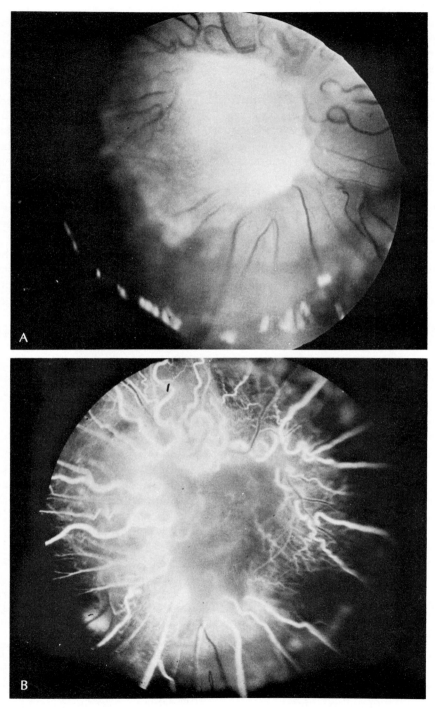

Fig. 7–8. **A.** An elevated lesion involving the optic disc in a 6-year-old child. **B.** Fluorescein angiogram of lesion seen in **A**, showing marked vascularity. The diagnosis was hamartoma vs toxocara lesion.

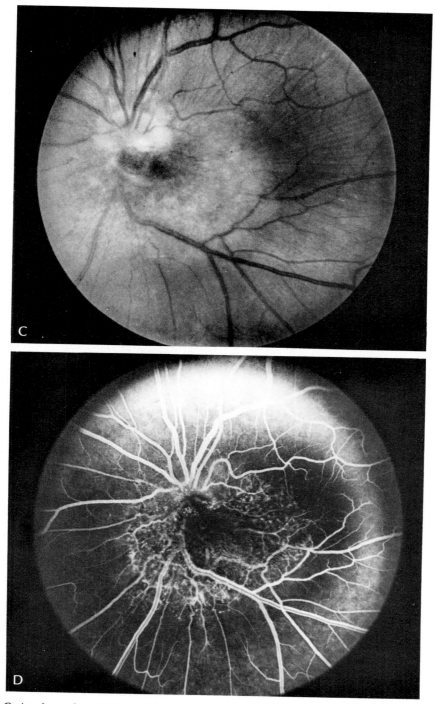

Fig. 7–8. **C.** An elevated partially pigmented elevation over the lower disc in a 19-year-old white male. **D.** Fluorescein angiogram of lesion seen in **C**, showing fine vascular channels. The diagnosis was hamartoma. The patient has been followed for 11 years.

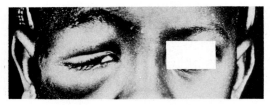

Fig. 7–9.   A young boy with neurofibromatosis with lid involvement.

toma of the cerebellum, leading to cerebellar cyst and increased intracranial pressure; angioma of the retina (angiomatosis retinae), leading to retinal detachment and blindness; and peripheral organ hematomas, such as hypernephroma of the kidney and pheochromocytoma of the adrenal gland. Multiple organ cysts, adenomata, and hemangiomas occur. Nevi, café-au-lait spots, and hemangioma are cutaneous manifestations of this syndrome.

Historic Background

The disease is named for the investigators who emphasized the pathologic features.

1. von Hippel (1867-1939), the ophthalmologist from Halle, Germany, described angiomatosis retinae in his classic paper of 1904.
2. Lindau (1892–1958), the neurologist and pathologist, described the central nervous system involvement in 1926 and recognized the association of the two as a complete syndrome.
3. Previous recognition of features of this syndrome before von Hippel and Lindau should include the names of D.J. Wood, Treacher Collins, Hughlings Jackson, and Harvey Cushing.

Basic Pathology

Hemangioblastomas (capillary angiomas, capillary hamartomas) occur in the cerebellum, medulla, spinal cord, and retina. Histologic evidence of reticulin network is gained by silver nitrate stain (Cushing) in basic lesions of the cerebellum and retina. Peripheral organ hamartomas in-

clude hypernephroma and pheochromocytoma.

Heredity

Autosomal dominant inheritance shows low penetrance and variable expressivity.

Brain Involvement

Almost always below the tentorium, the classic lesion is a hemangioblastoma of the cerebellum with cyst formation (Plate 7–I, Fig. 3; and Fig. 7–10). Involvement of the medulla may lead to syringobulbia, whereas spinal cord involvement, although occasionally causing syringomyelia or spastic paraplegia, is often asymptomatic and found only on autopsy.

Eye Involvement

Angiomatosis retinae is probably the most classic example of fundus involvement in a heredofamilial system disease. The classic retinal lesion is a peripheral angioma fed by a dilated and tortuous artery and vein (Plate 7–I, Fig. 4). Although usually in the periphery, the angioma may occur in the posterior pole (Fig. 7–11) or at the optic disc. Gass has referred to these lesions as endophytic or exophytic, de-

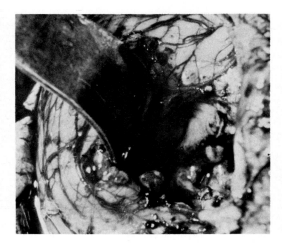

Fig. 7–10.   Patient with von Hippel-Lindau disease (see Plate 7–I, Fig. 3) with retractor in left cerebellar cyst showing mural hemangioblastoma medially.

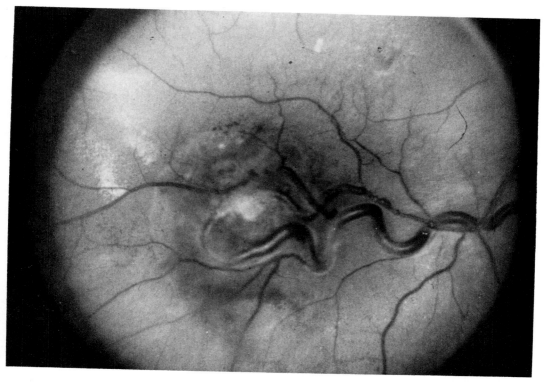

Fig. 7–11. Typical von Hippel angioma lower temporal to the macula in a 26-year-old white male.

pending on the area of the retina from which they arise. When involving the disc or peripapillary area, dilated feeder vessels are usually absent. Although uncommon, it shoud be recognized that angiomas may involve the optic nerve in the retrobulbar region.

The classic literature on angiomatosis retinae has divided the retinal disease into four stages: stage I, angiomas with dilated and tortuous arterial and venous feeders; stage II, angiomas with the development of hemorrhage and exudation; stage III, angiomas with retinal detachment; and stage IV, glaucoma with uveitis and loss of the eye. From my study of this disease, I have reclassified the stages of retinal involvement to include a preclinical or dormant stage, in which ophthalmoscopy or angioscopy reveals tiny angiomas without demonstrable feeder vessels (Fig. 7–12; Plate 7–I, Fig. 5). The clinical stages are:

stage I, small angiomas or capillary clusters with small undilated feeder vessels (Fig. 7–13); stage II, prominent angiomas with dilated and tortuous feeder vessels; stage III, angiomas with hemorrhage, surrounding lipid deposition, and localized detachment, as well as lipid formation in the macula; stage IV, extensive retinal detachment with subretinal lipid deposition; and stage V, end stage deterioration of the eye from glaucoma, inflammation, or phthisis bulbi. Fluorescein angioscopy and photography may be of value in recognizing early lesions as well as a documentation of the angiomatous makeup of the lesion (Fig. 7–14). Disc involvement may be subtle (Fig. 7–15), and the possibility of retrobulbar involvement should not be forgotten.

Skin Lesions

Cutaneous involvement is not a prominent feature of this syndrome, but heman-

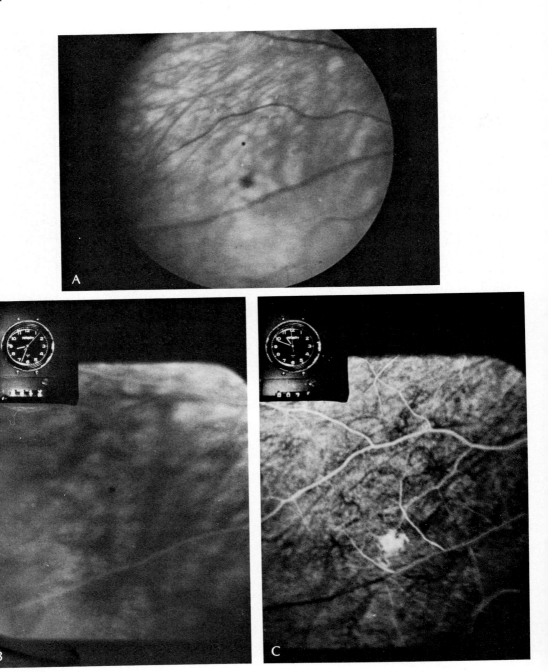

Fig. 7–12. **A.** A preclinical or dormant stage of angiomatosis retinae in a 21-year-old white male. A small reddish nodule is seen in the mid-periphery of the right eye (small black dot is an artifact); no demonstrable feeder vessels. **B.** Fluorescein angiogram of lesion seen in **A** failed to demonstrate feeder vessels. **C.** The same lesion 21 months later now shows definite feeder vessels and fluorescence of the angioma (see Plate 7–I, Fig. 5 for clinical appearance).

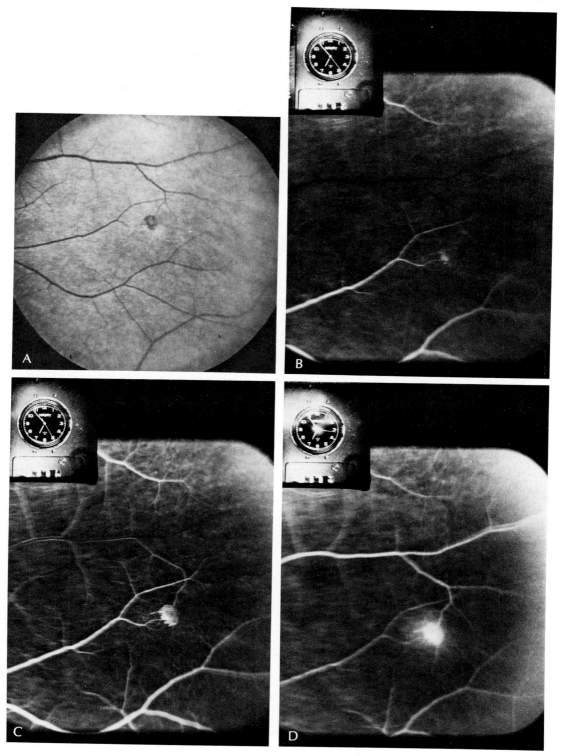

Fig. 7–13. **A.** Stage I angiomatosis retinae (capillary clusters with small undilated feeder vessels) in a 30-year-old white female. **B, C, D.** Sequential fluorescein angiograms showing filling of the lesion.

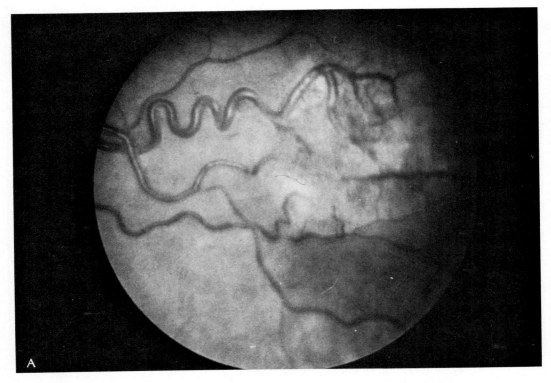

Fig. 7–14. **A.** A large angioma in a 15-year-old white female with stage III angiomatosis retinae.

giomas and café-au-lait spots may occasionally be found.

Bone Involvement

Although this feature is an uncommon aspect of the syndrome, cysts and hemangiomatous involvement have been reported.

Peripheral Organ Involvement

Hypernephroid tumors are a distinctive feature of this disease and include epididymal tumors as well as hypernephroma (renal cell carcinoma) of the kidney. The pheochromocytoma of the adrenal gland is perhaps the most important of all visceral tumors and may be a prominent feature of many pedigrees (Plate 7–I, Fig. 6). Adenomata and cysts may also occur in the pancreas, ovary, spleen, liver, and other organs.

Diagnostic Evaluation

Today, the advancement of computerized axial tomography has made feasible an evaluation of patients for pheochromocytoma and renal cell carcinoma (Fig. 7–16) and cerebellar hemangioblastoma (Fig. 7–17).

Notable Points

1. This heredofamilial disease (in 20% of cases) of autosomal dominance shows low penetrance and variable expressivity. The basic lesion is the multicentric hemangioblastoma (capillary hamartoma) occurring especially in the cerebellum and retina.
2. Hemangioblastomas of the brain make up 2% of all intracranial vascular tumors (Cushing).
3. Twenty-five percent of patients with retinal involvement develop central

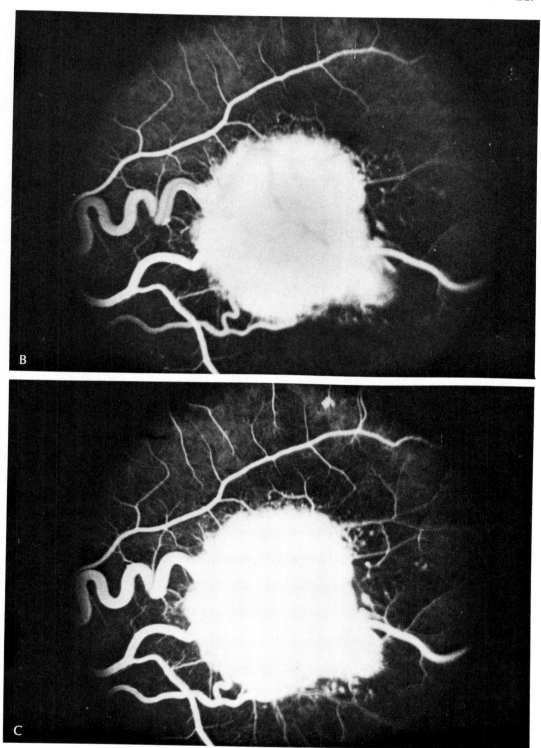

Fig. 7–14. **B, C.** Fluorescein angiograms of the lesion seen in **A.**

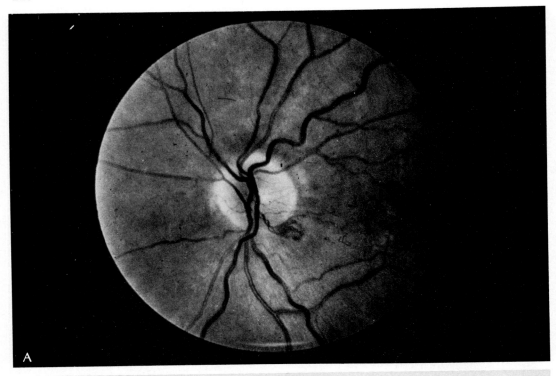

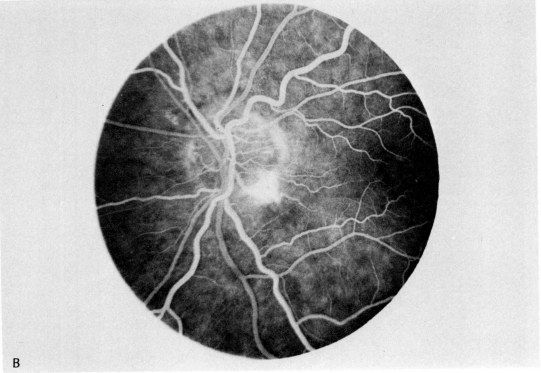

Fig. 7–15. **A.** A small angioma off the disc at 5:30 in a patient with von Hippel-Lindau disease. **B.** Fluorescein angiogram shows filling of the angioma seen in **A.**

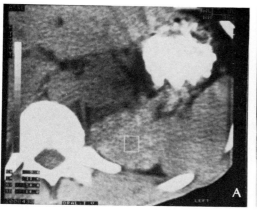
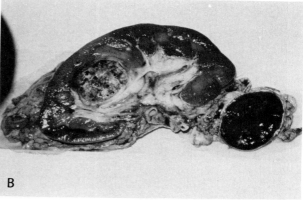

Fig. 7–16. **A.** Body CT of patient with von Hippel-Lindau disease, showing kidney mass and adrenal mass. **B.** Surgical specimen from patient in **A** showing kidney with renal cell carcinoma and adjacent pheochromocytoma.

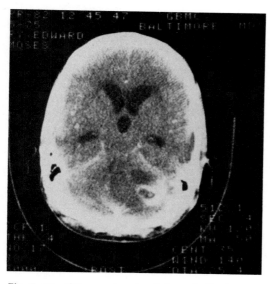

Fig. 7–17. CT scan showing left cerebellar hemangioblastoma.

nervous system disease. The average age for cerebral symptoms is 36 years.

4. Spinal cord hemangiomas are common, but may be asymptomatic and found only on autopsy.

5. The average age for eye symptoms is 25 years; but they may become manifest in childhood or not until the seventh decade.

6. Retinal angiomas are bilateral in 50%

of the cases and multiple angiomas occur in 33% of the cases.

7. Early lesions have often been overlooked, but indirect ophthalmoscopy and fluorescein angioscopy have increased ophthalmic detection.

8. Visceral organ involvement is common, and pheochromocytoma and hypernephroma should always be considered.

9. Cutaneous lesions are not as important as in other phakomatoses, yet hemangiomas of the skin and café-au-lait spots are encountered.

Differential Diagnosis

Lesions with Retinal Lipid Deposition. Since lipid deposition in the fundus is a prominent feature of angiomatosis retinae, every retinal disease process in which this condition may be an associated factor should be considered in the differential diagnosis. Careful attention to details and the entire clinical picture usually make differentiation possible.

1. *Coats' disease (Leber's miliary aneurysms).* In 1908, Coats published his classic paper on forms of retinal disease with massive exudation. From his personal study of six patients, from both clinical and pathologic viewpoints, as well as from a review

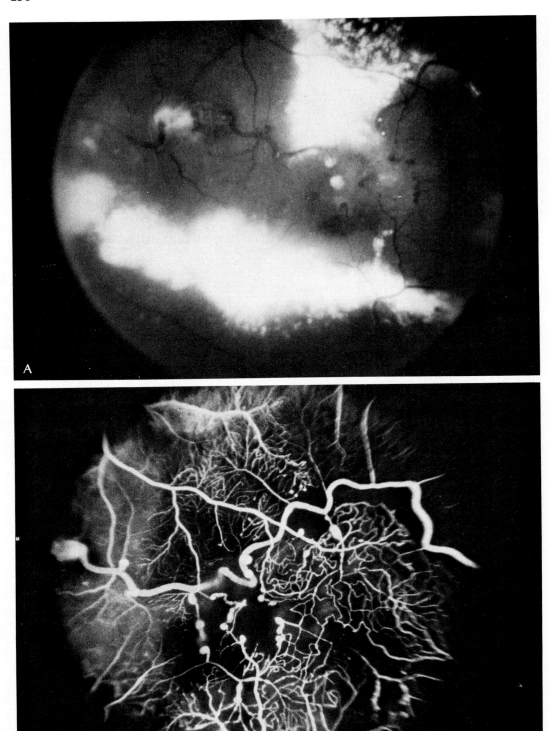

Fig. 7–18. A 19-year-old white male with decreased vision of the left eye from Coats' disease. **A.** Fundus photograph showing telangiectasis and aneurysms. **B.** Fluorescein angiogram of the same area.

of case reports in the literature, he was able to assemble a number of patients whom he divided into three groups: group I, cases without gross vascular disease; group II, cases with gross vascular disease; and group III, cases with arteriovenous communication. All were characterized by the presence, in some parts of the fundus, of an extensive mass of exudation. Coats recognized the similarity of his first two groups in that the disease was almost always found in young people (age 20), with a marked preponderance of males; the right eye was more often affected and it was usually unilateral. His group III, which would soon become recognized as patients with angiomatosis retinae (von Hippel's disease), was different from the other groups, and Coats commented upon this difference. Although the group III conditions occurred in young people, they were

usually bilateral, with no predominance of the male sex. Even in his original article, Coats recognized that the group III cases might well be another entity. Leber and Coats (in a later publication) recognized that group III was a separate entity, thus narrowing the concept of this disease.

My concept is that the designation, Coats' disease (Leber's miliary aneurysms in cases with limited involvement), should be reserved for those cases with a primary retinovascular telangiectasis and aneurysm formation that emanates primarily from the arterial side of the retinal circulation and shows lipid deposition and varying degrees of serous retinal detachment. The abnormality is nonhereditary, probably congenital, usually unilateral, and most commonly found in young males (Plate 7–II, Fig. 1; Fig. 7–18). (Since classic cases are found in females, the latter point

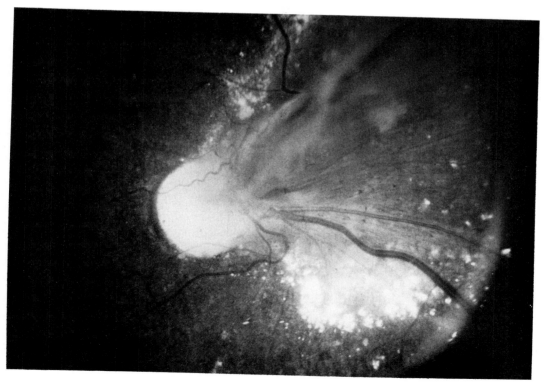

Fig. 7–19. An unusual appearance in the fundus of a patient with sickle cell anemia (SS). Vascular proliferation led to an angiomatous proliferation with a dragged disc and vessels and lipid deposition in the retina.

should not be overemphasized.) Such terms as "Coats' response," "secondary Coats' disease," and "vasculopathy of the Coats' type" are often used in ophthalmic parlance and sometimes criticized by ophthalmic purists. To me, they are good descriptive terms when used by those knowledgable in retinal disease and reflect a true understanding of George Coats' original article.

2. *Pars planitis-like syndrome*. The majority of those with pars planitis do not develop secondary vascular abnormalities that lead to lipid exudation. Nevertheless, certain patients are seen with typical "snow banks" over the peripheral retina and with angiomatous tumefactions, dilated feeder vessels, and subretinal lipid deposition. Some of the patients we have seen appear to have a familial condition, and familial exudative vitreoretinopathy described by Criswick and Schepens may be related. Although some investigators consider neovascularization and lipid deposition a complication of pars planitis, I feel that these cases most often represent another entity.

3. *Intraocular Toxocara canis*. Whether at the posterior pole or in the periphery, discrete lesions do not usually have lipid exudation surrounding them. Typical cases in the periphery with secondary feeder vessels and lipid are occasionally seen, however; and in nematode endophthalmitis with total detachment, lipid is common and the differentiation between Coats' disease and retinoblastoma may be difficult.

4. *Retrolental fibroplasia*. Although not a common feature, a number of these cases develop pseudoangiomatous masses and subretinal lipid depositions.

5. *Retinoblastoma*. Exophytic retinoblastoma with retinal detachment and secondary telangiectasis may simulate an extensive Coats' disease Ultrasonography and evidence of telangiectatic vessels dipping into the subretinal space may help to differentiate the true Coats' disease.

6. *Retinitis pigmentosa with vasculopathy of the Coats' type*. The condition is rare, but has been seen in some 15 cases in the literature.

7. *Congenital retinoschisis*. Hemorrhage into a schisis cavity may lead to circinate lipid surrounding the schisis, with involvement of the macula.

8. *Diabetic retinopathy*. Pseudo-Leber's miliary aneurysms with circinate lipid retinopathy may be a feature of diabetic retinopathy.

9. *Radiation retinopathy*. Another pseudo-Leber's aneurysm, this one shows circinate retinopathy.

10. *Branch vein occlusion*. This occlusion may lead to a pseudo-Leber's picture with circinate lipid involving the macula.

11. *Sickle cell disease*. Lipid exudation is not a feature of the vascular proliferation (sea fans) in sickle cell hemoglobin-C disease or in the vascular proliferation occasionally seen in sickle cell anemia (SS); but rarely, a pseudoangiomatous mass may form with dilated feeder vessels and retinal lipid deposition. (Fig. 7–19).

12. *Retinal macroaneurysms*. These may masquerade as macular degeneration.

13. *Other vascular abnormalities*. These disorders may occur with lipid deposition, such as in sarcoid.

Lesions without Lipid Deposition.

1. *Racemose aneurysms of the fundus*. The dilated vessels are reminiscent of angiomatosis retinae, but no intervening angioma is present (Plate 7–II, Fig. 2). The aneurysms do not leak. This condition is part of the Wyburn-Mason syndrome.

2. *Cavernous hemangioma of the retina (mulberry hemangioma)*. These hamartoma have a characteristic appearance and may be associated with systemic involvement. Fluorescein shows they are somewhat isolated from the retinal vasculature, with slow and incomplete filling (Plate 7–II, Fig. 3; Fig. 7–20).

3. *Lesions associated with arteriosclerosis and hypertension*. Both pseudoan-

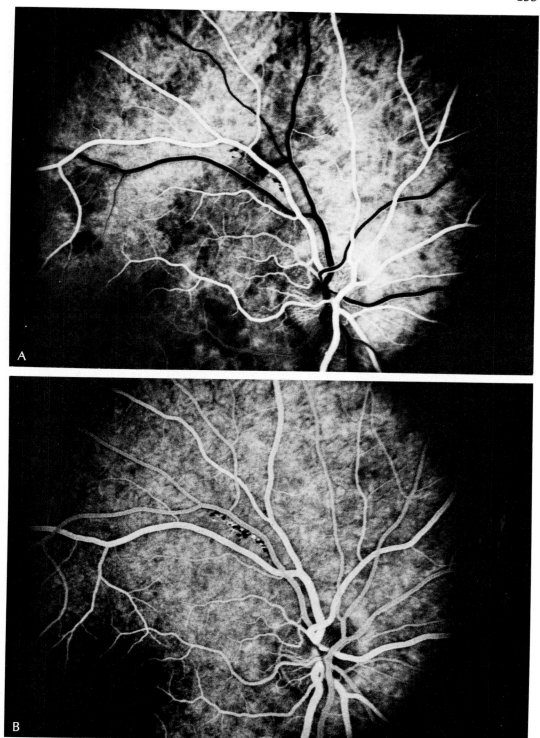

Fig. 7–20. Fluorescein angiograms of a 22-year-old white male with small cavernous hemangioma of the retina (see Plate 7–II, Fig. 3). **A, B, C.** Sequential fluorescein angiograms showing late and incomplete filling of the hemangioma.

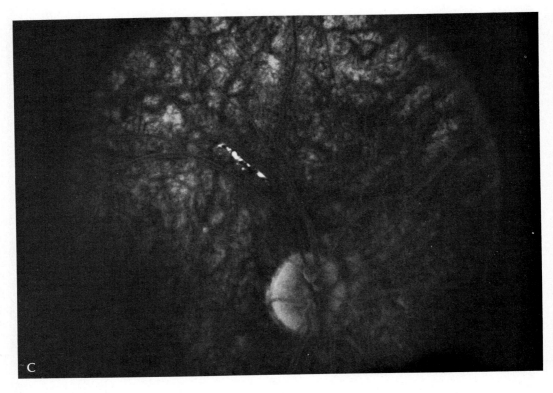

Fig. 7–20 *Continued.*

giomas and microaneurysms may be found and may mimic true angioma or cavernous hemangioma of the retina.

4. *Choroidal hemangiomas.* These lesions may mimic exophytic angiomatosis retinae, especially when they are peripapillary. Fluorescein angiography may help in differentiation.

5. *Peripheral subhyaloid hemorrhage from peripheral disciform lesions.* Hemorrhagic initially, this lesion may become a yellow, tumor-like lesion and persist for years.

6. *Sickle cell disease with pseudoangioma.* large, round hemorrhages under the internal limiting membrane often simulate a retinal angioma (Plate 7–II, Fig. 4). These hemorrhages may also occur intraretinally over a sea fan (Fig. 7–21).

Encephalotrigeminal or Encephalofacial Angiomatosis (Sturge-Weber Syndrome)

The final syndrome to be included as a member of the phakomatoses by van der Hoeve is probably not a heredofamilial disease as are the others. Its characteristic features include (1) port wine stain of the face (nevus flammeus), (2) ipsilateral angiomatous malformation of the meninges and brain with intracranial calcifications and contralateral jacksonian seizure, (3) ipsilateral choroidal hemangioma (both localized and diffuse), and (4) ipsilateral congenital glaucoma.

Historic Background

1. Schirmer in 1860 mentioned buphthalmos and facial hemangioma.
2. Sturge in 1879 described the triad of buphthalmos, facial hemangioma

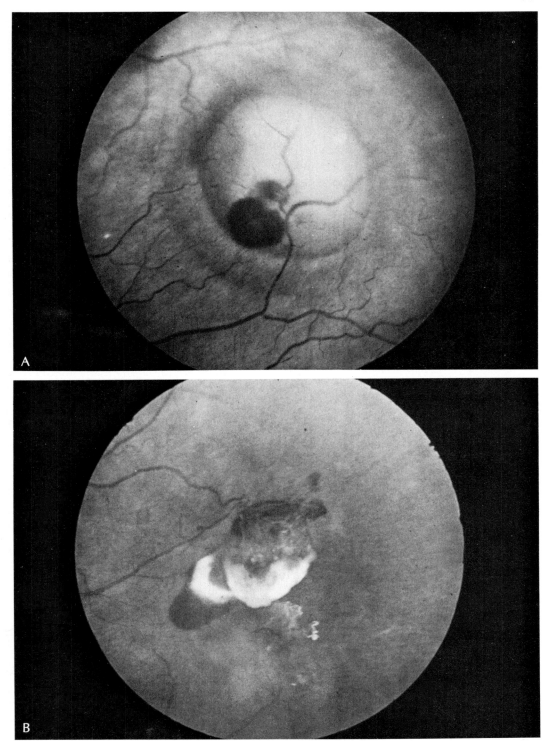

Fig. 7–21. Two patients with sickle cell hemoglobin C disease with pseudoangiomas. **A.** A patient with intraretinal hemorrhage. **B.** A patient with a hemorrhage over a sea fan.

(same side), and contralateral epileptic attacks.
3. Weber correlated the features of the syndrome.

Basic Pathology

Sturge-Weber syndrome is an angiomatous developmental abnormality of mesodermal elements embryologically involved in the development of the vasculature of the face, meninges, and choroid.

Heredity

Unlike the other phakomatoses, no clearcut evidence shows hereditary transmission. Chromosome abnormality has been suggested but not proven.

Brain Involvement

Racemose angiomatous malformations involve the meninges and cortex. These leptomeningeal hemangiomas usually involve the parietal and occipital regions. They occur on the same side as the facial involvement. Calcification of the cortex causes the characteristic "railroad track sign" on roentgenogram. Convulsions are the most common sign of cerebral involvement and contralateral jacksonian seizures usually occur. Mental deficiency may or may not be present.

Eye Involvement

Congenital glaucoma with accompanying angiomatous involvement of the lids is well established. The classic fundus lesion is caused by a choroidal hemangioma, which may be of two types. (1) The most common is the diffuse hemangioma of the choroid, which manifests itself as an overall red velvet texture to the fundus with loss of normal choroidal markings (Plate 7–II, Fig. 5; Fig. 7–22). (2) Localized hemangiomas are less common and are associated with secondary serous detachment of the retina with shifting fluid (Fig. 7–23). Conjunctival and episcleral dilated vessels and heterochromia of the iris also occur (Fig. 7–24).

Skin Lesions

The facial angioma (nevus flammeus) or port wine stain is the hallmark of this syndrome. It involves the areas of the first and second division of the trigeminal nerve and is often associated with telangiectasia of vessels as the patient ages. Hemihypertrophy of the face may be associated (Fig. 7–25).

Peripheral Organ Involvement

Hemangiomas of the orbit and nasal cavities may occur, but widespread organ involvement is not a feature of this disease.

Notable Points

1. The facial angioma (nevus flammeus or port wine stain) is the hallmark of this disease. It may be associated with facial hemihypertrophy.
2. Cerebral involvement is owing to racemose angiomatous malformation of the leptomeninges of the parietal and occipital areas. These disorders may lead to contralateral jacksonian epilepsy.
3. The eye may be involved by congenital glaucoma.
4. The fundus shows choroidal hemangiomas, which may be localized or diffuse. When diffuse, the fundus shows a characteristic red velvet texture.
5. Unlike the other phakomatoses, this syndrome shows little evidence of being a hereditary disease.

Differential Diagnosis

1. Congenital glaucoma occurs in both Sturge-Weber syndrome and neurofibromatosis. Differentiation should not be difficult.
2. Choroidal hemangiomas of the localized type may occur without evidence of Sturge-Weber syndrome.
3. This syndrome is rarely confused with the other phakomatoses.

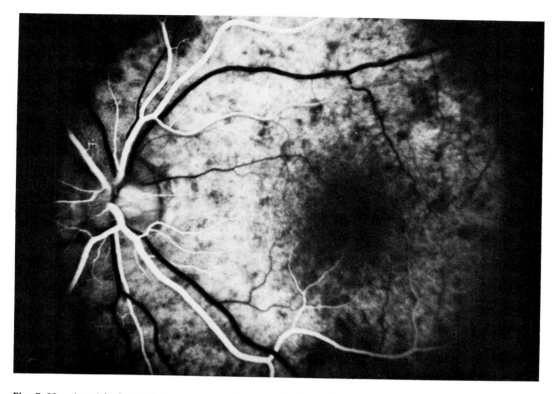

Fig. 7–22. Arterial phase of fluorescein angiogram in left eye of patient with diffuse hemangioma of the choroid. (Plate 7–II, Fig. 5B). Note marked choroidal fluorescence.

EXPANDED PHAKOMATOSES

In recent years, various syndromes have been added to the list of phakomatoses. The inclusion of some seems justified, while others, although of interest, do not really fit into this group.

1. Ataxia-telangiectasia (Louis-Bar syndrome)
2. Arteriovenous aneurysms of midbrain and retina (Wyburn-Mason syndrome).
3. Cavernous hemangioma of the retina (and brain)
4. Klippel-Trenaunay-Weber syndrome
5. Hereditary hemorrhagic telangiectasia (Osler-Rendu-Weber syndrome)
6. Riley's syndrome

A brief comment on some of these diseases seems appropriate from a differential diagnostic viewpoint.

Ataxia Telangiectasia (Louis-Bar Syndrome)

This syndrome is characterized by progressive cerebellar ataxia, oculocutaneous telangiectasis, and chronic infection of the respiratory system. A defect in the immune system is the basic cause of infections, and malignant lymphomas and leukemia are associated findings. Inheritance is autosomal recessive.

Conjunctival telangiectasia is a constant feature. Other telangiectasia may involve the face, ears, and extremities. The neurologic defect begins early in life. This syndrome does not simulate any of the classic phakomatoses.

Arteriovenous Aneurysms of Midbrain and Retina

Racemose aneurysm, cirsoid aneurysm, and Wyburn-Mason syndrome are other

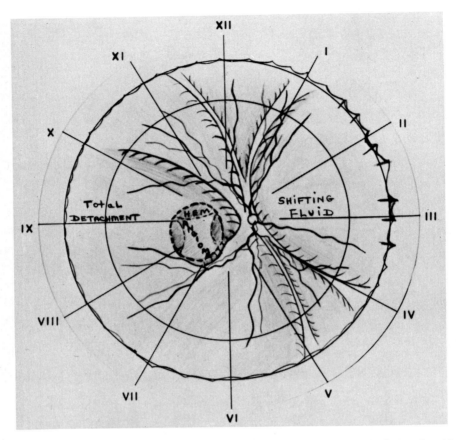

Fig. 7–23. Fundus drawing of a focal hemangioma of the choroid of an 8-year-old white male with Sturge-Weber disease. A total detachment with shifting fluid had occurred.

names used to describe these arteriovenous aneurysms.

The association of racemose hemangioma of the retina and midbrain was emphasized by Wyburn-Mason in 1943. He stated that a high association existed between retinal and brain involvement. Others feel this association has been overemphasized.

The fundus picture consists of unilateral dilated and tortuous arteries and veins that anastomose directly (Plate 7–II, Fig. 2). Vision is often not affected, and the vessels do not leak fluorescein. These patients have been erroneously classified as cases of angiomatosis retinae because of improper fundus evaluation. Epilepsy and intracranial hemorrhage are manifestations of the central nervous system lesions. Arteriovenous malformations of the face, orbit, and maxilla on the ipsilateral side may occur.

Cavernous Hemangioma of the Retina and Optic Disc

This entity is characterized by a mulberry-like cluster of aneurysmal dilations in the retina without demonstrable feeder vessels (Fig. 7–26; Plate 7–II, Fig. 3). The blood within the angiomatous malformation is dark and venous in appearance, and the lesion appears to be isolated from the mainstream retinal circulation by both appearance and fluorescein evaluation (Fig. 7–20). With fluorescein, filling is incomplete, and often the aneurysms show blood

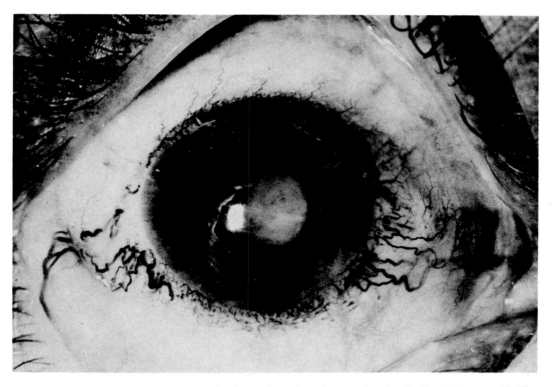

Fig. 7–24. Dilated conjunctival and episcleral vessels in the right eye of patient in Fig. 7–23 at age 19. The eye is blind with cataract, glaucoma, and rubeosis iridis.

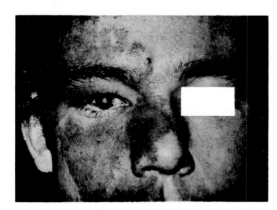

Fig. 7–25. 19-year-old white male with Sturge-Weber disease showing nevus flammeus of the face. Note blind right eye from hemangioma of the choroid with secondary glaucoma and rubeosis iridis.

plasma levels. No surrounding lipid deposition occurs in the retina, and the lesions rarely lead to difficulty other than occasional vitreous hemorrhage. The optic disc may be involved. The condition may be familial (autosomal dominant) and associated with intracranial cavernous hemangiomas as well as angiomatous hamartomas.

Isolated early cases of Leber's miliary aneurysms (before lipid exudation) should enter into the differential diagnosis, but it is unlikely to be confused with Coats' disease, angiomatosis retinae, or racemose angioma. It is easily differentiated by its characteristic fluorescein pattern.

Klippel-Trenaunay-Weber Syndrome

This syndrome is closely related to Sturge-Weber disease. It is inherited as an autosomal dominant and is characterized by angiomatous hamartomas over the

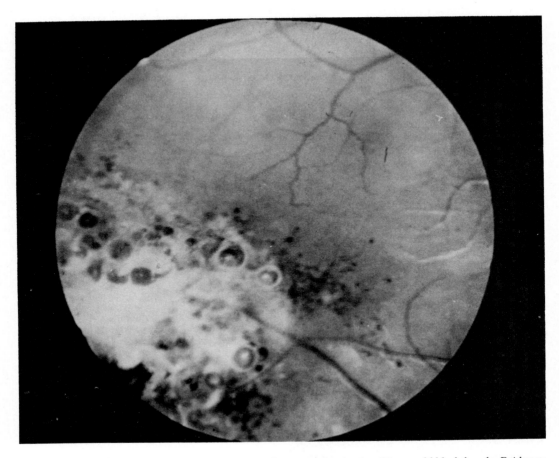

Fig. 7–26. A large cavernous hemangioma of the right temporal retina in a 15-year-old black female. Evidence showed previous hemorrhage with blood in the vitreous.

limbs, with associated varicosities and hypertrophy of bone and soft tissues. Conjunctival telangiectasis and congenital glaucoma have been reported. The hallmark of the disease is angiomatous hamartomas and hypertrophy of the arm or leg.

Hereditary Hemorrhagic Telangiectasis (Osler-Rendu-Weber Syndrome)

This autosomal dominant disease is characterized by telangiectasis of conjunctiva, face mucous membranes, bladder, gastrointestinal tract, lungs, and brain. Conjunctival and cutaneous lesions do not occur until adolescence. Fundus involve-

ment is rare but should be remembered. Bleeding from involved sites alerts attention to the disease.

Riley Syndrome

This autosomal dominant disease is characterized by widespread cavernous hemangiomas associated with macrocephaly and pseudopapilledema.

SUMMARY OF PHAKOMATOSES

The phakomatoses, both the classic four and the expanded group, illustrate most graphically the need for the cooperation of various medical disciplines to fully appreciate a disease entity. In addition to drawing together various specialties of medicine, they also affect every ophthalmic subspecialty, thus reminding us that ophthalmology is still a field of medicine in spite of present day emphasis on various ophthalmic surgical procedures that reflect the rapid advances in technology today. Indeed, it is the very fact of technological advance, as illustrated by such techniques as computerized tomography and ultrasonography that has enhanced the capabilities of the ophthalmologist and kept him in the mainstream of diagnostic medicine.

DISEASES AFFECTING THE OPTIC NERVE AND ITS VASCULATURE
(with common interest to both retinal specialist and neuro-ophthamologist)

Although there should be no sharp delineation between the various subspecialties of ophthalmology, extraordinary technological advances have furthered the trend toward fragmentation of the specialty. The retinal specialist and the neuro-ophthalmologist have, in effect, assumed the role of ophthalmic diagnostician, and since both are primarily referral specialties and since both deal with patients with decreased vision, there is considerable overlap of disease entities referred to each. Thus, the retinal specialist frequently deals with a case of nuclear cataract, optic neuritis, or optic nerve atrophy that is referred to him as a case of "macular disease" with an accompanying request for fluorescein angiography. By the same token, the neuro-ophthalmologist sees patients with bilateral detachments or retinoschisis as cases with "neurologic field defects," and cases of pars planitis as intracranial lesions with papilledema.

The common denominator of interest to both specialties remains the optic nerve and its vasculature, which may reflect a variety of both local and systemic diseases. Because some are life-threatening while others are sight-threatening, this subject should always be at the forefront of differential diagnosis.

Central Retinal Vein Occlusion and Related Conditions

Terminology has caused considerable confusion in this area. Hayreh has divided so-called central retinal vein occlusion into two groups with different clinical and prognostic features. The first is central retinal vein occlusion with retinal ischemia, which he calls hemorrhagic retinopathy, and the second is venous stasis retinopathy, which is self-limited and comparatively benign. Others have referred to this more benign form as partial, incomplete, or impending central retinal vein occlusion (Fig. 7–27). To add to the confusion is the fact that Kearns and Hollenhorst had originally introduced the term venous stasis retinopathy in 1963 to describe the fundus picture associated with carotid artery occlusion. In this incidence, the venous distension, hemorrhages, and cotton-wool spots in the retina may closely mimic the picture of partial or central retinal vein occlusion caused by local disease within the optic nerve as demonstrated by Green in his prospective histopathologic study. In the case of carotid artery occlusion, the differentiation is easy if one considers the possibility that the slightest digital pressure on the globe will cause the central retinal artery to collapse. (Plate 7–III, Fig. 1.)

When evaluating a case of central retinal vein occlusion, it is important to remember that a significant number of individuals will show the presence of glaucoma. In addition, it should be noted in following the patient, that he may develop secondary glaucoma from rubeosis iridis in a far shorter time than the traditional 90-day glaucoma. Since laser therapy may now regress rubeosis, more frequent follow-up visits in the first 90 days seem warranted.

A high percentage of patients with central retinal vein occlusion have hypertension. In addition, a myriad of systemic diseases have been reported to be associated.

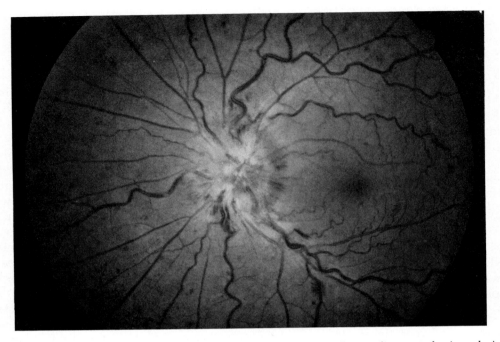

Fig. 7–27. A 67-year-old patient followed for 1½ years, with a picture of impending central vein occlusion.

These range from simple iron-deficiency anemia to more exotic defects in fibrinolytic activity. Whatever the cause, the physician seeing a patient with clinical manifestations of central retinal vein obstruction should touch all bases, but above all, he should rule out carotid artery disease, which may lead to stroke or death.

If the hemorrhagic retinopathy of Hayreh is at one end of the spectrum, then the condition of papillophlebitis described by Lyle and Wybar in 1961 is at the other. This syndrome occurs in young adults and shows variable degrees of optic nerve swelling, engorged retinal veins, retinal hemorrhages, and cotton-wool spots. Visual acuity usually remains good, and the condition resolves spontaneously in most cases. The cause is unknown. Although many think it is an inflammatory vasculitis, others feel it is related to thrombotic and ischemic factors. (Plate 7–III, Fig. 3).

Anterior Ischemic Optic Neuropathy

This condition is basically caused by decreased blood supply to the optic nerve and may be associated with diffuse or local atherosclerosis, diabetes, collagen vascular diseases, temporal (giant cell) arteritis, raised intraocular tension, arterial hypotension, and the post-cataract syndrome. Clinically, the disc is often swollen, and altitudinal defects comprise the most common deficits in visual fields. Although Hayreh distinguishes between anterior ischemic optic neuropathy and posterior ischemic optic neuropathy, the important entity to remember is giant cell arteritis and the fact that it may present in various ways. (Plate 7–III, Fig. 2). History, sedimentation rate, and temporal artery biopsy are small inconveniences compared with the prevention of blindness and, indeed, death.

Chronic insidious decrease in blood supply to the eye has usually been pointed out as a part of the picture of Takayasu's disease or the aortic arch syndrome, with arteriovenous shunts forming around the optic nerve. This disease is rare in this country and anastamotic shunts on the disc that we see usually occur in elderly patients

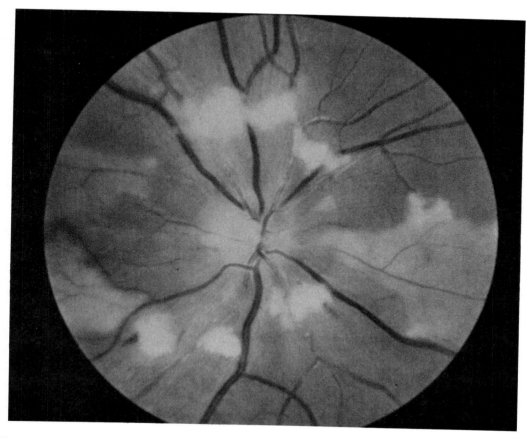

Fig. 7–28. A young patient showing retinal ischemia and cotton wool spots following IV drug injection.

with arteriosclerotic disease (Plate 7–III, Fig. 4) One should always remember the possibility of meningioma, because this may be a cause of opticociliary shunt vessels.

Central Retinal and Branch Arterial Occlusions

The causes of central retinal and branch arterial occlusions are many, but one should always be alert to carotid artery disease with Hollenhorst plaques or platelet emboli, myxomas of the heart, calcific aortic stenosis, cardiac valve involvement, mural thrombi in the heart, giant cell arteritis, hemoglobinopathies (sickle cell disease) and drug abuse or parenteral therapeutic administrations (Fig. 7–28).

SUMMARY OF THE OPTIC NERVE AND ITS VASCULATURE

The optic nerve not only reflects diseases of the central nervous system but also is involved in various vascular and inflammatory diseases, local to the nerve as well as a manifestation of systemic disease. Of primary importance are carotid artery disease and temporal (giant cell) arteritis. One should always think of these entities and perform the simple tests available to rule them in or out. History, which is so often given a short cut in today's technological world, is still a "test" that matches or exceeds CT scans, ultrasonography, or fluorescein angiography on many occasions. The true ophthalmic diagnostician of today uses technology as an adjunct to and not a replacement for basic clinical expertise.

BIBLIOGRAPHY

Berg, H.: Vererbung der tuberösen sklerose durch zwei bzw. drei generationen.Z.Gesamte Neurol. Psychiatrie *19*:528, 1913.

Bird, R.M., et al.: A family reunion: a study of hereditary hemorrhagic telangiectasia. N. Engl. J. Med. *257*:105, 1957.

Bourneville, D.M.: Sclérose tubéreuse des circonvolutions cérébrales: idiote et epilepsie hemiplegique. Arch. Neurol. (Paris) *I*:81, 1880.

Coats, G.: Forms of retinal disease with massive exudation. R. Lond. Ophthalmol. Hosp. Rep. *17*:440, 1907-1908.

Coats, G.: Üeber Retinitis exudativa (Retinitis hemorrhagica externa). Arch. f. Ophthalmol. *81*:275, 1912.

Collins, E.T.: Intraocular growths 1. Two cases, brother and sister with peculiar vascular new growth, probably primarily retinal, affecting both eyes. Trans. Ophthalmol. Soc. U. K. *14*:141, 1894.

Criswick, V.G., and Schepens, C.L.: Familial exudative vitreoretinopathy. Am. J. Ophthalmol. *68*:578, 1969.

Cushing, H., and Bailey, P.: Hemangiomas of cerebellum and retina (Lindau's disease). A.M.A. Arch. Ophthalmol. *57*:447, 1928.

Davies, W.S., and Thumin, M.: Cavernous hemangioma of the optic disc and retina. Trans. Am. Acad. Ophthalmol. Otolaryngol. *60*:217, 1956.

Davis, D.G., and Smith, J.L.: Retinal involvement in hereditary hemorrhagic telangiectasia. Arch. Ophthalmol. *85*:618, 1971.

Duke-Elder, S.: System of Ophthalmology. Vol. X. Diseases of the Retina. St. Louis, C.V. Mosby Co. 1967.

Gass, J.D.M.: Cavernous hemangioma of the retina. Am. J. Ophthalmol. *71*:799, 1971.

Gass, J.D.M.: Angiomatosis retinae (von Hippel's disease. *In* Differential Diagnosis of Intraocular Tumors. A Stereoscopic Presentation. St. Louis, C. V. Mosby Co., 1974.

Gorlin, R.J., et al.: Multiple mucosal neuromas, pheochromocytomas and medullary carcinoma of the thyroid—a syndrome. Cancer *22*:293, 1968.

Green, W.R., et al: Central retinal vein occlusion: A prospective histopathologic study of 29 eyes in 28 cases. Trans. Am. Ophthalmol. Soc. *79*:371, 1981.

Hayreh, S.S.: So-called "central retinal vein occlusion." I. Ophthalmologica (Basel) *172*:1, 1976.

Hayreh, S.S.: So-called "central retinal vein occlusion." II. Ophthalmologica (Basel) *172*:1, 1976.

Hayreh, S.S.: Ischemic optic neuropathy. Concilium Ophthalmologicum, Kyoto *23*:313, 1978.

Jackson, J.H.: A series of cases illustrative of cerebral pathology. Cases of intracranial tumor. Med. Times Gaz. *2*:541, 568, 1872.

Kearns, T.P., Hollenhorst, R.W.: Venous stasis retinopathy of occlusive disease of the carotid artery. Mayo Clin. Proc. *38*:304, 1963.

Klippel, M., and Trenaunay, P.: Naevus variquex osteohypertrophique, J. Pact. *14*:65, 1900.

Lagos, J.C., and Gomez, M.R.: Tuberous sclerosis: reappraisal of a clinical entity. Proc. Staff Meet. Mayo Clin. *42*:26, 1967.

Leber, T.: Über eine durch Vorkommen multipler miliaraneurysmen charakterisierte form von Retinaldegeneration. Arch. f. Ophthal. *81*:1, 1912.

Lindau, A.: Angiomatosis retinae (V. Hippelsche Krankheit). Acta. Pathol. Microbiol. Scand., Suppl. 1, p. 77, 1926.

Louis-Bar, D.: Sur un syndrome progressif comprenant des telangiectasies capillaires cutanées et conjunctivales symétriques a disposition navoide et des trouble cérébelleux. Confin. Neurol. (Basel) *4*:32, 1941.

Lyle, T.K., Wybar, K.: Retinal vasculitis. Br. J. Ophthalmol. *45*:778, 1961.

Miller, N.R.: Walsh and Hoyt's Clinical Neuro-Ophthalmol. 4th Ed. Baltimore, Williams & Wilkins, 1982.

Nyboer, J.H., Robertson, D.M., and Gomez, M.R.: Retinal lesions in tuberous sclerosis. Arch. Ophthalmol. (Chicago) *94*:1277, 1976.

Riley, H.D., Jr., and Smith, W.R.: Macrocephaly, pseudopapilledema, and multiple hemangiomata: A previously undescribed heredofamilial syndrome. Pediatrics *26*:293, 1960.

Schinner, R.: Ein Fall von teleangiekstasie. Arch. f. Ophthalmol. *7*:119, 1860.

Sherlock, E.B.: The Feeble-Minded. A Guide to Study and Practice. London, MacMillan and Co., Ltd., 1911.

Sipple, J.H.: Association of pheochromocytoma with carcinoma of thyroid gland. Am. J. Med. *31*:163, 1961.

Spalter, H.F.: Retinal macroaneurysms: A new masquerade syndrome. Trans. Am. Ophthalmol. Soc. *80*:113, 1982.

Sturge, W.A.: A case of partial epilepsy apparently due to a lesion of one of the vaso-motor centres of the brain. Trans. Clinical Soc. Lond. *12*:162, 1879.

Vail, D.: Angiomatosis retinae, eleven years after diathermy coagulation. Trans. Am. Ophthalmol. Soc. *55*:217, 1957.

van der Hoeve, J.: Eye symptoms in tuberose sclerosis of the brain. Trans. Ophthalmol. Soc. U.K. *40*:329, 1920.

van de Hoeve, J.: Eye diseases in tuberose sclerosis of the brain and in Recklinghausen's disease. Trans. Ophthalmol. Soc. U.K.*43*:534, 1923.

van der Hoeve, J.: The Doyne Memorial Lecture: eye symptoms in phakomatoses. Trans. Ophthalmol. Soc. U.K. *52*:380, 1932.

Vogt, H.: Zur Diagnostik der tuberösen Sclerose. Z. Erforsch Benhandl Jugendl Schwachsinns *2*:1, 1908.

Von Hippel, E.: Euber eine sehr seltene erkrankung der netzhaut. Arch. f. Ophthalmol. *59*:83, 1904.

von Recklinghausen, F.D.: Ueber die multiplen fibrome der Haut und ihre Beizehung zu den multiplen Neuromen. Berlin, A. Hirschwald, 1882.

Walsh, F.B., and Hoyt, W.F.: Clinical Neuro-ophthalmology, 3rd Ed. Baltimore, Williams & Wilkins, 1969.

Weber, F.P.: A note on the association of extensive

haemangiomatous naevus of the skin with cerebral (meningeal) haemangioma, especially cases of facial vascular naevus with contralateral hemiplegia. Proc. Roy. Soc. Med. 22:431, 1928.

Weber, F.P.: Angioma-formation in connection with hypertrophy of limbs and hemihypertrophy. Br. J. Dermatol. 19:231, 1907.

Welch, R.B.: Von Hippel-Lindau disease: the recognition and treatment of early angiomatosis retinae and the use of cryosurgery as an adjunct to therapy. Trans. Am. Ophthalmol. Soc. 68:367, 1970.

Wood, D.J.: Retinal detachment with unusual dilatation of retinal vessels and other changes. Trans. Ophthalmol. Soc. U. K. 12:143, 1892.

Wyburn-Mason, R.: Arteriovenous aneurysm of midbrain and retina, facial naevi and mental changes. Brain 66:163, 1943.

Chapter *8*

Radiology

STEPHEN L.G. ROTHMAN

This chapter is intended to provide a systematic approach to the radiologic evaluation of neuro-ophthalmologic disorders rather than to be an atlas of orbital radiology. To accomplish this purpose, the chapter is divided into a section on normal roentgen anatomy as seen on conventional radiographs, tomograms, orbital angiograms, and computerized tomograms and a section on differential diagnosis of neuro-ophthalmologic disorders. The second section is arranged so as to suggest a sequence of radiographic procedures useful in the evaluation of the various symptom complexes commonly seen in the practice of neuro-ophthalmology.

NORMAL ROENTGEN ANATOMY

The first roentgenographic examination of a patient with possible disease of the orbit usually consists of a series of roentgenograms of the entire skull. These routine views can be supplemented by specialized orbital projections designed for optimal visualization of the orbital walls, optic canals, and superior orbital fissures. Such radiographic projections are frequently named for those who first described them. They are more precisely described, however, by the angle produced

by the central ray of the x-ray beam and the canthomeatal line and the midsagittal plane.

Examination of the Skull

Routine roentgenographic examination of the skull should include at least a posteroanterior projection with the central ray angled 15 to 20° downward with respect to the canthomeatal line (Caldwell projection); a lateral projection; an anteroposterior projection angled downward 25 to 30° to the canthomeatal line (Towne projection); a posteroanterior axial view with the central ray 90° to the mid-sagittal plane (Pfeiffer projection) to visualize the optic canal and superior orbital fissure; and a posteroanterior projection angled 37° downward to the canthomeatal line (Water's view) for visualization of the paranasal sinuses and inferior and lateral margins of the orbit.

(1) Posteroanterior View With a 15 to 20° Caudal Angulation (Caldwell Projection) (Fig. 8–1). This projection permits visualization of the superior orbital structures unobstructed by the petrous ridges. The lesser and greater sphenoidal wings, the superior orbital fissures, the ethmoid sinuses, and the medial orbital wall are seen to advan-

166

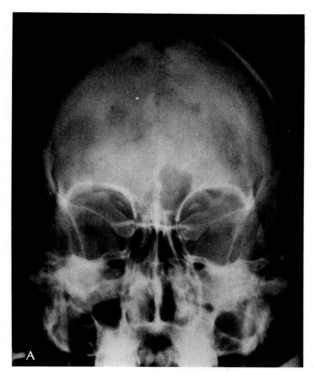

Fig. 8–1. Caldwell projections of the skull. **A**, Radiograph. **B**, Line drawing. (From Meschan, I.: An Atlas of Anatomy Basic to Radiology. Philadelphia, W.B. Saunders Co., 1975.)

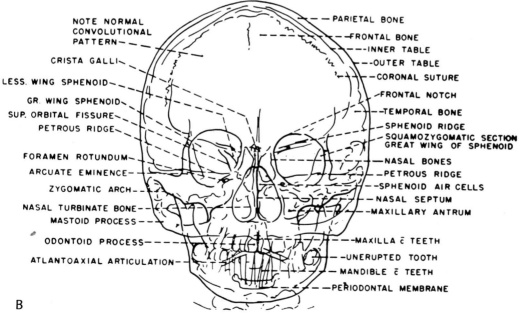

tage. The orbital floors are, however, obscured by the superimposed petrous bones. Intraorbital distance measurements are made in this projection by drawing a horizontal line between the lacrimal bones. Frontal laminography may be required for visualization of the cribriform plate, orbital floor, paranasal sinuses, and superior orbital fissures.

(2) Anteroposterior View With a 25- to 30° Caudal Tube Angulation (Towne Projection) (Fig. 8–2). In this projection, the facial structures are thrown forward off the cranial vault, and the foramen magnum and occipital bones are seen free of overlying bone. The dorsum sellae and posterior clinoid processes project into the foramen magnum and can be clearly identified. The inferior orbital fissure, which is bounded by the orbital surface of the greater sphenoidal wing and the posterosuperior surface of the maxillary sinus, is seen on end. Tumors that arise within the maxillary sinus and invade the orbit and middle cranial fossa frequently destroy the boundaries of the inferior orbital fissure and are best documented in this projection.

(3) Posteroanterior 90° Axial View (Base Projection) (Fig. 8–3). This view is designed for visualizing the base of the skull and its traversing foramina. We can identify the entire length of the ethmoid and sphenoid sinuses as well as the medial and posterolateral surfaces of the maxillary sinuses. The posterior wall of the maxillary sinus is seen as an S-shaped line continuous with the zygoma. Superimposed on the maxilla are two other surfaces. The first, a crescentic line, represents the cranial surface of the greater sphenoidal wing, marking the anterior boundary of the temporal lobes. The second is a flat surface demarcating the orbital face of the sphenoid bone (the posterior orbital wall). Laminography in this projection is the procedure of choice for the assessment of subtle erosive changes of the optic canal, since the entire length of both canals can be seen on a single laminographic section.

(4) Lateral Projection (Fig. 8–4). The lateral view demonstrates the bones of the calvarium, the cranial sutures, and vascular grooves. The sella turcica, one of the most important mirrors of intracranial disease, is evaluated in this position. The zygoma, which forms the lateral orbital rim, and the orbital plates of the frontal bone are also identified. Lateral laminography is most suited for the assessment of the earliest roentgen changes of pituitary tumors and of diffuse increased intracranial pressure. These sections are also important in the evaluation of the floor of the anterior cranial fossa for the presence of meningiomas.

(5) Special Orbital Oblique View (Fig. 8–5). Because of the medial and oblique position of the optic canal, it cannot be seen on the routine views. In the orbital oblique projection, the central ray of the x-ray beam traverses the length of the canal and projects it into the outer inferior quadrant of the orbit. The roof of the optic canal is formed by the lesser sphenoidal wing, and the floor by the optic strut. The size, shape, and configuration of these structures are important in the assessment of diseases of the optic nerve and orbital apex. The optic canal is a tubular structure approximately 8 mm long with a bean-shaped orbital opening and an oblong intracranial end. For optimal visualization, laminographic sections along the full length of the canal may be required.

On occasion, it may be difficult to identify the optic canal in the projection because of the variations in sphenoid pneumatization. A systematic analysis of the radiograph generally minimizes this difficulty. One should begin the search of this film by identifying the planum sphenoidale. It can be seen as a curvilinear structure sweeping across the upper third of the radiograph. In this projection, the planum sphenoidale ends at the anterior clinoid process; the optic canal lies below the planum sphenoidale approximately 0.5 cm proximal to the tip of the anterior clinoid

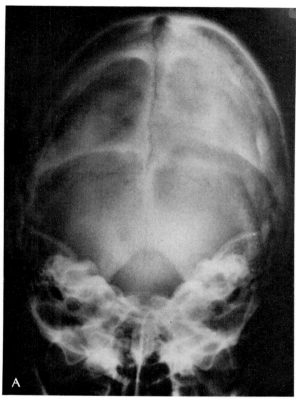

Fig. 8–2. Towne projection of the skull. **A,** Radiograph. **B,** Line drawing. (From Meschan, I.: An Atlas of Anatomy Basic to Radiology. Philadelphia, W.B. Saunders Co., 1975.)

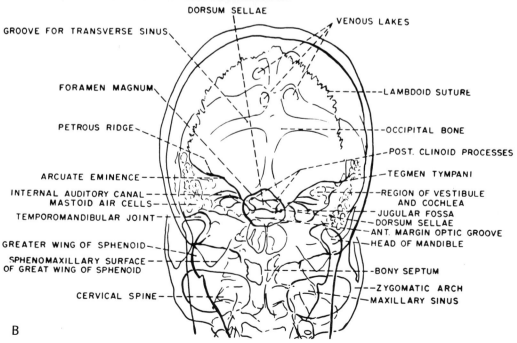

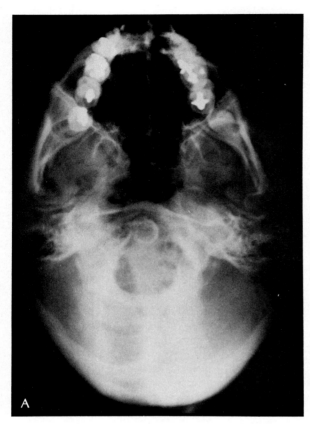

Fig. 8–3. Axial view of the skull. **A,** Radiograph. **B,** Line drawing. (From Meschan, I.: An Atlas of Anatomy Basic to Radiology. Philadelphia, W.B. Saunders Co., 1975.)

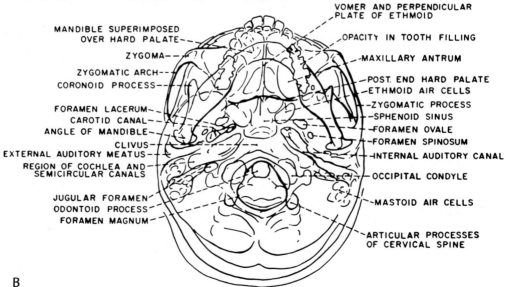

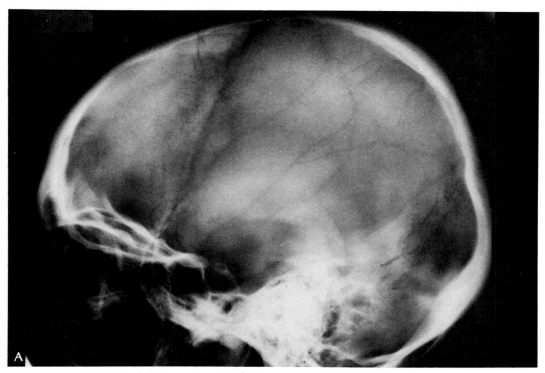

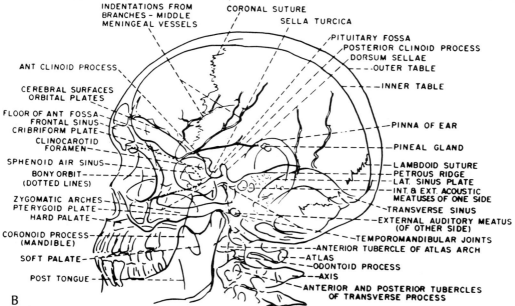

Fig. 8–4. Lateral view of the skull. **A,** Radiograph. **B,** Line drawing. (From Meschan, I.: An Atlas of Anatomy Basic to Radiology. Philadelphia, W.B. Saunders Co., 1975.)

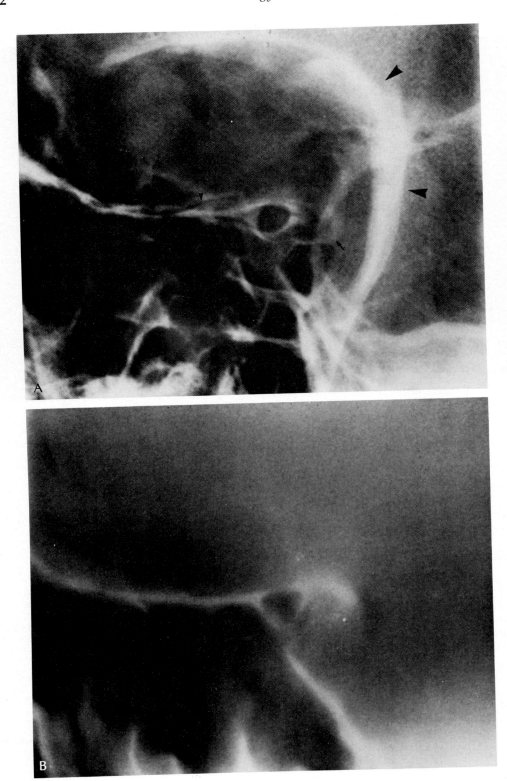

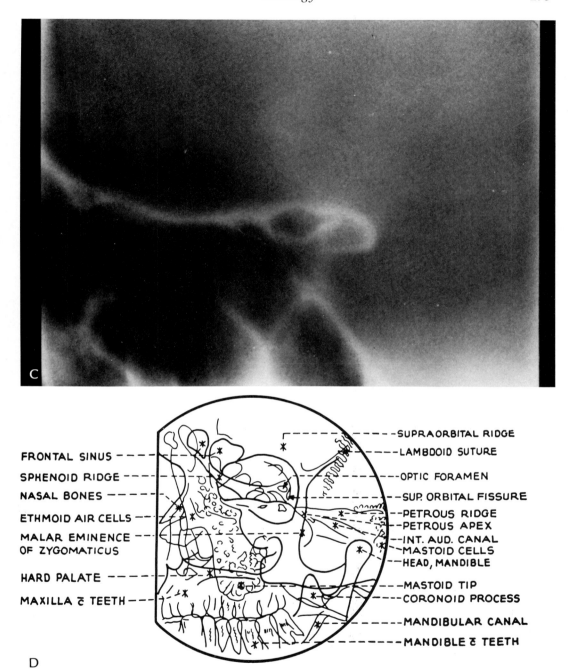

FRONTAL SINUS
SPHENOID RIDGE
NASAL BONES
ETHMOID AIR CELLS
MALAR EMINENCE OF ZYGOMATICUS
HARD PALATE
MAXILLA c̄ TEETH

SUPRAORBITAL RIDGE
LAMBDOID SUTURE
OPTIC FORAMEN
SUP. ORBITAL FISSURE
PETROUS RIDGE
PETROUS APEX
INT. AUD. CANAL
MASTOID CELLS
HEAD, MANDIBLE
MASTOID TIP
CORONOID PROCESS
MANDIBULAR CANAL
MANDIBLE c̄ TEETH

D

Fig. 8–5. Normal orbital oblique projection. **A,** The superior and lateral orbital rims appear as a dense curvilinear structure in the upper outer quadrant of the film (▲). To identify the optic canal, first locate the gentle sweeping curve of the planum sphenoidale (▲). Follow it laterally to its termination in the anterior clinoid process (↑). The optic canal lies approximately 0.5 cm from the end at the anterior clinoid just below the planum sphenoidale. The floor of the optic canal is formed by the optic strut. Just lateral to the optic strut is the superior orbital fissure. Laminograms performed in the oblique projection demonstrate the orbital opening of the optic canal to be bean-shaped, **B,** and the intracranial opening to be oblong, **C.** Labeled diagram, **D.** (From Meschan, I.: An Atlas of Anatomy Basic to Radiology. Philadelphia, W.B. Saunders Co., 1975.)

process. Circular structures closer to the end of the planum sphenoidale usually represent pneumatization of the anterior clinoid process or an ossified caroticocavernous canal.

(6) Posteroanterior View With 37° Angulation (Water's Projection) (Fig. 8–6). This projection is designed for evaluation of the maxillary and frontal sinuses, the fronto-zygomatic sutures, and the orbital floors. Stereoscopic Water's views are ideal for the diagnosis of fractures of the orbital floor and of maxillary tumors.

The next step in the roentgen evaluation of patients with neuro-ophthalmic disorders requires both specialized machinery

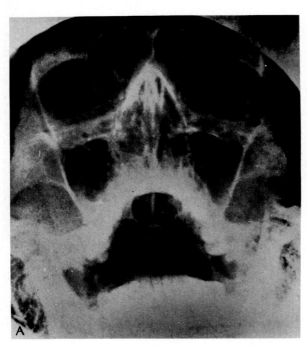

A

Fig. 8–6. Water's projection of the skull. **A,** Radiographs. **B,** Line drawing. (From Meschan, I.: An Atlas of Anatomy Basic to Radiology. Philadelphia, W.B. Saunders Co., 1975.)

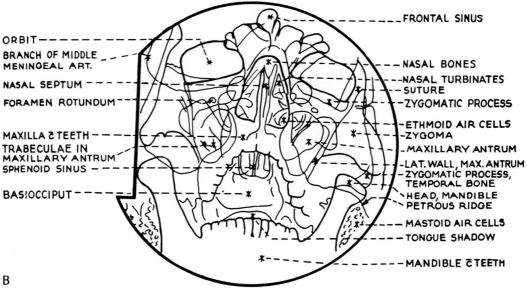

ORBIT
BRANCH OF MIDDLE MENINGEAL ART.
NASAL SEPTUM
FORAMEN ROTUNDUM
MAXILLA C̄ TEETH
TRABECULAE IN MAXILLARY ANTRUM
SPHENOID SINUS
BASIOCCIPUT

FRONTAL SINUS
NASAL BONES
NASAL TURBINATES
SUTURE
ZYGOMATIC PROCESS
ETHMOID AIR CELLS
ZYGOMA
MAXILLARY ANTRUM
LAT. WALL, MAX. ANTRUM
ZYGOMATIC PROCESS, TEMPORAL BONE
HEAD, MANDIBLE
PETROUS RIDGE
MASTOID AIR CELLS
TONGUE SHADOW
MANDIBLE C̄ TEETH

B

and personnel. The two most important procedures are computerized tomography and cerebral angiography. Orbital ultrasound frequently provides useful information on intraorbital structure; however, not being a radiologic procedure, it is not discussed in this chapter.

Normal Computerized Tomogram

With computerized tomography (CT), detailed axial images of the orbit can provide excellent visualization of the intraorbital structures. Generally, two or three 1-cm thick axial sections are produced (Fig. 8–7), clearly defining the globe of the eye, the optic nerves, ocular muscles, intraorbital fat, and the bony orbital walls. CT sections of the brain identify intracranial masses as well as the shape and size of the cerebral ventricles. Properly performed, CT scanning is probably the most important diagnostic procedure in the evaluation of structural disease causing neuro-ophthalmologic symptoms. It has greatly reduced the necessity for other more complex neuroradiologic procedures such as orbital venography and orbital angiography.

Normal Orbital Angiogram

The intraorbital vasculature is evaluated by cerebral angiography. This procedure is usually performed by transfemoral selective catheterization of both internal and external carotid arteries. Complete examination of the orbit generally requires filming in the frontal, lateral, and axial projections (Fig. 8–8) in order to visualize both the cerebral and orbital vasculature.

The normal anatomy of the ophthalmic artery and its branches has been detailed by Vignaud and co-workers. The ophthalmic artery complex is divided into three sections, the first two extraorbital, consisting of an intracranial and intracanalicular segment, and a third intraorbital segment.

The intracranial segment is 0.7 to 9.4 mm in length, arising in most cases from the anteromedial or superomedial aspect of the internal carotid artery, intradurally, approximately at the level of the anterior clinoid process. Rarely, it originates more proximally from the intracavernous portion of the internal carotid artery, in which case it enters the orbit through a separate canal in the optic strut.

The intracanalar segment is that portion within the optic canal that lies in relation to the inferior lateral surface of the optic nerve. Roentgenographically, this portion is usually seen as a straight segment with only minimal undulation. On rare occasions, the extraorbital segment of the ophthalmic artery may be totally absent. The orbital structures are then vascularized via collaterals through the superior orbital fissure by other meningeal arteries.

Of the several schemes for classifying the intraorbital segment, that presented by Vignaud et al. is most suited for a topographic analysis of orbital masses. In this scheme, the intraorbital segment is subdivided into three portions. The first or infraoptic portion runs below the optic nerve within the muscle cone and extends for approximately 10 to 15 mm. It appears as a direct extension of the intracanalicular segment, extending anteriorly and inferolaterally in a straight or slightly undulating course.

The second portion of the intraorbital segment crosses the optic nerve. For pur-

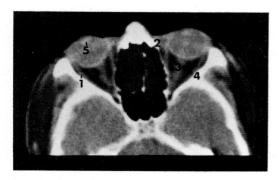

Fig. 8–7. Normal computerized tomogram of the orbits. Computerized tomographic scan through the orbits demonstrate: (1) lateral rectus muscle, (2) medial rectus muscle, (3) optic nerve, (4) orbital fat, (5) lens of eye.

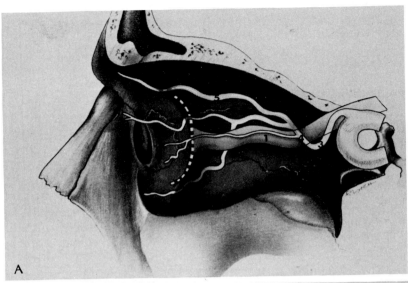

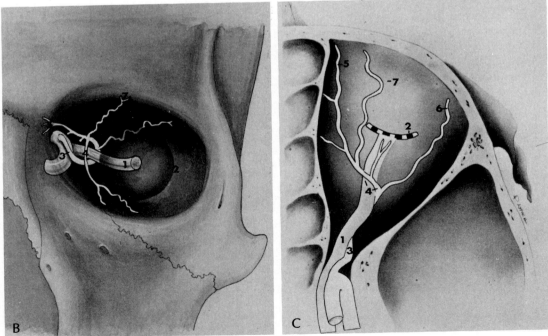

Fig. 8–8.   A, B, C, Diagrammatic representation of the anatomic relationships of the ophthalmic artery. **A,** lateral, **B,** frontal, and **C,** basal projection. (1) optic nerve, (2) choroidal blush, (3) infraoptic portion, (4) circumneural portion, (5) angular artery, (6) lacrimal artery, (7) supraorbital artery. (From Rothman, S.L.G., et al.: Am. J. Roentgenol. *122*:607, 1974.)

poses of later discussion I have proposed the term "circumneural" for this part of the ophthalmic artery. This circumneural portion may have one of three configurations. The most common type is a supraoptic loop in which the ophthalmic artery emerges from beneath the optic nerve on its lateral aspect and ascends around the superior surface of the nerve, ultimately emerging on the medial side where it continues forward perforating the muscle cone to extend along the medial wall of the orbit. On the lateral roentgenogram this loop has the classic "bayonet" appearance. In the frontal view, a well-formed medially directed concave loop is visible. Less commonly, the circumneural portion may present as two varieties of an infraoptic loop. In the first, the ophthalmic artery emerges from below the nerve and ascends directly along the medial side of the nerve. In the lateral view, the ophthalmic complex has an L shape rather than the more usual bayonet. In the frontal projection, no loop entwines the nerve.

In the other variety of infraoptic loop, the ophthalmic artery again emerges on the medial side but ascends in a semicircular direction to the superior surface of the nerve, thereby forming a loop about the medial half of the nerve. In the lateral projection, the bayonet appearance is maintained, but in the frontal view, the circumneural loop is concave laterally.

The third intraorbital portion of the ophthalmic artery is variable and is the most tortuous. The majority of the visualized branches arise from this portion. With certain exceptions, it is difficult to distinguish the small intraorbital branches that arise from the ophthalmic artery owing to the two-dimensional nature of the roentgenogram. The anterior and posterior ethmoidal arteries, the largest medially directed branches, can be detached in the lateral and submentovertical projections. The lacrimal artery, which ascends to vascularize the lacrimal gland, can also be identified in the submentovertical and an-

teroposterior projections where it is seen arising near the first loop of the ophthalmic artery and extending to the superolateral quadrant of the orbit.

When prominent, the supraorbital artery can be recognized because of its egress from the orbit via the supraorbital canal. The main trunk of the ophthalmic artery continues as the angular artery, which can be seen in all three projections. It makes a characteristic loop at the level of the trochlea of the superior oblique muscle where it continues forward and medially.

The characteristic crescentic blush of the choroid layer of the eye was first described by Schurr in 1951 and can be visualized on nearly all cerebral angiograms. No accurate measurements for the position of the choroidal blush are available, and marked variation in position exists. This variability is due in part to the effect of small degrees of rotation on the spatial relationship of the choroid to the more lateral zygomatic arches and more medial tuberculum sellae. The crescentic blush usually appears 3 to 4 seconds after injection of the contrast medium into the internal carotid artery and fades within 4 seconds. The choroidal blush may be seen in the frontal projection. Usually, only the superior and medial surfaces are visualized, but on occasion, the entire circle is seen. In my experience, the choroidal blush is frequently demonstrated in the submentovertical projection. Lateral and medial displacement as well as compression of the globe can be evaluated from this projection. The degree of proptosis is difficult to evaluate in this projection because small changes in the angulation of the head affect the relative position of the choroid.

DIFFERENTIAL DIAGNOSIS

Diseases of neuro-ophthalmologic importance can affect the eye in a variety of ways. Two of the more important presenting signs are exophthalmos and oculomotor dysfunction. The great majority of

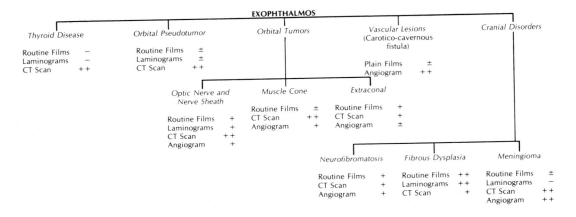

EXOPHTHALMOS

Thyroid Disease	*Orbital Pseudotumor*	*Orbital Tumors*	*Vascular Lesions (Caratico-cavernous fistula)*	*Cranial Disorders*

Thyroid Disease:
Routine Films −
Laminograms −
CT Scan ++

Orbital Pseudotumor:
Routine Films ±
Laminograms ±
CT Scan ++

Vascular Lesions:
Plain Films ±
Angiogram ++

Orbital Tumors → *Optic Nerve and Nerve Sheath*, *Muscle Cone*, *Extraconal*

Optic Nerve and Nerve Sheath:
Routine Films +
Laminograms +
CT Scan ++
Angiogram +

Muscle Cone:
Routine Films ±
CT Scan ++
Angiogram +

Extraconal:
Routine Films +
CT Scan +
Angiogram ±

Cranial Disorders → *Neurofibromatosis*, *Fibrous Dysplasia*, *Meningioma*

Neurofibromatosis:
Routine Films +
CT Scan +
Angiogram +

Fibrous Dysplasia:
Routine Films ++
Laminograms ++
CT Scan +

Meningioma:
Routine Films ±
Laminograms −
CT Scan ++
Angiogram ++

− = Not helpful
± = Rarely helpful
+ = Usually helpful
++ = Most important

disorders initially have at least one of these abnormal findings.

EXOPHTHALMOS

Orbital disorders usually present as exopthalmos or disturbances in orbital motility; however, they may present as both.

Thyroid Disease

Thyroid ophthalmopathy is the most common cause of unilateral exophthalmos. Plain films with laminograms are almost always normal. The diagnosis can be made with a high degree of accuracy on computed tomograms. The hallmark of this disorder is enlargement of the extraocular muscles, seen most prominently as asymmetric expansion of the medial and lateral rectus muscles (Fig. 8–9). Swelling of the superior rectus muscle is somewhat less reliable but may be demonstrated on coronal tomographic sections. The apex of the muscle cone is frequently abnormal as well. This abnormality is best described as a poorly demarcated density at the orbital apex, causing blurring of the normally sharp borders seen between the optic nerve, orbital fat, and extraocular muscles. In the most severe cases, the optic nerve may also be enlarged.

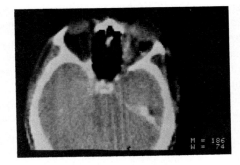

Fig. 8–9. Thyroid ophthalmopathy. Computerized tomographic scan demonstrates asymmetric enlargement of the (1) lateral and (2) medial rectus muscles. These findings are characteristic of thyroid disease.

The clinical severity of the ophthalmopathy appears to closely relate to the muscular changes seen on the CT scan.

Orbital Pseudotumor

Orbital pseudotumor is a heterogeneous group of disorders that may affect any of the orbital structures. Routine roentgenograms and laminograms are generally normal, although rarely, diffuse orbital enlargement can be noted. CT may be extremely helpful in diagnosing this group of disorders and in distinguishing it from Graves' ophthalmopathy. Because of the heterogeneous nature of pseudotumoral

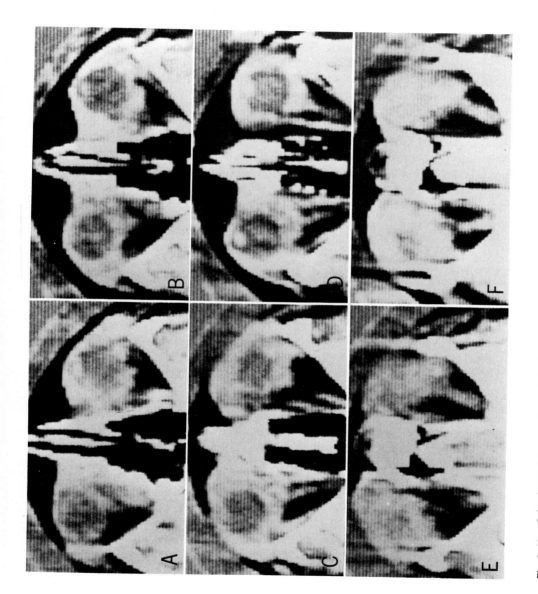

Fig. 8–10. Orbital pseudotumor. Computerized tomography demonstrates well-demarcated masses behind the eye. These masses involve the optic nerve and extraocular muscles as they insert into the globe. (From Enzmann, P., et al.: *Radiology 120:597, 1976.*)

conditions, the CT scan abnormalities are variable. Abnormalities are often asymmetric and are characterized by soft-tissue densities within the orbit. These densities may be attached to the globe of the eye or to the extraocular muscles, or they may fill the retro-orbital space, obliterating normal intraorbital landmarks (Fig. 8–10). These lesions are frequently multiple and involve different portions of the orbit simultaneously. Common sites are the junction of the extraocular muscles and optic nerve with the globe.

When the retro-orbital space is diffusely dense, the roentgen appearance may be indistinguishable from intraorbital neoplasm. Making the distinction is most troublesome in the unilateral form of this disorder.

Orbital Tumors

These tumors can conveniently be divided into three categories: optic nerve and nerve sheath lesions, lesions within the muscle cone, and extraconal muscles.

Optic Nerve and Nerve Sheath Lesions. Concentric enlargement of the optic canal without bony erosion usually indicates an expanding lesion within the canal (Fig. 8–11A). Optic gliomas are the most common lesions causing this deformity. In a series of 41 patients, standard optic canal views were normal in 36%, including several cases in which the tumor was found to invade the hypothalamus grossly. It is therefore suggested that, when an intracanalicular lesion is seriously considered in the differential diagnosis, pluridirectional tomograms be performed, generally in the orbital oblique and base projections. The oblique laminograms provide individual cross-sectional slices along the entire length of the canal, allowing the distinction between the orbital and cranial ends of the canal. Base laminograms are advantageous in that both optic canals are seen simultaneously throughout their entire length and subtle erosive changes can

be detected where none were seen on standard views.

CT demonstrates concentric expansion of the optic nerve by the tumor. Following intravenous injection of iodinated contrast media, the tumor is seen to increase in density (contrast enhance). This examination allows evaluation of intracranial spread of the tumor and can be used with great reliability in following the course of the disease (Fig. 8–11B).

Because of the intimate relationship of the proximal portion of the ophthalmic artery to the optic nerve, lesions of the optic nerve and nerve sheath cause characteristic angiographic changes. The most prominent abnormality is widening of the arterial loop around the optic nerve (Fig. 8–11C, D). The normal range for the width of the loops is from 3 to 7 mm. The muscular branches of the ophthalmic artery may be splayed apart and the vascular blush of the choroidal layer of the eye compressed by the retro-orbital mass.

The differential diagnosis of concentric enlargement of the optic canal includes optic gliomas, meningiomas, neurofibromas, retinoblastomas, neurofibromatosis without intracanalicular tumor, and several other rare causes. The most difficult of these to differentiate are optic gliomas and nerve sheath meningiomas. Occasionally, however, this differentiation is possible. Angiographically, meningiomas may demonstrate tumor neovascularity; on CT, their density increases prominently with intravenous contrast media somewhat more than would be expected with optic gliomata.

Muscle Cone Lesions. Lesions within the muscle cone, especially in children, may produce symmetric enlargement of the orbit because their central location produces centrifugal pressure on growing orbital walls. The most common of these lesions are hemangiomas and neurofibromas. Orbital enlargement is best evaluated on frontal radiographs or laminograms in the Caldwell projection. The orbits are normally symmetric structures, and the width of both orbits, as measured from zygoma to lacrimal bone, should not vary by more than 2 mm. Malignant tumors of the orbit—retinoblastomas, melanomas, and rhabdomyosarcomas—are rapidly growing lesions that rarely cause orbital enlargement. These tumors may escape the muscle cone and invade the orbital walls, causing local irregular destruction.

CT usually demonstrates masses of relatively high density within the orbit separate from the normal extaocular muscles. The optic nerve should be definable as a distinct structure being displaced or distorted by the intraorbital mass.

Angiography demonstrates that the relation of the ophthalmic artery to the optic nerve is maintained within the orbital apex. The circumneural loop is not widened, although the distal intraorbital branches are displaced around the tumor mass. Superior vessels are elevated, interior branches depressed, and lateral branches bowed laterally (Fig. 8–12).

Extraconal Lesions. These lesions produce the most prominent plain film abnormalities because of their proximity to the bony confines of the orbit. This class of tumor can be divided into those that invade from the paranasal sinuses or other distant sources. Some benign processes such as orbital dermoid and lacrimal gland tumors demonstrate characteristic plain film abnormalities. Dermoid and epidermoid tumors usually occur in the superolateral portion of the orbit and occasionally produce a characteristic circumscribed sphenoidal defect with sclerotic margins (Fig. 8–13). Benign lacrimal gland tumors tend to enlarge the lacrimal fossa in the superior lateral quadrant of the orbit. The infiltrative destruction caused by malignant lacrimal gland tumors can occasionally be distinguished from this benign deformity. Other malignant tumors such as neuroblastoma, lymphoma, and metastatic tumors from many sources can cause destruction of orbital bones as they do to bones elsewhere in the body.

Orbital impingement by benign and malignant lesions of the paranasal sinuses can best be evaluated by conventional and computerized tomography. Mucoceles of the frontal or ethmoid sinuses expand these structures with concomitant encroachment upon the orbit. Laminography may demonstrate the presence of inflammatory disease of the paranasal sinuses as well as ballooning of the sinus into the orbit (Fig. 8–14).

Carcinoma of the paranasal sinuses destroys bone. This bony destruction and the associated soft tissue mass are best evaluated by frontal and base tomography (Fig. 8–15B). Orbital extension of these tumors is deduced by this bone destruction, but the extent of intraorbital soft tissue mass can only be seen on CT.

CT performed in the axial and coronal planes is extremely helpful in visualizing the extent of extraconal orbital lesions. The soft tissue extension of sinus carcinomata is easily seen within the orbit (Fig. 8–15C).

Internal and external carotid arteriography has a definite place in the assessment of extraconal lesions. Most paranasal sinus tumors are hypovascular and hence can be visualized only by occlusion and displacement of maxillary and ophthalmic artery branches. When they are hypervascular, tumor stain outlines the intraorbital and intracranial spread of the lesion (Fig. 8–16).

Vascular Lesions

Proptosis owing to orbital venous enlargement has been divided into primary and secondary varices.

Primary   Congenital venous malformation
              Traumatic varices
              Varices in association with a hemangioma

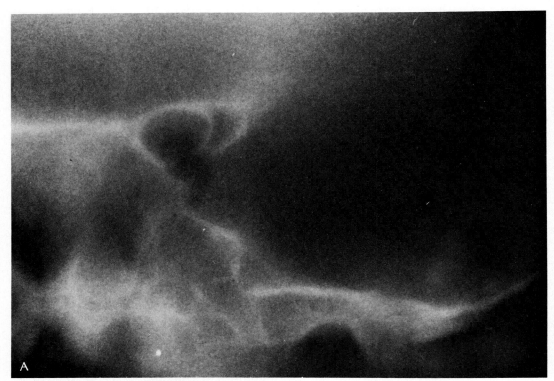

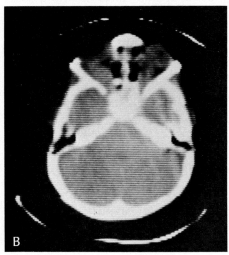

Fig. 8–11.   Optic glioma. **A,** Orbital oblique laminogram. The optic canal is symmetrically expanded by an intracanalicular optic glioma. **B,** Computerized tomographic scan demonstrates bilateral expansion of the optic nerves (↑).

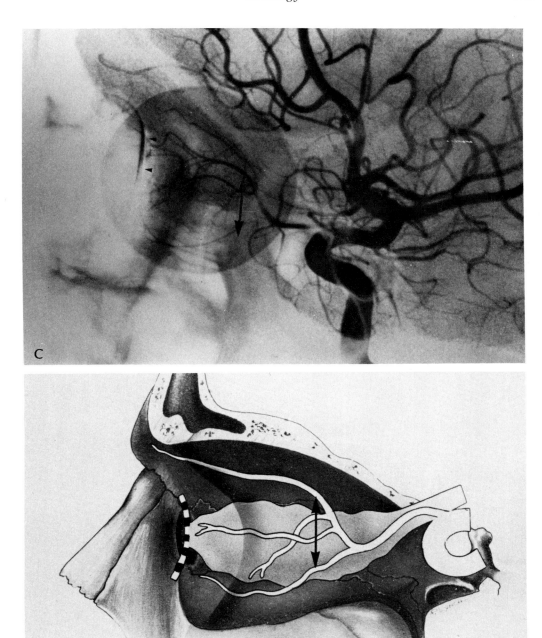

Fig. 8–11. **C, D,** Carotid angiogram. The infraoptic portion of the ophthalmic artery is normal and the circumneural loop is widened (↑). The major branches are swept around the mass, and the choroidal blush (▲) is displaced forward and flattened. The extent of the lesion is delineated by multiple stretched vessels. (From Rothman, S.L.G., et al.: Am. J. Roentgenol. *122:*607, 1974.)

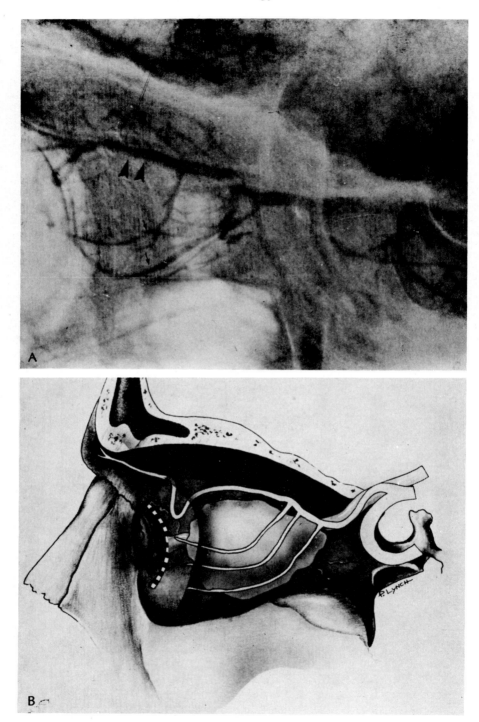

Fig. 8–12.   Muscle cone lesion. Lateral angiogram. **A, B,** The first portion of the ophthalmic artery is normal. The inferior branches (↑) and angular artery (▲) are straightened and stretched, indicating the central position of the mass. (From Rothman, S.L.G., et al.: Am. J. Roentgenol. *122*:607, 1974.)

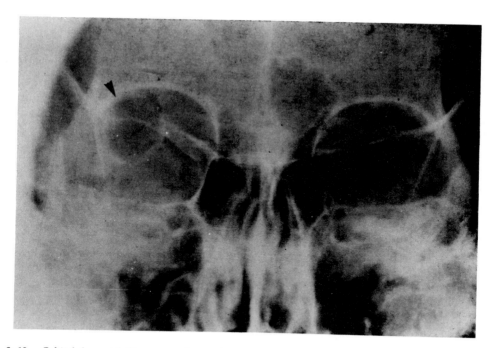

Fig. 8–13. Orbital dermoid. These growths produce a well-marginated lucency in the upper outer quadrant of the orbit (▲). This abnormality is seen in a minority of cases but is characteristic when present.

Secondary   Carotico-cavernous fistula
               Arteriovenous malformation

Congenital Venous Malformations. Congenital venous malformations, the most common primary varices, are usually seen in children and growing adults. A characteristic triad of plain film abnormalities, diffuse orbital enlargement, intraorbital phleboliths, and large venous channels in the frontal bone, are occasionally present.

The diagnosis is made on orbital venography where saccular dilatation of some or a majority of the tributaries of superior or inferior ophthalmic veins is diagnostic.

Orbital Hemangiomas. Orbital hemangioma is the most common intraorbital tumor and, like congenital venous malformation, usually occurs in children and growing adults. Most of these lesions occur within the muscle cone and therefore may cause diffuse orbital enlargement. Tumors outside the muscle cone may cause asym-

metric enlargement with local bone destruction.

CT scanning demonstrates contrast-enhancing masses within the orbit indistinguishable from other intraorbital tumors.

The afferent arterial supply to hemangiomas is usually sparse and, not uncommonly, is normal. Intraorbital vascular displacement depends on the precise location of the tumor. The venous phase of the arteriogram may reveal enlarged, tortuous venous channels that remain filled for a prolonged period of time (Fig. 8–17). Occasionally, the abnormal venous channels fail to fill on cerebral angiography and require orbital venography to opacify the lesions.

Carotico-Cavernous Fistulas. Caroticocavernous fistulas may be traumatic, arteriosclerotic, or congenital. In the full-blown syndrome, marked enlargement of the superior ophthalmic vein accompanies expansion of the superior orbital fissure. The borders of the fissure, although enlarged,

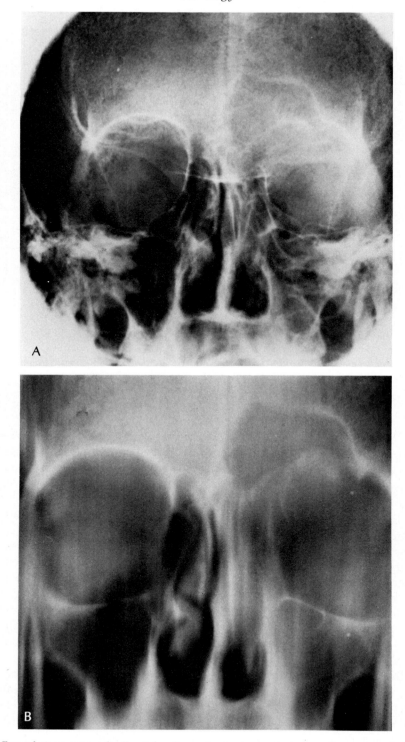

Fig. 8–14.   Frontal sinus mucocele. Frontal radiograph, **A,** demonstrates a well-marginated, irregular lytic area above the medial portion of the orbital rim. Laminographic section, **B,** shows destruction of the orbital roof by the expanding collection of pus under pressure.

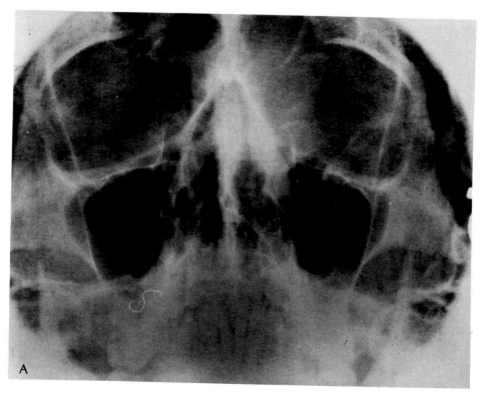

Fig. 8–15.   Carcinoma of the ethmoid sinus. Radiograph in the Water's projection. **A,** demonstrates opacity of the ethmoid sinus (▲).

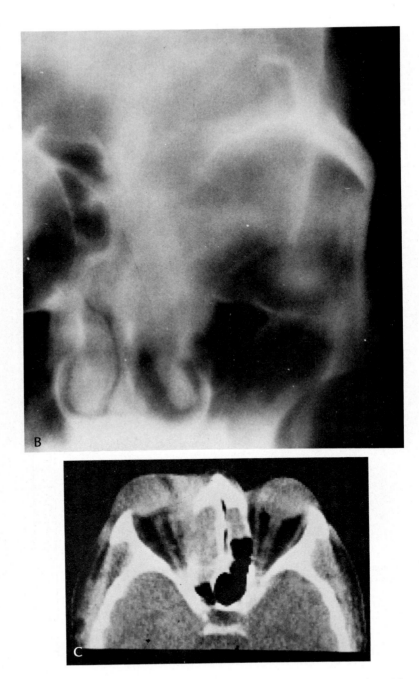

Fig. 8–15. Frontal laminography, **B,** defines destruction of the medial wall of the orbit and extension of the tumor into the frontal sinus. Computerized tomography, **C,** identifies a tumor mass displacing the globe of the eye, the optic nerve, and the medial rectus muscle laterally.

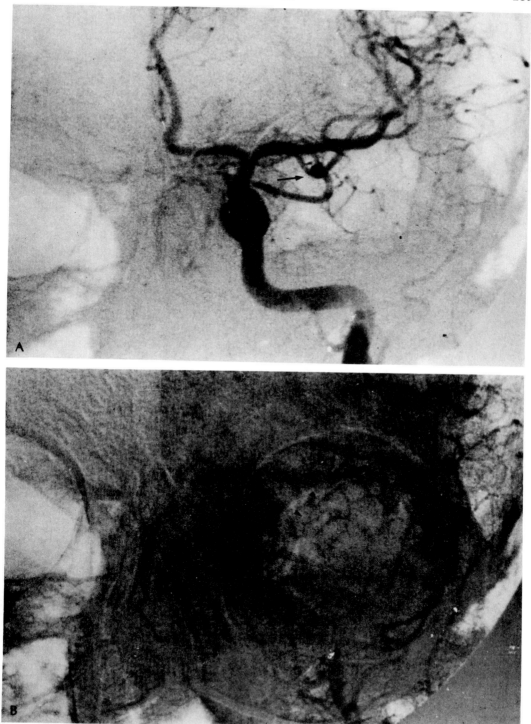

Fig. 8–16. Lymphoepithelioma of the ethmoid sinus. **A,** Arterial phase. The infraoptic portion of the ophthalmic artery is stretched and the circumneural loop is displaced laterally (▲). **B,** Venous phase. Tumor stain is present in the medial aspect of the orbit, and the choroidal blush is displaced laterally.

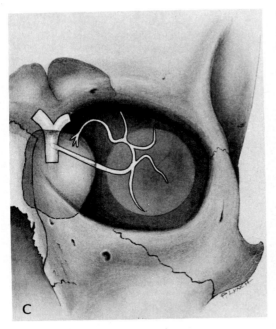

C

Fig. 8–16. C, Diagram of A. (From Rothman, S.L.G., et al.: Am. J. Roentgenol. *122*:607, 1974.)

are usually well seen and tend to be somewhat more prominent than usual (Fig. 8–18A). The diagnosis of carotico-cavernous fistula can be made on CT scan when the enlarged superior ophthalmic vein can be identified superiorly within the orbit. The vein is seen as a structure distinctly different from the optic nerve, extraocular muscle, or the orbital tumor masses. Cerebral angiography is usually required for complete evaluation of these lesions, because surgical therapy requires a detailed knowledge of the anatomic relationship between the carotid artery, the cavernous sinus, and the ophthalmic artery and vein. The angiographic features of carotico-cavernous fistula include early opacification of the cavernous sinus and superior ophthalmic vein and poor opacification of the cerebral vessels owing to marked shunting of blood from the intracranial vessels (Fig. 8–18B, C). Recently, superselective catheterization of the actual fistula has been performed, using extremely small catheters with balloon tips. These catheters can be positioned within the cavernous sinus and the balloons inflated, thereby occluding the fistula.

Cranial and Intracranial Disorders

Proptosis owing to encroachment upon the orbit by either congenital skull deformity or secondary bone expansion occurs in a variety of disorders. The most important of the congenital causes is neurofibromatosis.

Neurofibromatosis. Proptosis in this disorder may be caused by intraorbital tumors (optic nerve gliomas, orbital meningiomas, and diffuse orbital neurofibromas) or by dysplasia of the sphenoid bone with or without herniation of the temporal lobe into the orbit.

The most frequent plain film abnormality is concentric enlargement of the optic canal. Although this pattern is usually caused by intracanalicular tumors, it may be caused by a diffuse mesodermal dysplasia.

The skull in neurofibromatosis is commonly asymmetric owing to temporal or sphenoid bone dysplasias. The sphenoid dysplasia is characterized by unilateral enlargement or absence of the greater sphenoidal wing, which is best demonstrated in the Caldwell and lateral projections. The orbit appears asymmetrically expanded and the innominate line, representing the temporal surface of the greater sphenoidal wing, is distorted or absent. This change is manifest in the lateral view as anterior displacement of the bony border of the temporal lobe (Fig. 8–19A, B).

CT scanning is extremely helpful in the evaluation of these patients because it allows differentiation of those patients who have proptosis owing to intraorbital tumors and hence are surgical candidates from those patients with sphenoid expansion or agenesis with intraorbital herniation of the temporal lobe. It is possible to distinguish between lesions of the optic nerve and diffuse orbital neurofibromatosis as well as to assess the presence and

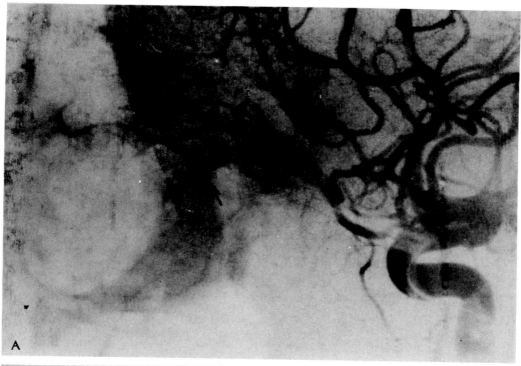

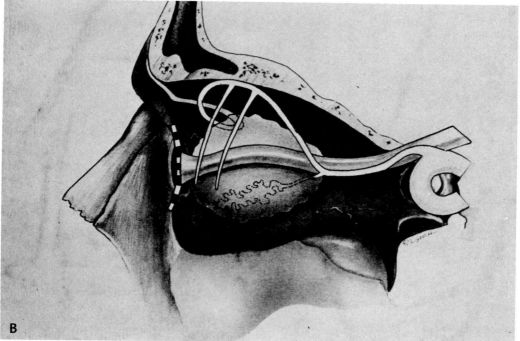

Fig. 8–17. Hemangioma of the orbit. **A** and **B,** The ophthalmic artery (▲) and its distal branches (↑) are elevated and stretched. An abnormal venous structure (▲) is noted draining the hemangioma. (From Rothman, S.L.G., et al.: Am. J. Roentgenol. *127*:607, 1974.)

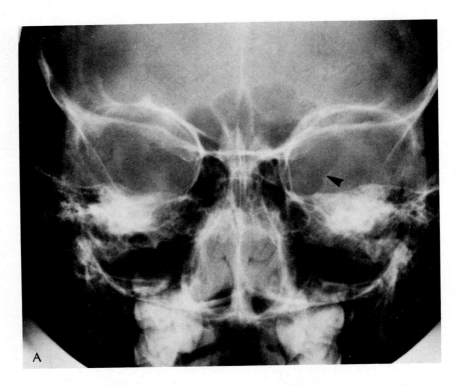

Fig. 8–18. Carotico-cavernous fistula. **A,** Caldwell projection. The left superior orbital fissure is expanded and its margins are unusually distinct (▲).

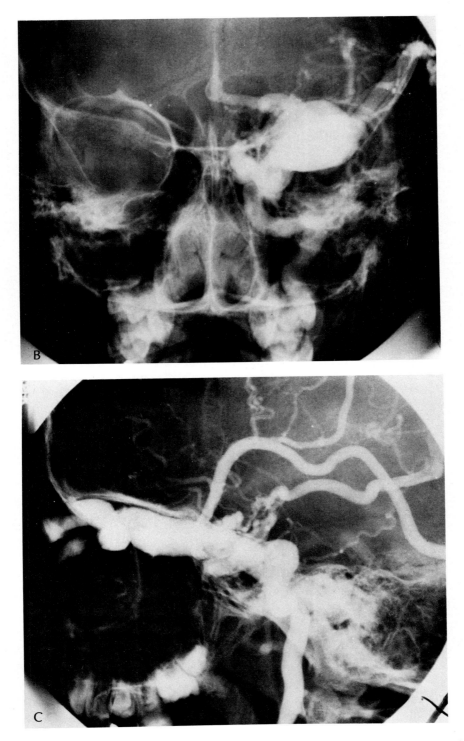

Fig. 8–18. Frontal, **B,** and lateral, **C,** projections of an internal carotid angiogram demonstrate early filling of a dilated superior ophthalmic vein. The front projection shows the venous mass filling the superior orbital fissure.

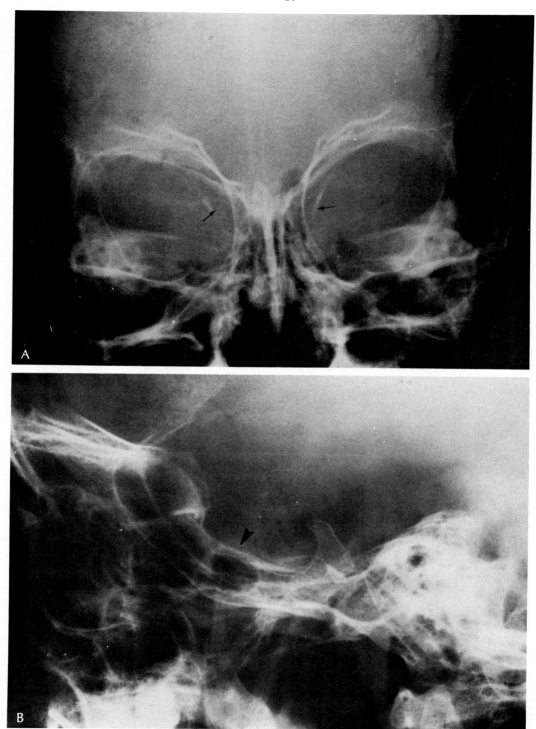

Fig. 8–19. Neurofibromatosis. Frontal projection, **A,** of a patient with neurofibromatosis and bilateral optic gliomas. The orbits are expanded. The optic canals (↑) can be identified in the Caldwell projection only when they are enlarged. Lateral projection, **B,** reveals expansion of the sella turcica with destruction of the chiasmatic sulcus (▲), indicating intracranial extension of the optic gliomas.

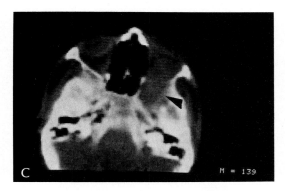

Fig. 8–19. C, CT scan in a different patient with neurofibromatosis. The posterior wall of the orbit is missing (▲), and intraorbital herniation of the temporal lobe has occurred.

extent of diffuse brain malformation (Fig. 8–19C).

Fibrous Dysplasia and Meningioma. Bony expansion of the sphenoid causing proptosis is commonly seen in fibrous dysplasia and sphenoid ridge meningioma. Although totally different disorders, their radiologic appearance is occasionally similar. The affected bone is thickened and hyperostotic. In the localized form, fibrous dysplasia may be impossible to differentiate from meningioma, although it is said that the bone of fibrous dysplasia has a characteristic ground-glass homogeneous appearance (Fig. 8–20). In the diffuse form, the disorder may affect a large portion of

the facial skeleton and is not a diagnostic problem. Meningiomas tend to incite a sclerotic reaction in the bone adjacent to the tumor mass. Common sites include the planum sphenoidale, the parasellar area, and the sphenoid ridge (Fig. 8–21). Hyperostotic reaction is most commonly associated with sphenoid ridge lesions although the tumor mass may be small. Planum sphenoidale lesions cause bone reaction less often, but tend to produce larger intracranial masses.

CT and cerebral angiography are required in the assessment of these lesions. They allow differentiation between the benign bone enlargement of fibrous dysplasia and the tumor mass of meningioma. Meningiomas are vascular tumors that produce a characteristically dense tumor stain on internal carotid arteriography. The hallmark of these lesions is vascular supply to the tumor from meningeal branches of the external carotid artery.

DIPLOPIA

Trauma

Diplopia caused by orbital trauma may be owing to a direct compressive blow to the eyeball or to involvement of the orbit in complex facial fractures. Routine radiographs are occasionally adequate to define

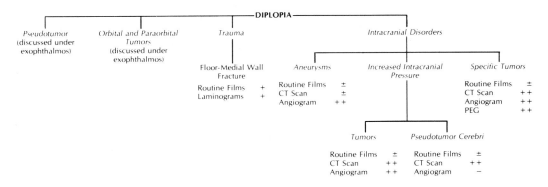

- = Not helpful
± = Rarely helpful
+ = Usually helpful
+ + = Most important

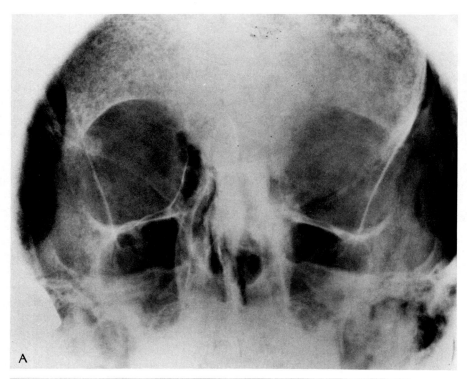

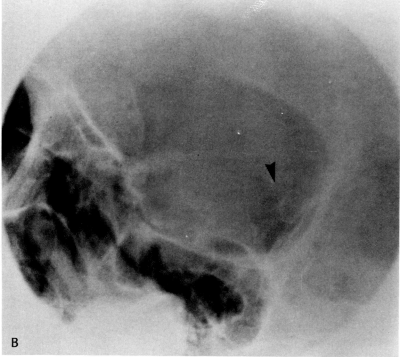

Fig. 8–20. Fibrous dysplasia: Frontal, **A,** and orbital oblique, **B,** views of a patient with fibrous dysplasia of the frontal, ethmoid, and sphenoid bones. The involved bones have a ground-glass appearance and are more dense than the remainder of the skull. In the oblique projection, the optic canal is compressed by the hyperostotic bone (▲).

the extent of orbital injury, but laminography is required in the more subtle cases.

The roentgenographic signs of orbital trauma are varied. The continuity of the orbital bones is interrupted and fracture fragments are displaced. The overall density of the orbit may be increased by soft tissue swelling and hematoma. Air is occasionally seen within the orbit when fractures extend into one of the paranasal sinuses. Adjacent sinuses may be totally opaque or may contain air-fluid levels owing to the presence of blood.

Blow-Out Fractures. Fractures owing to direct ocular trauma usually involve the orbital floor or medial orbital wall. The blow produces a rapid increase in orbital pressure, which is dissipated by outward explosion of the extremely thin lamina papyracea or orbital floor. Orbital fat and extraocular muscles herniate into the involved sinus and become entrapped, causing diplopia. Orbital emphysema is produced by air dissecting into the orbit from the involved sinus. In the Water's projection, a small soft-tissue bulge representing the herniated orbital contents is frequently noted projecting down into the maxillary sinus. Frontal laminograms are usually required for full evaluation of these lesions, especially those involving the lamina papyracea (Fig. 8–22).

Complex Facial Fractures. A diagram for classifying complex facial fractures is beyond the scope of this chapter. For simplicity, they can be divided into fractures involving the zygoma and lateral orbital wall and those primarily involving the maxilla and medial and posterior orbital walls. The most important lateral wall fracture is the "tripod fracture." In this entity, there is fracture or separation of the zygomatico-frontal suture, fracture of the inferior orbital rim and floor, of the zygomatic arch, and of the lateral wall of the maxillary sinus. Antral air-fluid levels are frequently observed. Depression or rotation of the free zygomatic fragment can cause facial deformity and diplopia requir-

ing surgical correction. The Water's projection usually demonstrates the fracture fragments, but preoperative laminograms may be required to evaluate the amount of rotation and bony overlap (Fig. 8–23).

Fractures of the medial orbital wall tend to be part of complex facial trauma commonly associated with nasal, frontal, ethmoidal, maxillary, and sphenoid fractures. The LaForte classification describes three maxillofacial injuries. The simplest is the LaForte I, a horizontal maxillary fracture that does not affect the orbit. LaForte II fractures involve the nasofrontal area and extend across both orbits. The maxillae lie free, disconnected from the rest of the facial skeleton. The most severe form, LaForte III, is a total craniofacial separation. The fractures cross both orbits and extend posteriorly into the sphenoid bone (Fig. 8–24). These fractures may be asymmetric and involve one portion of the face more than another, depending on the cause and severity of the trauma. They frequently are disfiguring injuries, requiring maxillofacial operations for correction of the deformity.

Intracranial Disorders

Diplopia owing to cranial nerve palsies can be caused by a variety of intracranial disorders. The most important ones from a neuroradiologic point of view are intracranial aneurysms, diffuse increased intracranial pressure, benign intracranial hypertension (pseudotumor cerebri), and a variety of intracranial tumors causing brain stem dysfunction.

Aneurysms. Cerebral aneurysms are localized dilatations of major cerebral vessels, classified according to their shape and origin. The most common sites include the origins of the anterior communicating artery (30%), posterior communicating artery (25%), and the main branches of the middle cerebral artery (13%). They most frequently occur with devastating subarachnoid hemorrhage. Large, unruptured aneurysms cause local mass effect and can compress the cranial nerves. Posterior

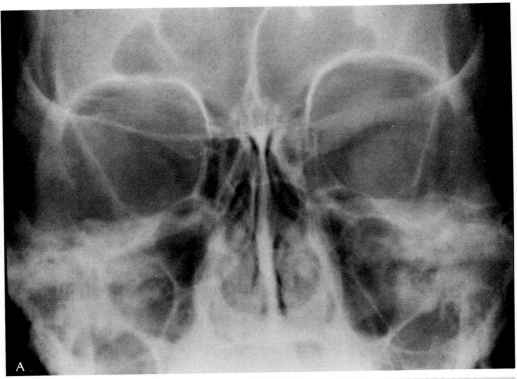

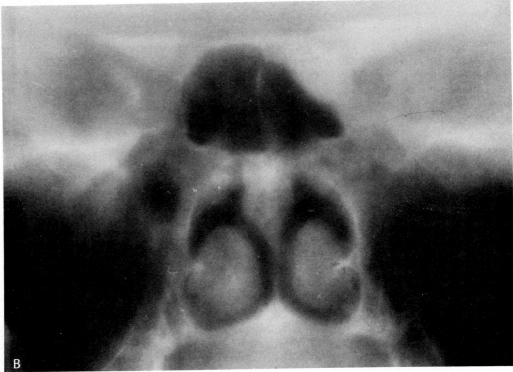

Fig. 8–21. Sphenoid ridge meningioma. Caldwell view, **A,** reveals hyperostosis of the greater and lesser sphenoidal wings. The superior orbital fissure is seen unusually well on the involved side. Frontal laminogram, **B,** further defines the extent of the involvement of the sphenoid bone. The orbital oblique view, **C,** demonstrates sclerosis of the bony confines of the optic canal. This condition may be indistinguishable from fibrous dysplasia.

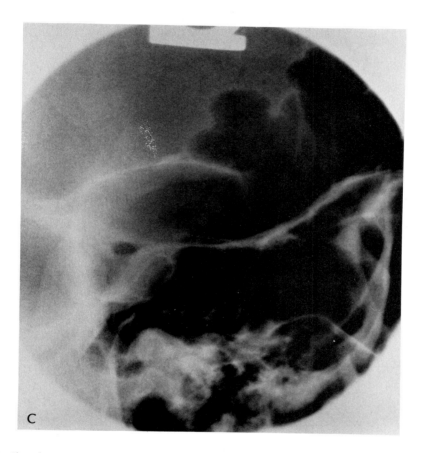

Fig. 8–21 *Continued.*

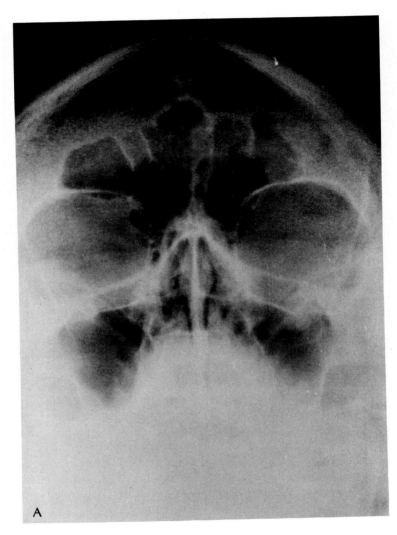

Fig. 8–22. Blow-out fracture. Water's view of the skull, **A,** reveals a small soft-tissue mass protruding down from the roof of the sinus. Fracture fragments cannot be identified.

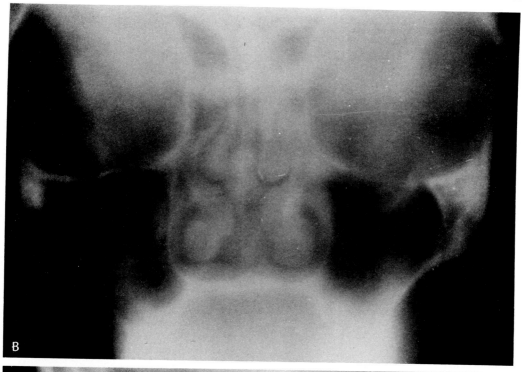

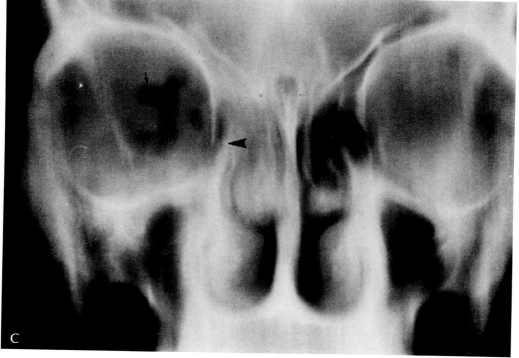

Fig. 8–22. B, Frontal laminogram is necessary to visualize the fracture. Compare the normal right to the abnormal left orbital floor. **C,** Frontal laminogram on a second patient with fracture of the lamina papyracea (▲). The ethmoid sinus is opaque and air is seen within the orbit (↑).

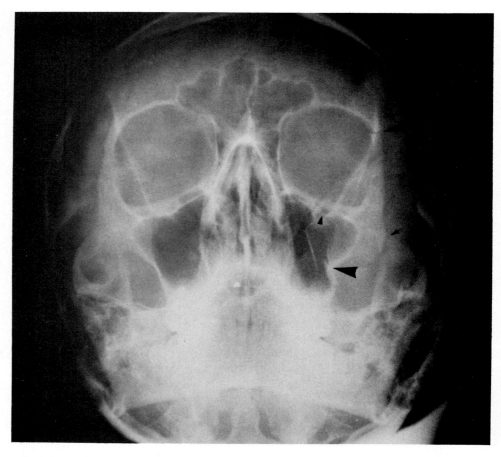

Fig. 8–23. Tripod fracture. Water's projection reveals fractures of the lateral wall of the maxilla (▲), orbital floor (▲), zygomatic arch (↑), and frontozygomatic suture (⇌). The zygoma is free of all supporting bony attachments.

communicating and intracavernous carotid aneuryms frequently affect the third cranial nerve within the basal cisterns, and intracavernous lesions compress the third, fourth, and sixth nerves within the cavernous sinus, producing total ophthalmoplegia.

Routine roentgenograms occasionally demonstrate a rim of calcification within the wall of the aneurysm (see Fig. 8–26A). Localized plain film abnormalities occur in approximately 10% of carotid aneurysms arising within the cavernous sinus. They include enlargement of the superior orbital fissure (Fig. 8–25), expansion of the sella turcica, and localized destruction of portions of the sphenoid bone. Bony abnor-

malities are less commonly seen with aneurysms in other locations.

CT is helpful in several ways. It allows evaluation of the presence, extent, and location of subarachnoid and intracerebral hemorrhage owing to aneurysm rupture. The iron in hemoglobin attenuates x-rays far more than brain tissue or cerebrospinal fluid, so blood appears denser on the CT scan. The lumina of aneurysms fill with the iodinated contrast medium, further enhancing the visualization of that portion of the aneurysm containing flowing blood.

The most important diagnostic examination is transfemoral selective cerebral angiography. Complete arterial examination includes visualization of both carotid and

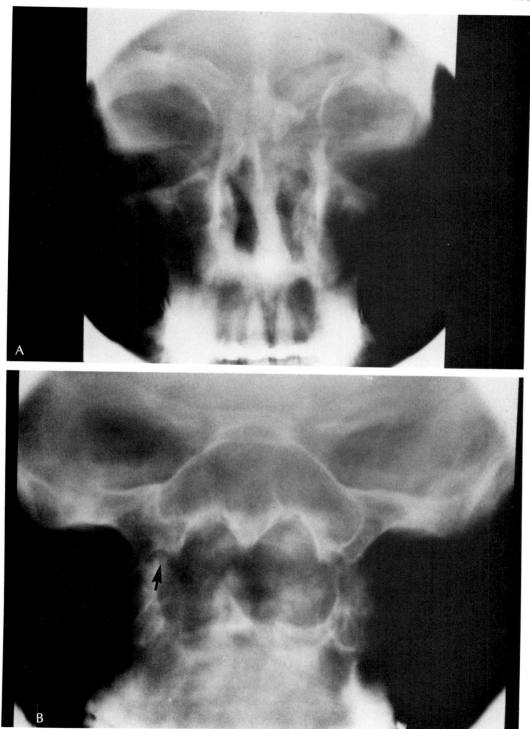

Fig. 8–24. Complex facial fracture. Frontal laminograms of a patient with a complex facial fracture. On the more anterior laminograms, **A,** note breaks in the orbital roof and medial walls bilaterally. On the more posterior, **B,** the body of the sphenoid is opacified and the fracture is seen to extend into the pterygoid plates (▲).

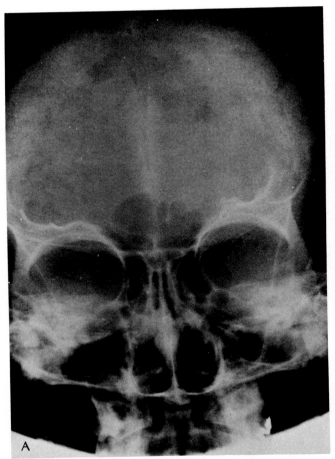

A

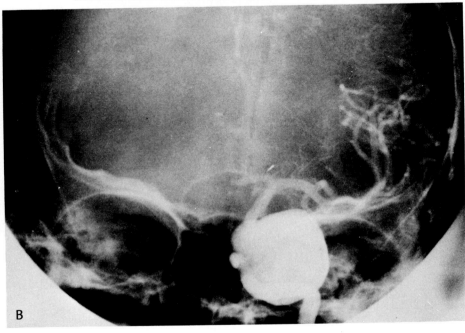

B

at least one vertebral artery in at least two projections (Fig. 8–26 B, C). High-resolution magnification angiograms with the aid of subtraction techniques (a photographic method for eliminating the image of the bony calvarium, leaving only the opacified vessels) permit the most precise localization of these lesions.

Increased Intracranial Pressure. Paralysis of one or both lateral rectus muscles owing to sixth nerve compression is commonly caused by diffuse increased intracranial pressure and the syndrome of benign intracranial hypertension (pseudotumor cerebri). The diagnosis of increased intracranial pressure in childhood can be made on routine roentgenograms by a combination of abnormalities, including widening of the cranial sutures and prominence of the digital markings of the inner table of the skull. These pathologic changes are caused by direct pressure of the expanding intracranial contents.

After closure of the cranial sutures, increasing intracranial pressure manifests itself by erosion of various portions of the skull bones. The most commonly visualized abnormality in adults and older children is demineralization of the floor of the sella turcica. The cortical bone of the floor of the sella is termed the lamina dura. It normally appears as a clearly defined dense bony line adjacent to the pneumatized sphenoid sinus and a somewhat thinner line above portions of nonpneumatized sphenoid bone.

After a period of sustained increased intracranial pressure, the bony margin of the sella becomes indistinct. This process is seen earliest in areas where no sinus pneumatization occurs, but progresses anteriorly into the floor above the pneumatized

sinus if the pressure is not relieved (Fig. 8–27A). In very long standing cases the entire floor of the middle fossa, the anterior clinoid processes, and the optic canal all may become markedly demineralized (Fig. 8–27 B,C). All the preceding changes are manifestations of the effect of pressure on the skull. They do not relate directly to the cause of the pressure elevation. Disease-specific abnormalities, such as hyperostosis in patients with meningiomas and pineal shift owing to intracranial tumors, are occasionally observed.

CT is the crucial neuroradiologic procedure in this entire class of disorders. It is the most sensitive, noninvasive diagnostic modality for evaluation of intracranial contents. It easily distinguishes those patients in whom increased pressure is caused by the presence of tumor mass from those with hydrocephalus. It allows assessment of the extent of tumor spread, the amount of midline shift, and occasionally, the actual cell type of the lesion.

It further allows differentiation of those patients in whom hydrocephalus is caused by obstruction of the ventricular system by colloid cysts, pinealomas, brain stem gliomas, and other posterior fossa neoplasms from those with communicating hydrocephalus, aqueductal stenosis, and cerebral atrophy.

The diagnosis of pseudotumor cerebri can be made on the basis of a CT scan demonstrating no intracranial mass and normal or small cerebral ventricles in the presence of sustained intracranial pressure elevation.

In the pre-CT era, cerebral angiography was the most sensitive screening process for serious intracranial pathology. Its role has somewhat changed, although its im-

---

Fig. 8–25. Aneurysm of the carotid artery within the cavernous sinus. Caldwell view, **A,** reveals expansion of the superior orbital fissure. Cerebral angiogram, **B,** demonstrates a large aneurysm expanding into the sphenoid sinus and superior orbital fissure.

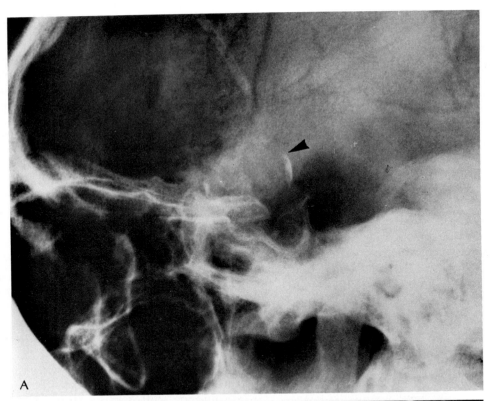

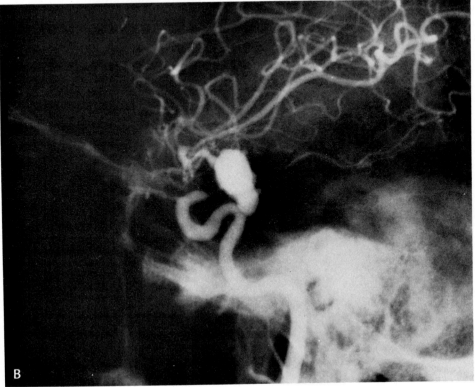

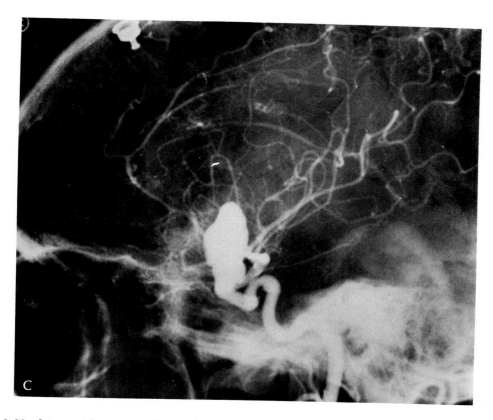

Fig. 8–26. Intracranial aneurysm. Routine lateral radiograph, **A,** demonstrates a curvilinear calcification in the suprasellar region and another above the dorsum sella (▲). Right carotid angiogram, **B,** reveals a large aneurysm arising from the posterior communicating artery with severe spasm of the intradural portion of the carotid artery. **C,** Left carotid angiogram reveals a second aneurysm arising from the origin of the ophthalmic artery.

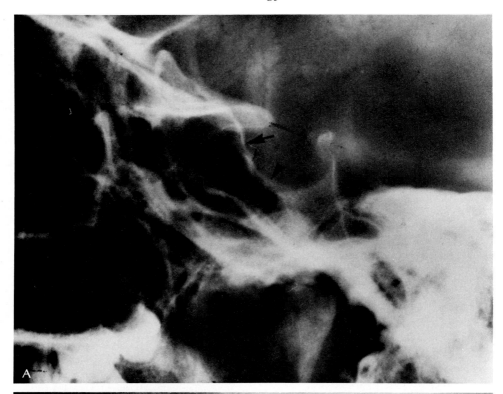

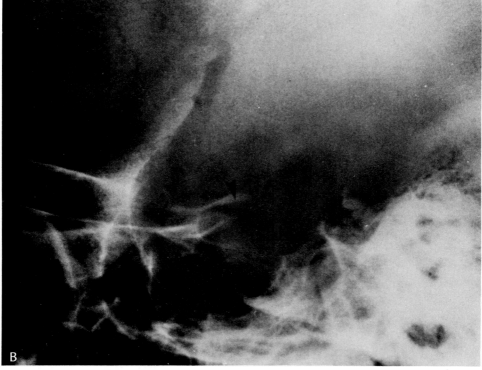

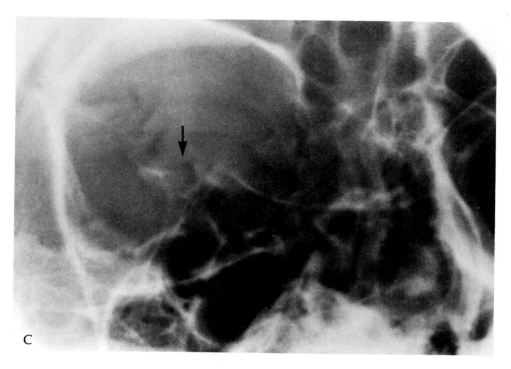

Fig. 8–27. Increased intracranial pressure. **A,** Long-standing increased pressure causes loss of the lamina dura over nonpneumatized sphenoid (▲); normal lamina dura (↑). **B,** Extreme case of increased pressure. The floor of the sella is totally missing and the anterior clinoid is eroded (▲). **C,** In the orbital oblique projection, the borders of the optic canal are indistinct. Only a ghost of the canal is visible (▲).

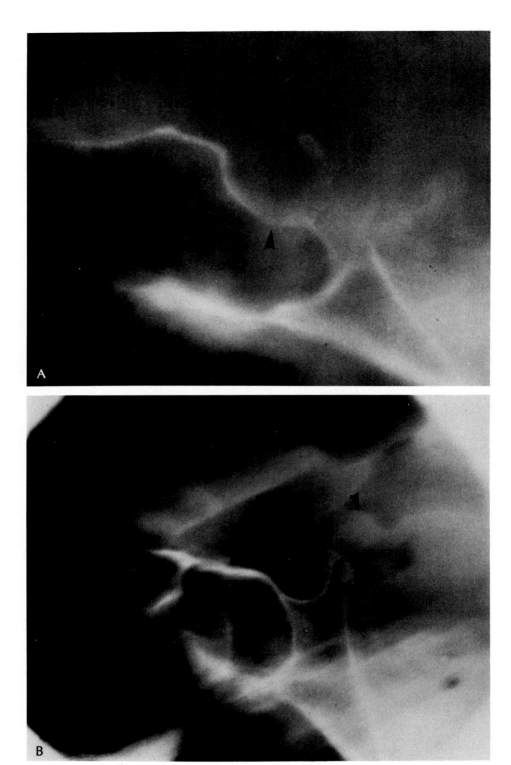

Fig. 8–28.   Pituitary and suprasellar tumors. **A,** Microadenomas of the pituitary causing subtle erosion of the floor of the sella turcica (▲); conventional roentgenograms were normal. **B,** Midline laminogram during pneumoencephalography. The sellar contents are normal. Gas within the suprasellar cisterns outlines a normal optic nerve (↑). A soft tissue mass is seen indenting the anterior recesses of the third ventricle (▲). The anterior and inferior surfaces of this small suprasellar mass are seen owing to the presence of gas in the interpeduncular and suprasellar cisterns (▲).

portance has not. It is now used as a second-line procedure following CT in an attempt to identify tumor cell type more exactly and to describe for the neurosurgeon tumor vascularity and important surgical landmarks. A detailed analysis of the angiographic abnormalities in cerebral tumors and hydrocephalus is beyond the scope of this chapter. The interested reader is referred to the encyclopedic work of Newton and Potts for a complete review of cerebral angiography.

Intracranial Tumors. A variety of intracranial tumors can cause eye signs owing to cranial nerve or brain stem dysfunction. Expanding lesions of the pineal body frequently compress the quadrigeminal plate, causing paralysis of upward gaze. Tumors at the foramen magnum may also produce a fairly specific type of nystagmus. Other posterior fossa lesions likewise affect the nerves or their nuclei. CT scans, angiography, and occasionally, pneumoencephalography are the procedures of choice for the diagnosis of specific lesions compressing the visual system intracranially.

Pituitary Tumors. These tumors frequently result in visual disturbance owing to suprasellar extension. Diplopia may be present with lateral extension, but the classic neuro-ophthalmologic finding is bitemporal visual field cut owing to suprasellar mass compressing the optic chiasm.

From the radiologic standpoint, pituitary tumors can be classified into two types—those confined to the sella turcica and those that have grown to a size sufficient to escape from the confines of the sella.

Small intrasellar tumors (microadenomas) may first appear clinically in several ways, depending on cell type. The rarest, the basophilic adenoma, occurs with Cushing syndrome; eosinophilic adenomas occur as gigantism or acromegaly; and chromophobe adenomas, usually as disturbance in reproductive function and lactation. The sella turcica is frequently normal on conventional radiographs. Thin-section pluridirectional tomograms at 1-mm intervals are required to visualize areas of minimal bone erosion along the sellar floor (Fig. 8–28A). Larger tumors cause characteristic ballooning of the sella. This expansion frequently produces a "double floor" appearance on the radiograph, indicating asymmetric growth of the tumor.

Preoperative evaluation usually includes CT scan and cerebral angiography to assess the extent of suprasellar mass and to exclude intrasellar aneurysms. The most sensitive method for evaluation of the suprasellar region and optic chiasm is pneumoencephalography. It should be performed with frontal and lateral tomograms in order to evaluate the diaphragm sella, the optic nerves and chiasm (Fig. 8–28B).

BIBLIOGRAPHY

Allen, W.E., III, Kier, E.L., and Rothman, S.L.G.: The maxillary artery in craniofacial pathology. Am. J. Roentgenol. *121*:139, 1974.

Enzmann, D., et al.: Computed tomography in Graves ophthalmopathy. Radiology *118*:615, 1976.

Enzmann, D., et al.: Computed tomography in orbital pseudotumor. Radiology *120*:597, 1976.

Geehr, R.B., Allen, W.E., Rothman, S.L.G., and Spencer, D.D.: The significance of pluridirectional tomography in the evolution of pituitary tumors. Am. J. Roentgenol. *130*:105, 1978.

Gerald, B.E., and Silverman, F.N.: Normal and abnormal interorbital distances with special reference to mongolism. Am. J. Roentgenol. *95*:154, 1965.

Harwood-Nash, D.C.: Optic gliomas and pediatric neuroradiology. Radiol. Clin. North Am. *10*:83, 1972.

LeFort, R.: Étude experimentale sur les fractures de la machoire superieure. Rev. Chir. *23*:208, 1901.

Lloyd, G.A.S.: Pathological veins of the orbit. Br. J. Radiol. *47*:570, 1974.

Locksley, H.B.: Report on the cooperative study of intracranial aneurysms and subarachnoid hemorrhage. Section V, Natural history of subarachnoid hemorrhage, intracranial aneurysm and arteriovenous malformations, based on 6368 cases in the cooperative study. J. Neurosurg. *25*:219, 321, 1966.

Lombardi, G.: Radiology in Neuro-ophthalmology. Baltimore, Williams & Wilkins, 1967.

Michotey, P., et al.: The contribution of computerized axial tomography to ophthalmology. J. Neuroradiol. *3*:257, 1976.

Moss, H.M.: Expanding lesions of the orbit. Am. J. Ophthalmol. *54*:761, 1962.

Newton, T.H., and Troost, B.T.: Arteriovenous malformations and fistulae. *In* Radiology of the Skull and Brain, 2nd Ed. Edited by T.H. Newton and D.G. Potts. St. Louis, C.V. Mosby, 1974.

Potter, G.D., and Trokel, S.L.: The optic canal. *In* Radiology of the Skull and Brain, Edited by T.H. Newton and D.G. Potts. St. Louis, C.V. Mosby, 1974.

Reese, A.B.: Expanding lesions of the orbit. Trans. Ophthalmol. Soc. U.K. *91*:85, 1971.

Reese, A.B.: Tumors of the Eye. New York, Harper & Row, 1963.

Rothman, S.L.G., et al.: Arteriographic topography of orbital lesions. Am. J. Roentgenol. *122*:607, 1974.

Schurr, P.H.: Angiography of normal ophthalmic artery and choroidal plexus of eye. Br. J. Ophthalmol. *35*:473, 1951.

Shapiro, R., and Robinson, F.: Alterations of the sphenoidal fissure produced by local systemic processes. Am. J. Roentgenol. *101*:814, 1967.

Vignaud, J., Clay, C., and Aubins, M.L.: Orbital arteriography. Radiol. Clin. North Am. *10*:30, 1972.

Zizmor, J., and Noyek, A.M.: Orbital trauma. *In* Radiology of the Skull and Brain, 1st Ed. Edited by T.H. Newton and D.G. Potts. St. Louis, C.V. Mosby, 1971.

Chapter **9**

Computed Tomography in the Evaluation of Retrobulbar Extracranial Causes of Visual Loss

CHARLES M. CITRIN, AND MELVIN G. ALPER

The combined art and science of computed tomography has now completed an approximate 10-year course in clinical development. We have advanced from the earliest form of scanners, which required more than 5 minutes to produce images derived from approximately 29,000 bits of information and were presented in an 80 × 80 matrix, to a point at which we can now produce scans in 2 seconds that are presented in a 512 × 512 matrix derived from a base of over 1,000,000 data points. This has obviously resulted in added sophistication, more accurate diagnosis, and presentation of data in orthogonal projections.

The price that is being paid for this advance in technology is both financial, with CT scanner prices now running well over $1,000,000, and in radiation dosage, which has, in some cases, trebled. This increased cost is mitigated by the greater accuracy, greater comfort, and reduced risk to the patient because of the lesser need for such studies as orbitography, superior orbital venography, and arteriography.

The nature of this chapter necessitates the use of scans that have been obtained over the past 9 years. Images employed in this work have been derived from first, second, third, and fourth generation CT scanners. The image matrices vary from 160 × 160 to 512 × 512. Scan times are as long as 5 minutes in the older, first generation scanner, and as short as 5 seconds in the more recent fourth generation scanner. Those cases depicting neoplastic and inflammatory processes have been proven by either biopsy or surgical intervention. The other disease entities have been diagnosed by endocrinologic methods, case history, or angiography. These cases were accumulated during the past decade from over 50,000 scans of the head and orbits.

A variety of disease entities cause visual field defects or loss of visual acuity. Within this chapter, we will discuss those types of disease states arising behind the globe and anterior to the optic canal that can be responsible for loss of vision. Congenital, developmental, traumatic, endocrinologic, inflammatory, and neoplastic causes can be responsible for either a loss of visual acuity or a visual field cut. Scans will be presented in both transaxial and coronal orientations. In all cases, the patient's right side will be on the left, and vice versa.

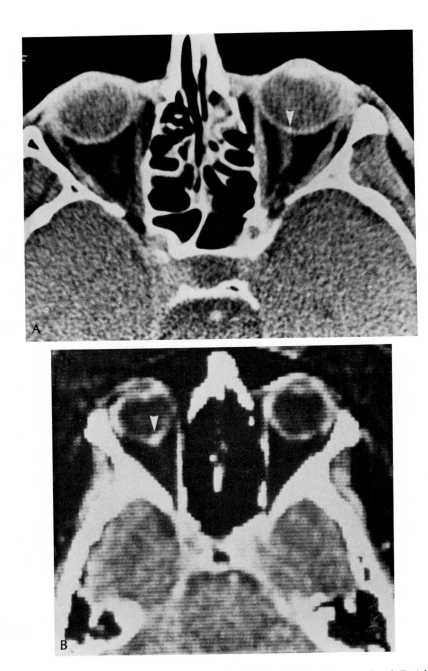

Fig. 9–1. **A.** A small calcified drusen (arrowhead) is identified in the left optic nerve head. **B.** A large calcified drusen can be identified with first or second generation CT scanners (arrowhead).

LESIONS INVOLVING THE OPTIC NERVE HEAD

Drusen

A common observation at the level of the optic disc is a calcific deposit, usually of approximately 1 to 2 mm in dimension, which represents an optic nerve drusen (Figs. 9–1A, B). These drusen are composed of a calcific/hyaline substrate and are invariably situated at or anterior to the lamina cribrosa. They present to the ophthalmologist as an elevated disc at funduscopic examination, and when buried deep within the disc their hyalinized nature may not be appreciated. In these cases of "pseudopapilledema/pseudoneuritis," the demonstration of a calcific deposit in the optic nerve head verifies the diagnosis of drusen and virtually excludes any other cause of an elevated disc. Decreased visual acuity is a common manifestation of drusen. Drusen may be either unilateral or bilateral in distribution. Drusen should not be confused with calcifications occurring off the disc such as choroidal osteoma, phthisis bulbi, retrolental fibroplasia, or choristoma.

Coloboma

A second cause of an abnormal-appearing disc is the ocular coloboma (Fig. 9–2), a posterior pit of lamina cribrosa at the level of the optic nerve junction, commonly associated with buphthalmic globe and associated chronic myopia. Visual acuity is generally decreased and optic atrophy can also simultaneously be appreciated on CT scans in this entity. This is a common malformation secondary to abnormal closure

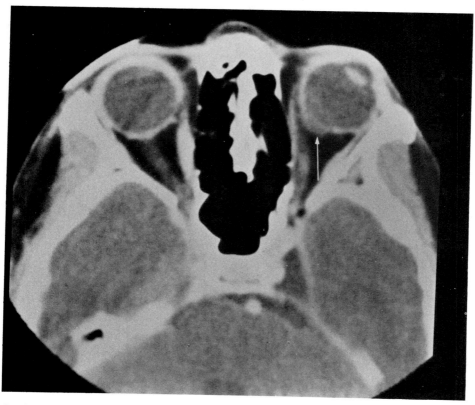

Fig. 9–2. A posterior pit (coloboma) is identified at the posterior aspect of the left globe (arrow). An associated retinal cyst is not present.

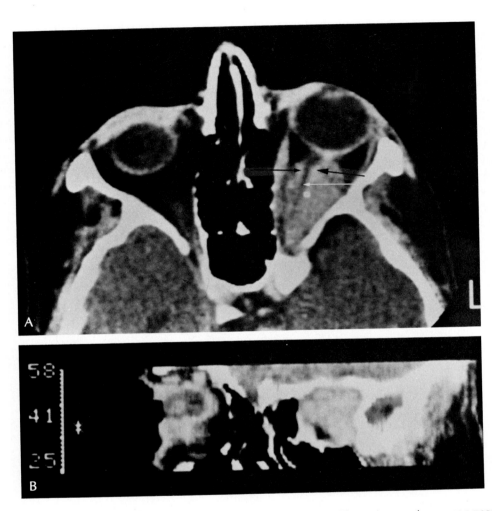

Fig. 9–3. **A.** Fusiform thickening of the optic nerve sheath is identified. The optic nerve is seen as a negative defect (arrow) amidst the hyperdense tumor. A "region-of-interest" box lies along the most medial aspect of the nerve and does not represent a portion of the tumor. Hyperdensity greater than that of the tumor, immediately adjacent to the optic nerve, is a sign that has been described only in meningioma (black arrows). **B.** An oblique reconstructed image perpendicular to the optic nerve meningioma.

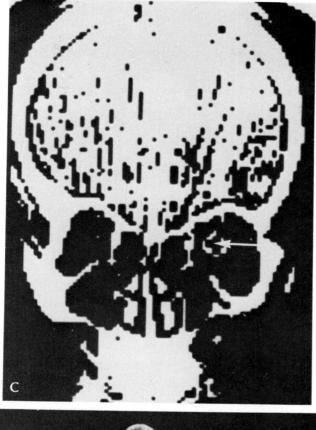

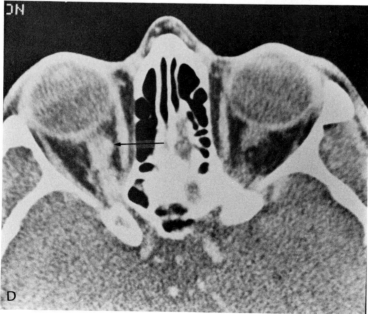

Fig. 9–3.   **C.** A direct coronal scan (not reconstructed) demonstrates the optic nerves seen as a negative shadow (arrow) surrounded by a hyperdense meningioma. This is an image from a second-generation scanner. **D.** Irregularity and focal bulging of the tumor as seen in the right optic nerve (arrow) is indicative of extradural invasion.

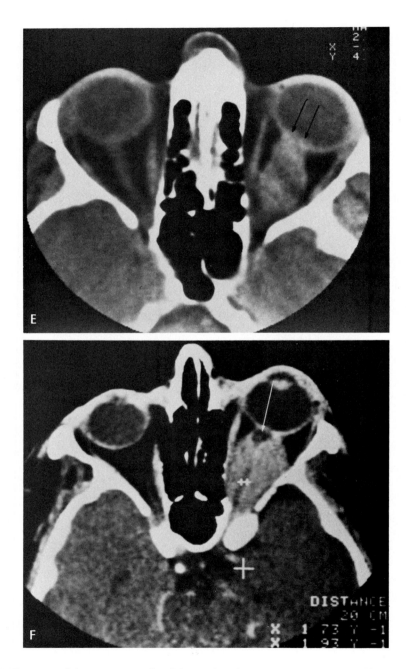

Fig. 9–3. **E.** Elevation of the optic nerve head (arrows) is due to tumor invasion. **F.** Elevation of the optic nerve head in this case is due to focal edema of the distal optic nerve sheath (arrow).

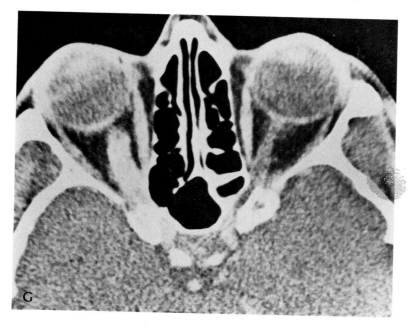

Fig. 9–3.   G. Scan obtained after contrast infusion demonstrates enhancement of the right optic nerve, a sign highly suggestive of the presence of optic nerve meningioma.

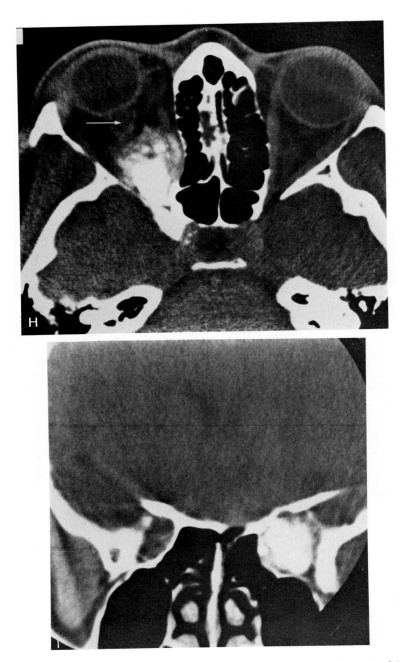

Fig. 9–3.   H, I. Transaxial and coronal scans of the same patient demonstrate a densely calcified right-sided retrobulbar mass. This finding is also highly suggestive of the presence of a meningioma. Focal edema of the distal optic nerve (arrow) is identified on the transaxial section and is similar to that seen in Figure 9–3 F.

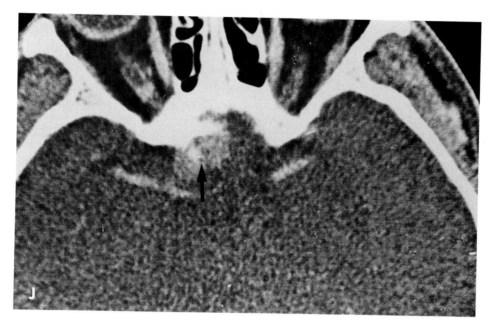

Fig. 9–3. **J.** Extension of meningoma through the optic canal is common and should be looked for during the orbital study (arrow).

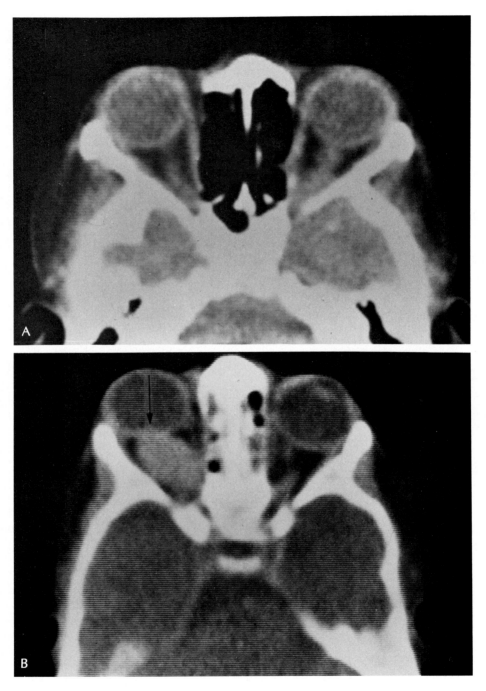

Fig. 9–4. **A.** A diffusely thickened left optic nerve is identified. The density of the nerve is homogeneous. (Case courtesy of Dr. David Brallier.) **B.** This large right-sided optic nerve glioma is flattening the posterior aspect of the globe and elevating the optic nerve head (arrow). (Case courtesy of Dr. David Brallier.) **C.** Bilateral optic nerve gliomas were identified in this child with neurofibromatosis. (Case courtesy of Dr. David Brallier.) **D.** Extension of an optic nerve glioma through the optic canal has resulted in marked involvement of the optic chiasm, hypothalamus, and the right optic tract (arrow). (Case courtesy of Dr. David Brallier.)

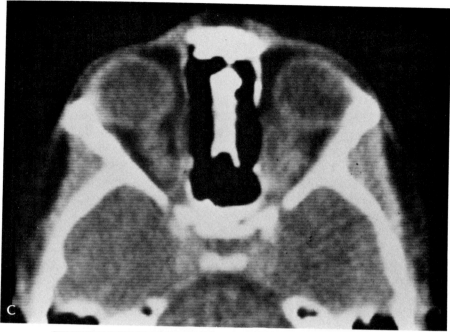

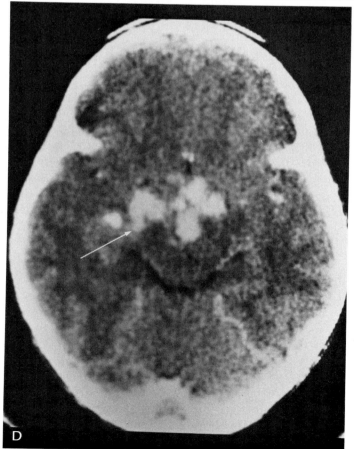

of the optic fissure. It may or may not be associated with retinal cysts. The cysts can become large enough to result in ex-ophthalmos. These cysts, when present, have CT numbers identical to the vitreous.

LESIONS PRIMARILY INVOLVING THE OPTIC NERVE

A thickened optic nerve, as seen on CT scanning, is almost invariably associated with visual loss. The causes of a thickened optic nerve are either neoplastic (menin-gioma, glioma, or metastatic disease) or in-flammatory (papilledema, optic neuritis, orbital pseudotumor).

Meningioma

Optic nerve meningiomas usually arise from the surrounding arachnoid but are at-tached to the dura. Histologically, the cells are similar to fibroblasts. Characteristically, these tumors present with the complaint of a decrease in visual acuity. Proptosis is common.

In patients with meningioma, the distri-bution of the thickening of the optic nerve is most commonly fusiform (Fig. 9–3A) with almost total involvement of the nerve, but it can be focal or cylindrical. Visual-ization of the optic nerve as a negative de-fect amid a perineuronal mass is suggestive of the diagnosis of meningioma but is not pathognomonic of this entity. Coronal, sagittal, and oblique reconstructions are excellent for demonstrating the distribu-tion of the mass but do not have the re-solving power of direct coronal scans (Figs. 9–3B, C). Commonly seen in meningiomas is the presence of focal expansions of the optic nerve at either the proximal or distal aspect within the orbit. Focal bulging of the tumor implies extradural invasion, as do irregular margins (Fig. 9–3D). Elevation of the optic nerve head may be caused by di-rect tumor invasion or edema of the optic nerve sheath (Figs. 9–3E,F). Meningiomas may enhance after contrast infusion and therefore appear denser than the contra-lateral uninvolved optic nerve (Fig. 9–3G).

Bony hyperostosis at the level of the planum sphenoidale or greater wing of the sphenoid bone is supportive of the diag-nosis of meningioma. A negative optic nerve seen through the density of the tumor excludes the diagnosis of glioma. Calcification within the tumor mass helps to make the diagnosis but is not absolutely specific for a meningioma (Figs. 9–3H,I). A specific sign is the presence of hyper-density greater than that of the tumor, seen immediately adjacent to the negative optic nerve (Fig. 9–3A). This may be indicative of subdural spread of mass and has, to date, been seen only in meningioma.

Meningiomas may extend through the optic canal and present within the intra-cranial cavity at the level of the tuberculum sellae or cavernous sinus (Fig. 9–3J). En-largement of the optic canal on plain roent-genographic films, CT, and polytomes can be appreciated.

Optic Nerve Glioma

These rare tumors represent less than 5% of all orbital tumors, and the vast majority of these present in the first decade of life. These tumors arise from astrocytes and oli-godendroglioma cells. Their pattern of growth is that of concentric enlargement, without invasion of neighboring tissues. Clinical presentation may be via exophthal-mos; although more commonly, a com-plaint of decreased visual acuity is the pre-senting complaint in this disease. Optic atrophy and a Marcus Gunn pupil can be found on physical exam.

The CT manifestations of optic nerve glioma are those of a finely defined and encapsulated mass that usually cannot be distinguished from the optic nerve, since the nerve and tumor have identical den-sities (Fig. 9–4A). When the optic nerve is apparent on CT, it may usually be seen as an area of noncalcified increased density relative to the tumor. This is in contradis-tinction to the relative decreased density of the optic nerve in meningioma. Approxi-mately 10 to 20% of optic nerve gliomas present as a diffuse fusiform enlargement of the nerve, which can make distinction from other processes difficult. It may raise the optic nerve head and flatten the posterior aspect of the globe (Fig. 9–4B). A close relationship exists between optic nerve gliomas and neurofibromatosis (von Recklinghausen's disease). The histology of the tumor is identical whether it arises in a solitary fashion or as part of the neurofibromatosis complex. In the overall spectrum of optic nerve gliomas, bilateral optic nerve gliomas occur frequently. For this reason, when evaluating for the presence of optic nerve glioma, it is equally important to examine the assumed uninvolved eye, as well as to include in the area of reconstruction the parasellar areas and posterior fossa, to search for the presence of concomitant neoplastic changes in these areas (Fig. 9–4C), which have a predilection for tumor development in neurofibromatosis. Extension through the optic canal and involvement of the optic chiasm is a frequent occurrence in optic nerve glioma (Fig. 9–4D).

Optic Neuritis

The optic nerve is usually identified as a cylindrical structure, the total length of which measures approximately 4.5 cm, with an intraorbital component of approximately 25 to 30 mm. The width of the nerve should be approximately 4.5 mm as seen in the transaxial plane, but may actually measure approximately 5 mm when seen in the coronal plane. This is owing to the fact that the nerve is imaged obliquely in coronal scans. In cases of an acute inflammation of the optic nerve, which is often a manifestation of multiple sclerosis, diffuse enlargement of the optic nerve in a cylindrical fashion will be appreciated (Fig. 9–5A), owing to a generalized edema of the nerve. This is easily appreciated in cases of unilateral neuritis. In cases of bilateral optic neuritis, the nerves must be measured and compared with the normal standard in order to make the determination of optic nerve widening (Fig. 9–5B). Enhancement

of the optic nerve in optic neuritis is unusual but has been reported, presumably as a result of increased vascular permeability. CT scans in the coronal plane simply demonstrate a widened nerve with a homogeneous density throughout its width (Fig. 9–5C). In cases of optic neuritis owing to inflammatory conditions such as syphilis, toxoplasmosis, tuberculosis, or to viral infections, the CT findings are similar to those seen in the acute demyelinating process. The findings are usually totally reversible following appropriate medical treatment. In patients presenting with acute papillitis only, a normal CT scan may be obtained.

Papilledema

The appearance of papilledema on computed tomographic scans is virtually identical to that of optic neuritis. The nerve is diffusely enlarged in a cylindrical fashion from the level of the papilla to the optic canal (Fig. 9–6A). There is, however, no evidence for the presence of enhancement of the optic nerve in papilledema. In individuals with increased intracranial pressure, the optic nerve may or may not be enlarged. This depends on the patency of the subarachnoid space at the level of the optic canal. In individuals with continuity of the subarachnoid space into the orbit, increased intracranial pressure can be transmitted and can dilate the subarachnoid space that surrounds the optic nerve. This can be beautifully demonstrated during CT performed after an intrathecal injection of metrizamide (Fig. 9–6B). If, however, this connection is nonpatent, the optic nerve will appear normal. Patency of the subarachnoid space into the perineuronal subarachnoid space is commonly a unilateral observation; therefore, the presence of unilateral optic nerve thickening does not exclude the diagnosis of papilledema. A thickened optic nerve silhouette is much more commonly seen in patients with benign intracranial hypertension than in patients with hydrocephalus. Trauma

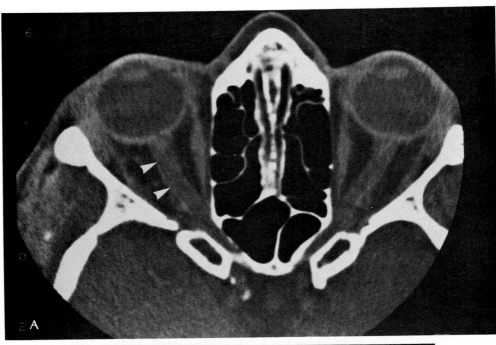

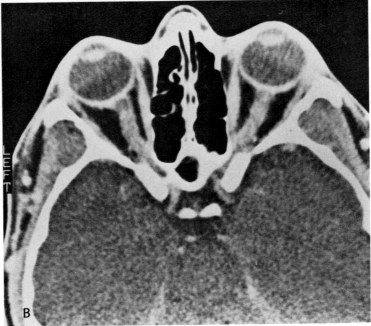

Fig. 9–5. **A.** A mild but definite cylindrical-type thickening of the right optic nerve is apparent (white arrowheads) in optic neuritis. **B.** An example of bilateral cylindrical optic nerve thickening. The symmetry of this finding makes it more difficult to diagnose than unilateral disease. These optic nerves must be measured to determine whether or not they are greater than 4.5 mm in transverse diameter.

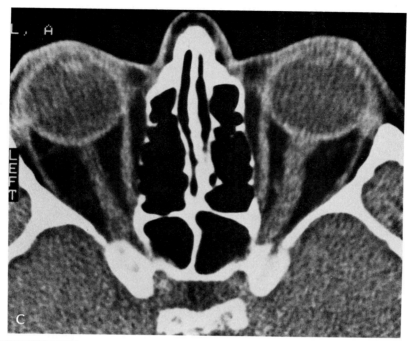

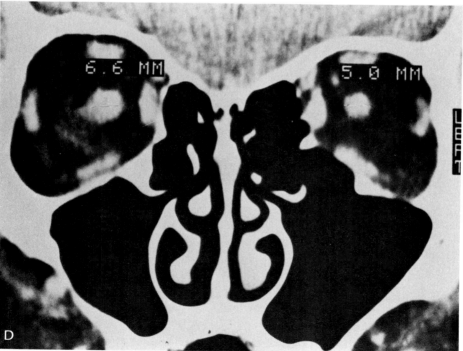

Fig. 9–5. **C.** Transaxial (top) and **D** coronal (bottom) scans show that thickening of the optic nerve is easily demonstrable in either plane. The involved optic nerve has a homogeneous density in optic neuritis.

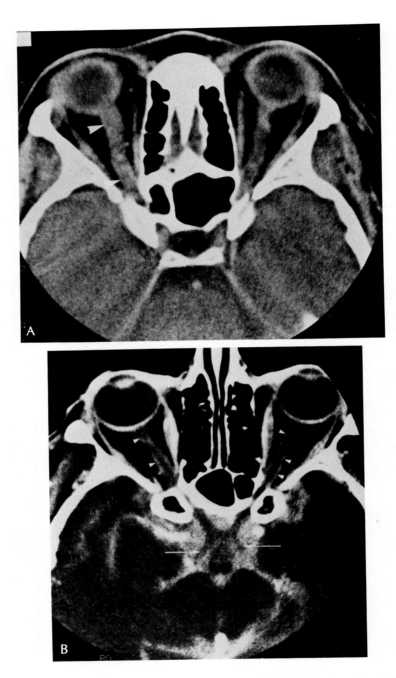

Fig. 9–6.   **A.** Diffuse thickening of the right optic nerve is noted. This thickening extends from the level of the papilla to the optic canal, a finding that is typical of papilledema (arrowheads). **B.** Scans obtained following intrathecal injection of metrizamide identify opacification of the perineuronal subarachnoid space, proving the continuity of this space with the cerebral subarachnoid space (arrowheads). Also note visualization of the optic tracts bilaterally (arrows).

and central retinal vein occlusion may also be responsible for this type of diffuse cylindrical optic nerve thickening. Papilledema often results in a decrease in visual acuity, and chronic papilledema can ultimately result in optic atrophy.

Orbital Pseudotumor

A nonspecific inflammatory process that is frequently observed within the orbit may present in a variety of ways. If the distribution of the inflammatory process is perineuronal in nature, then the optic nerve will appear as a diffusely thickened, irregularly margined structure (Fig. 9–7A). The process can be unilateral or bilateral. If the contralateral orbit is involved, it may have a different distribution of involvement than the side with the thickened optic nerve. Involvement of the optic nerve may or may not be associated with a generalized increase in retrobulbar fat density secondary to edema within the fat (Fig. 9–7B). In addition, the classic finding of uveal scleral rim enhancement may or may not be present in this process (Fig. 9–7C). The nerve is not only irregular in its thickening, but the edges of the nerve are ill-defined, as strands of edematous tissue extend out into the retrobulbar fat. These observations are highly specific for orbital pseudotumor and, in conjunction with the usual clinical presentation and the rapid response of this disease entity to steroid therapy, the diagnosis should be made without surgical intervention. There are times, in cases of orbital pseudotumor, when the optic nerve is not involved despite extensive involvement of the perineuronal retrobulbar fat. In these cases, the optic nerve is seen as a negative (low-density) defect relative to the increased density of the retrobulbar fat (Fig. 9–7D). Both examples of orbital pseudotumor, that is, direct involvement of the optic nerve and involvement of the perineuronal retrobulbar fat, can present with an acute loss of visual acuity and a painful, reddened eye.

Optic Atrophy

A variety of disease entities may result in attenuated, thinned optic nerves. Chronic pressure from mass lesions, congenital diseases, chronic papilledema, and burnt-out inflammatory and infectious processes may result in this end state. Since the optic nerve is essentially an extension of cerebral white matter, disruption anywhere along the axon will ultimately result in destruction along the entire axon. Therefore, in order to make the computed tomographic diagnosis of optic atrophy, the visualized nerve along its entire intraorbital length must be narrowed. In addition, very thin sections, preferably 1 mm in thickness, are recommended so as to exclude the possibility of averaging the optic nerve with retrobulbar fat (Fig. 9–8A). Optic atrophy may occur unilaterally or bilaterally. Calcification of the optic nerve centrum can be seen in cases of chronic atrophy (Fig. 9–8B). Rarely in cases of olfactory groove and frontal lobe lesions, one atrophic and one papilledematous optic nerve can be observed (Foster-Kennedy syndrome).

INTRAORBITAL EXTRANEURONAL CAUSES OF LOSS OF VISION

An extensive list of lesions, which are not derived from a neural origin, can be responsible for a loss of vision. They can be broken down into two major categories: those lesions that arise within the orbit and those that arise outside the orbit. Lesions arising within the orbit may be neoplastic, endocrinologic, congenital, or infectious in origin. Those lesions arising outside the orbit are mainly neoplastic or infectious in nature. A multitude of intraorbital extraneuronal masses may result in a loss of vision owing to increased pressure within the orbit or to direct optic nerve compression. A review of the most common of these is appropriate.

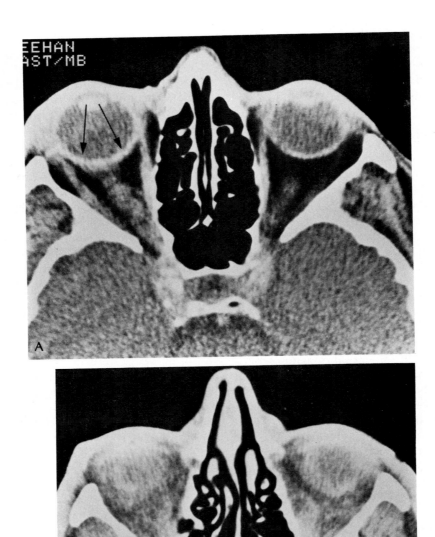

Fig. 9–7. **A.** An irregularly thickened right optic nerve is identified in this patient with orbital pseudotumor. Also note mild thickening and enhancement of the uveal scleral rim (arrows), a finding that is highly suggestive of the diagnosis of orbital pseudotumor. **B.** A generalized increase in the density of the retrobulbar fat is identified bilaterally, indicating diffuse edema.

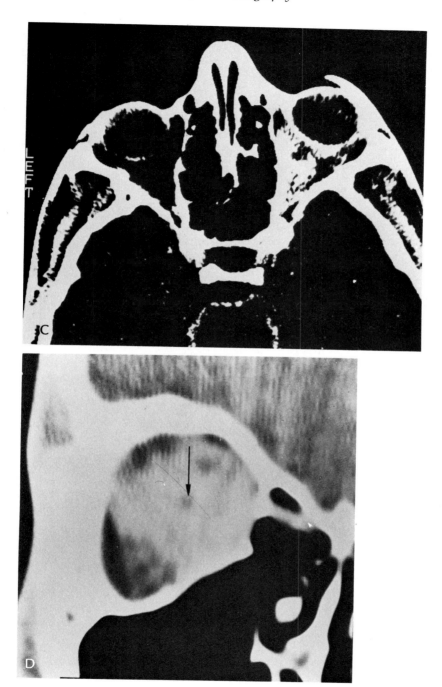

Fig. 9–7. **C.** Thickening of the uveal scleral rim, with enhancement of that rim seen involving the left globe. This is a low window-width picture that has exaggerated the thickened rim and has also demonstrated the generalized increased density of the retrobulbar fat involving the left retrobulbar area compared with the right retrobulbar area. **D.** A coned-down view of the right retrobulbar region demonstrates the optic nerve as a negative defect (arrows) amidst the markedly inflamed retrobulbar fat.

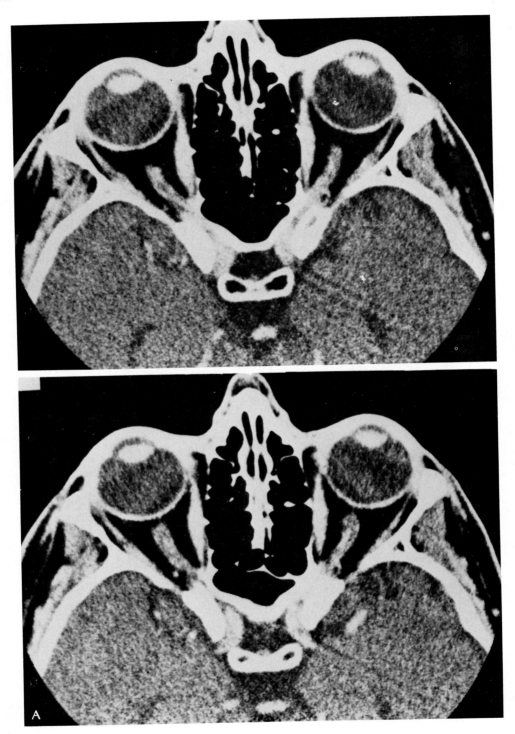

Fig. 9–8. A. Bilateral optic atrophy. Transaxial sections are presented, separated by 1 mm. Both sections demonstrate very thin optic nerves bilaterally, excluding the possibility of volume averaging as the cause of the thin optic nerves.

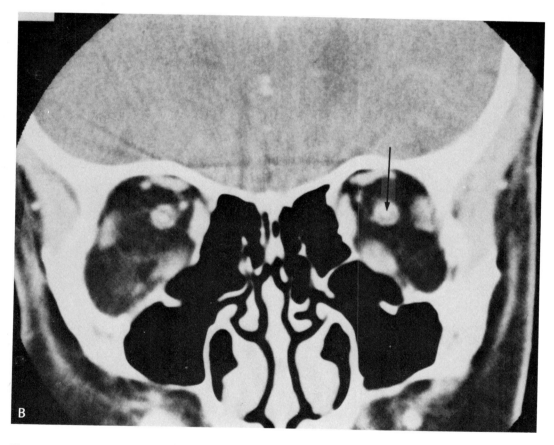

Fig. 9–8. B. Calcifications seen within the centrum of the optic nerves bilaterally is a finding that can rarely be seen in optic atrophy (arrow indicating right optic nerve calcification only).

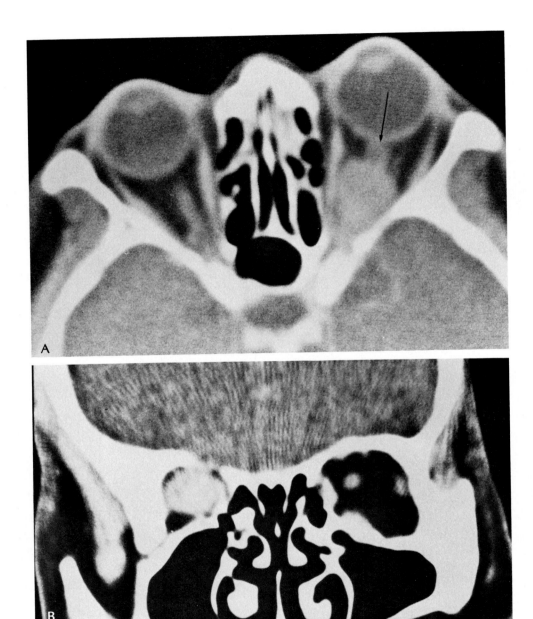

Fig. 9–9. **A.** A left-sided, perineuronal cavernous hemangioma is identified and is noted to lose its spherical configuration where it conforms to the bony margin of the orbit at its apex. Near the optic nerve head, a small amount of tumor surrounds the lateral aspect of the nerve, and the nerve can be seen as a relative negative density (arrow). **B.** A coronal scan demonstrates the central position of the left-sided apical cavernous hemangioma. The optic nerve lies in the midst of the tumor and, at this location, cannot be distinguished from the tumor.

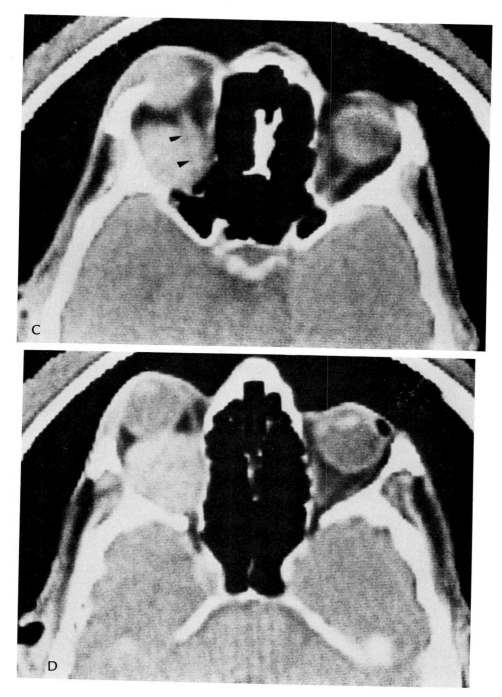

Fig. 9–9. C. Another example of a perineuronal cavernous hemangioma with the optic nerve seen as a negative defect (arrowheads). This is a scan obtained on a second generation CT scanner. **D.** Expansion of the right orbit laterally and medially is apparent, and is due to the presence of a slow-growing cavernous hemangioma.

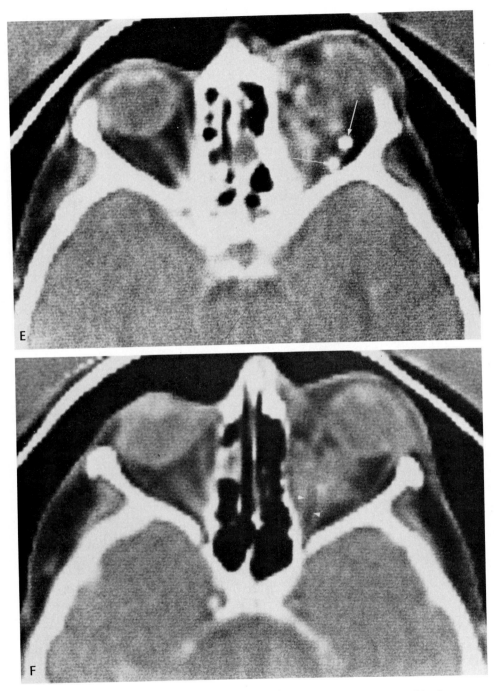

Fig. 9–9. **E.** In telangiectatic hemangiomas, phleboliths presenting as calcifications within the mass may be present (arrows). **F.** In telangiectatic hemangiomas, the optic nerve may also be seen as a negative defect (arrowheads).

Neoplastic Causes

Cavernous Hemangioma. The most common intraorbital neoplasm is the cavernous hemangioma. It is usually intraconal in origin but is not limited to this space. Cavernous hemangiomas are mostly spherical in configuration but can conform to the orbit at its apex (Figs. 9–9A,B). They surround the optic nerve but usually do not compress it. Scotomata may result from compression, but more commonly than not the lesions present mainly as exophthalmos without visual loss. They are slow-growing lesions, which enhance after contrast infusion, and rarely the optic nerve can be visualized as a negative defect within the mass (Figs. 9–9A,C). Because of their slow rate of growth and insidious nature, deformity of the bony orbit owing to chronic pressure may be observed (Fig. 9–9D).

A variant of this entity is the high-flow telangiectatic hemangioma. This type of hemangioma is associated with larger vessels and lacks the lake-type expanses within the tumor in which relatively static blood may pool. This lesion can result in visual loss from ischemia. Calcifications are common (Fig. 9–9E). The optic nerve may also be viewed as a negative density in the vascular lesion (Fig. 9–9F).

Cavernous Lymphangioma. On histologic sectioning, the lesion may contain lymph rather than blood. Such tumors are called cavernous lymphangiomas, and they may be seen in the elderly as well as in infants. One third of the cases is congenital. Like cavernous hemangiomas, they are slowly growing, benign tumors. Diminution of vision owing to pressure of the tumor on the optic nerve may occur.

On CT scans, these lesions demonstrate an irregularly enhancing mass, commonly consisting of both solid and cystic components. They may extend anteriorly into the orbit to involve the lid, and this is a common presentation both clinically and on CT. The mass is usually poorly defined and involves the optic nerves secondarily. When lid involvement is present, it is common for the mass to appear in both the intra- and extraconal compartments (Figs. 9–10A,B). Owing to its chronic nature, bony remodeling may also be seen in this entity.

Orbital Osteoma. Osteoma, composed of lamellated bone, may occur and recur in regions of cancellous bone formation. Osteoma are commonly located in the frontal sinus, but on occasion, they can occur primarily within the orbit. If osteoma do occur at the orbital apex, optic nerve compression is an almost invariable consequence and will result in loss of vision. Surgical intervention is necessary to decompress the optic nerve (Figs. 9–11A,B).

Lacrimal Gland Tumors. A wide variety of lacrimal gland tumors develop in the superolateral aspect of the orbit. They may be benign or malignant. Involvement of the optic nerve most commonly does not occur in lesions that originate in this area, since the orbit at this point is its widest and the lacrimal gland lies anteriorly to the optic nerve head. In situations when large masses arise within the lacrimal gland, however, optic nerve compression can occur on an indirect basis. Direct involvement of the optic nerve by a primary lacrimal gland tumor, whether benign or malignant, is unusual (Figs. 9–12A,B).

Orbital Metastases. Several primary metastatic tumors may metastasize to the intraorbital contents or to the bony walls of the orbit. Carcinoma of the breast and lung commonly spread to the orbit, and several cases of prostatic metastatic disease involving the orbit have been reported. If the optic nerve is directly involved, the appearance of the condition is similar to that of the perineuronal type of orbital pseudomotor. The optic nerve is thickened and irregular; no enhancement of the uveal scleral rim occurs, but elevation of the optic nerve head may be observed (Fig. 9–13A). The perineuronal fat is usually normal in cases of metastatic disease to the optic

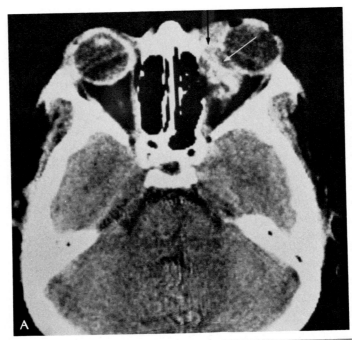

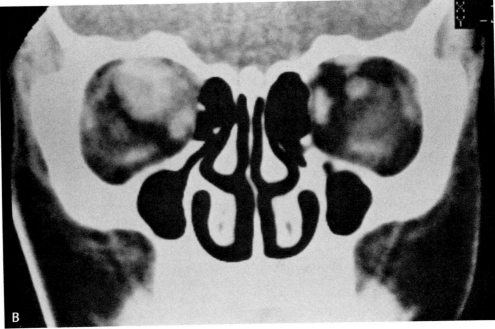

Fig. 9–10. A, B. Transaxial (top) and coronal (bottom) scans show an intraconal and extraconal cavernous lymphangioma, extending from the lid into the retrobulbar compartment and surrounding the optic nerve. The extraconal component is seen as a mass under the eyelid on the transaxial scan. This is an irregular, heterogeneously enhancing mass with both solid (black arrow) and cystic (white arrow) components being present.

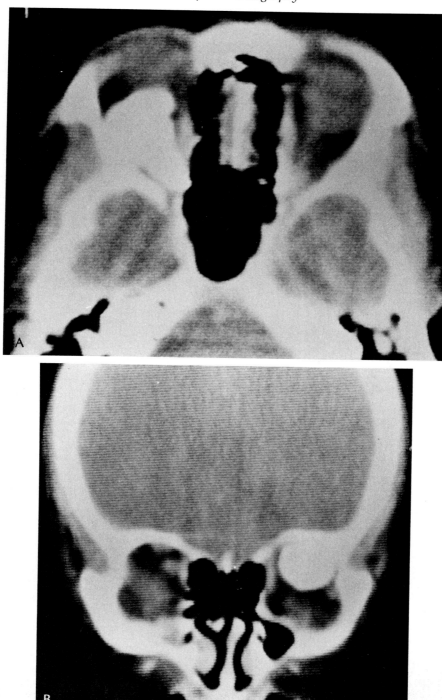

Fig. 9–11. A, B. Transaxial (top) and coronal (bottom) scans show a right orbital osteoma composed of lamellated bone, which extends into the orbital apex and is responsible, in this individual, for optic nerve compression and visual loss. Note, on the transaxial scan how the osteoma has conformed to the orbital shape. (Case courtesy of Dr. John Susac.)

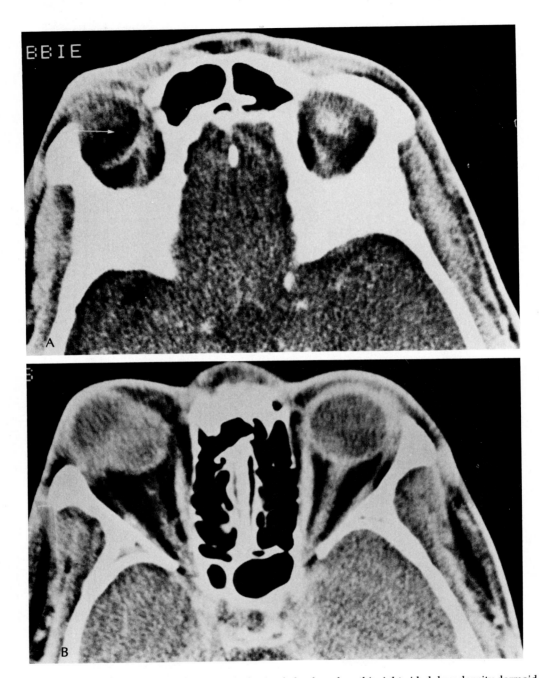

Fig. 9–12.   A, B. Large lesions arising within the lacrimal gland, such as this right-sided, low-density dermoid tumor (arrow), can, on rare occasions, cause a decrease in visual acuity. Scan **A** is through the superior orbit and scan **B** is approximately 6 mm lower. The lesion is located in the superolateral aspect of the orbit, indicating its lacrimal-gland origin.

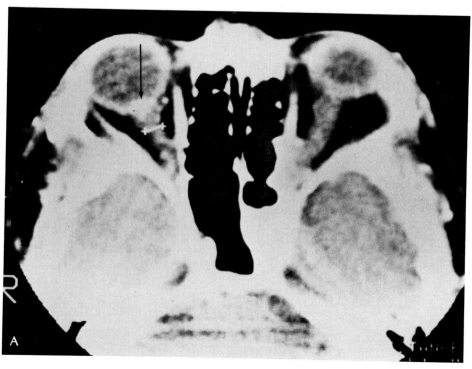

Fig. 9–13. **A.** Bilateral metastatic disease has resulted in thickened optic nerves. The appearance bears a marked similarity to orbital pseudotumor, but there is no evidence of an increase in the density of retrobulbar fat, a common finding in inflammatory processes. Also note elevation of the optic nerve head on the right side, indicating distal tumor spread (arrow).

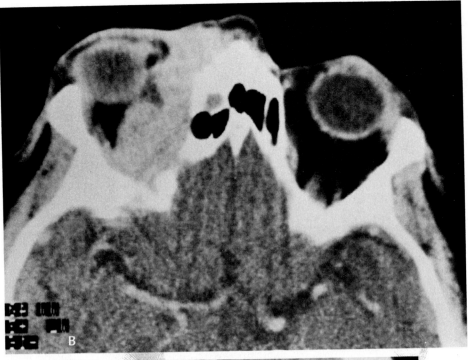

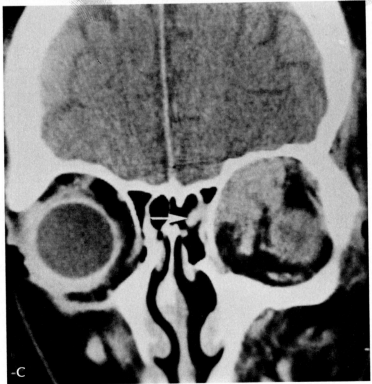

Fig. 9–13. B, C. A transaxial and a coronal scan. A right-sided, intraconal and extraconal, irregular retrobulbar mass with associated exophthalmos is seen. This picture is a common presentation of metastatic disease to the orbits. Involvement of the ipsilateral ethmoid sinus (**B,** arrow), indicating spread of the tumor through the lamina papyracea is a further sign of metastatic disease. Involvement of the retrobulbar fat manifested by increased density around the optic nerve is seen in **C.**

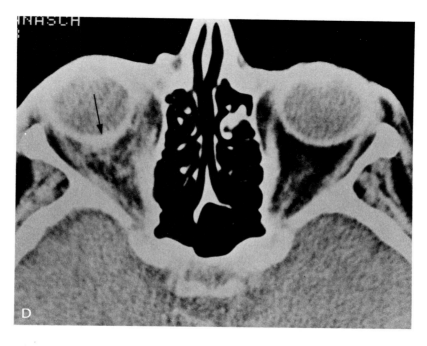

Fig. 9–13. **D.** Although it is unusual for metastatic disease to simultaneously involve the optic nerve and retrobulbar fat, it is not at all atypical for metastatic lesions to spread to the retrobulbar fat alone. This is well seen on the right side in this picture and has an appearance that is highly reminiscent of orbital pseudotumor. Thickening of the uveal scleral rim (arrow) in metastatic disease can further mimic the appearance of orbital pseudotumor.

nerve. In some cases, bilateral involvement may be present (Fig. 9–13A). More commonly, metastatic disease spreads to the non-neuronal components of the orbit or the bony walls of the orbit. It presents as an irregular, poorly defined mass lesion, not confined to either the intra- or extraconal compartments. Exophthalmos is common and is associated with pain (Fig. 9–13B,C).

Depending on the type of tumor, postcontrast enhancement may be present. Tumor can spread directly to the retrobulbar fat, and in these cases it has an appearance similar to that of diffuse orbital pseudotumor or a post-traumatic retrobulbar orbital hemorrhage (Fig. 9–13D). When the retrobulbar fat, is involved, extension of the tumor onto the posterior aspect of the globe is common, and the appearance further mimics pseudotumor; that is, thickening of the uveal scleral rim associated with enhancement following contrast infusion. This type of distribution of metastatic disease is virtually indistinguishable from an inflammatory orbital process.

In the pediatric age group, metastatic tumor to the orbit from neuroblastoma is second in frequency only to retinoblastoma. Uveal metastasis most commonly occurs from the breast, with the lung being the second most common site of origin. Tumors to the remainder of the orbit in the adult are also most commonly from the breast, with lung and prostate being the second and third most common causes. Although these manifest themselves in their earliest form with diplopia owing to muscle involvement, progression of pain may quickly follow. Compression of the optic nerve is a common consequence, and diminution of vision is a resulting clinical symptom. Metastatic disease directly to the optic nerve, of course, leads to diminution of vision much more rapidly than metastatic disease to the remainder of the orbit. The breast is also the most common site of origin for this metastatic disease to the optic nerve.

Inflammatory Disease

Wegener's Granulomatosis. Wegener's granulomatosis is a disease process with an unknown cause that results in a systemic vasculitis and commonly manifests itself with ocular complications. Necrotizing granulomatous lesions are found in the involved region associated with arteritis.

Direct orbital involvement is frequently perineuronal in distribution and manifests itself on CT scans as a high-density area located within the intraconal compartment, with CT numbers greater than that of vitreous and brain parenchyma (Fig. 9–14A).

When the optic nerve is completely surrounded by the inflammatory mass, it usually cannot be visualized (Fig. 9–14B). Although isolated cases of orbital involvement in Wegener's granulomatosis have been reported, it is much more common for orbital manifestations to be present concomitantly with abnormalities within the nose and paranasal sinuses (Fig. 9–14C,D). Underlying bony structures are frequently involved by this inflammatory process, and this may result in destruction or hyperostosis of these osseous structures (Fig. 9–14E,F).

Sarcoid. Sarcoidosis is a second granulomatous inflammatory disease that can present with orbital manifestations. Although most commonly manifested as a uveitis, it can involve the lacrimal gland. Involvement of the optic nerve is rare, but sarcoid can be an etiologic agent of visual loss from involvement of either the optic nerve or chiasm (Fig. 9–15A,B). Uveal scleral rim enhancement and thickening can be observed, usually not associated with visual loss. When there is systemic retrobulbar involvement, the mass is similar in appearance to that of Wegener's.

Pseudotumor. This nonspecific inflammatory process has been discussed earlier in this chapter. It can involve only the extraocular muscles or retrobulbar fat, as

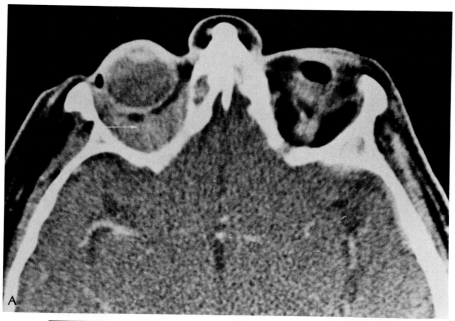

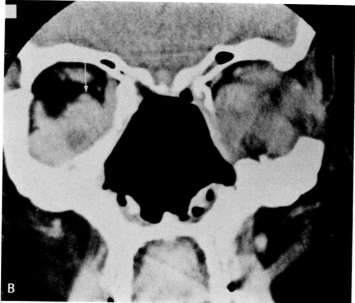

Fig. 9–14. **A.** Wegener's granulomatosis. A high-density mass is seen within the retrobulbar compartment of the right orbit (arrow). Note that the density of this lesion is higher than that of both vitreous and brain. **B.** Large retrobulbar masses are identified bilaterally. The left optic nerve (arrow) is visualized because it is not completely surrounded by inflammatory mass. The right optic nerve, as is typical in Wegener's, is obscured by the encompassing mass.

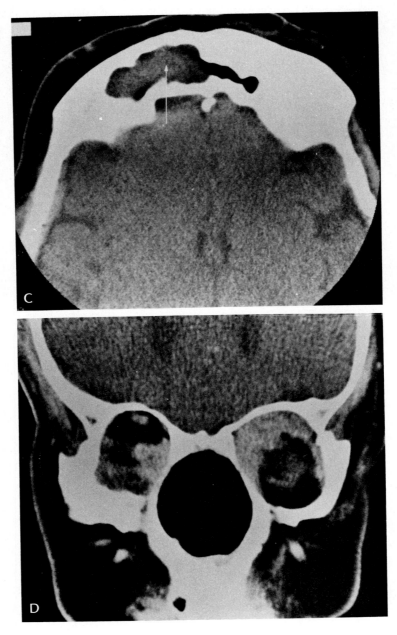

Fig. 9–14. **C.** A soft-tissue mass is identified in the right frontal sinus and represents sinus involvement by Wegener's granulomatosis (arrow). **D.** This patient has had a complete resection of his ethmoid sinuses due to chronic involvement by Wegener's. Retrobulbar involvement is identified bilaterally.

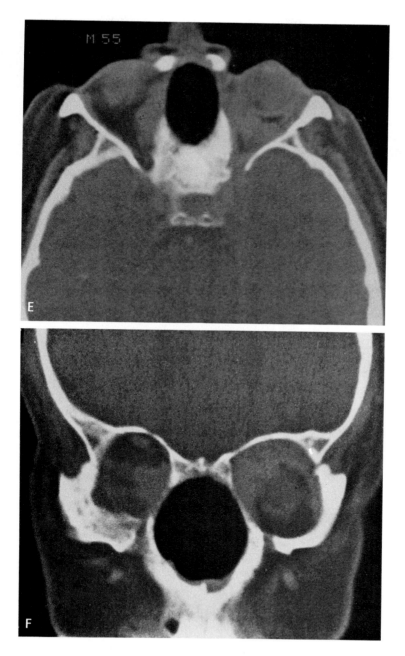

Fig. 9–14. **E, F.** Wide-window images demonstrate the bony hyperostosis that is commonly seen in Wegener's granulomatosis. Involved in this individual are both orbital and sinus bony margins.

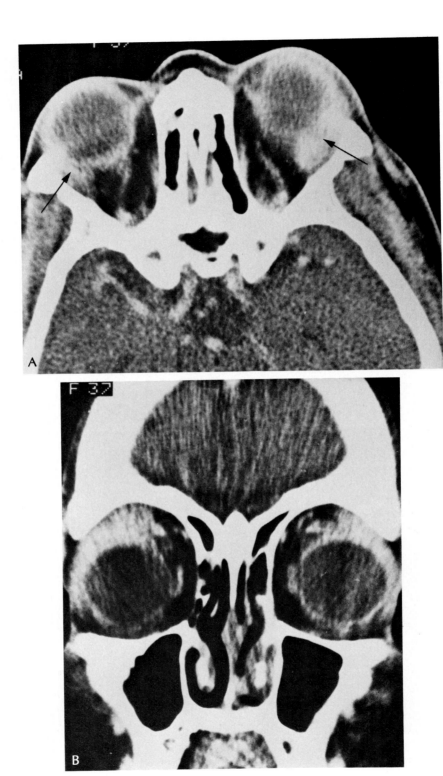

Fig. 9–15. Transaxial (top) and coronal (bottom) scans demonstrate that sarcoid has involved the lacrimal glands bilaterally and has markedly enlarged them (**A,** arrows). The coronal scan (**B**) shows an increase in lacrimal-gland size bilaterally, manifested by mass lesions above both globes. Involvement of the optic nerves by sarcoid may also occur, but was not present in this case.

seen on CT scanning, but still result in decreased visual acuity.

Endocrinologic Causes

The patient presenting with exophthalmos, either unilaterally or bilaterally, will most likely have Graves' disease. In individuals presenting with Graves' ophthalmopathy, a loss of visual acuity is a common finding. In addition, they may simultaneously present with a limitation of extraocular movement. A normal endocrinologic evaluation may result in the diagnosis of euthyroid Graves' disease.

A loss of visual acuity in individuals with Graves' disease may result from one of two causes. Not uncommonly, patients may present with marked exophthalmos owing to a generalized increase in retrobulbar fat. In these individuals, if the optic nerve is stretched sufficiently, it may result in a loss of visual acuity or a decrease in color discrimination. Obvious exophthalmos will be appreciated clinically and during CT scanning; the optic nerves will be markedly straightened and areas of optic nerve thinning can be seen (Fig. 9–16A). The extraocular muscles may be normal in patients with visual loss. In these cases, the amount of retrobulbar fat is increased, and one may easily appreciate fat infiltrating between the medial rectus muscles and lamina papyracea. Scans in the coronal plane (Fig. 9–16B) will demonstrate that the optic nerves may be discriminated from the surrounding extraocular muscles even at the orbital apex. In addition, on these coronal scans, it can be seen that the extraocular muscles are of normal size.

A more common manifestation of thyroid orbitopathy is that of diffuse muscular enlargement involving the extraocular muscles, in either a symmetric or asymmetric pattern. Figures 9–16C and 9–16D demonstrate transaxial and coronal scans with involvement mainly of the right orbit, with almost exclusive involvement of the medial rectus muscle on the right side. In this type of situation, in which there is a rather localized infiltration of extraocular muscle, a loss of visual acuity or visual field defect usually does not occur; however, in situations in which there is acute muscular enlargement, which often occurs bilaterally, the optic nerve is commonly compressed at the orbital apex (Fig. 9–16E,F). In Figure 9–16F, which is taken several millimeters anterior to the orbital apex, it can easily be appreciated that the optic nerve will be subjected to increased pressure from the enlarged extraocular muscles that are completely surrounding the nerve, especially well seen on the right side.

In cases of optic nerve thinning, which may result in demyelination secondary to marked exophthalmos owing to an increase in retrobulbar fat, and in cases of optic nerve compression owing to marked infiltration of extraocular muscles, surgical intervention may be necessary to relieve the situation in order to preserve sight. Figure 9–16G demonstrates herniation of intraorbital fat through a surgical defect in a patient with thyroid ophthalmopathy, manifested by both muscular infiltration and an increase in retrobulbar fat. Figure 9–16H, which is a coronal scan in the same individual, further demonstrates this herniation and also reveals a finding that is virtually pathognomonic of thyroid disease: that is, fatty infiltration into the inferior rectus muscle. Orbital decompression is often effective and can be used to maintain visual acuity and, in some cases, to improve it. Radiation therapy is an alternative treatment to surgical decompression.

BONY LESIONS

Abnormalities involving the bones of the orbit may or may not result in loss of visual acuity. If the origin of the bony change is neoplastic and the mass associated with this bony change is large enough, then optic nerve compression from an extraconal origin may result.

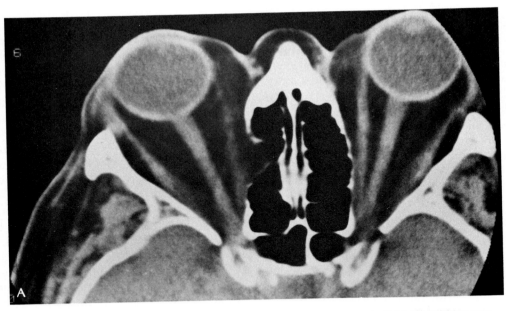

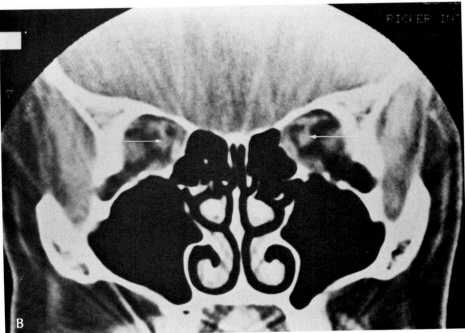

Fig. 9–16. **A.** The otpic nerves are stretched and attenuated due to an increase in retrobulbar fat bilaterally. **B.** Discrimination of the optic nerves from the extraocular muscles at the orbital apex is the normal situation, as can be seen in this patient (arrows).

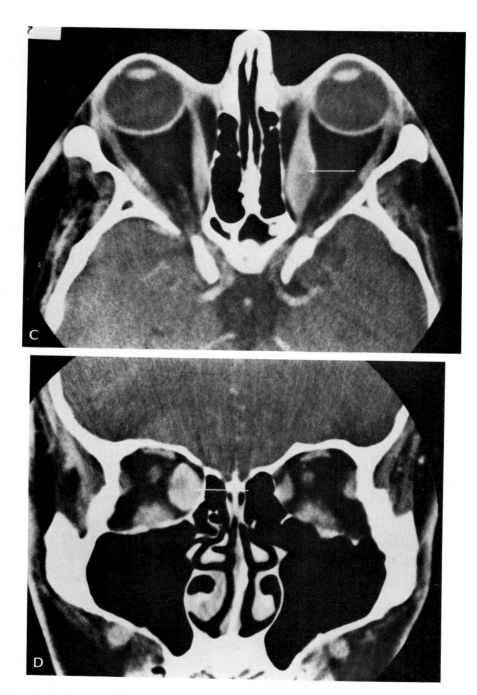

Fig. 9–16. C, D. Transaxial (**C**) and coronal (**D**) scans demonstrate marked infiltration of the medial rectus muscle (arrows). This type of muscular infiltration usually does not result in visual loss.

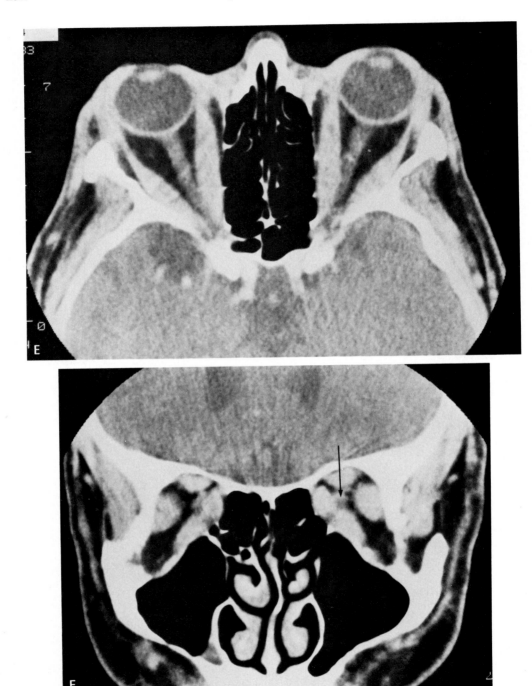

Fig. 9–16. E, F. Transaxial (**E**) and coronal (**F**) scans demonstrate diffuse extraocular muscle thickening in a patient with bilateral thyroid ophthalmopathy. The coronal scan, in particular, which was obtained several millimeters anterior to the orbital apex, indicates almost certain compression of the right optic nerve at the apex (arrow).

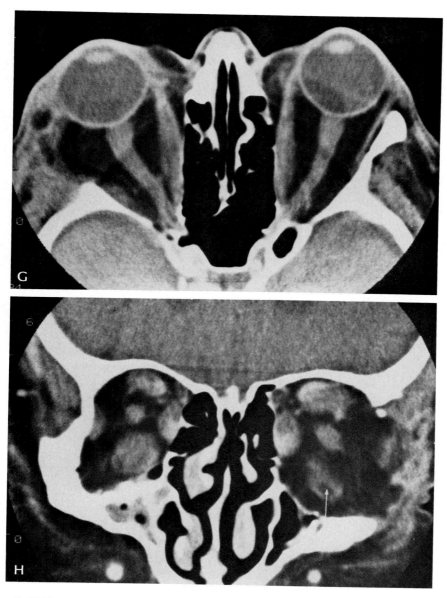

Fig. 9–16. **G, H.** Transaxial (**G**) and coronal (**H**) scans in a patient who has had a surgical orbital decompression owing to marked exophthalmos and visual loss, secondary to a generalized increase in retrobulbar fat with associated muscular thickening. Herniation of orbital contents out of the normal confines of the orbit is identified on both scans. In addition, a finding that is virtually pathognomonic of thyroid disease is identified on the coronal scan (arrow); a fatty deposition within the inferior rectus muscle has not been described in any other entity.

Carcinoma

In Figure 9–17A, carcinoma of the prostate has metastasized to the lateral wall of the orbit and extended along the greater wing of the sphenoid bone on the left side. This is causing a mild compression of the optic nerve at the orbital apex. A coronal reconstruction (Fig. 9–17B) demonstrates the degree of orbital narrowing owing to the hyperostotic bone. This type of change may be seen in cases of intracranial meningioma with invasion of the planum,

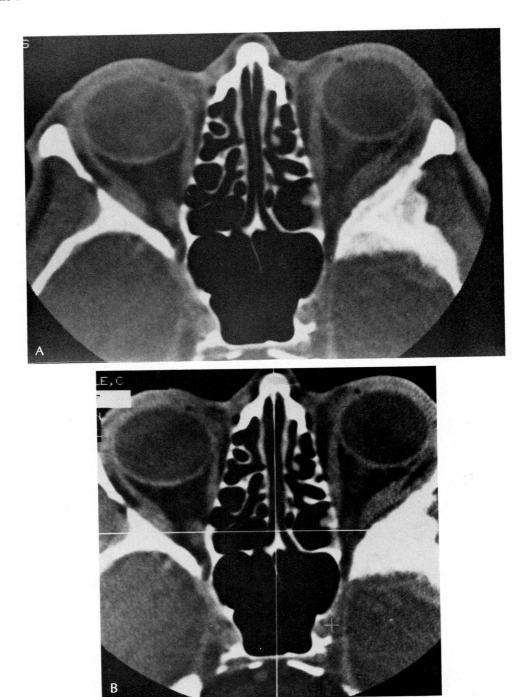

Fig. 9–17.   A, B. Two transaxial scans. Metastatic carcinoma of the prostate to the lateral wall of the orbit has caused a decrease in visual acuity owing to narrowing of the orbital apex.

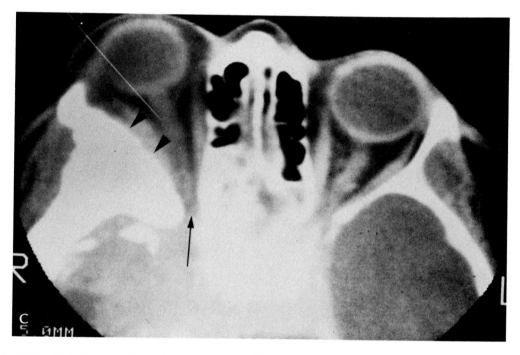

Fig. 9–17. **C.** An intracranial meningioma has caused hyperostosis of the greater wing of the sphenoid bone on the right side, and has narrowed the region of the orbital apex (arrow). Tumor is seen to occupy the temporal fossa on the right side. The thickened lateral wall of the orbit is also apparent (arrowheads).

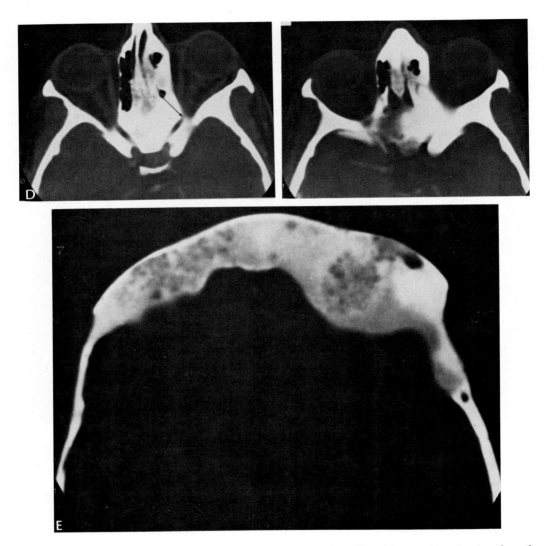

Fig. 9–17.   D, E. Fibrous dysplasia involving the frontal bones bilaterally, with posterior extension along the orbital roof on the left side and narrowing of the optic canal at the orbital side (arrows). This common complication of orbital fibrous dysplasia can result in visual loss and requires surgical treatment for relief.

optic strut, sphenoid ridge, or greater wing of the sphenoid bone. In these cases, there is usually an associated soft-tissue mass within the intracranial compartment, which may be associated with calcification within the tumor (Fig. 9–17C).

Fibrous Dysplasia

In fibrous dysplasia, the bone of the orbit may have an appearance similar to that of invasion from intracranial meningioma. In the instance of replacement of normal osseous medulla by fibrous components shown in Figure 9–17, poorly developed trabeculae occur from osseous metaplasia. This newly formed "bone" offers poor support, but has enough inherent strength to cause compression of the optic nerve at the orbital apex or optic canal (Fig. 9–17D). Usually, more than just the orbit is involved, and, in this figure, involvement of the left ethmoid sinus, anterior clinoid process, orbital roof, and frontal bone can be appreciated (Fig. 9–17D, E, and F).

Trauma

Other bony lesions that are non-neoplastic in origin may also result in loss of visual acuity or a decrease in visual field. Most of these are related to trauma. In cases of direct orbital trauma with a resultant loss in visual acuity, it may be possible to identify a bony fragment that is directly compromising the optic nerve, as seen in Figure 9–18A. Figure 9–18B shows the result of a compound fracture involving the medial wall of the orbit, as well as the frontal bone superiorly. In this case, a bony fragment has been displaced against the most distal aspect of the optic nerve. Compound fractures of the orbit may present with orbital emphysema, retrobulbar hemorrhage, and thickening of the extraocular muscles owing to hemorrhage within the muscle cone. Concomitant fractures may be observed on the same scan (Fig. 9–18C, D). Many orbital traumas can be evaluated by pluridirectional tomography; however, the relationship of the bony structures to the optic nerve and extraocular muscles can only be visualized employing computed tomography.

Figures 9–18E and 9–18F demonstrate a comminuted fracture of the orbital floor, orbital roof, and lateral wall of the orbit. In cases of diffusely comminuted orbital fractures, especially when the orbital roof is involved, examination of the brain parenchyma above the fracture site should be performed in order to evaluate for the presence of intracranial hemorrhage, as can be appreciated on these images. The coefficients of absorption of blood within the brain and within the orbit are similar. In addition, when performing CT scans of the orbit in cases of obvious orbital trauma, the remainder of the facial structures should be evaluated, since the presence of various facial fractures in association with orbital trauma is common. In some cases of visual loss following trauma, no demonstrable fracture may be appreciated on CT, and in these particular cases, pluridirectional tomography of the optic canals is recommended to evaluate for optic canal fracture.

The localization of foreign bodies in the orbit is also best performed with CT. The exact relationship of the foreign body to the sinuses, extraocular muscles, optic nerve, and sella region is best appreciated employing CT (Fig. 9–18G,H). In these figures, the metallic foreign object is not clearly related to the optic nerve; it does bear a close relationship to the medial rectus muscle and ethmoid sinus. In Figure 9–18I, however, it can clearly be appreciated that there is an intimate relationship between the metallic foreign object and the optic nerve.

Another sequela of trauma, which may not manifest itself with bony abnormality, is the development of carotid artery–cavernous sinus fistulae. Visual loss may occur from the process and is usually the result of optic nerve injury during head trauma. In untreated cases of cavernous carotid artery fistula, approximately 90% develop visual loss. This is usually attrib-

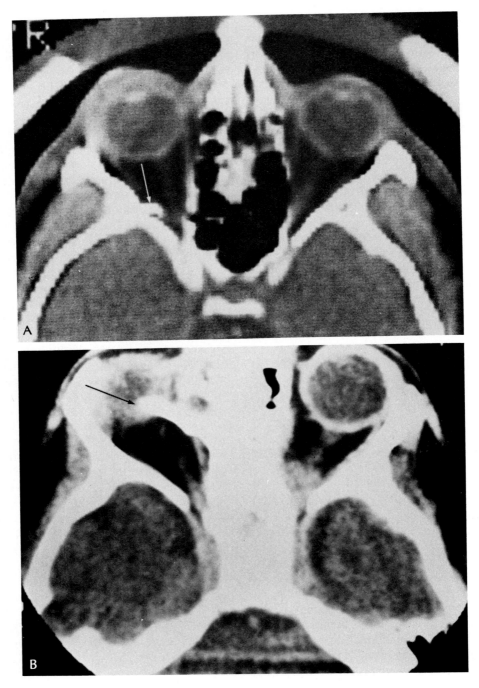

Fig. 9–18. **A.** Direct orbital trauma has resulted in a bony fragment causing direct compression of the right optic nerve (arrow). **B.** Medial wall fracture and fracture involving the roof of the orbit have resulted in a bony fragment compressing the optic nerve at the level of the papilla.

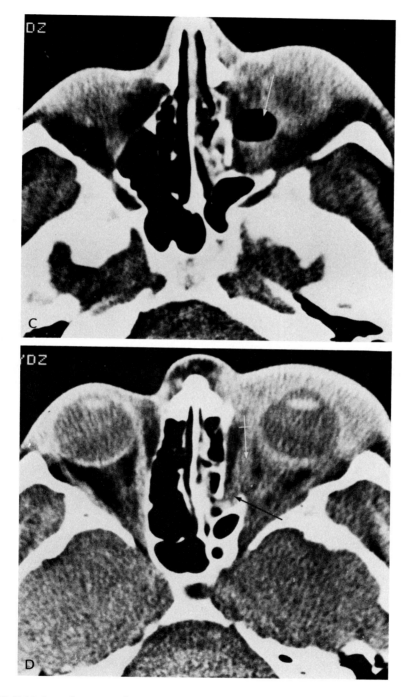

Fig. 9–18. C. Orbital emphysema (white arrow) is identified in this patient owing to a medial wall fracture. **D.** Thickening of the medial rectus muscle owing to hemorrhage (crossed white arrow) and hemorrhage within the eyelids is apparent. There is, in addition, a generalized increase in retrobulbar fat density, indicating hemorrhage and edema in this area. The medial wall fracture is also apparent (black arrow).

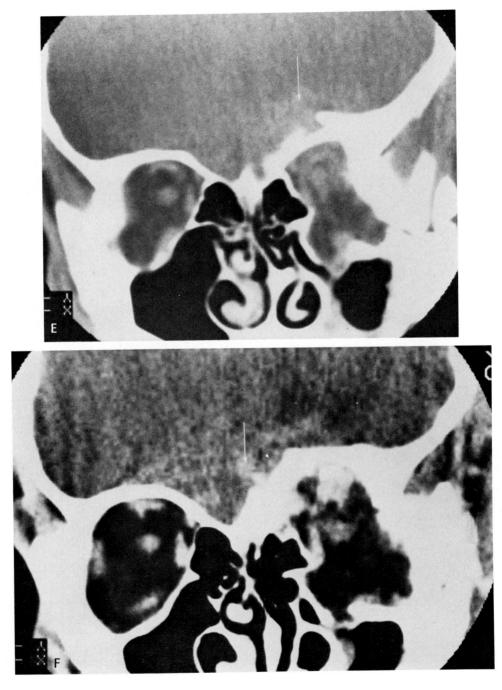

Fig. 9–18. E, F. Multiple fractures involving the right orbit are identified. Hemorrhage within the intracranial compartment is apparent (white arrows).

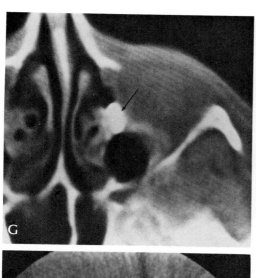

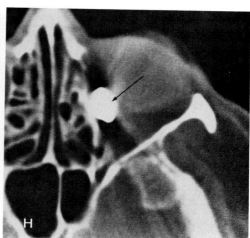

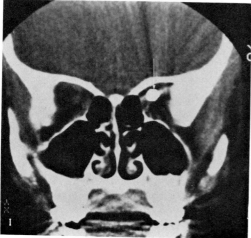

Fig. 9–18.   G, H. CT scanning accurately delineates the position of foreign objects relative to the optic nerves. In this particular case, it is clear that the metallic foreign object (arrow) does not bear a relationship to the optic nerve. **I.** This image demonstrates the close relationship of a metallic foreign object (arrow) to the optic nerve.

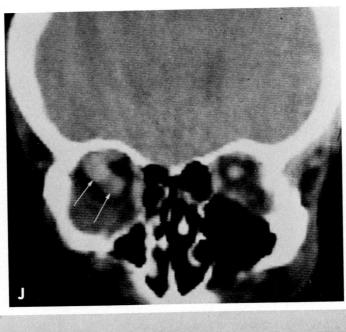

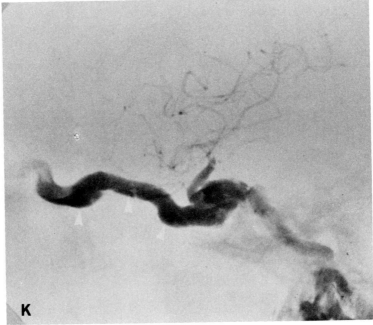

Fig. 9–18. J. An enlarged superior ophthalmic vein (arrow) is seen in this patient with recent head trauma and pulsating exophthalmos. An internal carotid artery angiogram (**K**) confirms the presence of a cavernous sinus-carotid artery fistula, with marked dilatation and opacification of the superior ophthalmic vein (arrowheads).

utable to a decrease in circulation to the retina. The computed tomographic diagnosis is made by the presence of an enlarged superior ophthalmic vein and, possibly, enlarged inferior ophthalmic vein. Exophthalmos is usually present, and an enlarged cavernous sinus on the ipsilateral side to the enlarged superior ophthalmic vein may be appreciated. Definite diagnosis is through angiography (Fig. 9–18J,K).

EXTRAORBITAL DISEASE

The extent and variety of extaorbital disease that may affect the orbits includes lesions arising from the nasopharynx, the cranial contents, the nasal structures, and the paranasal sinuses. The variety of diseases is extensive and includes inflammations, malignant tumors, and benign neoplasms. When visual loss has occurred secondary to one of these processes, there is usually evidence of frank bony destruction or extensive remodeling of bone. Visual loss may occur secondary to direct optic nerve compression and invasion, or may be secondary to stretching and attenuation of the optic nerve, or the presence of a large mass invaginating itself into the orbit. Conventional roentgenograms are often helpful. When exophthalmos is apparent, a unilateral decrease in extraocular motility can be expected. Coronal reconstructions are helpful, but direct coronal scanning, as in evaluating the orbit, is more informative.

Inflammatory Disease

Sinus infections may easily involve the orbit by rupture through the orbital floor, in the case of maxillary sinus disease, and through the lamina papyracea, in the case of ethmoid sinus disease. Exophthalmos is common, and opacification of the responsible sinus is invariable. In the pediatric age group, involvement of the orbit from an ethmoid sinusitis is the most common site (Fig. 9–19A). In the adult population, involvement from disease within the maxillary sinus is more common. This may ex-

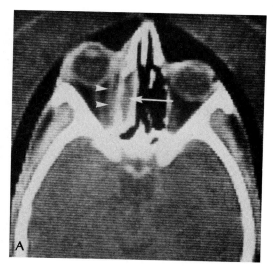

Fig. 9–19. A. An opacified, infected right ethmoid sinus (arrow) has ruptured through the lamina papyracea and formed an extraconal mass, displacing the right medial rectus muscle laterally (arrowheads).

tend either directly up through the orbital floor or, more commonly, via cellulitis involving orbital soft tissues, with subsequent involvement of the extraconal compartment and development of exophthalmos (Fig. 9–19B,C). The pathogens may be either bacterial or fungal. As is illustrated in Figures 9–19B and 9–19C, in a diabetic individual, mucormycosis should be placed high on the list of differential diagnoses. Either chronic or acute sinus disease can be the site of origin of orbital infection. When the frontal sinuses are involved, evaluation of the brain parenchyma should also be performed to exclude the presence of an intracranial abscess. Epidural spread may also develop from frontal sinus infection.

Mucoceles

When the normal communication between a sinus and the nasal cavity is obstructed and infected or aseptic, a mucocele may develop. The most common location is the frontal sinus, and the second most common is the sphenoid, but the ethmoid and maxillary sinuses can also be the sites of origin of mucoceles. They are char-

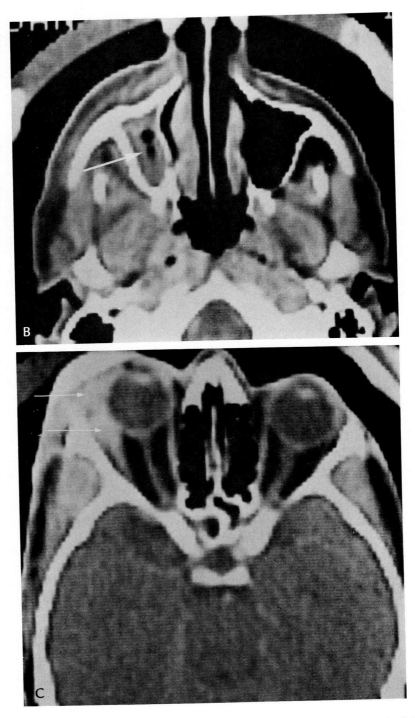

Fig. 9–19.   B. The right maxillary sinus is infected and opacified (arrow), and (**C**) associated cellulitis involving the lid and extraconal compartment is identified (small arrows).

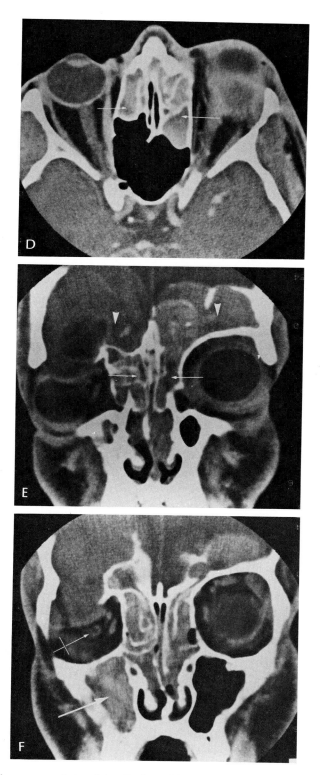

Fig. 9–19. D, E, F. A large mucocele involving the frontal (arrowheads), ethmoids (short white arrows), and left maxillary sinuses (large white arrow) is identified. Obvious deformity of the left optic nerve (crossed white arrow) is identified, explaining decreased visual acuity in this eye. Mucoceles are unpredictable in their mode of extension, and orbital involvement is common.

acterized by the presence of mucous secretions. Conventional roentgenographs demonstrate deformity of bone and loss of normal scalloping of the frontal sinus. Most commonly, they involve only a single sinus. Figure 9–19D demonstrates the presence of a mucocele that is involving almost all of the paranasal sinuses. In addition, intracranial rupture and intraorbital rupture are apparent. Deviation and deformity of the optic nerve in this individual are responsible for visual loss (Fig. 9–19D,E, and F).

Neoplasms

Malignant neoplasms involving the paranasal sinuses are most commonly squamous cell carcinomas. Adenocarcinoma also occurs in the paranasal sinuses, and sarcomas arising from the supporting structures, such as rhabdomyosarcoma, chondrosarcoma, and osteogenic sarcoma, are also known to arise within the sinuses. These carcinomas are well differentiated, and their mode of spread is usually local in nature, with distant metastases occurring late in the disease process. Visual loss as a result of sinus carcinomas is caused either by exophthalmos and attenuation of the optic nerve (Fig. 9–20A,B) or by direct invasion from the sinus into the retrobulbar compartment and direct involvment of the optic nerve (Fig. 9–20C,D). As in inflammatory disease, there is invariable involvement of the sinus, indicating the cause of the retrobulbar abnormality. Unlike infectious disease, frank destruction of the bony septa separating the orbits from the sinuses is common in the squamous cell carcinomas, as can be seen in Figure 9–20D.

Often difficult to differentiate from primary sinus carcinomas are the squamous cell carcinomas that arise in the nasopharynx. They may invade the sinuses and extend into the orbit and cause visual loss in a fashion similar to that of primary sinus carcinomas. They are somewhat more aggressive in their pathologic appearance, and tend to metastasize distally more often and earlier than the sinus carcinomas. Figures 9–20E and 9–20F demonstrate a squamous cell carcinoma that has extended into the orbital apex from a primary nasopharyngeal orgin. The maxillary sinus on the ipsilateral side is also involved by tumor invasion. Frank destruction of both the lateral wall and the medial wall of the sinus is apparent. Figures 9–20G and 9-20H are CT images of a young female who suffered from bilateral decreased visual acuity. A large mass lesion arising from the region of the frontal sinuses, with invasion into the orbit, is apparent. Histologic diagnosis was chondrosarcoma.

Inverting Papilloma

A benign neoplasm that can mimic a more aggressive tumor is an invaginating or inverting papilloma. It arises most commonly from the nasal cavity, but may originate from the ethmoid or maxillary sinus. It is a slow-growing, benign neoplasm, which can reach enormous size. Differentiation from a more aggressive malignant tumor can be difficult, since extreme thinning of the bone can, on CT scans and polytomography, appear identical to frank bony destruction. It may invade the orbit, or simply displace the globe and attenuate and stretch the optic nerve. Simultaneous involvement of the nasal cavity and adjacent paranasal sinuses is common in this disease process. Unilateral exophthalmos, with attenuation and stretching of the optic nerve, is apparent on Figures 9–21A and 9–21B. Inverting papillomas, despite surgical intervention, tend to recur locally; less than 10% of them may convert to squamous cell carcinoma.

COMMENT

The extent and variety of lesions arising outside the intracranial cavity that may cause visual loss is great. The preceding pages have discussed a variety of lesions, but have purposely excluded abnormalities arising anterior to the optic nerve head and

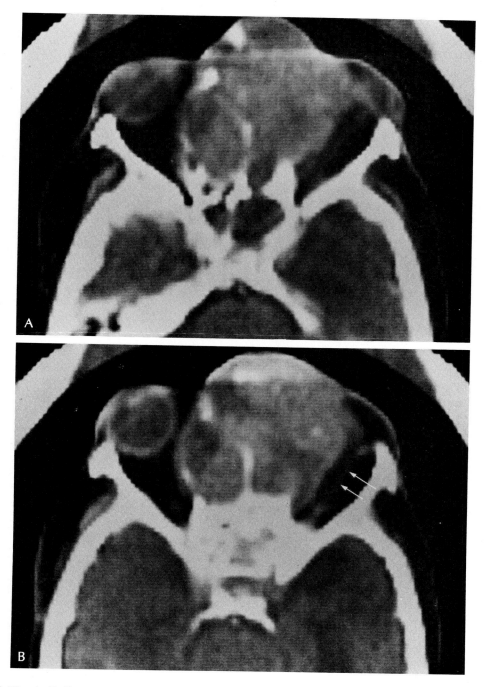

Fig. 9–20. A, B. Two transaxial scans; scan **A** (top) was obtained 6 mm below scan **B** (bottom). **A** shows that the center of the mass is within the ethmoid sinuses and has extended bilaterally. Bilateral exophthalmos with stretching and attenuation of the left optic nerve (arrows) has resulted in a decrease in visual acuity of the left eye in this patient with squamous cell carcinoma of the ethmoid sinuses.

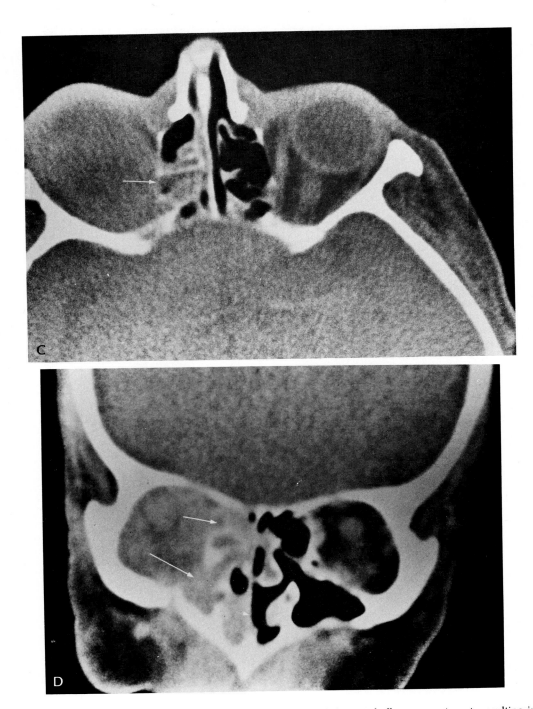

Fig. 9–20. C, D. Ethmoid sinus carcinoma has directly invaded the retrobulbar compartment, resulting in direct optic nerve compression and visual loss. Disruption of the lamina papyracea is apparent at several levels (arrows). The optic nerve is not defined amid this tumor.

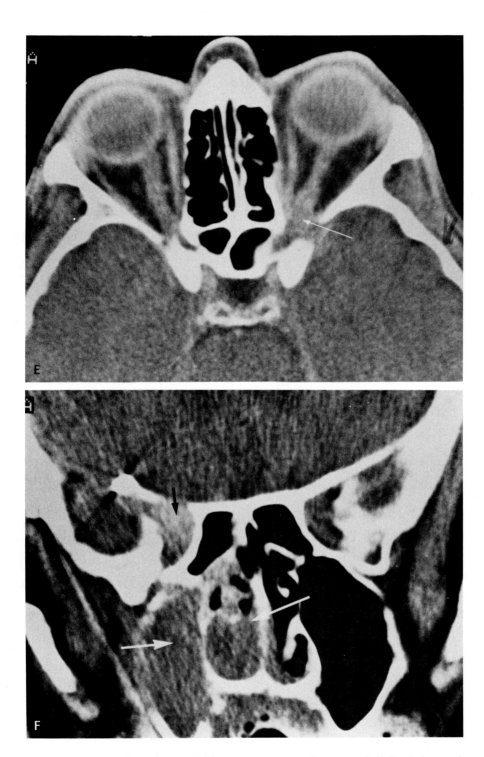

Fig. 9–20.   E, F. Transverse (**E**) and coronal (**F**) scans demonstrate invasion of a left-sided nasopharyngeal carcinoma into the orbital apex. Circumferential involvement of the optic nerve at the apex is apparent on the transaxial scan (arrow). On the coronal scan, involvement of the ipsilateral maxillary and nasal cavity is apparent (large arrows). The optic nerve on the coronal scan cannot be separated from the tumor mass (black arrow).

269

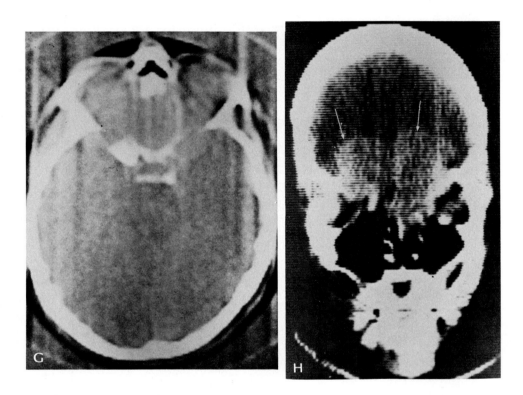

Fig. 9–20. **G, H.** These scans demonstrate the presence of a large, bifrontal chondrosarcoma. Involvement of both orbits with subsequent decreased visual acuity bilaterally was present. These images are from a first generation CT scanner. The mass of chondrosarcoma within the brain is indicated by white arrows.

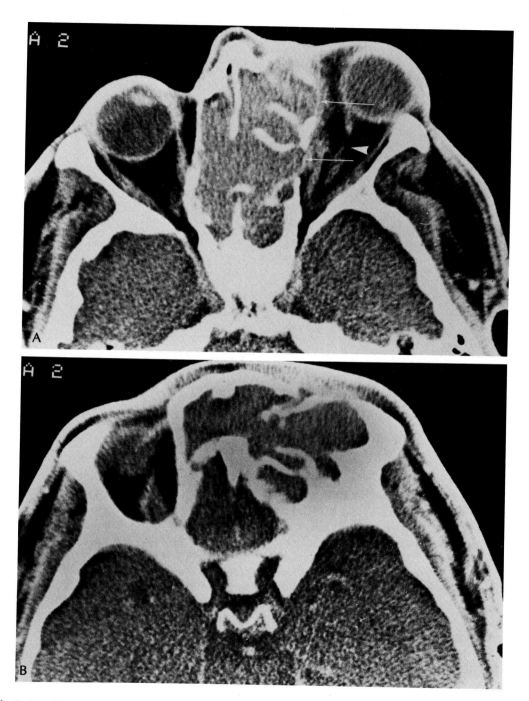

Fig. 9–21.   A, B. An invaginating papilloma has involved both ethmoids and both frontal sinuses. Disruption of the medial wall of the left orbit is apparent (white arrows). Deformity of the optic nerve is apparent on this scan and is the cause of a mild decrease in visual acuity in this individual (arrowhead). **B** reveals extension into the left orbit superiorly, as well as involvement of the frontal sinuses.

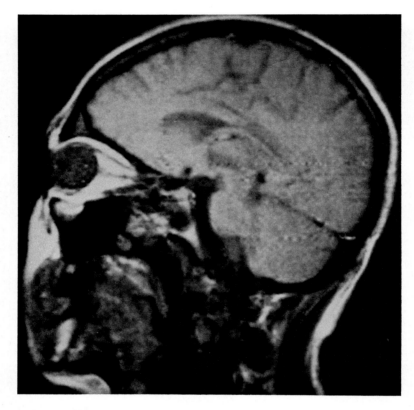

Fig. 9–22. A nuclear magnetic resonance scan obtained in a plane parallel to the course of the optic nerve. The inferior and superior rectus muscles can be seen. The sella is not seen. Note that no signal is coming from the maxillary sinus except in the superior anterior aspect, at which point a small polyp is present.

posterior to the optic canal. Computed tomography does not always delineate the exact histologic diagnosis, but is of undeniable importance in outlining the extent of disease, the amount of bony involvement, the direct or indirect effect upon the optic nerve, and is often valuable in adding information as to the vascularity of the abnormality.

Hovering on the horizon of medical imaging is the new modality of nuclear magnetic resonance (NMR). This imaging device employs the combined technologies of high magnetic field, radio frequency modulation, and computer manipulation of obtained data. This method results in an image similar to computed tomography in appearance, but representing entirely different information, which has been obtained in an entirely different fashion, employing strictly non-ionizing radiation. The last image in this chapter (Fig. 9–22) is a single NMR scan representing the state of this technology at the end of 1983. This NMR scan is obtained in the semi-sagittal plane, parallel to the optic nerve. The optic nerve itself is beautifully visualized, and careful scrutiny will demonstrate the ophthalmic artery as it is swinging lateral to the nerve to arrive at a supraneuronal position. The globe and a portion of the inferior oblique and inferior rectus muscles can be seen. Although nuclear magnetic resonance will almost certainly have its place in the future evaluation of orbital disease, it will probably be several years more before it develops the high spatial resolution necessary to demonstrate the discrete orbital anatomy that can now be visualized employing CT scanning. This new modality will certainly excite clinicians and radiologists, but will probably have less impact than computed tomography on the diagnosis of orbital disease.

BIBLIOGRAPHY

Bernardino, M.E., Danziger, J., Young, S.E., and Wallace, S.: Computed tomography in ocular neoplastic disease. Am. J. Roentgenol. *131*:111, 1978.

Bernardino, M.E., Zimmerman, R.E., Citrin, C.M., and David, D.O.: Scleral thickening: a CT sign of orbital pseudotumor. Am. J. Roentgenol. *129*(4):703, 1977.

Byrd, S.E.,et al.: Computed tomography of intraorbital optic nerve gliomas in children. Radiology *129*(1):73, 1978.

Cabanis, E.A., et al.: Computed tomography of the optic nerve: Part II. Size and shape modifications in papilledema. Journal of Computer Assisted Tomography *2*(2):150, 1978.

Citrin, C.M., and Alper, M.G.: Computed tomography of the visual pathways. Computerized Tomography *3*(4):305, 1979.

Daniels, D.L., et al.: CT recognition of optic nerve sheath meningioma: Abnormal sheath visualization. Am. J. Neuroradiol. *3*(2):181, 1982.

Edeiken, J., and Hodes, P.J.: Roentgen Diagnosis of Diseases of Bone. Baltimore, Williams & Wilkins Co., 1967.

Enzmann, D.R., Donaldson, S.S., and Kriss, J.P.: Appearance of Graves' disease on orbital computed tomography. Journal of Computer Assisted Tomography *3*(6):815, 1979.

Hammerschlag, S.B., Hesselink, J.R., and Weber, A.L.: Computed Tomography of the Eye and Orbit. Norwalk, CT, Appleton-Century-Crofts, 1983.

Hasso, A.N., et al.: High resolution thin section computed tomography of the cavernous sinus. Radiographics *2*(1):83, 1982.

Hesselink, J.R., and Weber, A.L.: Pathways of orbital extension of extraorbital neoplasms. Journal of Computer Assisted Tomography *6* (3):593, 1982.

Hesselink, J.R., et al.: Computed tomography of the paranasal sinuses and face. Part II: Pathological anatomy. Journal of Computer Assisted Tomography *2*:(5):568, 1978.

Hesselink, J.R., et al.: Evaluation of mucoceles of the paranasal sinuses with computed tomography. Radiology *133*(2):397, 1979.

Hesselink, J.R., et al.: Radiological evaluation of orbital metastases, with emphasis on computed tomography. Radiology *137*(2):363, 1980.

Howard, C.W., Osher, R.H., and Tomsak, R.L.: Computed tomographic features in optic neuritis. Am. J. Ophthalmol. *89*(5):699, 1980.

Hurwitz, B.S., and Citrin, C.M.: Use of computerized axial tomography (CAT scan) in evaluating therapy of orbital pseudotumors. Ann. Ophthalmol. *11*(2):217, 1979.

Jakobiec, F.: Personal communication, 1983.

Jacoby, C.G., Go, R.T., and Beren, R.A.: Cranial CT of neurofibromatosis. Am. J. Roentgenol. *135*(3):553, 1980.

Johns, T., Citrin, C.M., Black, J.L., and Sherman, J.: The optic nerve as a negative defect: A non-specific sign. Submitted for publication, Am. J. Neurol.

Lloyd, G.A.: CT scanning in the diagnosis of orbital disease. Computerized Tomography *3*(4):227, 1979.

Lobes, L.A., Jr.: Computed tomography in the detection of intraocular foreign bodies. Int. Ophthalmol. Clin. *22*(4):219, 1982.

Momose, K.J., and Grove, A.S., Jr.: Computed tomography for evaluation of sinus disorders involving the orbit. Int. Ophthalmol. Clin. *22*(4):181, 1982.

Moseley, I.F., and Sanders, M.D.: CT scanning in neuro-ophthalmology: Optic nerve compression. *In* Topics in Neuro-ophthalmology. Edited by H.S. Thompson, R. Daroff, J.S. Glaser, and M.D. Sanders, Baltimore, Williams & Wilkins Co., 1979; Section 5.3 pp. 302–17.

Peyster, R.G., Hoover, E.D., Hershey, B.L., and Haskin, M.E.: High-resolution CT lesions of the optic nerve. Am. J. Roentgenol. *140*(5):869, 1983.

Salvolini, U., et al.: Computed tomography of the optic nerve: Part I. Normal results. Journal of Computer Assisted Tomography *2*(2):141, 1978.

Salvolini, U., Menichelli, F., and Pasquini, U.: Computer assisted tomography in ninety cases of exophthalmos. Journal of Computer Assisted Tomography *1*(1):81, 1977.

Simmons, J.D., LaMasters, D., and Char, D.: Computed tomography of ocular colobomas. Am. J. Roentgenol. *141*(6):1223, 1983.

Swenson, S.A., Forbes, G.S., Younge, B.R., and Campbell, R.J.: Radiologic evaluation of tumors of the optic nerve. Am. J. Neuroradiol. *3*(3):319, 1982.

Trokel, S.: Computed tomographic scanning of orbital inflammations. Int. Ophthalmol. Clin. *22*(4):81, 1982.

Vermess, M., Haynes, B.F., Fauci, A.S., and Wolff, S.M.: Computer assisted tomography of orbital lesions in Wegener's granulomatosis. Journal of Computer Assisted Tomography *2*(1):45, 1978.

Walsh, F.B., and Hoyt, W.F.: Clinical Neuro-ophthalmology, 3rd Ed. Baltimore, Williams & Wilkins Co., 1969.

Wende, S., et al.: Computed tomography of orbital lesions: A cooperative study of 210 cases. Neuroradiology *13*(3):123, 1977.

Zimmerman, R.A., and Bilaniuk, L.T.: CT of orbital infection and its cerebral complications. Am. J. Roentgenol. *134*(1):45, 1980.

Chapter **10**

Facial Nerve Paralysis

PETER D. WILLIAMSON

ANATOMY

Pathologic conditions affecting the seventh cranial or facial nerve are frequently associated with ophthalmologic findings. Accurately evaluating these conditions requires a fundamental understanding of the functional anatomy of the region in question.

The seventh cranial nerve has four important anatomic characteristics. (1) It is composed of two different anatomic and functional components, the facial nerve and the intermediate nerve (nervus intermedius of Wrisberg). (2) It is encased in bone for a considerable distance. (3) The course of the nerve from the facial motor nucleus to its exit from the brain stem follows an unusual circuitous pathway. (4) The motor nucleus receives contralateral and ipsilateral input from the corticobulbar tracts. These characteristics have clinical implications.

The facial nerve proper is the motor nerve for the muscles of facial expression. Its nucleus is located in the dorsolateral caudal pons (Fig. 10–1). This nucleus receives its major input from the contralateral corticobulbar fibers. The contralateral input supplies the entire facial nucleus, whereas the ipsilateral fibers are concen-

trated on the cells that innervate the upper facial muscles. The nucleus also receives input from various sensory nuclei associated with reflex mechanisms, for example, the fifth nerve nucleus for the corneal reflex. Motor fibers leaving the nucleus travel medially, dorsally, and slightly rostrally to a position just beneath the floor of the fourth ventricle in the vicinity of the sixth or abducens nucleus. At this point, the motor fibers sweep over the sixth nerve nucleus, forming the facial colliculus in the floor of the fourth ventricle. The facial nerve fibers then travel in a ventrolateral direction, exiting from the brain stem at the caudal border of the pons just medial to the eighth cranial or acoustic nerve. The facial nerve leaves the cranial cavity with the eigth nerve through the internal auditory meatus to begin its long bony course (Fig. 10–2). At the lateral end of the internal auditory meatus, the facial and acoustic nerves part and the facial nerve enters the smaller facial canal. In this bony canal, the facial nerve continues laterally to the medial wall of the tympanic cavity, then turns abruptly backwards and down, forming the genu or bend of the facial canal. The nerve passes downward to the posterior wall of the tympanic cavity and exits at the

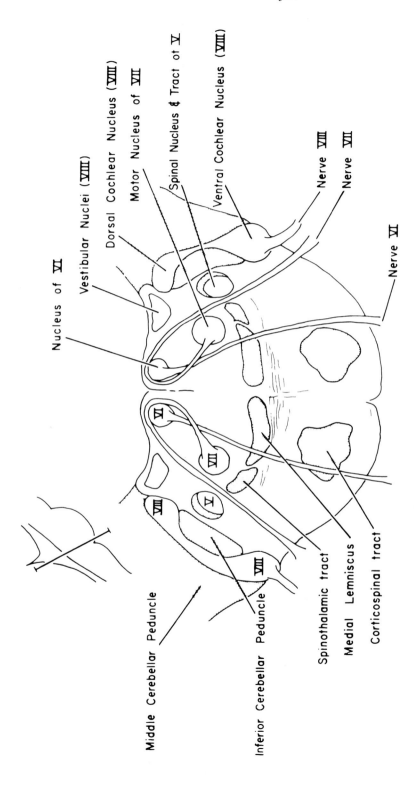

Fig. 10–1. Cross section through the lower pons demonstrating the relationship of the seventh nerve nucleus and motor fibers to other brain stem structures. Note particularly the relationship with the sixth nerve nucleus.

base of the skull through the stylomastoid foramen. After exiting from the skull, the facial nerve enters the parotid gland and divides into many branches, which in turn, travel to the various muscles of facial expression.

The intermediate nerve or sensory portion of the facial nerve is a combined visceral efferent and sensory afferent nerve. The visceral efferent components are parasympathetic fibers that regulate secretory functions in the salivary and lacrimal glands. The cells of origin of these nerves are in the superior salivatory nucleus of the brain stem. The sensory components of the intermediate nerve subserve primarily taste sensation for the anterior two thirds of the tongue, but a small somatosensory component also conveys sensory impulses from the external auditory meatus and a variable area of the external ear. The geniculate ganglion, which is located at the genu or bend in the facial canal, is the sensory nucleus for taste and somatic sensation. The central connections for taste fibers are to the solitary nucleus, and to the fifth nerve nucleus for somatosensory fibers. The intermediate nerve lies adjacent to the facial nerve at its point of exit from the brain stem and travels with this nerve as a separate entity for a variable distance before the two nerves fuse.

A number of branches exit from the facial nerve during its course in the facial canal (Fig. 10–2). Only those with clinical significance are described. The greater superficial petrosal nerve leaves the facial nerve in the region of the geniculate ganglion. This visceral efferent nerve subserves secretory function for the lacrimal gland and for the nasal and palatine glands. The stapedial nerve is a small motor twig that leaves the facial nerve in the posterior tympanic cavity and innervates the stapedius muscle. The function of this muscle is to dampen low-frequency sounds. The chorda tympani is a large branch of the facial nerve that leaves the parent trunk just prior to its exit from the skull at the

stylomastoid foramen. The chorda tympani traverses the tympanic cavity, after which it emerges from the skull to join the lingual branch of the fifth nerve. It carries taste sensation from the anterior two thirds or one half of the tongue and provides visceral motor fibers for the sublingual and submaxillary glands.

DYSFUNCTION

Facial nerve function can be altered by lesions anywhere in the central controlling pathways or in the peripheral distribution of the nerve. The signs of facial nerve dysfunction vary depending on the site of the lesion.

Central Lesions

Lesions within the central nervous system can be divided into those that affect the corticobulbar fibers above the level of the seventh nerve nucleus and those that affect the nucleus and emerging fibers. The former are referred to as supranuclear lesions and can occur from the motor cortex to the mid pons. The latter are referred to as nuclear lesions and are confined to the region of the seventh nerve nucleus in the lower pons.

Supranuclear facial paralysis can be easily differentiated from a nuclear or peripheral lesion. As mentioned previously, the portion of the nucleus that receives both ipsilateral and contralateral innervation is strongly biased in favor of the upper facial muscles. As a result, following contralateral supranuclear lesions, volitional control of the frontalis and to a lesser extent the orbicularis oculi muscles is preserved. The eyes can be closed, the eyebrows raised, and the forehead wrinkled. Minimal weakness in these muscles can be detected only by testing their strength against forced contraction. Weakness in the lower facial muscles following supranuclear lesions is much more pronounced, but some volitional control is often maintained. The involved side of the face droops slightly, the palpebral fissure is slightly widened owing to sag-

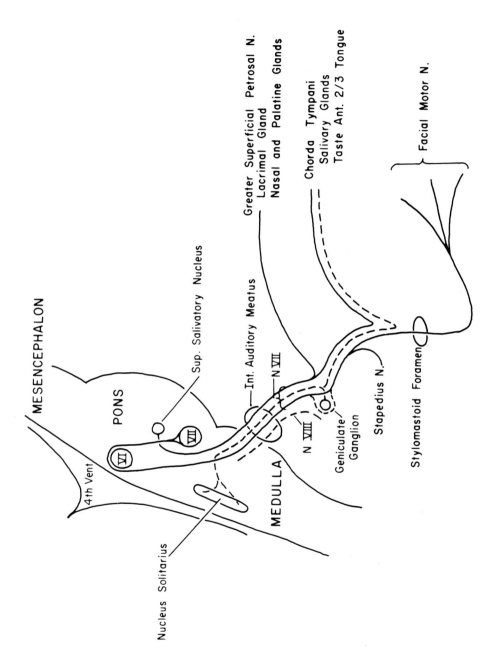

Fig. 10–2. Diagram showing the anatomic relationships and functional components of the central and peripheral facial nerve.

ging of the lower lid, and the nasolabial fold is flattened. Attempts to move the mouth, as in smiling or grimacing, accentuate the weakness of the lower facial muscles. Often, a dissociation exists between volitional and emotional motor control. Asking the patient to show his teeth or grimace reveals a definite motor asymmetry, while spontaneous emotional responses such as laughing or crying produce a more symmetric motor response. The reverse can be seen, but is much less common. Taste, lacrimation, and salivation are not altered by supranuclear lesions. Supranuclear facial weakness rarely occurs in isolation. Hemiparesis, hemisensory loss, language disturbance, and visual field defects are seen in various combinations, depending on the site of the lesion.

Lesions that involve the facial motor nucleus or its exiting fibers usually produce a complete facial paralysis on the same side as the lesion. This paralysis is identical to complete peripheral facial paralysis, which will be described in detail in the section dealing with peripheral facial paralysis. The upper and lower facial muscles are paralyzed, in contrast with the paralysis of lower facial muscles associated with supranuclear lesions. Taste and secretory functions are rarely affected. When the paralysis is not complete, the usual pattern is weakness in both upper and lower facial muscles. Occasionally, in partial nuclear lesions, lower facial muscles may be affected to a lesser or greater degree than the upper facial muscles. When the latter possibility occurs, the weakness resembles that seen with supranuclear lesions. Because of the relatively small size of the brain stem and the compactness of structures, however, nuclear facial paralysis does not occur in isolation. Associated findings such as involvement of other cranial nerves, particularly the fifth, sixth, and eighth, serve to differentiate the occasional nuclear facial palsy with lower facial weakness from that which occurs with supranuclear lesions (Fig. 10–1). Associated brain stem findings

also prevent confusion between nuclear and peripheral nerve lesions. These associated findings are described in greater detail when considering specific diseases.

Peripheral Lesions

These lesions can occur in any location along the course of the facial nerve, from the exit from the brain stem at the lower border of the pons to the terminal motor branches. Again, clinical manifestations depend on the extent and the site of the lesion. Lesions involving terminal branches produce regional paralysis of the muscles supplied by those branches. Severe damage to the facial nerve at any point along its course prior to branching into terminal motor nerves produces complete facial paralysis. At rest, the involved side of the face sags, and wrinkles are flat. The nasolabial fold is absent or greatly diminished. The lower lid sags, producing a wider palpebral fissure. Since loss of all voluntary and associated movements occurs, attempts at smiling or laughing result in the mouth being pulled to the opposite side. Eye closure is not possible, and attempts to do so result in upward rotation of the eye (Bell's phenomenon). Testing the corneal reflex on either side causes a blink only on the uninvolved side. The inability to close the eye results in corneal abrasions if the eye is left unprotected. Since the upper facial muscles are paralyzed, attempts to raise the eyebrows or wrinkle the forehead are successful only over the uninvolved side. Complete lesions in the region of the stylomastoid foramen produce only total facial paralysis as described. Incomplete lesions produce less severe but usually uniform weakness. The loss of peripheral sensory fibers produces no clinical findings, probably because of overlap with sensory fields from adjacent nerves. If the lesion is above the chorda tympani but below the nerve to the stapedius muscle, loss of taste sensation in the anterior two thirds of the tongue on the affected side occurs, in addition to the complete facial paralysis. The patient may also notice decreased salivation but this symptom is variable. Lesions at or above the site of the stapedius nerve are said to produce increased sensitivity to the low tones in addition to the foregoing findings. This hearing change is variable and is often difficult to demonstrate clinically without the aid of special audiometry techniques. Lesions from the geniculate ganglion to the brain stem produce all of the previously described findings, plus decreased lacrimation on the affected side. In addition, hearing loss and vestibular symptoms can be associated with facial lesions in the internal acoustic meatus. Central nervous system findings are not seen with uncomplicated peripheral facial palsy. Peripheral and central findings can occur in certain conditions, such as tumors between the brain stem and the skull, where both the brain stem and the facial nerve are invaded or compressed.

In summary, when a patient comes to the clinic with facial weakness, the region of the nervous system involved can be determined by the clinical findings. Supranuclear lesions between the motor cortex and the upper pons produce weakness in the lower facial muscles on the side opposite the lesion. Associated neurologic findings serve to localize the lesion more accurately. Nuclear lesions and peripheral lesions produce weakness in all the facial muscles on the same side as the lesion. Nuclear lesions are associated with other evidence of local brain stem dysfunction. Peripheral lesions can be associated with disorders of taste, salivation, lacrimation, and hearing. Evidence of central nervous system disease is usually lacking. Exceptions have been discussed.

Abnormal Movements

Certain conditions alter facial nerve function by producing abnormal movements with or without paralysis. These movements take the form of various tics, spasms, or muscular twitches. Hemifacial spasm consists of semirhythmic, brief contractions of all or various groups of the facial muscles, usually involving only one side of the face. Hemifacial spasm is involuntary and cannot be mimicked. Facial tics or habit spasms are contractions of facial muscles about the mouth or eyes. They are usually bilateral. They are of psychogenic origin and can eaily be mimicked. Paretic facial contracture consists of a continuous partial contracture of the facial muscles over one side. This condition produces an accentuation of the normal facial grooves and wrinkles. The eye is partially closed, and usually the corner of the mouth is elevated. Facial myokymia can describe several different entities. It has been used to describe those benign fasciculations commonly involving the eyelid that are enhanced with fatigue and relieved by rest. They are often seen in and complained of by medical students who have recently learned the clinical manifestations of motor neuron disease. Facial myokymia can be more extensive and persistent. In this situation, a large part, if not all, of the facial musculature reveals spontaneous activity that is arrhythmic and continuous producing a rippling movement in the overlying skin. This type of facial myokymia is associated with intrinsic diseases of the brain stem such as multiple sclerosis and infiltrating tumors. Focal motor seizures can occasionally produce isolated clonic activity in the facial muscles. The forceful repetitive type of facial muscular contracture readily differentiates focal seizures from other abnormal facial movements.

CAUSES

Central Nervous System

Supranuclear Lesions

The differential diagnosis of supranuclear lesions capable of producing a contralateral lower facial paresis is extensive and beyond the scope of this book. The most common causes are vascular accidents, cerebral trauma, brain tumors, and infection. If the lesion is a space-occupying process, increased intracranial pressure can occur, resulting in papilledema and, on occasion, unilateral or bilateral sixth nerve palsies. The sixth nerve palsies are an indirect effect of the increased intracranial pressure and are not caused directly by the space-occupying lesion.

Nuclear Lesions

Lesions affecting the motor nucleus of the facial nerve and adjacent regions imply brain stem disease. The vast majority of such lesions are vascular. An understanding of the blood supply to the brain stem is necessary for accurate interpretation of clinical findings. Each half of the brain stem receives a relatively independent blood supply. The innermost or medial aspect of the brain stem is supplied on both sides by multiple short paramedian branches from the vertebral and basilar arteries. The paramedian arteries vary considerably in distribution and number. The lateral regions are supplied by a limited number of short and long circumferential arteries that also provide the blood supply for the cerebellum. The compactness of the structures of the brain stem combined with its multiple blood supply result in numerous possible clinical combinations following vascular occlusion. Previous authors have combined various findings, attributed them to occlusion of specific arteries or to lesions in specific area of the brain stem, and have applied their names to these syndromes. A considerable variation, however, exists in the number of brain stem vessels, their exact distribution, and their degree of overlap of blood supply. In addition, in the case of vascular occlusive disease, the occlusion, either partial or complete, may be in one of the major vessels, such as the vertebral or basilar with the lesion resulting from inadequate perfusion in one or more of the terminal blood vessels. As a result, specific syndromes are rarely seen. It is therefore easier to understand the findings associated with brain stem lesions with respect to areas or zones involved. Only those conditions associated with alteration of facial nerve function have been described.

In the medial region of the lower pons, paramedian vessels from the vertebral and basilar arteries supply the corticospinal tract prior to pyramidal decussation, the abducens and para-abducens region, the seventh nerve fibers as they arch over the abducens nucleus, part of the olivo-dento-rubral tracts, and part of the medial lemniscus (Fig. 10–1). Clinical findings depend on the extent of the lesion in this area. Typically, the facial paralysis involves the upper and lower face equally. Taste and secretory function are not altered. The sixth nerve on the side of the lesion is involved. A variable hemiparesis of the arm and leg occurs on the opposite side of the body. If the para-abducens area is involved, a paresis of conjugate gaze occurs on the side of the lesion. This paresis can be seen in the absence of sixth nerve palsy or in combination with it. Involvement of the olivo-dento-rubral tracts can result in rhythmic contractions of the palate (palatal myoclonus). If the medial lemniscus is involved, position and vibratory sense on the contralateral side are altered.

The lateral area of the mid and lower pons is supplied by short and long circumferential branches from the basilar artery. The structures in this region include the eighth nerve nucleus, the seventh nerve nucleus, the sensory nucleus of the fifth nerve, descending sympathetic fibers, spinothalamic tract, vestibular nuclei, and part of the cerebellar hemisphere (Fig. 10–1). Extensive lesions in this territory produce ipsilateral complete facial paralysis, hearing loss, loss of sensation over the face, Horner syndrome, nystagmus, cerebellar signs, and contralateral loss of pain and temperature sensation over the extremities and the trunk. In practice, as with other brain stem syndromes, this one is seldom complete but occurs with a variable combination of the preceding findings.

Many conditions other than vascular occlusion can produce brain stem and seventh nerve findings. These disorders include infection, hemorrhage, trauma, congenital abnormalities, and neoplasms. The most common primary neoplasm of the brain stem, the pontine glioma, is of particular interest to the ophthalmologist because the patient often has visual symptoms. Pontine gliomas are seen most commonly, but not exclusively, in children and young adults. They are usually slow-growing, infiltrative lesions that frequently present with unilateral sixth nerve palsies.Facial weakness involving both the upper and lower half of the face often accompanies sixth nerve palsy. As the tumor continues to infiltrate the brain stem, other nuclear and long-tract structures are compromised, resulting in predictable clinical dysfunctiion. Facial myokymia, although more often associated with multiple sclerosis, is occasionally seen in patients with pontine gliomas. When myokymia is persistent, often over months or years, and associated with a paretic facial contracture, it is said to be a reliable indicator of a pontine glioma. This combination is occasionally seen with other brain stem lesions.

Peripheral Nerve Lesions

The entire spectrum of disease processes from traumatic and infectious to neoplastic and congenital can affect the peripheral seventh nerve anywhere in its course. Variable degrees of facial paralysis, often complete, are common in most of these conditions. The site of the lesion and the type of disease process serve to differentiate these various conditions. Peripheral seventh nerve palsies can be seen in association with general disease processes or with relatively specific syndromes or disease entities.

General Disease States

Various types of malignancies can produce peripheral seventh nerve palsies. These malignancies include primary bone tumors that directly compress the nerve; tumors of the posterior nasopharynx, which have a tendency to infiltrate the meninges and pick off cranial nerves in a sequential fashion; and meningeal leukemic infiltrations, which often produce multiple cranial and peripheral nerve palsies. Bacterial infections of the middle ear and mastoids can produce seventh nerve palsy. When this process spreads to involve the petrous portions of the temporal bone, a sixth nerve palsy can also be seen (Gradenigo syndrome). Suppurative or granulomatous meningitis can result in multiple cranial nerve palsies, including the seventh. Several viral infections have a predilection for peripheral nerve involvement. In the past, diphtheria and polio were often associated with bilateral or unilateral facial paralysis. Modern inoculation programs have reduced these to rarities. Herpes zoster (shingles) can involve the seventh nerve. This condition (Ramsay Hunt syndrome) produces complete facial paralysis with loss of taste sensation and secretory functions. In addition, pain occurs, followed by the typical vesicular eruptions of herpes zoster in the peripheral sensory distribution of the seventh nerve, namely, the external auditory meatus, the tympanic membrane, and the posterior aspect of the external ear. Tinnitus, decreased hearing, and vertigo are occasionally associated with this condition owing to involvement of the adjacent eighth nerve. Paralysis of cranial nerves can be seen in association with post-infectious polyneuropathy (Guillain-Barré syndrome). Bilateral facial palsy is commonly seen, whereas extraocular movements are only rarely involved. In this condition, facial diplegia can be the presenting finding and can, on occasion, occur in isolation. Usually, an associated wide-spread loss of peripheral nerve function occurs. Rare systemic conditions that can produce seventh nerve palsies include acute intermittent porphyria and heavy-metal intoxication.

Bell's Palsy

By far the most common disease producing isolated peripheral seventh nerve dysfunction is Bell's palsy. The precise etiology of this conditon remains unknown but it commonly follows exposure to cold. Possible familial predisposition and viral causes have been reported. The clinical signs are thought to be caused by swelling of the nerve or nerve sheath in the facial canal. The patient presents with a partial or complete facial paralysis. Any of the previously mentioned findings affecting taste, hearing, lacrimation, or salivation may be present, depending on the site and extent of the lesion. Although pain in the ear canal is commonly seen with herpes zoster, it is only occasionally seen with Bell's palsy. Recovery is spontaneous and complete in up to 90% of cases. Partial or incomplete recovery can be associated with the development of contractures in the involved facial muscles. Seventh-nerve misdirection and/or short-circuiting can occur following recovery, resulting in abnormal muscle activity, such as eye blinking when the mouth is moved. If this misdirection of nerve fibers involves parasympathetic fibers that control glandular function, stimulation of salivary glands can result in excessive tearing (crocodile tears). Rarely, generalized or asynchronous spasms of the facial muscles occur following recovery.

Trauma

After leaving the bony facial canal, the seventh cranial nerve and its branches are distributed superficially and are therefore vulnerable to injuries. These injuries are usually of penetrating varieties such as stab wounds. Occasionally, blunt trauma or prolonged compression can produce functional impairment. Trauma of the nerve within the facial canal is not uncommonly associated with basal skull fractures. In addition, surgery of the middle ear, mastoids, and fifth nerve can be complicated by seventh nerve damage.

Hemifacial Spasm

Although this type of spasm has been described in the section on symptoms of facial nerve dysfunction, it probably represents a specific condition reflecting facial nerve disease. In the past, hemifacial spasm was thought to be an idiopathic disorder, usually affecting older people. More recently, it has been described in children. Hemifacial spasm is thought to be caused, in most cases, by compression of the seventh nerve in its proximal portion near its origin from the brain stem, and the importance of a complete neurologic examination is emphasized. This compression has been attributed to vascular structures and tumors. A condition similar, if not identical, to hemifacial spasm occasionally follows incomplete recovery from Bell's palsy.

Uveoparotid Fever

Sarcoidosis is a systemic granulomatous disease of unknown cause. When sarcoidosis involves the parotid gland and the eye, it is referred to as uveoparotid fever. Approximately one third of these patients develop unilateral or bilateral peripheral facial palsies. More recently, it has been noted that uveitis, parotitis, or facial nerve palsies can exist alone or in combination. Isolated facial nerve paralysis is one of the common neurologic presentations of sarcoidosis.

Melkersson-Rosenthal Syndrome

This rare condition is characterized by recurrent episodes of facial paralysis and facial swelling. The facial swelling may precede, accompany, or follow facial paralysis. The condition is associated with a deeply furrowed tongue (lingua plicata) in approximately 30% of patients and migraine headache in approximately 10% of patients. The etiology is unknown; however, some cases may be caused by sarcoidosis. The course is usually benign, although repeated episodes of facial paralysis and facial swelling may lead to permanent disfigurement.

Möbius Syndrome

This rare, congenital disorder is apparent at birth. A bilateral facial palsy affects the upper part of the face more severely than the lower. Paralysis of abduction of the eyes and ptosis are common. Sagging and contracture of the facial muscles are not seen. Spontaneous or induced nystagmus are not present. The patient does not complain of diplopia. Pupillary reactions are normal, as are conjugate vertical gaze movements. A number of other findings suggesting cranial nerve involvement can also be seen, such as atrophy of the tongue, the muscles of mastication, and the sternomastoid muscles. Other occasional findings include syndactylism, foot deformities, and mental retardation. Postmortem examinations have revealed apparent aplasia of the involved cranial nerve nuclei but multiple causes have been suggested.

Acoustic Neuroma

Early symptoms associated with acoustic nerve tumors would only rarely prompt the patient to see an ophthalmologist; however, since the early symptoms and signs associated with acoustic neuromas are often subtle, diagnostic failure is common and the patient may develop significant neuro-ophthalmologic signs. The importance of early diagnosis of this condition is emphasized since it is directly related to therapeutic success.

Acoustic neuromas are benign tumors that begin in the internal acoustic meatus, originating in the nerve sheath. Initial symptoms usually relate to the eighth nerve, and consist of decreased hearing and tinnitus. Hearing loss may be mild. Progression can be so slow that it escapes detection by the patient even to the point of a complete unilateral deafness. Tinnitus can be intermittent or constant. Vestibular symptoms are rare initially and, when they do occur, are more often a vague sense of giddiness rather than true vertigo. As the tumor enlarges, it grows out of the internal acoustic meatus and begins to compress structures in the angle between the cerebellum and the pons. The seventh nerve, owing to its anatomic relationship with the eighth nerve, can also be involved early. It can present as a complete facial paralysis, but more often, the weakness is subtle and only careful examination will reveal mild facial weakness. Compression of the fifth nerve produces signs of facial sensory impairment. The patient may complain of paresthesias with no objective sensory loss or of a mild hypesthesia. More often, a depressed corneal reflex on the side of the lesion is the only early objective sign. The sixth cranial nerve exits from the base of the pons and is only rarely involved early in the disease. When involvement does occur, usually later in the course, the expected findings of diplopia and a lateral gaze palsy are seen. Compression of the cerebellar peduncles and hemisphere and vestibular nuclei produce ataxia with a tendency to fall to the side of the lesion, nystagmus that is accentuated with gaze toward the lesion, and often, true vertigo. Downward extension of the tumor affects the ninth, tenth, and eleventh cranial nerves, producing swallowing difficulties and weakness of the neck muscles. Upward extension can occlude the cerebral aqueduct and produce internal hydrocephalus with depressed mentation, headache, and papilledema. Medial extension compresses and distorts the brain stem and eventually compromises the long sensory motor tracts, producing spastic paresis and sensory loss on either or both sides of the body. The development of hydrocephalus, lower cranial nerve signs, and long-tract signs indicate that the tumor has reached considerable size.

TREATMENT

Those patients with central nervous system diseases that produce facial nerve signs would seek treatment from neurologists and neurosurgeons—an aspect beyond the scope of this book. The ophthalmologist is often consulted to assist in the evaluation of fundus changes, motility abnormalities, and visual field defects. The primary treatment, whenever possible, is directed at the cause. Often, in the case of highly malignant brain tumors or extensive vascular lesions, this treatment is a lesson in futility.

Diseases involving the peripheral distribution of the facial nerve are also primarily managed by physicians outside the realm of ophthalmology. When the peripheral facial palsy is of such severity that the cornea is in danger of being damaged, ophthalmologic assistance is often required.

Treatment of Bell's palsy is considered in greater detail. Although it is the most common cause of an isolated seventh nerve paralysis, therapy for this condition is controversial. Most would agree that incomplete paralysis that does not progress requires no treatment. In the past, surgical decompression of the facial nerve has been recommended for complete facial paralysis. Even those currently advocating a surgical procedure, however, admit that no diagnostic tests are capable of predicting which patients will not recover spontaneously. Furthermore, surgical decompression may be detrimental. Current evidence strongly suggests that complete recovery from acute Bell's palsy can be significantly increased with the judicious use of steroids.

BIBLIOGRAPHY

Adour, K.K., and Wingerd, J.: Idiopathic facial paralysis (Bell's palsy): factors affecting severity and outcome in 446 patients. Neurology (Minneap.) 24:1112, 1974.

Adour, K.K., et al.: Prednisone treatment for idiopathic facial paralysis (Bell's palsy). N. Engl. J. Med. 287:1268, 1972.

Aleksic, S.N., Budzilovich, G.N., and Lieberman, A.N.: Herpes zoster oticus and facial paralysis (Ramsay-Hunt syndrome). Clinico-pathologic study and review of literature. J. Neurol. Sci. 20:149, 1973.

Alter, M.: Familial aggregation of Bell's palsy. Arch. Neurol. 8:557, 1963.

Baker, A.B., and Baker, L.H. (eds.): Clinical Neurology. Vol. 3. Hagerstown, Md., Harper & Row, 1976.

Boghen, D., Filiatrault, R., and Descarries, L.: Myokymia and facial contracture in brain stem tuberculoma. Neurology 27:270, 1977.

Bucy, P.C., and Keplinger, J.E.: Tumors of the brain stem with special reference to ocular manifestations. Arch. Ophthalmol. 62:541, 1959.

Byl, F.M., and Adour, K.K.: Auditory symptoms associated with herpes zoster or idiopathic facial paralysis. Laryngoscope 87:372, 1977.

Djupesland, G., et al.: Viral infection as a cause of acute peripheral facial palsy. Arch. Otolaryngol. 102:403, 1976.

Eckman, P.B., Kramer, R.A., and Altrocchi, P.H.: Hemifacial spasm. Arch. Neurol. 25:81, 1971.

Ehni, G., and Woltman, H.W.: Hemifacial spasm: review of 106 cases. Arch. Neurol. Psychiatry 53:205, 1945.

Federman, R., and Stoopack, J.C.: Moebius syndrome. J. Oral Surg. 33:676, 1975.

Fisch, U.: Facial paralysis in fractures of the petrous bone. Laryngoscope 84:2141, 1974.

Fisch, U., and Wegmüller, A.: Early diagnosis of acoustic neuromas. Oral Surg. 36:129, 1974.

Groves, J.: Facial palsies: selection of cases for treatment. Proc. R. Soc. Med. 66:545, 1973.

Hallet, J.W., and Mitchell, B.: Melkersson-Rosenthal syndrome. Am. J. Ophthalmol. 65:542, 1968.

Henderson, J.L.: Congenital facial diplegia syndrome: clinical features, pathology and aetiology; review of 61 cases. Brain 62:381, 1939.

Isamat, F., et al.: Neurinomas of the facial nerve. Report of three cases. J. Neurosurg. 43:608, 1975.

Kettel, K.: Melkersson's syndrome: report of 5 cases, with special reference to pathologic observations. Arch. Otolaryngol. 46:341, 1947.

Korobkin, R., Berg, B.O., and Wilson, C.B.: Facial myokymia in association with medulloblastoma. Dev. Med. Child Neurol. 17:340, 1975.

Leibowitz, U.: Epidemic incidence of Bell's palsy. Brain 92:109, 1969.

Levin, P.M.: Neurological aspects of uveo-parotid fever. J. Nerv. Ment. Dis. 81:176, 1935.

Matthews, W.B.: Facial myokymia. J. Neurol. Neurosurg. Psychiatry 29:35, 1966.

McNeill, R.: Facial nerve decompression. J. Laryngol. Otol. 88:445, 1974.

Minderhoud, J.M.: Diagnostic significance of symptomatology in brain stem ischaemic infarction. Eur. Neurol. 5:343, 1971.

Negri, S., Caraceni, T., and DeLorenzi, L.: Facial myokymia and brain stem tumor. Eur. Neurol. 14:108, 1976.

O'Connor, P.J., Parry, W., and Davies, R.: Continuous muscle spasm in intramedullary tumours of the neuraxis. J. Neurol. Neurosurg. Psychiatry 29:310, 1966.

Pisanty, S., and Sharav, Y.: The Melkersson-Rosenthal syndrome. Oral Surg. 27:729, 1969.

Radü, E.W., Skorpil, V., and Kaeser, H.E.: Facial myokymia. Eur. Neurol. 13:499, 1975.

Revilla, A.G.: Neurinomas of the cerebellopontile recess. A clinical study of one hundred and sixty cases including operative mortality and end results. Bull. Johns Hopkins Hosp. *80*:254, 1947.

Rowland, L.P.: Merritt's Textbook of Neurology, 7th Ed. Philadelphia, Lea & Febiger, 1984

Rubinstein, A.E., et al.: Moebius syndrome in Kallmann syndrome. Arch. Neurol. *32*:480, 1975.

Ruby, J.R., and Jannetta, P.J.: Hemifacial spasm: ultrastructural changes in the facial nerve induced by neurovascular compression. Surg. Neurol. *4*:369, 1975.

Salding, J.M.K., and Nelson, E.: The autonomic nervous system. *In* Clinical Neurology. Vol. 4. Edited by A.B. Baker and L.H. Baker. Philadelphia, Harper & Row, 1983.

Schloss, M.D., and Bebear, J.P.: Hemifacial spasm: importance of a complete investigation. J. Otolaryngol. *5*:319, 1976.

Shaywitz, B.A.: Hemifacial spasm in childhood treated with carbamazepine. Arch. Neurol. *31*:63, 1974.

Siltzbach, L.E., et al.: Course and prognosis of sarcoidosis around the world. Am. J. Med. *57*:847, 1974.

Stevens, H.: Melkersson's syndrome. Neurology (Minneap.) *15*:263, 1965.

Storrs, T.J.: The Melkersson-Rosenthal syndrome: a case report. Br. J. Oral Surg. *13*:160, 1975.

Taverner, D.: Medical management of idiopathic facial (Bell's) palsy. Proc. R. Soc. Med. *66*:554, 1973.

Tenser, R.B.: Myokymia and facial contraction in multiple sclerosis. Arch. Intern. Med. *136*:81, 1976.

Tenser, R.B., and Corbett, J.J.: Myokymia and facial contraction in brain stem glioma. An electromyographic study. Arch. Neurol. *30*:425, 1974.

Truex, R.C., and Carpenter, M.B.: Human Neuroanatomy, 6th Ed. Baltimore, Williams & Wilkins Co., 1969.

Van Allen, M.W., and Blodi, F.C.: Neurologic aspects of the Möbius syndrome. A case study with electromyography of the extraocular and facial muscles. Neurology (Minneap.) *10*:249, 1969.

Walton, J.N.: Brain's Diseases of the Nervous System, 8th Ed. Oxford, Oxford Univ. Press, 1977.

Wiederholt, W.C., and Siekert, R.G.: Neurological manifestations of sarcoidosis. Neurology (Minneap.) *15*:1147, 1965.

Williams, D., and Wilson, T.G.: The diagnosis of the major and minor syndromes of basilar insufficiency. Brain *85*:741, 1962.

Wolferman, A.: The present status of therapy of Bell's paralysis: a critical evaluation. Ann. Otol. Rhinol. Laryngol. *83*:1, 1974.

Chapter 11

Chromosome Changes

RUFUS O. HOWARD

All human development from conception to death results from an interaction of genetic and environmental factors. All disease probably has a genetic component that is variable, from almost complete, to substantial, to insignificant in different conditions. Genetic factors have been the primary cause of blindness in a large proportion of individuals of all age groups (Table 11–1).

The transmission of hereditary factors from one generation to another may be classified in four groups:

1. Mutant hereditary factors (genes) of large effect, transmitted according to mendelian laws.
2. Multifactorial inheritance, requiring the interaction of multiple genes and environmental influences.
3. Cytoplasmic genes (not yet demonstrated in humans, but suggested as a possible basis of Leber's optic atrophy).
4. Chromosome aberrations.

CHROMOSOME STRUCTURE AND FUNCTION

In humans, most, if not all, hereditary traits are located within the cell nucleus in structures called chromosomes (κρωμα, or

Table 11–1. Genetic Factors as Cause of Blindness

Age	% Blind Owing to Hereditary Factors
0 to 5 years	64.6
6 to 19 years	47.7
> 19 years	13.2
all ages	16.7

color, and σωμα, or body). The chromosomes are small intranuclear, basophilic-staining, rod-like structures. The principal component of the chromosome is chromatin. Nuclear chromatin is formed from deoxyribonucleic acid (DNA), ribonucleic acid (RNA), histone, and the so-called residual protein, a high molecular weight material that has been poorly characterized. The chemical structure of DNA within the chromosome is precisely arranged: one phosphate, one sugar (deoxyribose), and one base [adenine (A), or guanine (G), or cytosine (C), or thymine (T)] are chemically joined to form a nucleotide (Fig. 11–1A). Several hundred nucleotides are joined by covalent bonds between the phosphate and sugar groups to form a linear polynucleotide, deoxyribonucleic acid (DNA). Two strands of DNA are arranged side by side in a right-hand double helix, with the base of one strand

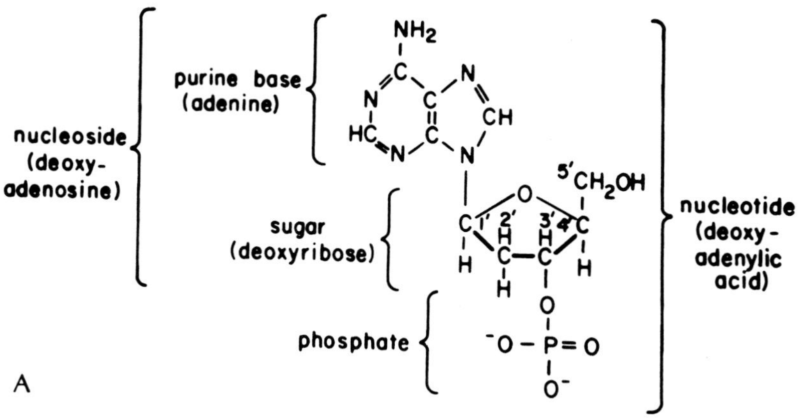

Fig. 11–1. **A.** Chemical structure of one nucleotide. The phosphate and sugar are constant, but the base may be adenine, guanine, cytosine, or thymine. (From Howard, R.O.: Classification of chromosomal eye syndromes. Int. Ophthalmol. 4:77, 1981. With permission from Dr. W. Junk, Publishers, The Hague, The Netherlands.)

opposed to the base of the second strand, and are stabilized in this position by the precise pairing of base A in one strand with T in the second strand, and of G with C (Fig. 11–1B). The diameter of the helix is approximately 20Å, and each strand makes one complete turn every 34Å. Aggregates of double helices form chromatin fibers, approximately 240 ± 50Å, and tightly packed chromatin fibers form a single chromosome.

One specific linear sequence of nucleotides determines one specific gene, a term introduced by Johannsen in 1909 to describe a single genetic unit. While the total number of genes is not known, it has been estimated that human chromosomes represent between 2000 and 100,000 or more (theoretical maximum of 10^7) genes. All genes are distributed in the normal human between 46 chromosomes, 22 pairs of autosomes, and 2 sex chromosomes. The sex chromosome complement in males is XY, and in females, XX. Each chromosome must, therefore, represent at least several hundred genes. The significance of the sequence of genes in a chromosome or of a change in the sequence of genes in a chromosome is not known.

The 6 feet of DNA in each cell nucleus is not crowded in randomly; precise compacting is achieved by means of larger structures. During interphase, 2 turns of the DNA superhelix are wound on a histone octamer to form the nucleosome. Adjacent nucleosomes compact under the influence of increasing ionic strength and other factors to form solenoids and dense 250Å chromatin strands (Fig. 11–1C). These structures are stabilized by the H1 histone. With one specific interphase configuration, some gene sites are hidden or shielded, while others are exposed and have the potential for biochemical action: translation and DNA replication.

HISTORICAL HIGHLIGHTS

Although the unambiguous identification of humans with chromosome error could not be made prior to 1956, when chromosomes could be counted accurately, chromosomally abnormal individuals have been recognized for centuries. The cyclops anomaly is associated with chromosome abnormality frequently, if not exclusively (Fig. 11–2). Descriptions of the cyclops deformity are recorded on Babylonian clay tablets of approximately 4000 B.C. In 1657, Thomas Bartholin probably described the first case of D trisomy. In 1838, Esquirol reported individuals with short stature, small heads and slanted eyes. Langdon

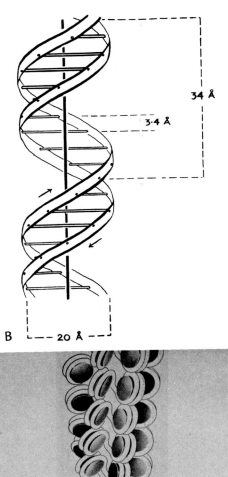

34 Å

3·4 Å

B

20 Å

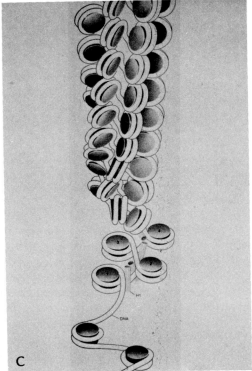

C

Fig. 11–1. **B.** Two linear polynucleotides are arranged side by side to form a right-hand double helix. This structure is extended during most of cell life, but is compacted at metaphase and can be seen with the light microscope. **C.** The nucleosome is formed by two full turns (166 nucleotide pairs) of the DNA superhelix wound about a histone octamer core. The nucleosomes compact to form a solenoid, a helix with about six nucleosomes per turn. (From Howard, R.O.: Classification of chromosomal eye syndromes. Int. Ophthalmol. 4:77, 1981. With permission from Dr. W. Junk, Publishers, The Hague, The Netherlands.)

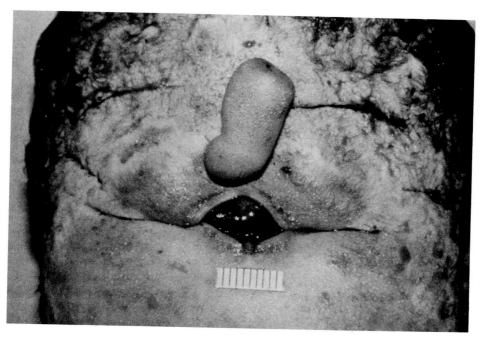

Fig. 11–2. Cyclopia, a single midline ocular defect, may be true cyclopia, represented by central unduplicated eye tissues, or synophthalmia, with partial fusion of two separate eyes, or by clinical anophthalmia. Cyclopia has been associated with 13 trisomy (this illustration), or B trisomy, or 18p-, 18r, 46XY/45G-, or 46XY/47XY + mar. (From Howard, R.O.: Classification of chromosomal eye syndromes. Int. Ophthalmol. 4:77, 1981. With permission from Dr. W. Junk, Publishers, The Hague, The Netherlands.)

Down in 1866 called this group of individuals Mongols because of their presumed oriental features. In 1932, P.J. Waardenburg suggested that Down syndrome might be the result of a chromosome abnormality, and even correctly proposed the mechanism translocation as one basis of this anomaly. In 1959, individuals with Down syndrome (Fig. 11–3) were shown to have an extra autosome of the G group, and the first chromosome disorder was proven. With adequate chromosome technology, it became possible to identify individuals with extra whole chromosomes (trisomies), deleted whole chromosomes (monosomies), as well as those with partial deletions and partial replications.

The ability to identify chromosomes became possible with the development of the microscope and histologic techniques. In 1857, Virchow described cell division in a histologic preparation. Subsequently,

chromosomes were observed in numerous preparations, and in 1880, Flemming correctly reported the longitudinal division of chromosomes. By 1880, chromosomes were recognized in human tumor cells. In 1882, cell division of corneal epithelium was described, and in 1883, Beneden noted reduction division. The term chromosome was introduced by Waldeyer in 1888. In 1891, Henking studied meiosis in the chromosomes of an insect. He was not sure of the function of one structure, and labelled it an 'X'. Later, when this structure was shown to determine sex, X was employed to designate the sex chromosome. In 1912, Winiwarter (incorrectly) counted 47 to 48 chromosomes in the human male, and 48 in the human female. Painter reported in 1921 in the "clearest equatorial plates so far studied only 46 chromosomes found," but, in 1923 he reevaluated his preparations and concluded that the human had 48 chro-

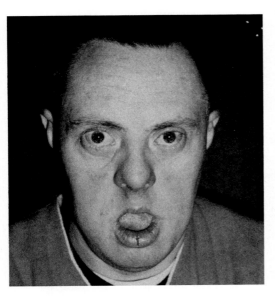

Fig. 11–3. In Down syndrome, or trisomy 21, numerous eye abnormalities occur, including blepharitis, strabismus, keratoconus, cataracts, and retinoblastoma. (From Howard, R.O.: Classification of chromosomal eye syndromes. Int. Ophthalmol. 4:77, 1981. With permission from Dr. W. Junk, Publishers, The Hague, The Netherlands.)

mosomes. This error in counting chromosomes was repeated by numerous others until 1956 when Tjio and Levan demonstrated the correct diploid number to be 46. This finding was confirmed the same year by Ford and Hammerton, who found 23 chromosomes in human germ cells.

TECHNIQUES TO DEMONSTRATE CHROMOSOMES

A chromosome is not seen with equal ease during all phases of the cell cycle; it is highly extended during most of cell life. However, prior to cell division (early prophase, prophase, and metaphase) the chromatin compacts and the chromosome can be seen with the light microscope.

Chromosome determinations can be made on any nucleated cell, but for convenience, venous blood, bone marrow biopsy, or fibroblasts from a skin biopsy are most often used to study chromosomes. Selected cells are placed into tissue culture,

colchicine is added to arrest cell division at metaphase, when the chromosomes have replicated, but prior to cell division. The cells are swollen with a hypotonic solution to separate the chromosomes, and stained to facilitate viewing. Different cytologic techniques reveal different qualities of individual chromosomes (orcein, autoradiography, Q, G, R, C, and banding. The chromosomes are displayed in a karyotype, "a systematized array of chromosomes from a single cell, prepared by a drawing or a photograph, and arranged in sequence from the largest to the smallest." The chromosome pairs 1, 2, and 3 are called Group A; pairs 4 and 5, Group B; pairs 6 to 12, Group C; pairs 13 to 15, Group D; pairs 16 to 18, Group E; pairs 19 and 20, Group F; and pairs 21 and 22, Group G. The unbanded X chromosome is not distinguished from C Group chromosomes and is usually grouped with them. A moderate variation occurs in size of the Y chromosome, but generally it is larger than either chromosome 21 or 22. In early chromosome preparation, because adjacent chromosomes had a similar size and shape, it was possible to identify only chromosomes 1, 2, 3, 16, and Y. In 1961, an autoradiographic technique was introduced, based on the fact that parts of chromosomes replicate at different times, and therefore, could show a differential uptake of tritiated thymidine. With this technique, it was possible to differentiate between chromosome 4 and 5, 13, 14 and 15, 17 and 18, and to identify all late-replicating X chromosomes. In 1970, Caspersson stained metaphase chromosomes with quinacrine or quinacrine mustard, and examined these preparations with ultraviolet light. He found fluorescence varied from chromosome to chromosome (Y chromosome fluoresced intensely; 19 and 22, weakly), and fluorescence varied along the length of each chromosome in a characteristic pattern, resulting in "bands" of greater and lesser fluorescence. This has been called 'Q' banding. With this technique it became possible to identify each chromosome precisely, and to recognize small deletions and duplications and translocations. However, fluorescent preparations fade and fluorescent microscopy was not generally available. Newer techniques using Giemsa stain have permitted permanent chromosome preparations with similar banding patterns (G banding). A 'C' banding pattern has permitted staining patterns of constitutive chromatin. Pretreatment of the chromosomes with controlled heat followed by staining with Giemsa results in staining patterns opposite to the usual Giemsa stains, and is called 'R' banding; this is particularly useful for examining the ends of the chromosomes. Many variations and different staining techniques have been introduced in an effort to assist with the morphologic identification of metaphase chromosomes. By common agreement at the Paris conference of 1971, the bands of each chromosome have been standardized and a total of 320 metaphase bands have been recognized (Fig. 11–4). More recently, extended chromosomes from early prophase or prophase have been stained with Giemsa. By this technique, 1256 distinct bands have been identified. Although approximately 5% of a metaphase chromosome must be absent or replicated before the change can be recognized using conventional chromosome techniques, it is apparent that very small chromosome errors can be identified with the G banding of prophase chromosomes. One important case report described a patient with retinoblastoma who had normal Q banding, but in whom a deletion of a very small fragment of 13q14 was shown by banding extended prophase chromosomes.

Chromosome abnormalities are usually separated into structural and numeric changes. As opposed to single-gene disease, in which the defect occurs in a single gene (polynucleotide sequence), and the associated abnormal structural protein or enzyme is the cause of the genetic disease, chromosome disease arises as the result of an abnormal number or sequence of normal genes, and the abnormality is generally not of defective genes, but of altered gene dosage.

Numeric abnormalities arise from errors in germ cell division during meiosis in either the father or mother. The numeric abnormality may be one of the following:

1. Absence of an entire sex chromosome (45,X or Turner syndrome) (Fig. 11–5).
2. Absence of an entire autosome (45,XY, -21, or 21 monosomy) is rare; usually lethal.
3. Extra entire sex chromosome (47,XXY or Kleinfelter syndrome).
4. Extra entire autosome (47,XX, + 13, or 13 trisomy) (Fig. 11–6).
5. Multiple extra entire chromosomes (48,XXY, + 21, or Kleinfelter Mongol).
6. 23 extra entire chromosomes (69,XXY, or triploidy) (Fig. 11–7).
7. Multiple cell lines from a single zygote lineage (46,XX/47,XX, + 21, or mosaic Mongol).
8. Chimera or organism whose cell lines derive from two or more distinct cell lines (46,XX/46,XY).

Structural chromosome abnormalities refer to an altered sequence of DNA along one or more chromosomes. The changes may be as follows:

1. Translocation or interchange between different chromosomes.
2. Isochromosome or asymmetric division of chromosome at cell division.
3. Inversion or alteration in the linear sequence of DNA in a single chromosome.
4. Deletion or loss of chromosome fragment (Fig. 11–8A, 11-8B, 11-8C).
5. Duplication or replication of a segment of a chromosome.

ENVIRONMENTAL INFLUENCE ON CHROMOSOMES

Structural chromosomal abnormalities are preceded by chromosome breaks.

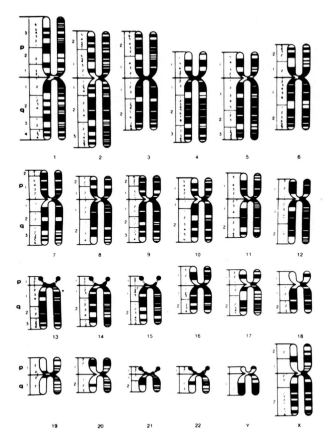

Fig. 11–4. Chromosome bands have been standardized, and 320 metaphase bands have been recognized (left of each chromosome). In expanded—prophase or prometaphase—chromosomes (right of each chromosome), 1256 or more distinct bands can be demonstrated. (From Yunis, J.J.: High resolution of human chromosomes. Science *191*:1268, 1976.)

Chromosome breaks may occur spontaneously, or several environmental factors may produce chromosome fracture. They include:

Physical agents—electromagnetic and particulate radiation, heat, cold.

Chemical agents—industrial chemicals, heavy metals, drugs.

Biologic agents—viruses.

INCIDENCE OF CHROMOSOME ABNORMALITY

Approximately 3.5 to 4% of all recognized conceptions are associated with some gross chromosome abnormality; most of the embryos with abnormal chromosomes abort in the first trimester of pregnancy (Table 11–2).

It is possible to collect amniotic fluid at 15 to 18 weeks of pregnancy and identify a fetus with abnormal chromosomes. This information would permit parents to consider a surgical abortion of the abnormal individual. Amniocentesis, especially just after the introduction of the technique, did involve a significant risk of complication by abruptio placenta, amniotitis, fetal hemorrhage, puncture of the fetus, and laceration of the spleen and eye. The use of ultrasound to localize the placenta and fetus has signficantly reduced the likelihood of a complication.

The incidence of chromosome error at

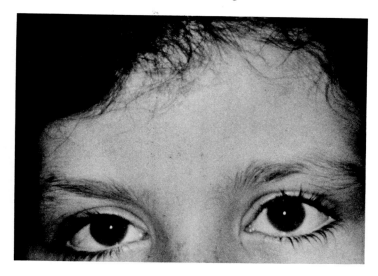

Fig. 11–5. Turner's syndrome individuals with a chromosome complement of 45X have an increased incidence of blepharoptosis, color blindness, and strabismus. (From Howard, R.O.: Classification of chromosomal eye syndromes. Int. Ophthalmol. 4:77, 1981. With permission from Dr. W. Junk, Publishers, The Hague, The Netherlands.)

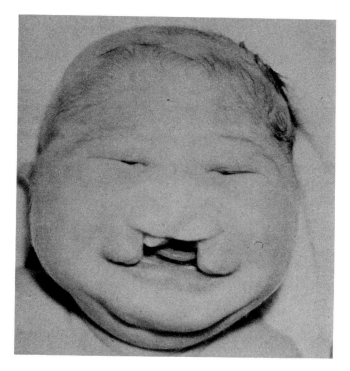

Fig. 11–6. Trisomy 13: the eyes are grossly abnormal, and may exhibit synophthalmia, cyclopia, anophthalmia, microphthalmia, cataracts, retinal dysplasia, and/or intraocular cartilage among numerous other defects. (From Howard, R.O.: Classification of chromosomal eye syndromes. Int. Ophthalmol. 4:77, 1981. With permission from Dr. W. Junk, Publishers, The Hague, The Netherlands.)

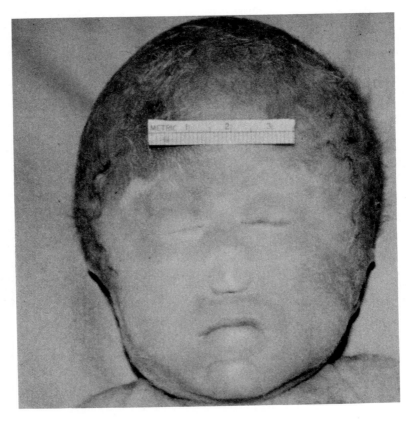

Fig. 11–7. Triploidy (69,XXY). This stillborn child with triploidy had blepharophimosis, iris coloboma, and microcornea. (From Howard, R.O.: Classification of chromosomal eye syndromes. Int. Ophthalmol. 4:77, 1981. With permission from Dr. W. Junk, Publishers, The Hague, The Netherlands.)

conception is not the same as at birth or in adult life because of fetal, embryonic, neonatal, and premature demise. (The data in Table 11–3 was obtained from prebanding studies, and probably represents low estimates).

Major ocular abnormalities such as anophthalmia, cyclopia, retinoblastoma, microphthalmia, corneal opacities (Fig. 11–9), colobomas, cataracts, intraocular cartilage, retinal dysplasia, and absent optic nerves, and minor abnormalities such as ptosis, abnormal eyelid fissures, and Brushfield spots are present in individuals with either normal or abnormal chromosomes. From one survey of educable blind children, no chromosome abnormalities were identified. From multiple chromosome surveys of children with retinoblastomas, with both sporadic and dominant patterns of inheritance, only a single child with abnormal chromosomes was identified. Yet retinoblastoma occurs in physically retarded and mentally retarded children, with partial deletion of the long arm of chromosome 13 (specifically band 13q14) and individuals with Down syndrome or Down syndrome plus multiple sex chromosomes. If the individual has a chromosome error, then presumably the defect is present in all body tissues, and it is likely that multiple somatic tissues will develop abnormally. Therefore, it is unlikely that a single ocular abnormality in an otherwise normal individual will be the result of a chromosome disorder. On the other hand, if numerous ab-

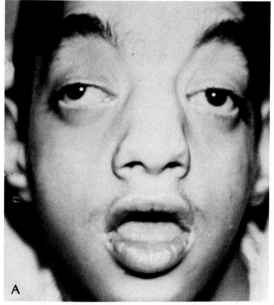

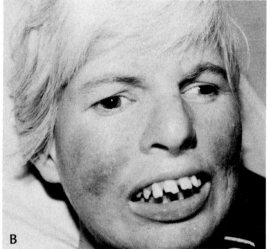

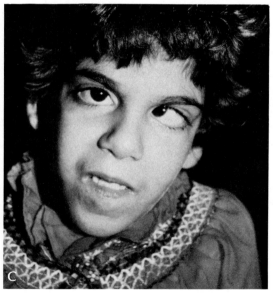

Fig. 11–8. **A.** Wolf syndrome (4p-). This severely retarded individual had blepharoptosis, exotropia, antimongoloid eyelid fissures and microcornea. **B.** Cri-du-chat syndrome (5p-). Premature graying of hair, exotropia, deafness, and optic nerve atrophy are present before age 30 in this retarded woman. **C.** 13q14 deletion. Almost all individuals with deletion of this segment of chromosome have had retinoblastoma. (From Howard, R.O.: Classification of chromosomal eye syndromes. Int. Ophthalmol. 4:77, 1981. With permission from Dr. W. Junk, Publishers, The Hague, The Netherlands.)

normalities exist, especially mental retardation, in the individual with an ocular defect, the possibility of a chromosome disorder should be considered. If a karyotype is obtained, a chromosome abnormality can be established or excluded. It is important to examine multiple cells, and possibly multiple body tissue, blood and skin fibroblasts, in order to exclude mosaicism.

Specific ocular abnormalities have been listed with the corresponding chromosome error in Table 11–4. If a specific clinical abnormality (i.e., exotropia) is to be a feature of a chromosome error (i.e., 5p-), the abnormality must occur with greater frequency in the individual with the chromosome abnormality than in the general population. It should be recognized that

Table 11–2. Incidence of Specific Chromosome Abnormality

Study	Incidence of abnormal chromosomes
Embryo (conception to 3 months)	
spontaneous abortion 0 to 6 weeks	66%
spontaneous abortion 7 to 12 weeks	20%
Fetus (12 weeks to birth)	No Data
Newborn	0.6%
Perinatal mortality	6–12%
Liveborn with one congenital abnormality	4.3%
Liveborn with three or more abnormalities	8.0%
Mentally retarded or institutionalized	5.7%
Full term, low birth-weight, mentally retarded	9.1%
"Normal" adult population	0.5%

for many chromosome errors in this table, the case reports are too few to adequately document the true incidence of the clinical abnormality (Table 11–4).

The recurrence of a chromosome abnormality depends on several variables. If both parents have normal chromosomes, increased maternal age predisposes to increased incidence of chromosome error. Good empirical data show an increase in incidence of Down syndrome with increasing maternal age: <20 years, 1/2325; 20 to 24 years, 1/1612; 25 to 29 years, 1/1282; 30 to 34 years, 1/860; 35 to 39 years, 1/285; 40 to 45 years 1/100 and > 45 years, 1/45.

Other studies show increased incidence of trisomy 13 and trisomy 18 (Fig. 11–10) and XXX with increased maternal age. Paternal age does not appear to influence chromosome error. Some studies suggest that there may be a familial tendency for meiotic nondisjunction and increased chromosome error. When one parent is a balance carrier of a translocation, the recurrence of a chromosome error should be 1/4 or 25%. Experience indicates that this estimate is too high. Increased fetal wastage certainly explains part of this difference.

On the basis of present understanding, the following clinical and morphologic features characterize human chromosome disorders:

1. Deletion and duplication of part or all of each chromosome have now been identified (Fig. 11–11).
2. While none or rare chromosomal syndromes have truly pathognomonic clinical features, accurate diagnosis can be made with a karyotype determination.
3. The majority of chromosomal abnormalities resulting in an entire dupli-

Table 11–3. Frequency of Specific Chromosome Abnormality and Different Ages

Chromosome abnormality	Spontaneous abortions (Number/1000)	Live neonatal (Number/1000)	Perinatal mortality (Number/280)	"Normal" adult (Number/1000)
Monosomy G	1			
Triploidy	160		1	
Tetraploidy	51			
Trisomy A	17			
Trisomy B	8			
Trisomy C	85			
Trisomy D	113	0.14	2	
Trisomy E	199	0.11	5	
Trisomy F	8		1	
Trisomy G	105	1.06	3	
Translocation		1.94		4
47,XYY		1.21	1	
47,XXY		1.29	2	
47,XXX		0.89		
45,X	174	0.15		
46X, inr (Yp + q −)		0.27		
Others		0.41		

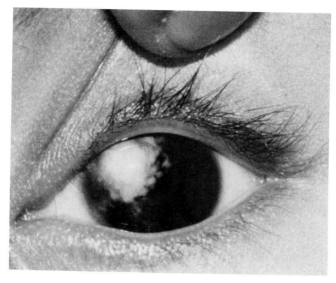

Fig. 11–9. A dense, elevated corneal opacity is present in a child with trisomy 8 mosaicism syndrome. (From Howard, R.O.: Classification of chromosomal eye syndromes. Int. Ophthalmol. 4:77, 1981. With permission from Dr. W. Junk, Publishers, The Hague, The Netherlands.)

cated or deleted chromosome are lethal.

4. Chromosome disease occurs because of a defect in the number or sequence of genes, and not in the quality of genes.

5. Significant abnormalites are usually present in multiple systems; only rarely will a single-organ abnormality be associated with a chromosome error.

6. Moderate to severe mental retardation is common in chromosome error, except for sex chromosome abnormalities.

7. In deletions, the phenotype may represent the unmasking of a recessive trait.

8. Missing genetic material (deletions) are more deleterious than extra chromosome material.

9. Duplications or deletions of late-replicating regions (positive Q or G bands replicate late) are less harmful than those involving earlier replicating regions.

10. Chromosomal syndromes have a high concentration of Q and G positive bands.

SUMMARY

Chromosome variation is one technique for natural selection in general evolution. An inaccuracy in the copying of chromosomes, however rarely it occurs, provides an alternative to the original specie. In the subsequent competition for survival, some of the variants will not survive, while others will live to reproduce, and produce offspring that can have comparable or superior qualities for survival. If the individual with the altered chromosomes has a selective advantage, even of minor degree, then over several generations, this will be effective in gradually transforming the chromosomes in the population.

The present human complement of 44 autosomes and 2 sex chromosomes represents the average, idealized arrangement for man at this period of time; for with this number, man is healthy, active, productive, and capable of interpreting and regulating his environment and employing its resources to his advantage. If the propo-

Table 11–4. Ocular Abnormalities with Specific Chromosome Errors

	Ocular abnormalities	Chromosome aberration
Facial, Orbits	hypoplasia	18 +
	eyebrow, high arch	9p −, 9r, 10p +, 10q +, 12p −
	eyebrow, low arch	4p +
	flat, supraorbital ridges	11p +
	hypotelorism	5p +, 6p +, 13 +, 13q +, 13q −, 14q +, 18p −, 21 +, 22 +, XXXXX
	hypertelorism	4p +, 4p −, 5p −, 7q +, 8 +, 9p +, 9p −, 10q +, 11p +, 11q −, 12p +, 13q −, 13r, 18p −, 18q −, 22 +, 22q +, XXXXX, XXXXY
Eyelids	entropion	13 +
	telecanthus	9p +, 13 +, 20p +, 21 +, 22q −
	epicanthal folds	4p −, 5p −, 9r, 12p +, 13 +, 13q −, 18 +, 18p −, 18q −, 21 +, 22q −, 22r, XO, XXXXX
	ptosis	4p −, 4q +, 10q +, 13 +, 13r, 18 +, 18p −, 18r, 22q −, 22r, XO, XXY, XYY
	mongoloid lid fissure	9p −, 9r, 10p +, 11q −, 15q +, 18p −, 20p +, 21 +, XXXX, XXXXX, XXXXY
	antimongoloid lid fissure	2q +, 4p +, 4p −, 5p −, 8 +, 9p +, 10q +, 11p +, 11q −, 12p −, 14q +, 15q +, 18p −, 21q −, 21r, 22 +, 22q +, XO
	horizontal lid fisssure	15q +
	blepharophimosis	4p +, 6p +, 7q +, 9 +, 10q +, 13 +, 14q +, 18 +, 21 +
	eyelashes, long and incurved	13q +
	blepharitis	21 +, XXX
	ectropion	21 +
Lacrimal	deficient tears	5p −
	stenosis nasolacrimal duct	4p −
Globes	anophthalmia	13 +, t(4,14)
	cyclopia	B +, 13 +, 18p −, G −
	microphthalmia	4p −, 5q +, 10q +, 13 +, 13q +, 13q −, 13r, 14q +, 16q +, 18 +, 18p −, 18q −, 18r, triploidy
	exophthalmia	4p −, 9p −, XXY
	enophthalmia	9 +, 9p +, 9q +, 11p +, 15q +, 18q −
	buphthalmia	13 +, XYY
Motility	nystagmus	4p −, 5p −, 11p +, 17p +, 18 +, 18q −, 18r, 21 +, XO, Dr, XXX
	strabismus	4p −, 5p −, 7q +, 8 +, 9p −, 11p +, 13 +, 13q +, 15q +, 18 +, 18p −, 18q −, 20p +, 21 +, 22 +
Refractive error	astigmatism	18q −, 21 +, XO, XXY
	myopia	5p −, 18q −, XO, NOONAN, XXY, XXXXY
	hyperopia	XO, XO/XX
Intraocular pressure	glaucoma	13 +, 13q +, 13q −, 18 +, 18q −, 21 +, XO, Cp − q +
Cornea	macrocornea	C +
	sclerocornea	4p −
	corneal leukoma	4p −, 4q +, 8 +, 13 +, 18 +, 18p −, 18q −, XO
	keratoconus	18p −, 21 +, 22 +
	microcornea	13 +, 18 +, 18q −, 18r, XO
	dysgenesis	XXY
Sclera	blue sclera	18 +
	coloboma	13 +

Table 11–4. *(Continued)*

	Ocular abnormalities	Chromosome aberration
Iris	anisocoria	18+
	atrophy	18p−, XXY
	aniridia	11p13−, XXXXY
	Brushfield spot	18q−, 21+, 22+, XXX
	ectopic pupil	9p+
	coloboma	4p+, 4p−, 5p−, 9p+, 10p+, 13+, 13q+, 13q−, 13r, 18+, 18q−, 18r, 22+, 22q+, G+, triploidy, XXXXX, XXY
	Iridoschisis	XXX
Lens	luxation	13+, XXY, XYY, triploidy
	aphakia	13+
	cataract	4p−, 10+, 13+, 13r, 15q+, 18+, 18p−, 18q−, 18r, 21+, 21q−, XO, triploidy, XYYYY, XXYY, XXX, XXXX, XXqi, XYY
Vitreous	persistent primary vitreous	13+
	vitreous membranes	13+
Retina	chorioretinitis	XXX, XYqi
	detachment	13+, 21+, XXY, XO
	retinal dysplasia	Dr, 13+, 13q−, 18+, 18r, triploidy
	retinoblastoma	13q14−, 21+, 21+/XXX, 21+/XXY
	tapetoretinal degeneration	5p−, 18p−, XO/XX
	lattice degeneration	XO
	coloboma	triploidy
Uvea	decreased pigment	18+
	coloboma	13+, 18+, XO, XXY, triploidy, XYY
Optic Nerve	absent nerve	18+
	atrophy	5p−, 13+, 18q−, 18r
	hypoplasia optic nerve	13+, 18+
	staphyloma	10+, 13+, XO
	coloboma	13+, 18+, XXXXY
Other	persistent primary vitreous	13+
	intraocular cartilage	13+, 18+
	albinism	XO, B+
	amblyopia	18q−, 21+
	color blindness	XO, XXY
	facial paralysis	18+
	cranial nerve 6 palsy	XO
Pupil	eccentric	XO
	ectopic	4p−, 9p+
	anisocoria	18+
Iridocorneal Angle	immature	13+, 13r, triploidy
	dysgenesis	XXY
	Canal of Schlemm absent	13+, 13r
Visual Field	central scotoma	XXXX
	constricted	XO

nents of an evolutionary change from 48 to 46 chromosomes should prove to be correct, then at some prior time, man's precursor had 48 chromosomes, and at some future date "man" may have a different number of chromosomes. Any future changes in the number of "normal" chromosomes will probably arise from numeric and structural changes similar to those described in this report.

With the present 46 chromosomes, man appears to have fewer deformities and less disease. With most chromosome aberrations, physical and mental development is restricted, and numerous body organs or tissues, including the eye, are deranged.

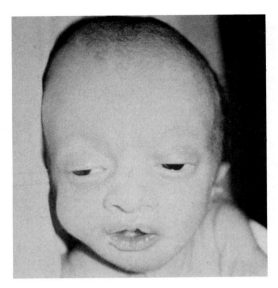

Fig. 11–10. Few major ocular defects are associated with trisomy 18. This patient had blepharoptosis. (From Howard, R.O.: Classification of chromosomal eye syndromes. Int. Ophthalmol. 4:77, 1981. With permission from Dr. W. Junk, Publishers, The Hague, The Netherlands.)

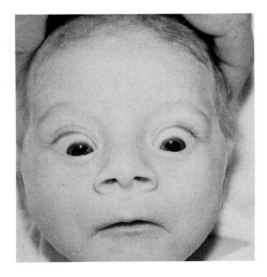

Fig. 11–11. Bilateral eyelid retraction was present in this child with deletion of the short arm of chromosome 13 and a giant satellite on chromosome 21. (From Howard, R.O.: Classification of chromosomal eye syndromes. Int. Ophthalmol. 4:77, 1981. With permission from Dr. W. Junk, Publishers, The Hague, The Netherlands.)

Chromosome abnormalities resulting in defects of one single organ or tissue are exceedingly rare.

BIBLIOGRAPHY

Abuelo, J.G., and Moore, D.E.: The human chromosome. Electron microscopic observations on chromatin fiber organization. J. Cell. Biol. 41:73, 1969.

Arrighi, F.E., and Hsu, T.C.: Localization of heterochromatin in human chromosomes. Cytogenetics 10:81, 1971.

Beneden, E.: Recherches sur la mutation de l'oeuf, la fécondation et la division cellulaire. Arch. Biol. 4:265, 1883.

Berner, H.W., Jr.: Amniography, an accurate way to localize the placenta: a comparison with soft tissue placentography. Obstet. Gynec. 29:200, 1967.

Boué, J.G., Boué, A., Lazar, P., and Gueguen, S.: Sur les durées de d'avortements spontanes précoces. C. R. Acad. Sci. Paris 272:2992, 1971.

Burnett, R.G., and Anderson, W.R.: The hazards of amniocentesis. J. Iowa Med. Soc. 58:130, 1968.

Caspersson, T., Zech, L., Johansson, C., and Modest, E.J.: Identification of human chromosomes by DNA binding fluorescent agents. Chromosome 30:215, 1970.

Chen, A.T.L. et al.: Chromosome studies in full term, low birth weight mentally retarded patients. J. Pediatr. 76:393, 1970.

Court Brown, W.M., et al.: Chromosome studies on adults. Eugenics Laboratory Memoirs XLII, 1966.

Creasman, W.T., Lawrence, R.A., and Thiede, H.A.: Fetal complications of amniocentesis. JAMA 204:949, 1968.

Cross, H.: Ocular trauma during amniocentesis. Arch. Ophthalmol. 90:303, 1973.

Day, R.W., Wright, S.W., Koons, A., and Quigley, M.: XXX, 21 trisomy and retinoblastoma. Lancet 2:154, 1963.

deGrouchy, J., Turleau, C., Roubin, M., and Colin, F.C.: Chromosomal evolution of man and the primates. In Chromosome Identification, Edited by T. Caspersson, and L. Zech. New York, Academic Press, 1973.

Denver Conference: A proposed standard system of nomenclature of human mitotic chromosomes (editorial comment by L.S. Penrose). Ann. Hum. Genet. 24:319, 1960.

Drets, M.E., and Shaw, M.W.: Specific banding patterns of human chromosomes (heterochromatin—giemsa stain—chromosome banding). Proc. Natl. Acad. Sci. U.S.A. 68:2073, 1971.

Dutrillaux, B., and Lejeune, J.: Cytogenetique humaine, sur une novelle technique d'analyse du caryotype humain. Comp. Rendu Hebd. Seances Acad. Sci. 272:2638, 1971.

Egley, C.C.: Laceration of fetal spleen during amniocentesis. Am. J. Obstet. Gynecol. 116:582, 1973

Enoch, J.M., and Novick, S.: Causes and Costs of visual impairment. In Vision and its Disorders. National Institute of Neurological Diseases and Blindness, U.S. Department of Health, Education and Welfare, Public Health Services, National Institute of Health, Monograph 4, 1967, pp. 23–28.

Esquirol, J.E.D.: Des maladies mentales considerees sous les rapports medical hygienique et mediolegal. Bailliere, Paris. 1838.

Flemming, W.: Beitrage zur kenntniss der Zelle und ihrer Lebenserscheinungen. Arch. Mikroskop. Anat. 18:151, 1880.

Flemming, W.: Beitrage zur kenntniss der Zelle und ihrer Lebenserscheinungen. III. Arch. Mikroskop. Anat. 20:1, 1882.

Ford, C.E., and Hammerton, J.L.: The chromosomes of man. Nature 178:1020, 1956.

Francois, J., Berger, R., and Saraux, H.: Les Aberrations Chromosomiques en Ophthalmologie. Paris, Masson et Cie, 1972.

Fraser, G.R., et al.: Karyotype studies among children with severe visual handicap. Br. J. Ophthalmol. 54:79, 1970.

Friedrich, U., and Nielsen, J.: Chromosome studies in 5,049 consecutive newborn children. Clin. Genet. 4:333, 1973.

Fulton, A.B., et al.: Ocular findings in triploidy. Am. J. Ophthalmol. 84:859, 1977.

German, J., and Bearn, A.G.: Asynchronous thymidine uptake by human chromosomes. Paper presented to Am. Soc. Clinical Investigators, Atlantic City, May 1961. J. Clin. Invest. 40:1041, 1961.

Howard, R.O.: Classification of chromosomal eye syndromes. Int. Ophthalmol. 4(1–2):77, 1981.

Howard, R.O.: Chromosomal abnormalities associated with cyclopia and synophthalmia. Trans. Am. Ophthalmol. Soc. 75:505, 1977.

Howard, R.O.: Ocular abnormalities in the cri-du-chat syndrome. Am.J. Ophthalmol. 73:949, 1972.

Howard, R.O., et al.: The eyes of embryos with chromosome abnormalities. Am. J. Ophthalmol. 78:167, 1974.

Howard, R.O., et al.: Retinoblastoma and partial deletion of the long arm of chromosome 13. Trans. Am. Ophthalmol. Soc. 76:172, 1978.

Imai, Y., and Moriwaki, D.: A probable case of cytoplasmic inheritance in man. A critique of Leber's disease. J. Genet. Hum. 33:163, 1936.

Johannsen, W.L.: Elemente der exakten Erblichkeitslehre. Jena, Gustave Fisher, 1909.

Kornberg, R.D., and Klug, A.: The nucleosome. Sci. Am. 244:52, 1981.

Ladda, R., Atkins, L., Littlefield, J., and Pruett, R.: Retinoblastoma chromosome banding in patients with heritable tumour. Lancet 2:506, 1973.

Langdon Down, J.H.: Observations on an ethnic classification of idiots. Clin. Lect. Reps. London Hospitals 3:259, 1866.

Lejeune, J., Gauthier, M., and Turpin, R.: Les chromosomes humains en culture de tissus. Comp. Rendu. Acad. Sci. 248:602, 1959.

Lele, K.P., Penrose, L.S., and Stallard, H.B.: Chromosome deletion in a case of retinoblastoma. Ann. Hum. Genet. 27:171, 1963.

Liley, A.M.: The technique and complications of amniocentesis. N.Z. Med. J. 59:581, 1960.

Machin, G.A.: Chromosome abnormality and perinatal death. Lancet 1:549, 1974.

McKusick, V.A.: Mendelian Inheritance in Man, 3rd Ed. Baltimore, John Hopkins Press, 1971.

Miller, R.W.: Neoplasma and Down's syndrome. Ann. N.Y. Acad. Sci. 171:637, 1970.

Murphy, E.A., and Chase, G.A.: Principles of Genetic Counseling. Chicago, Yearbook Medical Publishers, 1975.

Painter, T.S.: The Y chromosomes in mammals. Science 53:503, 1921.

Painter, T.S.: Studies in mammalian spermatogenesis. II. The spermatogenesis of man. J. Exp. Zool. 37:291, 1923.

Pardue, M.L., and Gall, J.G.: Chromosomal localization of mouse satellite DNA. Science 168:1356, 1970.

Paris Conference: Birth defects. Orig. Art. Ser. 3, No. 7, 1972.

Peterson, C.D., and Luzzatti, L.: The role of chromosome translocation in the recurrent risk of Down's syndrome. Pediatrics 35:463, 1965.

Polani, P.E.: Sex-chromosome anomalies: recent developments. In The The Scientific Basis of Medicine. Annual Reviews, British Post Graduate Medical Federation, University of London, Athlone Press, 1965.

Pruett, R.C., and Atkins, L.: Chromosome studies in patients with retinoblastoma. Arch. Ophthalmol. 82:177, 1969.

Rethore, M., et al.: Syndrome 48 XXY, +21 et retinoblastoma. Arch. Franc. Ped. 29:533, 1972.

Sanchez, O., and Yunis, J.J.: New chromosome techniques and their applications. In New Chromosomal Syndromes. Edited by J.J. Yunis. New York, Academic Press, 1977.

Shah, C.M.: Placental size and fetal outcome following intrauterine transfusion. Presented at the Fortieth Annual Meeting, Royal College of Physicians and Surgeons, Ottawa, January 21–23, 1971.

Shaw, M.W.: Human chromosome damage by chemical agents. Ann. Rev. Med. 21:409, 1970.

Stern, C.: Principles of Human Genetics, 2nd Ed. San Francisco, Freeman, 1960.

Stewart, A.L., Keay, A.J., Jacobs, R.A., and Melville, M.M.: A chromosome survey of the unselected liveborn children with congenitial abnormalities. J. Pediatr. 74:449, 1969.

Summitt, R.L.: Cytogenetics in mentally defective children with anomalies: A controlled study. J. Pediatr. 74:58, 1969.

Summer, A.T., Evans, H.J., and Buckland, R.A.: New techniques for distinguishing between human chromosomes. Nature New Biol. 232:31, 1971.

Taktikos, A.: Association of retinoblastoma with mental defect and other pathological manifestations. Br. J. Ophthalmol. 48:495, 1964.

Tjio, J.H., and Levan, A.: The chromosomes number of man. Hereditas (Lund) 42:1, 1956.

Toma, F., Koller, T., and Klug, A.: Involvement of historic H 1 in the organization of the nucleosome and of the salt dependent superstructures of chromatins. J. Cell. Biol. 83:403, 1979.

Virchow, R.: Uber die Theilung der Zellankerne. Virchows Arch. Pathol. Anat. 11:89, 1857.

Vogel, F.: A preliminary estimate of the number of human genes. Nature 201:847, 1964.

Waardenburg, P.J.: Mongolismus. *In* Das menschliche Auge und seine Erbanlagen. The Hague, Martinus Nijhoff, 1932.

Waldeyer, W.: Ueber keryokine und ihre Beziehung zu den Befruchtungsvorgangen. Arch. Mikroskop. Anat. *32*:1, 1888.

Warburg, M., and Mikkelsen, M.: A case of 13–15 trisomy or Bartholin-Patau's syndrome. Acta Ophthalmol. (Kbh) *41*:321, 1963.

Warkany, J.: Congenital Malformation. Chicago, Yearbook Medical Publications, 1971.

Watson, J.D., and Crick, F.H.C.: Molecular structure of nucleic acid: A structure for deoxyribose nucleic acid. Nature *171*:737, 1953.

Weiner, S., Reese, A.B., Hyman, G.A.: Chromosome studies in retinoblastoma. Arch. Ophthalmol. *69*:311, 1963.

Wilcox, L.M., Bercovitch, L., and Howard, R.O.: Wolf-Hirschhorn syndrome. Am. J. Ophthalmol. *86*:834, 1978.

Wilson, M.G., et al.: Chromosomal anomalies in patient with retinoblastoma. Clin. Genet. *12*:1, 1977.

Wiltchik, S.G., Schwarz, R.H., and Emich, J.P., Jr.: Amniography for placental localization. Obstet. Gynecol. *28*:641, 1966.

Winiwarter H. von: Études sur la spermatogenese humaine. Arch. Biol. *127*:91, 1912.

Yanagisawa, S.: Cytogenetic studies on the mentally retarded children. Acta Pediatrica (Japan) *10*:30, 1968

Yunis, J.J.: High resolution of human chromosomes. Science *191*:1268, 1976.

Yunis, J.J., and Ramsey, N.: Retinoblastoma and subband deletion of chromosome 13. Am. J. Dis. Child. *132*:161, 1978.

Chapter 12

Electrodiagnosis

NICHOLAS R. GALLOWAY

Attempts to measure electrical changes throughout the body have been going on for the past one hundred years or more and developments in electronics have allowed the appearance of highly sophisticated measuring devices. This has allowed the measurement of even minute changes, sometimes at a marked distance from the organ of origin. The visual pathway has been an important center for investigation in this respect, and minute electrical impulses can now be recorded from the eye and visual cortex in a manner that would have astonished our Victorian forebears. The basis of all these electrical changes is the bioelectrical potential; this may be defined as the electrical pressure difference between the inside and the outside of a cell. This is the potential difference across a cell wall. All cells show this resting potential; in some, a marked change in the potential may occur when the cell is stimulated and this may cause an electrical current to flow in the surrounding region. Because bioelectrical potentials are often very small, in the region of a millivolt or less, they must be magnified by means of an amplifier before they can be detected by a suitable recording instrument, such as a pen-writer or an oscilloscope.

The small size of the recorded potential is partly owing to the fact that it may have to be picked up from a site remote from its source. One can see that if, during the course of clinical investigation, we were able to insert microelectrodes into individual cells in the body, we would be able to learn some exact information about the function of that particular cell or group of cells. Such techniques have, so far, been limited to the laboratory, and in the clinic we must rely on placing electrodes at some point on the surface of the body as near as possible to the organ under investigation. The eye itself provides the clinician with a view of tissues that are normally covered by opaque skin, and with the ophthalmoscope one can examine, at first hand, blood vessels and nerves. It is also possible to place electrodes on and around the eye and record electrical changes that occur when light is flashed on the retina or the retina is exposed to different forms of light stimulus. So far, at least, the electrical changes in the optic nerve have not been exposed to such direct examination, and changes in the optic tracts, lateral geniculate bodies, and optic radiations still remain out of reach of the clinician; however, electrical changes over the visual cortex in response to visual stimuli can now be measured. These changes, especially when taken alongside the changes recordable from the eye, are becoming increasingly useful in clinical practice, and there would seem to be enormous scope for the development of this means of measuring body function in the future. It is important to understand that these tests are measuring function rather than structure. They should never be regarded as an alternative to ultrasound or CT scan or other ways of measuring structural changes in the body. Instead, they complement the subjective tests of visual function that are carried out in the clinic. By itself, an electroretinogram (ERG) or visual evoked response (VER) is about as useless as a lone phonograph in the desert, and the clinical reporting of these electrical changes needs to be backed up by a full history and knowledge of the results of all the other relevant tests in a particular case. Electrodiagnosis can usually provide one small piece of extra evidence which sometimes may be conclusive in reaching a firm diagnosis. In this chapter, the electrical changes that are recorded in relation to seeing will be discussed by considering firstly those recorded around the eye and, secondly, those recorded from the surface of the scalp over the occipital cortex.

ELECTRICAL CHANGES RECORDABLE IN RELATION TO SEEING

Electrical Changes Recordable from the Eye

The Electroretinogram

In the early years of electroretinography, studies were largely confined to experimental animals, but there is now an International Society of Clinical Electroretinography which has been in existence for over 20 years. The first work in this field was concerned with the corneo-retinal potential or the resting potential. This may be defined as the difference in potential between the cornea and the posterior pole of the

eye. It was first described by Emile Dubois Reymond, Professor of Physiology, Berlin. In 1849, he showed that the cornea is electrically positive with respect to the posterior pole. It was not until 16 years later, however, that Holmgren observed that the resting potential can be modified by the action of light shining on the retina. Shortly after this, Dewar and McKendrick, working in Edinburgh, discovered this light response independently. They were able to show that the changes in potential on impact of light amounted to 3 to 10% of the normal resting potential and were independent of the anterior portion of the eye. Initially, their experiments were carried out by placing electrodes on the cornea and the posterior pole of the eye, but they subsequently showed that the response to light could also be recorded between the exposed brain and the cornea, allowing the eye to be left in situ. They then found that the same electrical changes could be recorded by placing electrodes on the cornea and an adjacent area of skin. Having made this discovery, they were able to attempt to produce a human electoretinogram; this was achieved by using a clay trough filled with saline as the corneal electrode. These early attempts at human electroretinography were far from satisfactory, and it was not until the turn of the century that advances in recording techniques allowed more accurate records to be made. At this point, the stage had been reached when a wave form could be accurately recorded and measured (Fig. 12–1) and it was known beyond doubt that this wave form was produced by the retina, even though it was recorded through electrodes which were placed at some distance from the eye. In the early 1930s, attempts were being made to record a human electroretinogram using the valve amplifier but, at the same time, an important milestone was reached in the study of responses from animals. This was the classic work of Granit. He developed the idea put forward by previous workers, suggesting that the electro-

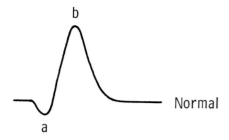

Fig. 12–1. A biphasic ERG. This is the type of response recorded from the human eye, using the simplest equipment and a relatively weak flash stimulus.

retinogram represents the sum of three wave forms which he termed "Processes." These he enumerated as PI, PII, and PIII. He showed that if the electroretinogram is recorded from a cat subjected to deepening levels of ether anesthesia, the wave form changes in a characteristic manner. This change in wave form was thought to be caused by the selective inhibition of each of the three processes PI, PII, and PIII in turn. Although they have been elaborated to some extent, these original ideas about the nature of the electroretinogram are still held to be true today. As soon as the knowledge of the basic components had become well established, much interest was centered on the relative contribution of photopic and scotopic mechanisms to the response; for example in 1940 it was noted that the flicker fusion frequency was not the same under photopic and scotopic conditions. This difference is now being used in many electrodiagnostic clinics to assess cone function.

Although these various advances in our understanding of the electrical responses from the eye were made from work on animals, investigations on human subjects had always been hampered by the technical problem of fixing the electrodes. A great step forward was made in 1941 when Riggs introduced the contact lens electrode. Until this time, clinical electroretinography did not really exist and little was known about alterations in disease. In fact, the use of the contact lens remained in abeyance during the war years until the pioneering work of Karpe began to be published from Stockholm in 1945. It soon became apparent that the contact lens electrode eliminated much of the interference caused by background noise. The late 1970s saw a further development in this respect: the introduction of a flexible electrode that hangs over the lower lid and allows good recordings to be made but at the same time enables the subject to view the stimulus directly rather than through a contact lens. This has certain advantages when a formed stimulus is required rather than a simple flash.

More Recently Discovered Components of the Electroretinogram. Using the method described by Karpe, the human electroretinogram could be recorded as a biphasic response, but it had previously been shown in other animals that a series of small wavelets could sometimes be seen on the 'b' wave. In 1954, Cobb and Morton decribed the phenomenon in man and named it the oscillatory potential. They counted four to six wavelets using a brief flash stimulus, and since then it has been shown that these wavelets may be selectively abolished by disease. The early receptor potential is another component, which can be seen at the very beginning of the response, immediately before the 'a' wave. Brown and Murakami first described it in 1964 and showed that it could be elicited only by an intense light stimulus. The latent period is very short, less than 60 microseconds and it appears as a small, positive peak followed by a larger, negative one. Its importance lies in the fact that it is thought to be an electrical manifestation of the bleaching of the photo pigment in the retina. These newer components can usually be seen in the human ERG if a photoflash stimulus is used; such a response can be seen in Fig. 12–2.

The Origin of the Electroretinogram. If the clinical value of the electroretinogram is to be fully realized in the future, a full understanding of the mode of production

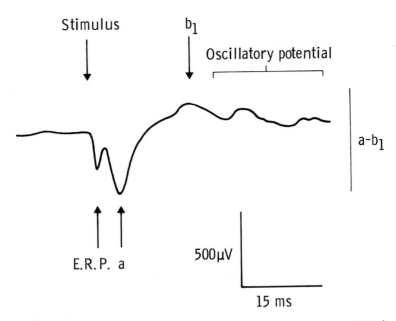

Fig. 12–2. ERG produced by a photoflash stimulus showing the early receptor potential and oscillatory potential.

of the waveform will be essential. A superficial inspection of the problem might lead us to search for an origin of the 'a' wave in one layer of the retina, a 'b' wave in another, and so on; however, the wealth of research that has been carried out so far indicates that the source of the response that we record must be looked for in two stages. First we must find out what component waves are added together to produce the final response; then, having isolated these components, their anatomic site of origin must be determined. A further question arises when we consider that the electroretinogram is a mass response; is it the sum of different kinds of response from different parts of the retinal sphere? Local responses from different parts of the retina can now be obtained at least in the laboratory, and it is perhaps surprising that the response from a small area of retina is similar to the mass response. Differences can be seen in the waveform of records from the fovea and the peripheral retina in the cynomolgus monkey, although they have not yet really been confirmed in man.

At the fovea, the 'b' wave is small whereas the 'a' wave is large. These differences are partly owing to the fact that the rods and cones do not produce exactly the same kind of response and partly because of the different anatomic configuration of the nerve elements at the fovea and the peripheral retina.

Analysis of the Response. In the electrodiagnostic clinic, the human electroretinogram is seen as a biphasic response, a negative 'a' wave followed by a positive 'b' wave. The 'b' wave is disturbed by the oscillatory wavelets in its ascending part. The other components of the electroretinogram can be elicited only by using special recording techniques. It is now widely accepted that the 'a' wave represents the leading edge of PIII, which is a negative wave derived from the inner segments of the receptors. PIII has a faster cut-off from cones than it does from rods, and this difference can explain differences between E.R.G.s from vertebrates with rod-dominated or cone-dominated retina (Fig. 12–3).

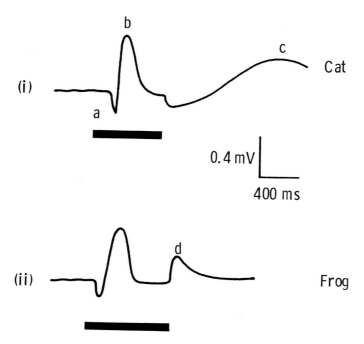

Fig. 12–3. Comparison of ERGs from a rod-dominated eye (cat) and a cone-dominated eye (frog). This diagram shows the absence of the 'c' wave and the presence of a 'd' wave in the cone retina.

Although the negative PIII continues for the duration of the E.R.G., its leading edge is all that is seen because PII appears and this positive wave is superimposed upon it. PII has recently been shown to arise in the Müller cells. That is, it comes from retinal supporting cells rather than from cells conducting visual information. There is, however, still some doubt about this because the rate of depolarization of the Müller cell is a little slow compared with the 'b' wave.

The 'c' wave, which is a positive wave following the familiar biphasic 'a'/'b' wave pattern, is not usually seen in the clinic because of the recording conditions, but it is thought to arise from the pigment epithelium. Fig. 12–4 shows how PI, PII and PIII summate to produce an E.R.G.

The Oscillatory Potential. It has been mentioned already that under suitable stimulus conditions, a number of small wavelets are seen on the 'b' wave. In the monkey, these wavelets are abolished in a striking manner by clamping the retinal circulation, and they are also abolished in the human eye after central retinal artery occlusion. The fact that their presence appears to depend on the integrity of the retinal circulation suggests that they may arise in the inner part of the retina, which receives its nourishment from this source. It is interesting, however, that the wavelets seem to be more susceptible to ischemic change than is the 'b' wave. Intraretinal microelectrodes have been used to record oscillatory responses from the inner nuclear layer of the frog's retina and the response can be produced only if a wide area of retina is stimulated. There is also some evidence that the wavelets are produced by tangentially orientated structures, and they are particularly well seen in vertebrates where there is a thick and well developed inner nuclear layer.

It has been suggested that the wavelets are related to observed cyclical changes in amplitude of the spike discharges in the

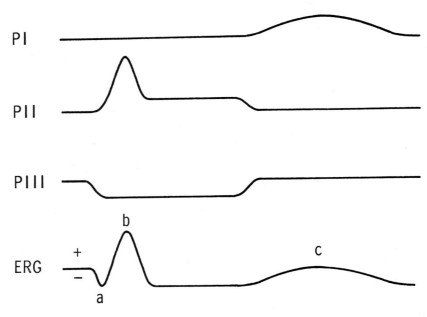

Fig. 12-4. Diagram to show how PI, PII and PIII summate to produce the ERG. Changes in the shape of PIII can account for the difference between rod- and cone-dominated retinas.

optic nerve, and hence their origin from the ganglion cells; but they are still present in optic atrophy, and antidromic stimulation of optic nerve fibers does not reset the rhythm of the wavelets. There is no doubt that the wavelets can best be produced by exposing the eye to double flashes spaced about 15 seconds apart. The second flash tends to produce a more well-defined response and this requirement for preadaptation becomes more marked when the eye is dark-adapted. The maximum chromatic sensitivity of the wavelets has been shown to be at the red end of the spectrum, and it has also been claimed that the wavelets are abolished in patients with congenital achromatopsia. Their exact site of origin is therefore still in doubt, although the evidence at present seems to point to the inner nuclear layer. In view of the fact that the wavelets show certain features in common with a response recordable from the amacrine cells, it has been suggested that they could reprsent a feedback mechanism from the amacrines to the bipolars.

More recently, it has been found that the last of the oscillatory potentials appears to behave in a different way from the others. Its timing alters with increase in stimulus frequency in a different manner. In fact, the last wavelet appears to be time-locked to the stimulus offset, whereas the others are not. The suggestion is that the last wavelet is part of the off-response, being generated by the retinal off-elements described in single-cell recordings.

The Early Receptor Potential. Although the latent period of the 'a' wave becomes much shorter with stronger stimuli, it is never less than about 2 msec and for some years before 1964 it was suspected that a response might exist that bridged the gap between the moment of excitation and the onset of PIII. In 1964, Brown and Murakami found that an electrical response of no detectable latency could be recorded from a microelectrode inserted into the inner segment of the receptors. It was then shown that this rapid biphasic response could be recorded with large electrodes outside the retina, and in fact, it can now be recorded as a routine clinical procedure in the human. The action spectrum of this response agrees with that for bleaching visual pigment. The early receptor potential has been elusive in the past because it is easily obscured by artifacts and a strong flash is required to elicit it. It is now known to be biphasic: a small positive component known as R_1 is followed by a larger negative component known as R_2 which leads directly into the 'a' wave. Because the latency is virtually zero, both R_1 and R_2 are thought to arise from the outer segments of the receptors, and it has been suggested that they are caused by movements of charge in visual pigment molecules. The early receptor potential is more resistant to disease than are the other components of the electroretinogram and, when recorded from the isolated retina, it is not much altered by formaldehyde or metal chelating agents. On heating the retina, it disappears at the same temperature at which the regular orientation of the pigment molecules is lost.

Variations in the Normal Electroretinogram. It is especially important that the clinician who interprets electroretinogram traces has a full understanding of all the different reasons why the normal electroretinogram may vary and all the different factors that may influence this. Without such knowledge, the reporting may be extremely misleading.

The factors that may influence a normal response can be summarized as follows:

1. Physiologic Variations
   State of dark adaptation
   Pupil size
   Diurnal rhythm
   Refractive error
   Age and sex
2. Variations owing to Type or Adjustment of Equipment
   Amplifier, setting of gain and time constant
   Type of recorder
   Electrode position
   Stimulus color, duration, and intensity
3. Variations in Response owing to Artifacts
   Blinking
   Tears
   Bubbles in contact lens
   Eye Movements
   Photoelectric and electrical artifacts

Types of Normal Electroretinogram

Photopic and Scotopic Electroretinogram. The electrical response of the dark-adapted retina to a white flash reflects both rod and cone activity, but in the clinic it is often useful to be able to separate these. This may be achieved in the following way:

1. If a flickering light is used with a frequency of 30 cycles per second, then a pure cone response results because the rod system cannot respond at this rate.

2. A pure cone electroretinogram can also be produced if the stimulus is superimposed on a steady background illumination. The background illumination serves to saturate the rods so that they cannot respond to brief flashes.

3. A rod response can be produced by stimulating the dark-adapted retina with a dim blue light which is below the cone threshold.

4. If a red light of suitable intensity is used, a double peak can be seen on the 'b' wave; and it has been widely accepted that the first peak represents a cone response and the second peak represents a rod response.

The Response to an Intense Flash. When an intense photoflash is used to produce an electroretinogram, certain special features appear in the response. Firstly, the early receptor potential can be seen immediately prior to the 'a' wave. The 'a' wave is abnormally large and the 'b' wave is small. However, if the 'b' wave is measured from the peak of the 'a' wave to the peak of the 'b' wave then the size of this wave is not very different from the 'b' wave obtained using the more classic technique of electroretinography described by Karpe. A further feature of this type of response is the prominence of the oscillatory potential. Finally, there is a pronounced refractory period after each response. If the stimulus is repeated half a minute after the first one, then the resulting response is half the size of the first; a repeat flash within 2 or 3 seconds of the first one produced no response whatsoever. Subjectively, a flash of this sort produces a dense afterimage which changes color over a period of one half to three quarters of a minute and then disappears.

Flicker. It has been shown that one method of obtaining a photopic electroretinogram is to present the eye with a rapid series of flashes. If a stimulus flash is repeated every few seconds, using a weak stimulus, then the second response resembles a normal electroretinogram. If the flash rate is increased to 2 per second, then the second response and successive responses have a photopic character and are reduced in amplitude. As the frequency is increased, the amplitude of 'a' and 'b' waves approach one another. Beyond a certain frequency, the trace becomes sinusoidal, and finally it flattens off altogether when the critical fusion frequency is reached. The critical fusion frequency varies with the intensity of the stimulus. If a graph is made of intensity values against critical fusion frequency, then the resulting curve has a kink in it at about 20 per second. This kink corresponds with the rod/cone break in the dark-adaptation curve and it suggests that the rods are not responding above the level of about 20 per second. With high intensities, a fusion frequency of 70 per second can be reached.

The "Off Effect." As a rule, the clinical electroretinogram is recorded using a brief stimulus flash whose duration is limited to less than 20 msec. If a more prolonged stimulus is used, however, a change in electrical activity is evident when the stimulus is discontinued. In animal experiments, this has been termed the "off effect" or 'd' wave, but it has never been exploited clinically. It is known that the human "off effect" is a negative going wave with a weak stimulus but becomes a positive wave as the stimulus is increased in intensity. The clinical applications of this have been limited, but it has been shown that the negative going wave elicited by a dim stimulus is absent in congenital stationary night blindness but present in patients with rod monochromatopsia. It has also been shown that a series of wavelets may be found on the "off effect" that bear a resemblance to the oscillatory potential. Nilsson has developed a DC registration technique which has allowed a more detailed study of the "off effect." After a very fast positive 'd' wave, a fast negative change occurs (the 'f' wave), a slower positive wave with a maximum at 0.9 to 1.5 sec after "off" (the 'g' wave), and a slow negative change with a maximum at 4 to 6 sec (the 'h' wave). The 'h' wave seems to be the "off" equivalent of the 'c' wave.

The Pattern ERG. Until recently it was assumed that the ERG produced by a pattern stimulus was similar to that produced by a flash stimulus if matched for luminance. Considerable interest ha been aroused by reports that the pattern ERG, unlike the flash ERG, is reduced in amblyopic eyes, and there is evidence that it may arise more deeply in the retina, perhaps from the ganglion cell layer. The ERG from a pattern stimulus is very small and for this reason its measurement is technically difficult, but as techniques improve the pattern response could be clinically helpful.

Let us now summarize the important features of the normal electroretinogram:

1. Although the electroretinogram can be recorded through electrodes placed outside and even at a distance from the eye, there is no doubt that it is produced by the retina, and other structures in and around the eye probably make no contribution to it.
2. The electroretinogram is made up of the following componets:
   the early receptor potential
   the 'a' wave

the 'b' wave

the 'c' wave

There is also an "off effect" whose position depends on the timing of the stimulus flash.

3. The early receptor potential is thought to arise from the outer segments of the receptors, the 'a' wave is part of Granit's PIII component, and this is thought to arise from the inner segments of the receptors. The 'b' wave corresponds to Granit's PII component, and this is thought to arise from the inner nuclear layer and possibly from the Müller cells. The 'c' wave, which corresponds with PI, probably arises from the pigment epithelium. Under suitable stimulus conditions, the 'b' wave is modified by the appearance of three or four small wavelets, which probably arise in the inner nuclear layer but not from the same source as the 'b' wave itself. These wavelets are particularly sensitive to pathologic changes in the retina.

The Electro-oculogram

So far we have been considering electrical responses that are produced by exposing the eye to a brief flash of light. Although a variety of light stimuli are used in electroretinography, they are all relatively short flashes, lasting for milliseconds rather than seconds. The electro-oculogram is a slightly different technique, which enables us to measure the electrical responses of the eye to a prolonged light stimulus lasting several minutes.

It is important to remember that there is a difference in potential between the cornea and the posterior pole of the eye, known as the corneo-retinal potential or the resting potential. It normally amounts to several millivolts but is of course modified to form the electroretinogram when the eye is exposed to a brief flash. Unfortunately, it is not easy to measure the corneo-retinal potential over long periods of time because in practice the steady response is obscured by blinks, random eye movements, and other artifacts. This problem can be resolved when performing electroretinography by using an AC coupled amplifier. This type of amplifier only responds to relatively rapid changes in potential, and a steady base line is more easily maintained. When the eye is exposed to a continuous light stimulus, a slow change in the corneo-retinal potential occurs. This would not normally be seen using an AC coupled amplifier, and the base line would be too unsteady to obtain accurate measurements if a directly coupled amplifier were used.

The electro-oculogram is a recording technique that allows an AC amplifier to be used to record these slow changes in the corneo-retinal potential; rapid changes of potential are produced by moving the eyes to and fro, and are fed through an AC amplifier to a pen recorder. These changes in potential have been shown to be related to the size of the corneo-retinal potential if the size of the eye movements is kept constant.

In order to perform the test, electrodes are placed on the skin on either side of the eye at the medial and the lateral canthi, and one indifferent electrode is usually placed on the forehead. The subject is seated, facing a screen that can be illuminated. In addition, two small red fixation lights are mounted on either side of the screen. The subject is then asked to look briskly from one fixation light to the other, thus making horizontal eye movements of a constant size.

The eye can be regarded as an electrical dipole, the cornea being positive with respect to the posterior pole. It can be seen from the diagram (Fig. 12–5) how eye movements in a horizontal direction can produce a modified square wave and how the vertical limbs of this waveform can increase and decrease in size, depending on the size of the corneo-retinal potential. The same method can, of course, be used to

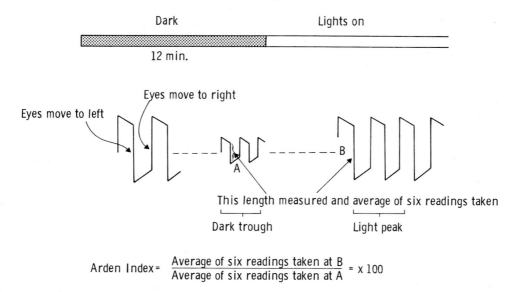

Fig. 12–5. Diagram to show electro-oculogram and measurement of the Arden index.

measure eye movements, but here we are concerned with changes in the corneo-retinal potential and the eye movements are kept at a constant value.

As long ago as 1929, it was shown that eye movements produce electrical changes that can be measured by skin electrodes, but at that time it was assumed that these electrical changes were related to muscle action potentials. It was later conclusively proved that the changes in potential were due solely to the existence of the standing potential. Furthermore, it was subsequently shown that the potential change exhibited by electro-oculography is directly proportional to the line of the angle of rotation of the globe.

Electro-oculography thus provides a means of monitoring long-term changes in the corneo-retinal potential and, in particular, a means of assessing the changes induced by light. In the clinic, the tests can be performed in an automated fashion so that only a nurse is needed to fix on the electrodes. A value known as the Arden Index is obtained at the end of the test. This value should be more than 180 in a normal subject, although some myopes have slightly lower values. In its most com-

monly used form, the test involves seating the subject in the dark and the corneo-retinal potential tends to fall in value during this period. In continued darkness, the potential remains at this low level but tends to wander up and down slightly. After 12 minutes, the light stimulus is applied. There is an initial electroretinographic response and then the potential falls for about 2 minutes, after which it begins to rise steadily over a period of about 7 minutes. The initial fall has been termed the transient and the rise has become known as the light rise. After about 7 minutes, the corneo-retinal potential reaches a peak value and then begins to fall in spite of the fact that the light stimulus is still being applied. This fall in potential is followed by a further rise, and it becomes apparent that the response is a form of damped oscillation.

Origin of the Electro-oculogram and its Relation to the Electroretinogram. The electro-oculogram recorded with skin electrodes is probably the resultant of several potentials. Potentials in the skin or other parts do not change as the eye rotates and therefore do not affect the results. Potentials arising in the eye itself, on the other hand, could be more important. For example, the cornea is thought to be polarized so that its anterior surface is negative; that is to say, it acts against the resting potential. If the corneal potential were to be abolished, then one might expect a corresponding increase in the resting potential. It is, therefore, interesting to find a considerable increase in the resting potential when the cornea is anesthetized. It is known that the standing potential and also the value of the dark trough of the electro-oculogram are markedly reduced by the administration of azide. This substance is known to produce selective damage to the pigment epithelium. Hence, this may be the site of origin of at least part of the electro-oculographic response. But the light rise is markedly impaired by occlusion of the central retinal artery, both in man and in experimental animals, and one might expect the response to be spared if it arose solely from the pigment epithelium. There is also some evidence that the absorption spectrum of the electro-oculogram matches that of visual purple. On the other hand, in a more recent investigation, blue and red lights were chosen to evoke equally large increases in the amplitude of the electro-oculogram. It was found that, in 5 totally color-blind subjects, the response to red light was below normal, whereas the response to blue light was within the normal range. These results suggest that both the rods and the cones contribute to the normal electro-oculogram. The time course of the rise in value of the standing potential in response to light suggests that it may be reflecting the chemical process of light adaptation. Perhaps the slow rise of the corneo-retinal potential over 7 minutes is a manifestation of the regeneration of photopigment. It has been suggested that the electro-oculogram is composed of 2 parts, a light-sensitive component arising in the receptors or perhaps more deeply in the retina, and a light-insensitive component arising in the pigment epithelium.

Whereas it is possible to detect differences in the shape and size of the electroretinogram in the light-adapted state, it has not so far been possible to demonstrate photopic and scotopic responses using the electro-oculogram, although spectral sensitivity measurements have indicated a predominantly rod response with some evidence of cone activity. In spite of all the differences in origin and behavior between the electro-oculogram and the electroretinogram, pathologic processes in the eye that cause alteration in one tend to cause similar changes in the other. This is probably because it is unusual for a disease process to be limited to one single layer of the retina. For example, a marked impairment of both the electro-oculogram and the electroretinogram is seen at an early stage in eyes suffering from retinitis pigmentosa. Claims have been made that in some instances either one or the other of these techniques shows the first changes, but this may depend on the accuracy of the particular equipment used rather than on the test itself. It has been claimed that in certain diseases the electroretinogram may be normal when the electro-oculogram is grossly abnormal or vice versa, and this may be of diagnostic value. Patients with vitelliform macula degeneration, for example may have a diminished light rise and a normal electroretinogram. It has also been shown that it may be possible to distinguish between a congenital retinal dysgenesis and a congenital retinal abiotrophy by the fact that, in the former instance, the electro-oculogram is normal, whereas both the electroretinogram and the electro-oculogram are affected in a congenital retinal abiotrophy. Although there are one or two instances where the changes in the electro-oculogram do not reflect changes in the electroretinogram and vice versa our knowledge of the meaning of these differences is still inadequate. In practice, the important differences between these two tests may be summarized as follows.

1. The electroretinogram measures

rapid changes in the resting potential in response to light, whereas the electro-oculogram measures slow changes.

2. A contact lens is not required for electro-oculography.
3. Less skill is required for electro-oculography and the equipment is more portable.
4. The electro-oculogram cannot easily be performed on patients who cannot fixate, and it is not suitable for testing retinal function in blind patients.

Electrical Changes Recordable from the Brain

Visually Evoked Potential (VEP). Recording the spontaneous electrical activity of the brain from electrodes placed on the scalp has been practiced as a clinical routine for many years. Only over the past 20 years has it become possible to record the electrical changes over the scalp evoked by peripheral stimuli. The visually evoked potential is one of several evoked potentials that can be recorded from scalp electrodes. Such electrical changes can be produced by sound, smell, and taste, as well as by sensory stimulation. The changes evoked by visual stimuli were recorded in animals directly from the surface of the pia mater in the 1930s. At that time, it was well recognized that the alpha rhythm seen on normal electroencephalographic traces could be accentuated by exposing the eyes to a light flashing at a similar frequency. When the eyes were exposed to repeated flashes at varying frequencies, the electrical changes recorded from scalp electrodes became small and more or less lost against the background of the normal spontaneous activity of the brain.

Signal Averaging. The problem of detecting these small electrical signals was largely solved by the introduction of the technique of averaging. Before the development of modern electronics, this simply entailed the superimposition of the repeated responses after each flash stimulus.

Examining the trace after a single flash revealed little or no sign of any waveform that one might relate to the flash, but when a sufficient number of traces had been superimposed, a response could be discerned that was not visible on the single record. This method of mechanical averaging has been supplanted by electronic averaging. The response following each consecutive stimulus is stored in the memory of a computer, and the average can be automatically displayed as a single trace on the face of an oscilloscope at the end of the operation. Figure 12–6 shows the effect of averaging on a raw EEG tracing obtained when the eyes were exposed to repeated light flashes.

If the responses to a large number of similar visual stimuli are averaged, the discrimination from irrelevant cortical activity can be improved greatly. From the clinical viewpoint, the introduction of averaging was an important breakthrough, because we can now record visually evoked potentials (VEPs) as small as 2 or 3 microvolts (μV). Furthermore, the nature of the response and its amplitude and waveform can be related to the type of visual stimulus in a way never before possible. As will be seen later, the development of the VEP offers the possibility of a true objective measurement of visual acuity and of the visual field.

From the time of the early recordings of the averaged evoked potentials to the present day, the research interest in this subject has gradually increased. The research possibilities have attracted the attention of neurologists, psychiatrists, and engineers, as well as of optometrists and ophthalmologists.

Methods of Recording the VEP. Many electrodiagnostic clinics throughout the world now investigate the VEP as a routine procedure; but because it is still in the stage of development, no successful attempts at standardization of the equipment have so far been made. By and large, the equipment and electrodes do not differ greatly,

EEG recorded with Scalp Electrodes during Repeated
Light Flashes of 1 ms duration at approx. 2 s Intervals

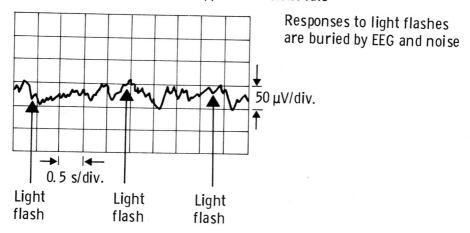

Responses to light flashes
are buried by EEG and noise

50 μV/div.

0.5 s/div.

Light
flash

Light
flash

Light
flash

The above Waveform after Analysis by a Signal
Averaging Instrument triggered from Light Flash

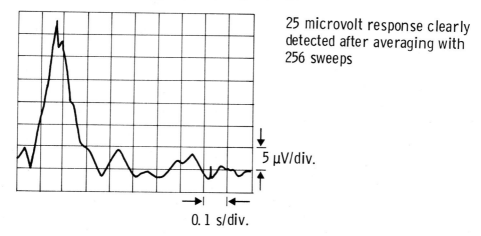

25 microvolt response clearly
detected after averaging with
256 sweeps

5 μV/div.

0.1 s/div.

Fig. 12–6. The figure shows how the technique of averaging can bring out hidden information from the raw trace.

but the type of stimulus used in different clinics varies considerably. The nature of response recorded from the scalp may vary widely from clinic to clinic and records must be interpreted with great care.

In order to record the VEP, four groups of equipment are needed: a repeated stimulus is required, electrical contact with the patient's scalp must be achieved by means of suitable electrodes, electrical changes in these electrodes must be magnified by means of a suitable system of amplifiers, and an averaging computer and readout system to display the information obtained.

1. Stimulus. This can be a diffuse flash of flight or a pattern displayed on a screen. The diffuse flash or unstructured stimulus may vary in frequency, intensity, size, or color. The patterned stimulus is most popularly a checkerboard of black and white squares, although for some purposes, lines, gratings, or other patterns are used. It is important to distinguish between pattern reversal and pattern appearance, because each produces a different response from the scalp. In pattern reversal, the luminosity of the black and white squares is reversed alternately, the black becoming white and the white becoming black. In pattern appearance, a black and white checkerboard is presented in an on-off sequence. It is also important to distinguish between a rapidly repeated stimulus and a slowly repeated stimulus. The rapidly repeated stimulus produces a sinusoidal type of response, referred to as the "steady state" response. Stimuli repeated less than two or three times a second produce a characteristic waveform known as the transient response.

2. Electrodes. Ideally, the skin electrodes must make good contact, be electrically inert, and have a low electrical resistance. The most popular ones are made of silver coated with silver chloride, a layer of electrode jelly being placed between the electrode and the scalp. It may be held in place by collodion or a head strap. Fitting the scalp electrode takes time and patience and should be performed by an experienced technician for best results. The exact positioning of the electrode is critical. The standard "10–20" system of electroencephalographers provides a useful variety of positions, although some prefer to state their electrode positions as direct measurements from the inion. In practice, the choice of electrode position depends on the particular aspect of the VEP being investigated.

3. System of Amplifiers. Usually two amplifiers are used, a preamplifier and a main amplifier, the system being designed to amplify the minute electrical signals from the scalp to a level acceptable for the computer and readout display. This must be done without causing undue distortion of

the signal and without danger to the patient.

4. Averaging Computer and Readout System. The design and function of electronic equipment are continually being improved. Whereas, until recently, a small computer designed only for signal averaging was used, it is now more common to find larger and more versatile computers in use. These allow the waveform of the response to be processed mathematically in a short space of time and provide a convenient way of storing records.

Normal VEP. The character of the normal VEP depends on the type of stimulus being used and the position on the scalp from which it is being recorded. It also varies greatly from one individual to another. In spite of these difficulties, reliable features, particularly of the transient response to a checkerboard stimulus, are beginning to be identified. Figure 12–7 shows the features of the response to a flash stimulus recorded from midline electrodes above the inion. The response to a pattern appearance stimulus is shown alongside it for comparison.

In general, three peaks are distinguishable on all these recordings: an initial positive peak at about 10 to 100 msec, a negative peak at about 100 to 130 msec, and a second positive peak at about 150 to 200 msec. This last positive peak is often prominent in pattern stimulus records and is especially sensitive to changes in contrast, it is favored by binocular stimulation. The timing of the peaks depends on the exact nature of the stimulus and also on the position of the scalp electrodes. The response to a plain flash stimulus is smaller and less well defined and cannot easily be compared with the patterned response, although as the check size of a patterned stimulus becomes very large or very small, the electrical response more closely resembles that produced by an unstructured flash stimulus.

The normal VEP has now been studied under a wide variety of stimulus conditions. Investigations of the effect of altering

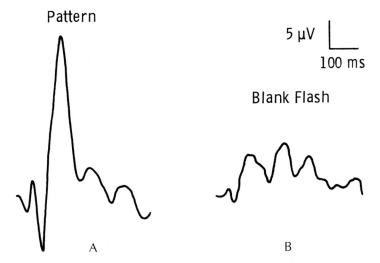

Fig. 12–7. Comparison of VEPs recorded (a) using a flash stimulus and (b) using a checkerboard stimulus.

the size of the stimulus indicate that most of the response is derived from the central macula area of the retina. The VEP shows a progressive increase in size with dark adaptation, and it is abolished by pressure blinding the exposed eye, recovering after about 90 seconds.

Many other types of stimulus have been used, and studies have been made on the effect of altering contours and the size of the pattern elements, the effect of eccentricity of retinal stimulation, and the effect of retinal disparity in binocular stimulation.

VEP and the Visual Field. If different parts of the visual field are stimulated by a small patterned stimulus and the VEP is measured from midline electrodes, the amount of information obtained is disappointing. This is not only because the response becomes very small when the stimulus is only a few degrees from fixation, but also because the method is not capable of detecting extensive defects in the visual field. Responses from the upper part of the field are always smaller than those from the lower part in normal subjects, using midline electrodes. Furthermore, all three components of the transient response show a polarity reversal when the stimulus

is changed from upper to lower half. The information obtainable from a single midline electrode when different parts of the visual field are stimulated is therefore limited, and numerous workers are now investigtating the detailed scalp topography of the response.

A more fruitful approach to the problem of relating the effect of stimulating different parts of the retina to the cortical evoked response has been gained from hemifield stimulation. By stimulating corresponding right or left half-fields of vision, and thereby presumably stimulating contralateral hemispheres, significant electrical changes can be measured from electrodes placed away from the midline on either side.

At first sight, results of the investigations of these and other workers appear to conflict with one another: some claim clear-cut contralateral responses with half-field stimulation; others claim, surprisingly, a large response over the ipsilateral hemisphere. The apparent difference in these results is probably owing to the different types of stimulus used, whether pattern reversal or pattern onset, and also to the fact that different peaks on the transient response were being measured. Thus, an early peak, measured 90 msec after the stimulus, is found contralaterally and well away from the midline with pattern onset stimulation, and a well developed peak at 25 msec is found over the ipsilateral hemisphere with a pattern-reversal response. The positive peak at 125 msec is largely ipsilateral, as is the negative peak at 165 msec using pattern reversal. The peak at 225 msec is largest in the midline in both pattern-onset and pattern-reversal stimulation, but the P125 is contralateral with pattern-onset stimulation.

VEP and the Meaurement of Visual Acuity. The fact that blurring the outline of a checkerboard stimulus or altering its size can greatly influence the latency and the amplitude of the VEP has led to attemps to use the test to measure visual acuity. The results of such tests are not likely to have much meaning when compared with the results of standard Snellen test types because a different aspect of visual acuity is being measured in each case. Psychophysical measurements of ability to detect changes in contrast can also be made and compared with the VEP, using contrast gratings. Here, the results of psychophysical testing can be more closely related to electrophysiologic findings.

The VEP has also been used in attempts to make an objective assessment of refractive error. Regan has shown that by rotating a stenopeic slit in front of the cornea of a subject viewing a checkerboard stimulus, the axes of astigmatism can be determined. Once these axes have been ascertained, the necessary lens power in each axis can be determined by a variable-power lens system. A graph of VEP amplitude versus slit angle and another of VEP amplitude versus lens power can be produced electronically within a few seconds of starting the tests.

The investigation of the electrical changes over the scalp has attracted the interest of research workers from many disciplines all over the world, because such electrical changes might give some indi-

cation of the working of the brain itself. A rudimentary knowledge of the pattern of changes over the scalp in response to certain repeated stimuli is beginning to emerge. As the results in normal subjects are beginning to be understood more clearly, investigations into the changes in disease are also taking place. It will be shown later that the VEP has an important place in the detection of healed retrobulbar neuritis, and is also used for assessing visual acuity and field defects in young children.

Factors Influencing the Normal VEP. The method of recording the VEP varies considerably from center to center. A major point of confusion arises from the fact that there is as yet no agreement as to which way up the trace should be recorded. In clinics that have previously been concerned largely with clinical electroencephalography, the convention is to have negative upwards, and in clinics with a background of pure science or ocular electrophysiology, the convention is to have positive upwards. To add to the confusion, a wide range of stimulus and recording equipment is used. The present lack of clinical standarization reflects a need for more research; in spite of this, some useful results are beginning to emerge concerning the nature of the normal response. Some of the factors that must be taken into account when reporting on a VEP are the stimulus, age and sex differences, the electrode position, and anatomic variations.

Stimulus. The VEP to a flash stimulus increases in amplitude with an increase in stimulus intensity, but a saturation point is reached. The latency is reduced with an increase in intensity. Dark adaptation can be demonstrated with a VEP, as it can with the ERG, and a rod/cone break has been shown. A possibly useful clinical application of the VEP was realized when it became known that the response to a flash was relatively large, with a small centrally located stimulus. This appeared to reflect the wide area of macula representation on the occipital cortex. The VEP can therefore be used as a test of macula function.

Even though the response to an unstructured stimulus has been proved to be of some clinical value, pattern stimuli are now widely preferred, because the response to a pattern is much larger and bears a closer relationship to the act of seeing. Thus, it has been shown that small patterns give a relatively large response when viewed by the macula area, whereas progressively larger patterns give a maximal response as the more peripheral parts of the retina are stimulated. It has already been mentioned that the frequency of the stimulus has a profound influence on the type of trace that can be obtained. Higher frequencies of stimulation, 10 Hz or more, make the test quicker and are probably more satisfactory to use from the technical point of view. On the other hand, low frequency stimulation produces a more detailed response (the so-called transient response), and it is likely that this will hold more useful clinical information. A completely different approach from the stimulus point of view has been made by recording the trans-scleral VER. This is elicited by light delivered through an optical probe on the lower lid. The method has some promise when investigating retinal function in the presence of opaque media.

Age and Sex Difference. The effect of age on the VEP has been extensively examined and the possible value of this type of test in the investigation of young children has produced many studies in infants. It appears that the pattern-reversal VEP resembles that of an adult at the age of 6 months. In premature infants, the VEP is limited to the occipital region and gradually spreads with increasing age. The waveform also changes, and it has been claimed that the diffuse-flash VEP of the premature infant can be distinguished from that of the full-term infant. During maturation, the occipital VEP shows a rapid increase in amplitude of most components. This is seen in early childhood and reaches a maximum in 6- to 8-year old children. At this age, the VEP may be more than twice as large as that obtained in older age groups. After this peak, there appears to be a decline in amplitude associated with increasing age until the 13- to 14- year-old age group, when an abrupt increase is seen, especially in the earlier components, occurring in the first 200 msec. The amplitude of the VEP seems to become stabilized about the age of 16, showing a subsequent gradual reduction throughout life and then a more rapid decline in old age. The difference between male and female responses is not great, although female responses appear to be larger during adolescence and in adults, whereas male responses are larger in children.

Electrode Position. Recording the VEP from a single electrode placed above the inion reveals only a small facet of the total response; for clinical purposes, it is essential that an array of electrodes be used across the back of the scalp. The electrical changes from each electrode vary from millisecond to millisecond in a different manner at each electrode. This means that the response over a period of 500 msec following the stimulus flickers across the scalp like light from moving water. Methods have now been worked out to represent this graphically or as spaciotemporal maps. Again, it must be remembered that these results depend on the type of stimulus being presented and may vary greatly depending on whether this is flashed pattern, pattern onset, or pattern reversal.

Anatomic Variations. The amplitude of the VEP differs markedly from subject to subject, and although not yet clearly shown, it is presumed that much of this variation is caused by anatomic differences such as the thickness of the skull or the orientation of the occipital cortex in relation to the scalp. This is borne out by studies on identical twins, who show similar responses, and by the fact that in a given individual the response is repeatable from day to day and hour to hour.

Other Factors that may Influence the Response. Unfortunately, accurate recording of the VEP depends on subject cooperation and may be influenced by attention, fixation, and focusing. A malingerer could fool the machine by deliberately defocusing his eyes from the pattern or by fixing on a point elsewhere in the room. The problem of fixation in children can be overcome by presenting a television image in the center of the screen to attract the child's attention. It is, of course, essential that the patient's correct spectacle prescription be worn at the time of the test.

Summary of VEP

1. Electrical changes can be recorded from the scalp that bear a relationship to a repetitive light stimulus presented to the eyes.

2. These electrical changes appear to be largely derived from the macula area of the retina, that is the central 5 to 10° of visual field on each side.

3. Specific changes in the response can be seen when a checkerboard pattern of differing size of checks is presented.

4. It is possible to make accurate measurements of the latency, that is the time taken from stimulus presentation to appearance of electrical response on the scalp, and such measurements have proved clinical usefulness.

CLINICAL APPLICATION OF ELECTRODIAGNOSTIC TESTS OF VISION

Inherited Retinal Disease

Since the late 1940s, it has been known that the electroretinogram shows marked changes in patients suffering from retinitis pigmentosa. Even at an early stage of the development of this type of retinal degeneration, the electroretinogram is more or less completely abolished; the light rise of the electro-oculogram is also similarly affected. The majority of patients who show the typical fundus changes of retinitis pigmentosa have an extinguished electroretinogram, and it has even been suggested that the response may be extinguished from birth. There is no doubt, though, that patients in early stages of the disorder have some response, and in fact, a close relationship probably exists between electroretinogram sensitivity and the functioning area of the retina. It seems that when the electroretinogram is relatively well preserved, the patients often give a history of a late onset of a mild form of the disease. In some series in which early cases have been examined, the electroretinogram has been almost normal, and the early changes are usually seen in the scotopic electroretinogram, particularly if this is recorded when a red-light stimulus has been applied. Electroretinography has also served to confirm the value of the genetic classification of retinitis pigmentosa. In the recessive type, the 'b' wave is practically always abolished, whereas in the dominant type it may be present to some degree. Carriers of retinitis pigmentosa often have subnormal electroretinograms, although this is not always the case. Often, of course, a firm diagnosis of retinitis pigmentosa can be achieved with the ophthalmoscope alone. In spite of this, one cannot claim that such a case has been properly documented until a record has been made of the visual field and electroretinogram. If the ERG is totally abolished, there is little point in repeating the test subsequently, unless some form of new treatment is being tried and it is necessary to monitor the disease objectively. When the visually evoked response is measured in patients with retinitis pigmentosa, this is found to be normal unless the disease is advanced or unless there is early macula involvement. Figure 12–8 shows a typical example of the ERG in a patient with retinitis pigmentosa.

Retinitis Pigmentosa and Associated Systemic Disease

A wide variety of diseases have been associated with retinitis pigmentosa and some of the other progressive degenera-

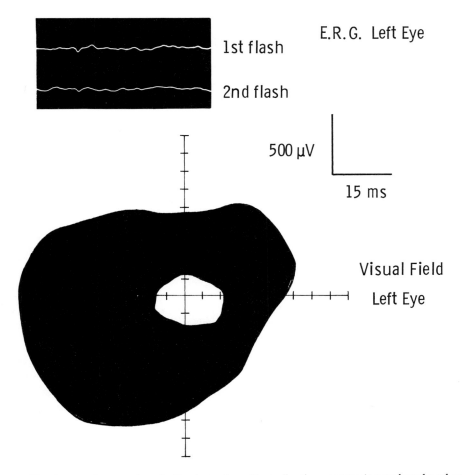

Fig. 12–8. The electroretinogram in retinitis pigmentosa. Typically, the response is greatly reduced or absent at an early stage. The constricted field and absent response are evident.

tions related to it. Although in their present state of development, electrodiagnostic investigations cannot distinguish between classic retinitis pigmentosa and that associated with disorders in the rest of the body, they have a particular value when applied to the latter. Sometimes, the fundus changes are minimal in these patients, and they may be referred from the neurologist or the physician with the question "Are eyes normal?" The electroretinogram and electro-oculogram can provide an immediate answer. Apart from this, the vision may be affected by other pathologic processes. Figure 12–9 shows the result from a patient with ill-defined peripheral constric-

tion of her visual fields and enlargement of the pituitary fossa. She also had polydactyly, having had the extra finger removed in infancy. The fundi showed one or two irregular flecks of pigment in the periphery. The problem was to decide whether the field defect was caused by chiasmal compression or early retinitis pigmentosa in association with polydactyly, the Laurence-Moon-Biedl syndrome being suspected.

A list of the systemic disorders associated with progressive retinal degeneration includes the following conditions:

1. Metabolic disorders:
    a. Lipid abnormalities:

⌂ MEDICAL PHYSICS DEPARTMENT
UNIVERSITY HOSPITAL & MEDICAL SCHOOL
NOTTINGHAM, NG7 2UH. tel 700111 Ex.3382

NAME   HOSPITAL NUMBER
WARD/DEPT.   INVESTIGATION NUMBER

REPORT

The electroretinogram was barely recordable from either eye
even when a bright stimulus flash was used.
The findings are consistent with retinitis pigmentosa.

EVOKED POTENTIALS REPORT

Fig. 12–9. The electroretinogram was barely recordable from either eye even when a bright stimulus flash was used. The findings are consistent with retinitis pigmentosa.

i. A-beta-lipoproteinemia
ii. Refsum's disease
iii. Familial amaurotic idiocy
2. Neurologic disorders:
a. Laurence-Moon-Biedl syndrome
b. Hereditary ataxias
c. Ocular myopathy
d. Syndromes involving mental retardation
3. Occasional associations:
a. Dermatologic disorders
b. Megacolon
c. Marfan syndrome
d. Familial nephropathies

Most of the listed conditions are associated with retinitis pigmentosa, but familial amaurotic idiocy, although characterized by progressive degeneration of the retina, is probably a completely separate entity. The electroretinogram in the infantile form has been reported as normal from several sources and this is in keeping with pathologic changes that are restricted at first to the ganglion cell layer and spare the outer parts of the retina whence the electroretinogram arises. In late infantile and juvenile amaurotic idiocy, however, the electroretinogram may be reduced or absent. All the other conditions listed are associated with retinitis pigmentosa and the electroretinogram and the electro-oculogram are affected accordingly. The main interest of these other conditions is that several of them show specific biochemical abnormalities that seem to throw some light on the cause of the pigmentary degeneration. For example, the association of a-beta-lipoproteinemia, retinitis pigmentosa, ataxia, and acanthocytosis of the red cells also involves a lowering of the blood level of the fat-soluble vitamins, including vitamin A. Recently it has been claimed that vitamin A supplements in sufficient dosage to raise the vitamin A level to normal will also lead to restoration to normal of the dark-adaptation curve and also the electroretinogram. In the mucopolysaccharidoses, vision may be impaired by infiltration of the cornea, and the fundus may not be visible. Electrodiagnostic tests may thus be the only way of detecting associated retinitis pigmentosa. It should be apparent that, because retinitis pigmentosa may sometimes present with minimal changes in the fundi, an electroretinogram is essential if any of the above conditions are suspected. Figure 12–10 shows the serial results in a patient with Refsum's disease. Here, the ERG has been recorded annually because the patient has been maintained on a special diet. It will be seen that no improvement in the response is visible. The electroretinogram and the electro-oculogram have been investigated in a wide variety of conditions related to retinitis pigmentosa, and for more details of this the reader is referred to more specialized textbooks (see the Bibliography).

Leber's Amaurosis

Leber's amaurosis was first described by Leber in 1869. He classed the condition with pigmentary degenerations of the retina even though the pigmentation was minimal or appeared at a late stage. The condition is usually congenital, the affected child being blind from birth, but some become blind during the first year of life. The fundi may appear normal, but a variety of minor changes have been described from fine pigment strippling to choroidal sclerosis. On occasion, the classical appearance of retinitis pigmentosa may be observed. The advent of electroretinography has made it possible to distinguish these children from those with optic atrophy and Tay-Sachs disease. Since it is usually necessary to examine the fundi under a general anesthetic, it is important to take the opportunity to perform electroretinography at the same time. If a general anesthetic is contraindicated, it is often surprisingly easy to insert a contact lens without an anesthetic in a child up to 3 or 4 months old. The electroretinogram is abolished or very small in all these cases.

Sometimes, these children present as having congenital nystagmus, and the electroretinogram under general anesthesia may be crucial in making the diagnosis. In such cases, it is important that the diagnosis be made as soon as possible in order that the parents can be properly advised about the future education of the affected child.

Heredomacula Dystrophies

This includes a group of diseases characterized by bilateral macula degeneration, a hereditary tendency, and the absence of associated disease in the central nervous system. These diseases have been classified and named eponymously according to the age of the onset, but it has been suggested that they are all one and the same condition. They may be listed as follows:

Infantile heredomacula dystrophy—Best's disease or "vitelline dystrophy"

Juvenile heredomacula dystrophy—Stargardt's disease

Adult heredomacula dystrophy—Behr's disease

Presenile and senile heredomacula dystrophies

As a general rule, these patients present with a gradual deterioration of their central vision. Children may have difficulty in reading or seeing the blackboard at school, which is not corrected by wearing glasses. The fundus appearance varies considerably from case to case; in Best's disease, a round or oval lesion is seen at the macula, which has a yellowish color and has been likened to the yolk of an egg—hence the term "vitelline dystrophy." The vitelline lesion evolves into a pigmented scar. Rather surprisingly, the vision of these patients may remain normal in spite of the fundus appearance. In Stargardt's disease, which usually appears between the ages of 8 and 11 years, the vision may be impaired when the fundus is still normal. The earliest change is disappearance of the normal foveal reflex and gray, yellow, or brown spots may appear at the macula. Eventually, an oval circle of pigment stippling is seen, and occasionally, this may spread to involve the entire posterior pole. Senile macula degeneration is associated with degenerative changes in the underlying choroid and

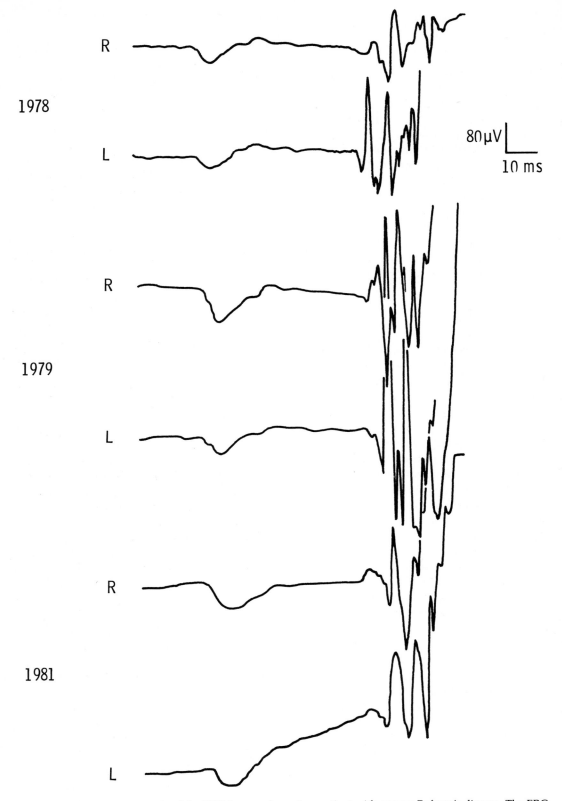

Fig. 12–10. Recordings made of the ERG from each eye in a patient with proven Refsum's disease. The ERG is being used here to monitor any possible effect of treatment.

Bruch's membrane, and although it may bear some resemblance to the types that occur at an earlier age, it may be complicated by the presence of hemorrhages and subretinal exudates. Sometimes, senile macula degenerations are divided into dry and wet types, or the degeneration of Haab and disciform degeneration, respectively.

Electrodiagnostic Investigations. It has been shown that if the macula area in the monkey is photocoagulated, the electroretinogram obtained from this damaged eye is normal. Furthermore, a normal electroretinogram has been described in cases of solar retinopathy. It is not surprising, therefore, that early reports reveal normal electrical responses in these cases; however, when examination is carried out using a red-light stimulus, a high percentage of patients show a reduced amplitude of the 'b' wave. The photopic electroretinogram has been shown to be normal, but the spectral sensitivity curve of the photopic electroretinogram may be displaced towards the shorter wavelengths.

The foveal electroretinogram has also been shown to be subnormal in all cases including those in which the visual acuity was still fairly good. The visually evoked response has also been shown to be normal. This might be expected when we consider the relatively large macula representation on the occipital cortex.

Some slightly unexpected changes have been described in the electro-oculogram in cases of macula degeneration. Several different sources report that the electro-oculogram may be markedly impaired as the sole sign of disturbed retinal function in patients with vitelline dystrophy. The electroretinogram in these cases is usually abnormal. In Stargardt's disease, the electro-oculogram is usually normal unless the retinal periphery is involved.

It is, therefore, no longer true to say that the electroretinogram and the electro-oculogram are normal in patients with macula degeneration, but the difficulty still remains that a physically minute lesion can cause a serious disturbance of vision where macula disease is concerned. Thus, one would expect to find relatively minor changes in the electrical responses even with severe impairment of visual acuity. The foveal electroretinogram is a promising technique but its value is limited when opacities in the media scatter the stimulus light; the use of averaging techniques and a weak stimulus may be more helpful in these cases. The visually evoked potential may be of some help in monitoring the progressive natures of these conditions. Figure 12–11 shows the VEP obtained from a child with a lesion at one macula with a doubtful history of contusion injury. In this particular patient the history of injury was probably irrelevant because there was a family history of macula disease, the child's brother being affected. The VEP shows specific changes that are repeatable from month to month.

Acquired Retinal Disease

Diabetes

It has been known for many years that the classic waves of the electroretinogram are not affected until a late stage in diabetic retinopathy, and even then, the reduction in amplitude does not show any features that might be specific for diabetes. However, a renewed interest in the subject was created by Yonemura and Kawasaki, and others, who described the selective disappearance of the oscillatory potential. Similar changes were also described in some other circulatory disturbances of the retina. A recent report involving a large series of eyes has shown beyond doubt that this component of the electroretinogram may be absent; furthermore, there is no doubt that early changes are seen in diabetic retinopathy. The exact point in the development of the retinopathy at which the wavelets are affected differs markedly in different series but this is probably owing to differences in the type of stimulus used.

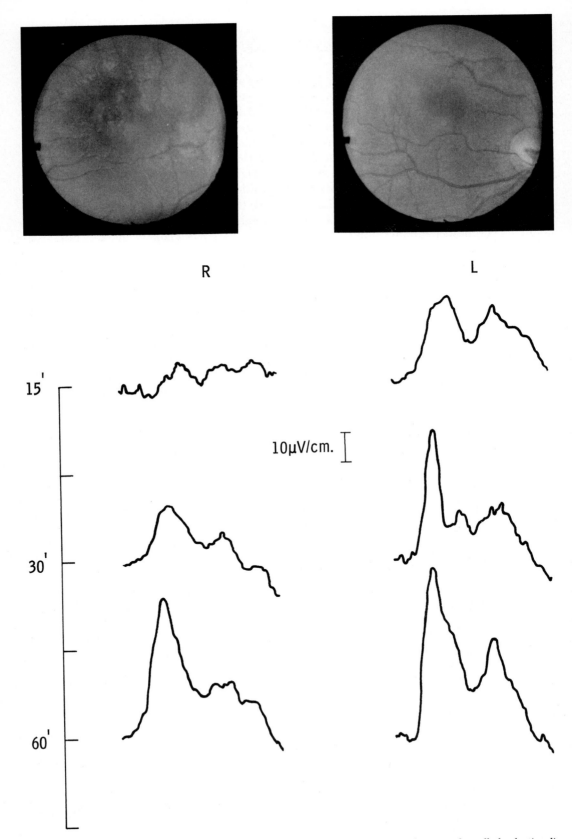

R   L

15′

10μV/cm.

30′

60′

Fig. 12–11. VEP from a patient with a right-sided macula hole. The response to large- and small-check stimuli can be seen. Note the impaired response to small checks in the affected eye.

It appears, therefore, that selective loss of the oscillatory potential is a feature of diabetic retinopathy (Fig. 12–12), but of course, this is often accompanied by a reduction in the size of the 'b' wave and the 'a' wave. In advanced diabetic retinopathy, a small 'b' wave alone may persist. Now that vitreous surgery has become better developed, it is often important to assess the function of the retina in advanced cases. The electroretinogram must be interpreted with great care under such circumstances because sometimes a small island of healthy retina may remain at the posterior pole and yet the electroretinogram may be poor. A very small 'b' wave is therefore not a contraindication to vitreous surgery, but a well-developed response would suggest a good prognosis. Changes in the VEP in diabetic cerebrovascular disease so far have not been accurately assessed.

Occlusive Vascular Disease

From the early days of clinical electroretinography an interest has been shown in the effect of retinal vascular disease on the electrical response. We have already seen that striking changes can be elicited in patients with diabetic retinopathy and it is now proposed to review the electroretinographic changes that may be seen in other types of vascular disease of the retina.

Occlusion of Central Retinal Artery. The retina may be regarded as having a double blood supply: the inner half being supplied by the central retinal artery and the outer half being nourished from the choroidal circulation. Obstruction of the circulation of the central retinal artery might, therefore, be expected to affect that part of the response derived from the inner half of the retina and spare the components of the electroretinogram that originate from the receptors and the pigment epithelium.

The two characteristic features of the electroretinogram in central artery occlusion are (1) loss of the oscillatory potential and (2) a "negative" type of electroretin-

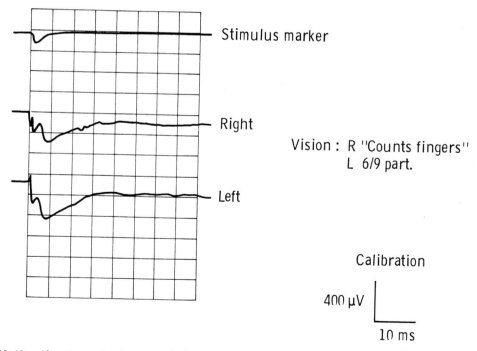

Stimulus marker

Right

Vision : R "Counts fingers"
L 6/9 part.

Left

Calibration

400 µV

10 ms

Fig. 12–12. Absent wavelets in a case of advanced diabetic retinopathy. Notice how the ERG does not reflect macula function but indicates diffuse disease in the retina.

ogram with enlargment of the 'a' wave and no change or slight diminution of the 'b' wave.

In general, the more severe types of occlusive episode, those with a poor prognosis, show a marked reduction in the size of the 'b' wave, whereas the milder types of occlusion may show a "negative" response. In branch artery occlusions, the electroretinogram may be normal or minimally affected. When the oscillatory potential is examined, a reduction in amplitude or abolition of it may be seen even in branch artery occlusions. It has been claimed that the wavelets give a good indication of the prognosis in any given case.

Occlusion of the Central Retinal Vein. The findings are similar to those in central retinal artery occlusion, the most common change being a subnormal negative response and diminution of the oscillatory potential. The changes, however, are milder than in arterial occlusion.

Sometimes, patients are referred to the electrodiagnostic clinic with unexplained field defects and systemic hypertension. The electroretinogram can help to decide whether these defects are caused by retinal ischemia or proximal changes in the optic nerve.

Disease of the Optic Nerve Head

For many years, it has been generally accepted and confirmed that damage to the optic nerve does not affect the electrical response from the retina. Histologic evidence also confirms this in that the part of the retina that is thought to give rise to the response is not damaged with optic atrophy. This fact creates a serious pitfall in the interpretation of electroretinogram traces; any eye may be completely blind from glaucoma and yet show a normal electroretinogram. In fact, minor changes in the photopic components of the electroretinogram have been described in chronic glaucoma, but these are slight. The visually evoked response may well prove to be an important supplementary test in these

cases. It has been shown that in cases of traumatic optic atrophy, the visually evoked response shows changes in proportion to the amount of visual loss, whereas the electroretinogram remains normal. The electroretinogram has also been reported as normal in patients with congenital unilateral hypoplasia of the optic nerve. The fact that some patients with optic nerve atrophy seem to have a supernormal response has excited some interest and there are several authentic reports of the phenomenon. It has been suggested that the increase in amplitude of the electroretinogram may be caused by the division of centrifugal fibers in the optic nerve; these fibers may normally have an inhibitory influence on the size of the response.

In general, any changes that are seen in the electroretinogram appear to be minimal and the visually evoked response provides a more valid clinical test.

VEP in Retrobulbar Neuritis

A high incidence of abnormal patterned VEPs in patients suffering from retrobulbar neuritis was described by Halliday, McDonald, and Mushin. This in itself would not have been of clinical interest were it not for the fact that more subtle changes in the VEP could be seen to persist long after the clinical signs of optic neuritis had subsided. A test of previously healed optic neuritis is of more value to the clinician than a test of active disease, which is already detectable by routine clinical methods. Therefore, it was of special interest when Halliday and several others showed that the latency of the major peaks in the transient VEP to pattern reversal is increased and may remain increased for several years following an acute attack. This delay in the response is best shown by comparing the response from the two eyes. During an acute attack of retrobulbar neuritis, when the visual acuity is severely impaired, the VEP is severely affected. In some cases, the response from the affected eye is abolished altogether. As the vision recovers, the amplitude of the VEP returns toward its normal value, but a characteristic slight delay in the response remains. It has also been shown that a surprisingly large number of patients with multiple sclerosis who have supposedly normal eyes give abnormal results when the VEP is checked. This delay in the response is not, of course, specifically seen in demyelinating disease; other possible causes of an altered response such as amblyopia or macula disease must be excluded. Other evoked responses have also been investigated in multiple sclerosis and measurement of a variety of evoked responses can provide diagnostic evidence in suspected cases. The VEP recorded from a patient with acute retrobular neuritis is shown in Figure 12–13. It can be seen that the response from the right side is greatly impaired.

The VEP recorded from the same patient 4 months later is also seen, and although the response from the right eye has apparently recovered, careful inspection shows a delay in the latency of all the major components. It is this slight change that enables the electrodiagnostician to say whether a patient has suffered from retrobular neuritis in the past, and the change may persist after other clinical evidence of the attack has disappeared.

VEP in Tobacco Amblyopia

The amplitude of the VEP is sensitive to changes in visual acuity during an acute attack of optic neuritis, in which the response may be abolished altogether. Similar findings have been recorded in patients with tobacco amblyopia, in whom it is possible to monitor the recovery by measuring the VEP at intervals when the patient has abstained from tobacco. In some of these patients, the normal positive peak at about 100 msec may be inverted.

VEP in Chronic Glaucoma

Successful attempts have already been made to relate VEP changes to visual field defects. A purely objective test for field changes in glaucoma could prove useful when the question of glaucoma surgery may depend on an increase in field loss. Clear-cut alterations in phase and amplitude have been demonstrated in patients with glaucomatous field defects. This was achieved by examining steady-state visually evoked responses to pattern-reversal stimulation of retinal areas corresponding to discrete field quadrants.

One of the problems in using the VEP to monitor chronic simple glaucoma or to detect early disease is the fact that the VEP only measures a small central area of the visual field. For this reason, patients with advanced chronic glaucoma may have a normal VEP (Fig. 12–14). In fact, the VEP is likely to be more useful in monitoring cases in which a change in response is sought over a period of months, than in detecting early cases. This is because the changes in the VEP are rather unpredictable; sometimes a severe case of glaucoma has few changes, and sometimes a fairly mild case may show more marked changes that do not always seem to comply with the type of field defect. The results, however, should remain the same over a period of a few months, providing that the glaucoma has not advanced (Fig. 12–15).

VEP and Other Diseases of the Optic Nerve

The VEP has been measured in Tay-Sachs disease: an absent VEP and a normal ERG are the usual findings. This is the result that one might expect from a lesion at the level of the retinal ganglion cells, which involve central vision.

It is possible to monitor the function of the optic nerve by means of the VEP, and this technique has been practiced in orbital surgery. Permanent loss of vision following surgery is a recognized risk, particularly when hypotensive anesthesia is being used. Wright, et al. have described a method of monitoring the function of the optic nerve that entails continuously stim-

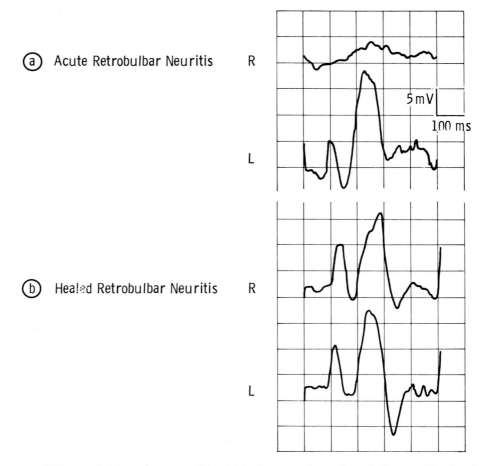

Fig. 12–13. VEP recorded from the same subject (a) in the acute phase of retrobulbar neuritis, showing the greatly diminished response on stimulation of the right eye, and (b) 4 months later, showing that although the response has recovered there is still a slight difference in latency between the main components from each eye.

ulating the retina with an unstructured stimulus and recording the VEP throughout the operation.

It can be seen that a knowledge of the electrodiagnostic changes in diseases of the optic nerve is essential when interpreting these responses in general. A surgeon who is encouraged to remove a cataract on the grounds of a normal electroretinogram alone may be unpleasantly surprised at the poor visual result if he has been led astray by an inadequate report.

Effect of Toxicity

A considerable amount of information is now available about the effect of various drugs on the electrical responses from the eye. These data have been provided both by animal experiments and by the results of over-dosage or accidental ingestion in human subjects. Electrodiagnostic tests have been applied in such circumstances to find out more about the nature and origin of the response and, in some cases, to help make a diagnosis. These techniques are also being used in an attempt to localize the site of action of drugs in the eye. Undoubtedly, the nature of these electrical changes is such that they can carry useful objective clinical information, but our knowledge is still limited and much of the

RIGHT EYE

Upper ½ response   Lower ½ response

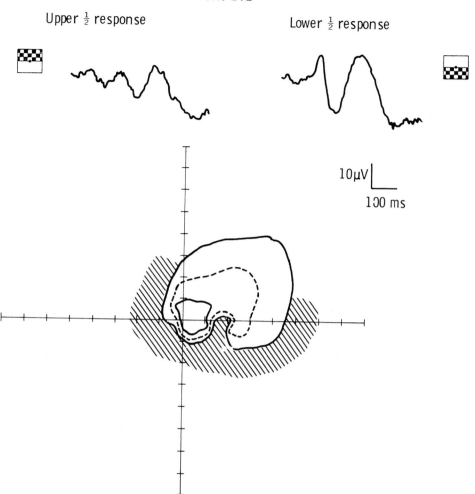

10μV

100 ms

Fig. 12–14. The VEP in a case of advanced chronic simple glaucoma. A checkerboard stimulus has been applied to upper and lower half-fields separately. The response is within normal limits in spite of the field loss. The response from the upper half-field normally shows a reduced amplitude.

work so far has concerned the electroretinogram rather than the visually evoked potential.

For many years, much interest has been centered on drugs used to produce selective damage to different layers of the retina. Sodium iodate, for example, causes selective damage to the pigment epithelium and abolishes the 'c' wave in rabbits. Another substance that has been used for localization studies is sodium glutamate. This causes loss of vision in mice and se-

lective loss of the inner layers of the retina with destruction of the bipolars and ganglion cells. Several drugs have been used to assess the site of origin of the electroretinogram. Table 12–1 shows the effect of some drugs on the electroretinogram.

Antimalarials

Quinine. Although the toxic effects of quinine have been well recognized for many years, there still exists a controversy

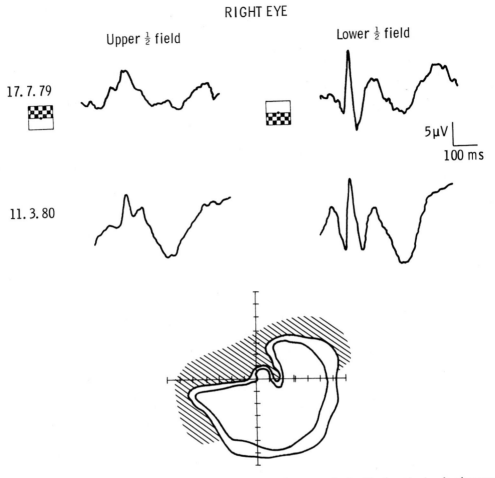

Fig. 12–15. The traces recorded on two separate occasions from a patient with chronic simple glaucoma to show the degree of consistency that can be obtained by the method. The visual field was also unchanged.

Table 12–1. Effect of some drugs on the Electroretinogram

Drug	Effect on Electroretinogram	Author
Ethyl alcohol	'b' wave increase	Manfredini and Trimarchi (1968)
Amyl acetate	Progressive reduction of 'a' and 'b' waves but return to normal after 45 days	Gorgone, et al. (1970)
Dichlorphenamide	55% increase in 'b' wave	Tota and Cavallacci (1970)
Carbon disulfide	Rapid and irreversible extinction of 'a' and 'b' waves	Malfitano, et al. (1972)
Triamterene	'b' wave incresed by 40% in rabbits	Tota and Cavallacci (1971)
Strychnine	'b' wave increased, but lowered in higher concentrations in rabbit	Vorkel and Hanitzsch (1971)

as to the exact mode of action of this poison; electrodiagnostic tests help to throw some light on the problem. An overdose of quinine is usually taken in an attempt to procure an abortion, but cases have been reported in which an overdose was ingested as a prophylactic for malaria. Symptoms may follow after taking as little as 1 g in sensitive individuals, but the usual dose to cause blindness is put at 1.5 to 4 g. The affected patient experiences deafness, tinnitus, and visual failure, and larger doses produce coma. The fundus appearance may be normal at first; but in some cases, there is retinal edema with a cherry red spot at the macula. The visual fields become grossly constricted. The symptoms and signs often improve over a period of weeks, and the fundus then begins to show optic atrophy and narrowing of the retinal arteries. For many years, arguments have been put forward to decide whether the toxic effect of quinine is primarily on the retinal vessels or whether it acts directly on the retina. The question of vascular spasm is not easy to answer because we know that almost any condition that causes optic atrophy also causes constriction of the retinal vessels. Investigation of the effect of acute poisoning in animals has shown that the electroretinogram is initially depressed but recovers in a matter of hours. After this, a further slow deterioration in the response occurs, but the relatively slight degree of these changes compared with the severe visual loss indicates primary damage to the ganglion cells and nerve fiber layer. In humans, the electroretinogram may show a gradual decline between 10 days and 10 months after intoxication; paradoxically, the vision may gradually improve during this period. The electro-oculogram has shown an absent light-rise during the first few days after intoxication, and this has then recovered parallel with the subjective improvements. The absence of a light rise on the electro-oculogram is not easy to explain in terms of a ganglion cell poison and more cases will have to be investigated in detail in the future in order to find the true answer to this conflicting evidence. The matter takes on more clinical importance when we consider that disseminated sclerosis can present in a young girl in a similar manner; the fundus in bilateral optic neuritis may be completely normal, then gradually vision recovers in association with optic atrophy and narrowing of the retinal vessels.

Chloroquine (Resochin). Chloroquine was used extensively but in small doses in World War II as a prophylactic treatment for malaria. Corneal changes resulting from this drug were described at the end of the war, but the more serious retinotoxic effects were not observed until large doses were employed in the treatment of disseminated lupus erythematosus and rheumatoid arthritis. Its value in the treatment of disseminated lupus erythematosus was described in 1954, and the first case of chloroquine retinopathy was described in 1957. Since then, reports from many different centers have confirmed that when the total annual dose of chloroquine exceeds 100 g there is a serious risk of visual disturbance with associated changes in the fundus. The earliest sign is a perimacula pigmentary disturbance described as a "bull's eye appearance." In more advanced cases, the arteries become attenuated and peripheral pigmentation may appear. By the time fundus changes appear, irreversible field defects can be detected and, in some cases, a progressive deterioration of vision occurs in spite of cessation of treatment. Histopathologic investigation of human eyes and animal experiments have shown that chloroquine accumulates in and damages the receptor layer and the pigment epithelium, thus confirming the cumulative nature of the toxicity.

Electroretinographic studies have shown a depression of the 'b' wave amplitude in patients who had had treatment for more than a year, but in some series the electroretinogram was normal in the presence of fundus changes. It does appear that the electroretinogram may be of some prognostic value in these cases. This has been shown in a long-term follow-up study of 15 cases of chloroquine poisoning. The changes in the electro-oculogram were first described by Arden and Kelsey in 1962. In a detailed study, Kolb showed that depression of the light rise of the electro-oculogram is often an early sign of toxicity, which may sometimes precede the fundus changes, but in a series of 47 cases there was considerable overlap between treated and control groups. Furthermore, it was shown that in a group of patients who had not received treatment but who suffered from collagen disease, the mean value of the Arden Index was below normal, but not so low as in the group that had been treated with chloroquine. A study of patients in whom the drug therapy had been stopped revealed a return to normal of the Arden Index in many cases.

Both chloroquine and hydroxychloroquine (Plaquenil) produce the same toxic effects, but the toxic and the normal dosage of hydroxychloroquine is much larger. The evidence now indicates clearly that these drugs should not be used if at all possible and if they are used the patients should be carefully monitored if the dose exceeds 100 g chloroquine base in any 1 year. If the electro-oculogram is depressed, the drug should be stopped even if there are no subjective signs of toxicity. Unfortunately, there is no doubt that some patients may develop severe toxicity although retaining a normal electro-oculogram. Figure 12–16 shows the results obtained from a patient receiving chloroquine. The patient had complained of the appearance of a dark "blob" in front of her vision and was advised to stop using the drug on the strength of the electrodiagnostic findings.

In spite of its obvious hazards, chloroquine is still being prescribed, but the ocular damage can be avoided if the toxic dose is not exceeded. Recently, it has been found useful in short courses for the treatment of pulmonary sarcoidosis, and ophthalmologists must be continually on their guard for the appearance of side effects.

Effect of Opacities in the Media

The response to a patterned stimulus is, of course, severely affected by the presence of even slight opacities in the media, depending on how greatly they affect the visual acuity, but in response to a flash, either a VEP or an ERG can still be obtained, even when dense opacities are present. Indeed, providing the stimulus is bright enough and the retina is normal, there is virtually no opacity that can prevent a response from occurring. This means that the ERG and flash VEP can be used to assess retinal and cortical function when the fundus of the eye is not visible with the ophthalmoscope; for example, a normal ERG may be obtained using the bright flash stimulus through a dense vitreous hemorrhage. This can be of help when assessing retinal function in patients with diabetic retinopathy. Similarly, some ideas of general retinal function may be needed before removing a dense cataract, and once again, a normal ERG and flash VEP may be helpful. One must remember that the ERG by itself is simply a measure of diffuse retinal function; small areas of the retina may be damaged and not impair the ERG. This means that there may still be macular degeneration, and in this respect, the ERG cannot foretell the outcome of cataract surgery. The VEP has been shown more recently to be an accurate predictor of visual outcome, and it is clear that the VEP and ERG should always be used together when assessing opacities in the media. Under these circumstances, the ERG can be used to indicate whether widespread retinal disease is present or whether the retina is severely ischemic, whereas the VEP can indicate something about the function of the macular area. There are certain special instances in which electrodiagnostic tests can be of value in the presence of opaque media; in particular, vitreous hemorrhage

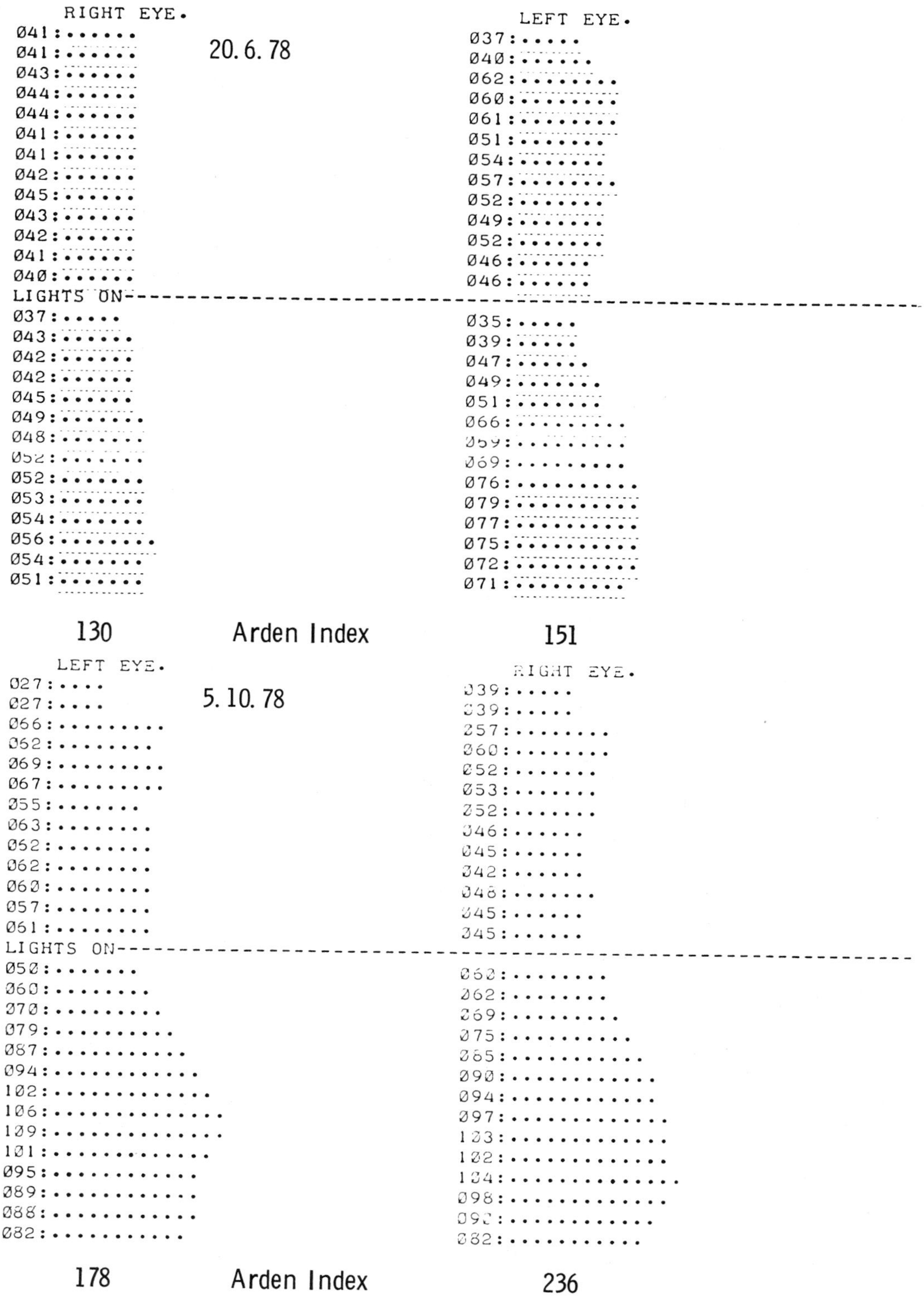

RIGHT EYE.   LEFT EYE.

041:. . . . . .   20. 6. 78   037:. . . . .
041:. . . . . .   040:. . . . . .
043:. . . . . .   062:. . . . .
044:. . . . . .   060:. . . . . . .
044:. . . . . .   061:. . . . .
041:. . . . . .   051:. . . . . . .
041:. . . . . .   054:. . . . . .
042:. . . . . .   057:. . . . . . .
045:. . . . . .   052:. . . . . .
043:. . . . . .   049:. . . . . .
042:. . . . . .   052:. . . . . .
041:. . . . . .   046:. . . . . . .
040:. . . . . .   046:. . . . . .
LIGHTS ON--
037:. . . . .   035:. . . . .
043:. . . . . .   039:. . . . .
042:. . . . . .   047:. . . . . .
042:. . . . . .   049:. . . . . . .
045:. . . . . .   051:. . . . . . .
049:. . . . . . .   066:. . . . .
048:. . . . . . .   059:. . . . .
052:. . . . . . .   069:. . . . .
052:. . . . . . .   076:. . . . .
053:. . . . . . .   079:. . . . .
054:. . . . . . .   077:. . . . .
056:. . . . .   075:. . . . .
054:. . . . . .   072:. . . . .
051:. . . . . . .   071:. . . . .

           130   Arden Index   151

LEFT EYE.   RIGHT EYE.
027:. . . .   5. 10. 78   039:. . . . .
027:. . . .   039:. . . . .
066:. . . . .   057:. . . . .
062:. . . . .   060:. . . . .
069:. . . . .   052:. . . . . . .
067:. . . . .   053:. . . . . . .
055:. . . . . . .   052:. . . . . . .
063:. . . . . . .   046:. . . . . .
052:. . . . . . .   045:. . . . . .
062:. . . . . . .   042:. . . . . .
060:. . . . . . .   048:. . . . . .
057:. . . . . . .   045:. . . . . .
061:. . . . . . .   045:. . . . . .
LIGHTS ON--
050:. . . . . . .   062:. . . . .
060:. . . . . . .   062:. . . . . . .
070:. . . . .   069:. . . . .
079:. . . . .   075:. . . . .
087:. . . . .   085:. . . . .
094:. . . . .   090:. . . . .
102:. . . . .   094:. . . . .
106:. . . . .   097:. . . . .
109:. . . . .   103:. . . . .
101:. . . . .   102:. . . . .
095:. . . . .   104:. . . . .
089:. . . . .   098:. . . . .
088:. . . . .   090:. . . . .
082:. . . . .   082:. . . . .

           178   Arden Index   236

Fig. 12–16. Electro-oculogram recorded from a patient who had taken chloroquine for 2 years and who complained of blurred vision but had no ophthalmoscopic or slit-lamp evidence of toxicity. The drug was stopped and 4 months later the EOG was within the normal range again.

following subarachnoid hemorrhage and head injury and also vitreous hemorrhage in which a retinal detachment is suspected. It is also extremely useful to determine whether the wavelets are present in a diabetic patient with dense cataracts.

Poor Sight with a Normal Optic Fundus

Several conditions in the eye or visual pathway may present to the ophthalmologist as poor vision with a normal fundus. Some of these have been mentioned already; in particular, retinitis pigmentosa in its early stages and the related condition Leber's amaurosis. In these cases, electroretinography may be diagnostic, and it is essential that this type of test be used. In the same way, patients with suspected healed retrobulbar neuritis require a measurement of their visually evoked potential as an effective means of confirming or denying the diagnosis.

Perhaps the most common condition in which the vision is impaired and the function is normal is amblyopia of disuse. Over the past 2 or 3 years, considerable interest has been centered on this condition. In elderly patients, the presence of a cerebrovascular lesion in a normal fundus may be confirmed by measuring the visually evoked potential. Also, the possibility of malingering or hysteria may be further elucidated by these tests.

Amblyopia of Disuse

The reduction of visual acuity that can be seen in association with squint or anisometropia with no visible abnormality in the retina would seem to be an ideal subject for VEP studies, especially if we assume that the VEP arises in the primary visual cortex. VEP studies might be expected to tell us something about the site of the defect in amblyopia. In general, the pattern VEP recorded by stimulating the affected eye shows a reduction in amplitude; this is in contrast to the electroretinogram as routinely recorded and the flash VEP, which are usually normal. At present it is

not possible to distinguish between the different types of amblyopia of disuse using the VEP, but some interesting facts are emerging. For example, a "binocular negative" effect has been described in which the binocular VEP is smaller than the VEP recorded from each eye individually. In normal subjects, the binocular VEP is usually larger than the response from the individual eyes and can be seen to represent the sum of the waveform of the two. This binocular negative effect would appear to represent some form of suppression, and it is found more frequently in strabismic amblyopia. Attempts to correlate the VEP with some of the psychophysical findings in amblyopia seem to indicate defects both peripheral to and "above" the primary visual cortex. In the normal eye, the VEP shows a maximum amplitude with 15-minute checks; the response is smaller when the stimulus is composed of either larger or smaller checks. In one careful study of an adult amblyope, the affected eye showed a maximum amplitude for the amblyopic eye with the 60-minute check stimulus, and there was a significantly larger signal for the 60-minute check from the amblyopic eye than from the normal eye. Furthermore, when a small-field 3° stimulus was used, there was no difference in amplitude between the normal and amblyopic eyes. It has been suggested that in the amblyope, the normal central 3° area is unable to exert sufficient lateral inhibitory effect on the surrounding retina and that the well-recognized increase in visual acuity with separate letter testing that is found with some amblyopes may be owing to the fact that they are looking at each letter in a manner equivalent to a small-field pattern stimulus.

A different light has been thrown on the study of this type of amblyopia by the examination of subjects with high degrees of astigmatism. It is known that the resolving power of the human visual system is better in the vertical and horizontal orientation than in the two oblique orientations. The same effect can be seen in the VEP. When astigmatic subjects are examined, a high proportion show a reduction in the amplitude of the VEP when a grating stimulus is oriented in the meridian with the lower refractive error. This impairment of the VEP occurs with full spectacle correction.

When a child with amblyopia is treated by occluding the sound eye, then interesting changes can be observed in the VEP as the vision of the weaker eye improves. These changes differ according to the check size of the patterned stimulus that is being applied. Figure 12–17 shows the improvement that occurs in the response. The VEP, therefore, provides the only objective way of measuring the results of treatment of amblyopia, and as such, it is likely to have some considerable importance in the future. It is well recognized that visual acuity measurements by themselves can occasionally be misleading.

Hemianopia

Sometimes, the ophthalmic surgeon may be puzzled by an apparent reduction in visual acuity and subsequently finds it is caused by a homonymous hemianopia. In the very young and the very old these defects may not be easy to pick up and so it is of special interest to consider some of the recently described VEP findings. The use of an unstructured flash stimulus together with laterally placed electrodes can give asymmetric responses from the two sides in hemianopic patients, but by and large such results have not proved reliable. The use of a patterned hemifield stimulus seems to be more promising. It has been shown that a hemifield pattern reversal stimulus produces a *larger* response from the electrodes placed over the ipsilateral hemisphere than over the contralateral hemisphere. A full-field pattern stimulus tends to produce the summed effect of the two half-field responses.

Full-field and hemifield stimulation of patients with homonymous and bitemporal hemianopias gives predictable results, using this technique. The exact position of the electrodes and the specifications of the stimulus appear to be important.

The rather surprising finding that a larger response is found over the inert hemisphere has been confirmed in a patient who had undergone an occipital lobectomy, which suggests that the electrical changes must be projected from the active side directly to the scalp rather than through the corpus callosum (Fig. 12–18).

The paradoxic response that seems larger when recording is made over the diseased side of the brain occurs only if the stimulus is flashed at a fairly high speed. If lower frequencies of stimulation are used with a pattern onset and the so-called transient response is examined, the response behaves predictably by being larger over the intact hemisphere and smaller over the diseased side; that is to say, using a low-frequency pattern-onset stimulus, we find a reduced response over the right occiput in a patient with a left homonymous hemianopia.

Cortical Blindness

We have seen that unilateral damage to the occipital cortex can cause unilateral impairment of the VEP. One might logically conclude that total loss of the occipital cortex and occipital blindness would always be associated with absence of any VEP. Unfortunately, the results from the limited number of published cases have been conflicting. VEPs have been recorded from patients with apparently complete cortical blindness; but in other cases, the VEP has been abolished. Cortical blindness must be carefully defined for this kind of study. The patient should have no perception of light and no blink reflex to a flashing light. The eyes themselves are normal as is the electroretinogram and the pupils also react normally both directly and consensually.

It is difficult to imagine how an electrical response can arise in a defunct part of the brain; but before revising our idea about

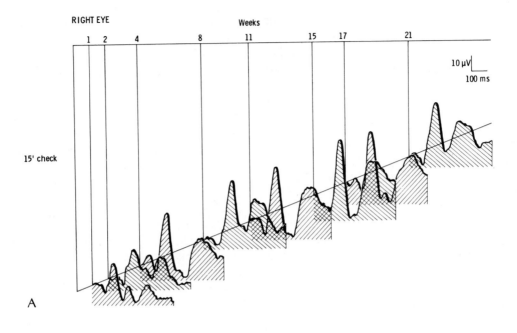

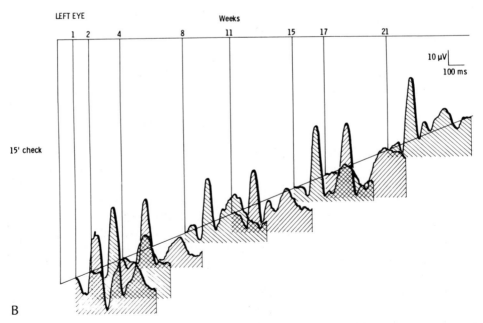

Fig. 12–17.   A. The serial recordings of the VEP produced by stimulating the right amblyopic eye during a period of left occlusion. Note the increase in size of the response with the passage of weeks. **B.** The response from the left (occluded) eye during treatment of amblyopia in the same child. Little change is seen other than a possible fall in the size of the response after 4 weeks.

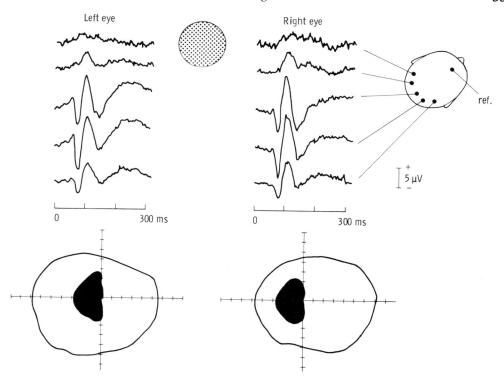

Fig. 12–18. Pattern reversal stimulation after subtotal occipital lobectomy. Note larger response from damaged side. (After Blumhardt, Barrett, and Halliday, *Br. J. Ophthalmol.* *61*:454, 1977.)

the origin of the VEP, it might be wiser to review a larger store of clinical data when it becomes available. Some patients with extensive cortical damage can be left with a very small area of central field. Such patients are behaviorally blind, being unable to walk about without knocking into furniture and being unable to read the Snellen test chart unless some time is spent locating it. Once the test chart has been found, they may have a surprisingly high level of visual acuity. The VEP in these cases should be tested, and no doubt the result of such tests will have clinical relevance in the future. We know that the stimulation of relatively small areas of the central field can produce a VEP, especially when a patterned stimulus is used.

Hysterical Blindness

Although in practice one might expect the VEP and the ERG to be ideal objective tests for the diagnosis of hysteria or malingering, in fact, such patients often refuse to cooperate during the tests, perhaps because they suspect that the results of the test will lose them the sympathy they so much require. In theory, of course, one would expect the results to be entirely normal both for the ERG and the VEP. In fact, one must remember that some patients have very small responses and yet are still within the normal range. This particularly applies to the VEP. It is essential in these cases that the VEP be measured to different sizes of pattern stimulus so that a clear-cut change can be noted, especially the increase in size of the second positive peak with smaller checks. Figure 12–19 shows the effect of altering the check size that one might expect to see in a normal subject.

Summary

The reader should now be aware that electrodiagnosis has something to offer the

Check size   V.E.R.

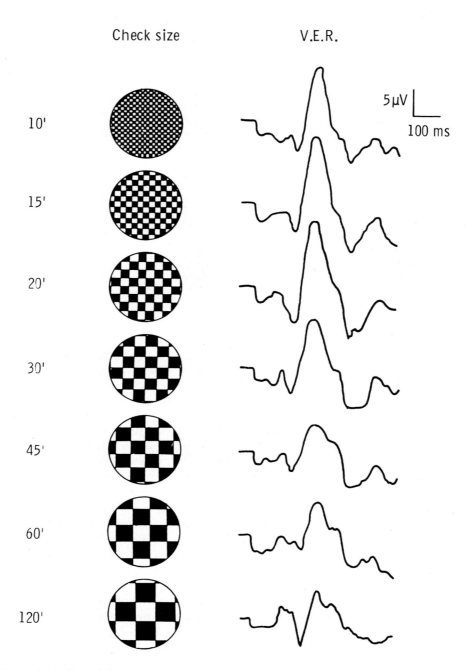

5 μV

100 ms

10'

15'

20'

30'

45'

60'

120'

Fig. 12–19. The effect of changing the stimulus check size on the VEP in a normal subject. Note especially the increase in size of the later positive peak with smaller checks.

neuro-ophthalmologist. The main advantage of this type of test is that it is purely objective and no one can argue about the result, providing that it is being accurately recorded. Better and more accurate recording methods are now available, and perhaps more importantly, they are becoming more portable. Both the VEP and the ERG, tend to show considerable inter-subject variation, but in a given subject the results are highly consistent when repeated from month to month. This makes the tests particularly useful for monitoring disease and for deciding whether treatment is being effective. The ERG is particularly sensitive in detecting diffuse retinal disease, and for this reason, it is used to help achieve a diagnosis in patients with early retinitis pigmentosa and especially in children with Leber's amaurosis. The VEP has a special value in detecting healed optic neuritis when the diagnosis of disseminated sclerosis is suspected, but it can also be used when an objective measure of visual acuity is needed, and perhaps its most interesting use in recent years is the monitoring of the treatment of amblyopia of disuse.

BIBLIOGRAPHY

Adrian, E.D.: The electric response of the human eye. J. Physiol. *104*:84, 1945.

Algvere, P.: Studies on the oscillatory potential of the clinical electroretinogram. Acta Ophthalmologica (København) (Suppl.) *96*:1, 1968.

Arden, G.B., and Kelsey, J.H.: Changes produced by light in the standing potential of the human eye. J. Physiol. *161*:189, 1962.

Armington, J.C.: The Electroretinogram. New York, Academic Press, 1974.

Barber, C. (ed.): Evoked Potentials. Lancaster, England, M.T.P. Press Ltd., 1980.

Berson, E.L.: Hereditary retinal diseases: classification with full field electroretinogram. Documenta ophthalmologica (Proceedings series) *13*:149, 1977.

Blumhardt, L.D., Barrett, G., and Halliday, A.M.: The asymmetrical visual evoked potential to pattern reversal in one half field and its significance for the analysis of visual field defects. Br. J. Ophthalmol. *61*:454, 1977.

Bodis Wollner, I.: Recovery from cerebral blindness: evoked potential and psychophysical measurements. Electroencephalogr. Clin. Neurophysiol. *42*:178, 1977.

Brown, K.T.: The electroretinogram, its components and their origins. *In*: The Retina. Morphology Function and Clinical Characteristics. Edited by R. Alba, F. Crescitelli, M. Hull, B. Straatsma. Los Angeles, University of California Press. 1969.

Brown, K.T., and Murakami, M.: A new receptor potential of the monkey retina with no detectable latency. Nature *201*:626, 1964.

Carr, R.E., and Siegel, I.M.: Visual Electrodiagnostic Testing: A Practical Guide for the Clinician. Baltimore, Williams and Wilkins, 1982.

Ciganek, L.: The electroencephalogram response to light stimulus (evoked potential) in man. Electroencephalog. Clin. Neurophysiol. *13*:165, l961.

Cobb, W.A., and Morton, H.B.: A new component of the human electroretinogram. J. Physiol. *123*:36, 1954.

Desmedt, J.E. (ed.): Visual Evoked Potentials in Man: New Developments. Oxford, Clarendon Press, 1977.

Deutman, A.F.: The Hereditary Dystrophies of the Posterior Pole. Assen, The Netherlands, Van Gorcum, 1971.

Dewar, J., and McKendrick, J.G.: On the physiological action of light. Trans. R. Soc. Edinburgh *27*:141, 1873.

Dustman, R.E., and Beck, E.C.: The effect of maturation and ageing on the waveform of visually evoked potentials. Electroencephalogr. Clin. Neurophysiol. *26*:2, 1969.

Francois, J., De Rouck, A., Cambiée et Zanen, A.: L'Électrodiagnostic des Affections Retiniennes. Paris, Masson et Cie, 1974.

Francois, J., Verriest, G., and De Rouck, A.: Modification of the amplitude of the human electro oculogram by light and dark adaptation. Br. J. Ophthalmol. *39*:398, 1955.

Galloway, N.R.: Ophthalmic Electrodiagnosis, 2nd Ed. London, Lloyd Luke, 1981.

Gorgone, G., Inserra, A., Barlotta, F., and Malfitano, D.: Electroretinogram in experimental intoxication with amyl acetate. Ann. Ottalmol. Clin. Oculista *96*:313, 1970.

Granit, R.: Sensory Mechanisms of the Retina. London, Oxford University Press, 1947.

Halliday, A.M.: Evoked Potentials in Clinical Testing. Edinburgh, Churchill Livingstone, 1982.

Halliday, A.M., McDonald, W.I., and Mushin, J.: Delayed visual evoked response in optic neuritis. Lancet *1*:982, 1972.

Harding, G.F.A., and Crews, S.J.: The VER in hereditary optic atrophy of the dominant type. *In*: Clinical Applications of Evoked Potentials in Neurology. Edited by, J. Courjon, F. Manguiere, and M. Revol. New York, Raven Press, 1982.

Harter, M.R., and White, C.T.: Evoked cortical responses to checkerboard patterns; effect of check size as a function of visual acuity. Electroencephalogr. Clin. Neurophysiol. *28*:48, 1969.

Harter, M.R., Deaton, F., and Vernon Odom, J.: Maturation of evoked potential and visual preference in 6-45 day old infants: effect of check size on visual acuity and refractive error. Electroencephalogr. Clin. Neurophysiol. *42*:595, 1977.

Holmgren, F.: Method att objectivera effecten av ljusintryck pa retina. Upsale Lackare foerenings Foerhandlingar *1*:177,. 1865.

Huber, C.: Pattern-evoked cortical potentials and automated perimetry in chronic glaucoma. *In*: Visual Pathways: Electrophysiology and Pathology. Edited by H. Spekreijse, and P. Apkarian. Documenta ophthalmologica (Proceedings Series) *27*:87, 1981.

Itzhak, C., Haimovic, I.C. and Pedley, T.A.: Hemifield pattern reversal visual evoked potentials. Electroencephalogr. Clin. Neurophysiol. *54*:121, 1982.

Jeffreys, D.A.: The physiological significance of pattern visual evoked potentials. *In* Visual Evoked Potentials in Man: New Developments. Edited by J.E. Dismedt. Oxford, Clarendon Press, 1977.

Karpe, G.: The basis of clinical electroretinography. Acta Ophthalmologica (København) Suppl. *24*, 1945.

Kolb, H.: Electro-oculogram findings in patients treated with antimalarial drugs. Br. J. Ophthalmol. *49*:573, 1965.

Krill, A.E.: Retinitis pigmentosa. A review. Sight Saving Review *42*:21, 1972.

Kubota, Y., Kubota, S., and Asanigi, K.: The ERG of chloroquine in clinical retinopathy. Documenta Ophthalmologica (Proceedings Series) *15*:95, 1978.

Landers, M.B., Wolbarsht, M.L., Dowling, J.E., and Laties, A.M. (eds.): Retinitis Pigmentosa: clinical implications of current research. *In* Advances in Experimental Medicine and Biology. New York, Plenum Press, 1977.

Lesevre, N., and Remond, A.: Potentials evoked by patterns: effect of pattern dimensions and contrast density. Electroencephalogr. Clin. Neurophysiol. *32*:593, 1972.

Maitland, C.G., Aminoff, M.J., Kennard, C., and Hoyt, W.F.: Evoked potentials in the evaluation of visual field defects due to chiasmal or retrochiasmal lesions. Neurology (N.Y.) *32*:986, 1982.

Malfitano, D., Barlotta, F., Inserra, A., and Gorgone, G.: Electroretinographic findings following experimental poisoning with carbon disulfide. Boll. Soc. Ital. Biol. Sper. *48*:113, 1972.

Manfredini, U., and Trimarchi, F.: L'azione dell'alcool etilico sull' electroretinogramma. Ann. Ottalmol. Clin. Oculista *94*:155, 1968.

Miller, R.F., and Dowling, J.E.: Intracellular responses of the Müller (glial) cells of mudpuppy retina: their relations to the b-wave of the electroretinogram. J. Neurophysiol. *33*:323, 1970.

Regan, D.: Evoked Potentials. London, Chapman and Hall, 1972.

Riggs, L.A.: Continuous and reproducible records of the electrical activity of the human retina. Proc. Soc. Exp. Biol. Med. *48*:204, 1941.

Sokol, S.: Visual evoked potentials to checkerboard pattern stimuli in strabismic amblyopia. *In* Visual Evoked Potentials in Man: New Developments. Edited by J.E. Desmedt, Oxford, Clarendon Press, 1977.

Spekreijse, H., Van der Tweel, L.H., and Suidema, T.: Contrast evoked responses in man. Vision Res. *13*:1577, 1973.

Thomspon, C.R.S., and Harding, G.F.A.: The visual evoked response in patients with cataracts. Documenta Ophthalmologica (Proceedings Series) *15*:193, 1978.

Tota, G., and Cavallacci, G.: The electroretinogram after administration of triamterene. Ann. Ottalmol. Clin. Oculista *97*:143, 1971.

Tota, G., and Cavallacci, G.: Changes in the electroretinogram produced by dichlorphenamide. Ann. Ottalmol. Clin. Oculista *96*:303, 1970.

Van der Tweel, L.H., and Verduyn Lunel, H.F.E.: Human visual responses to sinusoidally modulated light. Electroencephalogr. Clin. Neurophysiol. *18*:587, 1965.

Van Lith, G., and Balik, J.: Variability of the electro oculogram. Acta Ophthalmologica (København) *48*:1091, 1970.

Vörkel, W., and Hanitzch, R.: Effect of strychnine on the electroretinogram of the isolated rabbit retina. Experimentia, *27*:296–297, 1971.

Wildeberge, H.G.H., Van Lith, G.H.M., Wijngaarde, R., and Mak, G.T.M.: Visually evoked cortical potentials in the evaluation of homonymous and bitemporal visual field defects. Br. J. Ophthalmol. *60*:273, 1976.

Wright, J., Arden, G, and Jones, B.R.: Continuous monitoring of the VER during surgery. Trans. Ophthalmol. Soc. U. K. *93*:311, 1973.

Yonemura, D., and Kawasaki, K.: Electrophysiological study on activities of neuronal and non-neuronal retinal elements in man with reference to its clinical application. Jpn. J. Ophthalmol. *22*:195, 1978.

Chapter *13*

Blurred Vision

THOMAS J. WALSH

Blurred vision (and distorted vision) is a common complaint that has an extremely broad differential diagnosis. The complaint as expressed by the patient usually does not suggest any one particular diagnosis. This chapter outlines some of the tests and techniques employed in evaluating blurred vision and also reviews the more common causes of the condition to help the physician come to a rapid and correct diagnosis.

Evaluation of blurred vision requires more than the Snellen chart examination. It involves also examination of color vision, testing of the visual fields and pupillary function, and detailed examination of the retina.

EVALUATION OF THE SYMPTOM

Testing of Visual Acuity

Visual acuity is evaluated primarily by the Snellen chart at 20 feet and by a standard near card at 14 inches. It is assumed that the patient is wearing the full distance correction and appropriate add if needed for near vision.

Up to the present, the rule by which we have judged normal acuity has been the Snellen chart; however, even some patients with 20/20 acuity will say there is a difference. It appears that patients are more sensitive to small defects in vision than our standard tests can detect. Recent studies in many laboratories have shown that these patients have abnormal contrast sensitivity tests despite normal visual acuity and fields. Microelectrode studies have demonstrated that certain groups of cells in the visual system respond to different spacial frequencies, just as Zeki showed that some cells were color coded. Tests to measure the sensitivity gradient have been designed but are not in widespread clinical use outside of experimental laboratories.

Pinhole Test. In those situations in which an immediate refraction is not possible, a careful check of the pinhole vision may provide a valuable diagnostic clue. Improvement of vision by several lines on the Snellen chart (even if vision is not fully corrected to 20/20) by a single or multiple pinhole test suggests that the decreased acuity is the result of a refractive error. The vision of patients with retinal or optic nerve disease usually remains the same or is made worse by pinhole vision. The refractive error, however, may represent disease of the cornea, such as a keratoconus with increased astigmatism, or disease of the lens with increased myopia.

If the patient has hemianopsia, he may

read only half the line of Snellen letters. Repetition of this error in many lines strongly suggests a hemianopic field defect.

Sometimes, visual defects can be inferred in patients who cannot read a Snellen chart. For example, if the eyes of an infant are covered one at a time, the infant may show extreme resistance to the cover over one eye but not to the cover over the other eye. Lack of resistance to the cover may suggest poor vision in that eye.

A visual complaint in which the near acuity and the distance acuity are vastly different suggests a functional rather than an organic problem. The near and the distance acuity should be within one or two Snellen lines of each other, when corrected.

Complaints of decreased acuity after strenuous exercise (such as several games of tennis) or after warm baths suggests Uhthoff's sign, a phenomenon that occurs in nerves that have a conduction defect and that may be caused by a demyelinating process.

Testing with a Neutral Density Filter. The use of a neutral density filter may help to differentiate childhood amblyopia from organic optic nerve disease. The Kodak filter 96 ND #2 is the one recommended. Place the filter in front of the normal eye; the decrease in acuity should not be more than two Snellen lines. If the decrease in acuity is caused by organic optic nerve disease, a marked decrease in vision occurs.

Testing of Color Vision

Retinal disease, even of a significant degree, usually does not cause a severe loss of color vision as shown on the HRR plates. Most people with macular degeneration with a visual acuity of 20/200 can see most of the color plates. A slight decrease in acuity (even 20/30) owing to optic nerve disease causes a severe loss in recognizing the HRR plates. Thus, when a decrease in vision is minimal and when identification of a central scotoma with small white test ob-

jects is difficult, use of the HRR plates may point out the difference between retinal and optic nerve disease. This approach is valid also for patients who say they have had a color defect all their lives. It is the comparison of one eye with the other that is important. Women, particularly, are sensitive to subtle differences in color appreciation, and they may complain that colors now seem faded to them or that they have trouble working out the color scheme of their wardrobe.

Chronic progressive decrease of acuity associated with color changes may also be caused by brunescent cataract formation. (The changes in Gauguin's color style during his later years have been attributed to just such a cause.)

Afferent Pupillary Defect

This defect (Marcus Gunn pupillary escape phenomenon) is particularly valuable when only one optic nerve is involved. Occasionally, it is of value in bilateral but extremely asymmetric optic nerve involvement. (Directions for eliciting this sign are given in Chapter 3.) A subtle method of eliciting the sign may become apparent during the initial testing of acuity. When the involved eye is covered for the acuity test, the size of the pupil should show no significant change. When the uninvolved eye is covered, both pupils dilate because of decreased conduction of the involved optic nerve in the exposed eye. Acuity is usually tested in dim illumination, a factor that helps bring out the afferent pupillary defect.

The degree of the direct pupillary response is usually not an accurate guide to visual acuity. Severe visual loss secondary to retinal disease does not substantially affect the pupillary response. This is also true of mild decreases in acuity owing to optic nerve disease; however, a marked difference in the direct pupillary response to light can usually be considered the result of a decrease in acuity. The exception to this rule occurs when the pupil response itself has been altered, such as in cases of tonic pupil, Argyll Robertson syndrome, trauma, or the use of topical drugs.

Head Position

The position of the head is usually related more to ophthalmoplegia than to visual acuity. In congenital nystagmus, the visual acuity is at its best when the patient is allowed to turn his head so that his eyes are at the nul point (point of least nystagmus). Frequently, the patient is forced to read the acuity chart with his eyes straight ahead, which is not where the nul point is usually located. The nystagmus is worse in the straight ahead position and acuity decreases markedly. As a rule, the nul point is 10 to 15° lateral to the straight-ahead position. Another feature of congenital nystagmus is brought out when one eye is covered, no matter whether the eyes are turned to the nul point or not. When one eye is covered to check the acuity of each eye individually, an increase in the nystagmus drops the acuity even lower. In some instances at least, a slight blurring of one eye by a plus lens allows enough vision to suppress the latent nystagmus component, thus permitting the acuity to be measured in the other eye.

The position of the head may also be important if nystagmus is present in only one field of gaze. I have had several patients who have had vertical nystagmus only in down gaze. Their complaints regarding problems in reading had previously been called presbyopia, and the patients had been given many different prescriptions to correct their apparent problem. The patients all said that the strength of the glasses was adequate but that they had to either depress their heads or raise their reading material in order to see. Obviously they had not been examined carefully with their eyes in down gaze.

Photo Stress Testing

Visual function depends on the breakdown and regeneration of visual pigments at a steady rate, which ensures a smooth, continuous visual process. In retinal disease, this rate is disturbed. Bleaching the visual pigments with a steady bright light may further distort this process and prolong the recovery phase. This possibility can be demonstrated clinically by shining a bright light into the affected eye for a specified time (such as 2 minutes) and then measuring until the time elapsed acuity returns to the pretesting level. If a big difference exists in the pretesting to the post-testing recovery times of the two eyes, retinal disease, not optic nerve disease, is suggested. If the patient has only one eye, the physician can compare the response in the patient's eye with his own eye tested similarly. Unless the physician and the patient are the same age, this technique is not as accurate, since the time of recovery varies for different ages; however, if the difference in recovery time between the patient's eye and the physician's eye is great, retinal disease is certainly suggested.

Testing of the Visual Fields

The patient frequently has a difficult time distinguishing blurring in a particular field from an overall blurring. His complaint often is that he does not see well—as if his central acuity were blurred. A hemianopic defect is suspected when a patient reading the Snellen chart consistently misses half of a line of letters.

In informal testing of the fields, use color comparisons between nasal and central fields in the same eye. Present two bright red objects (such as the caps of two mydriatic bottles) simultaneously to the patient's nasal and temporal fields as the patient fixates centrally, and ask him to compare the colors. If a hemianopic defect is present, the patient reports that one cap has a faded or washed-out color and the other cap is bright red. If no hemianopic color difference exists, compare the color appreciation in one eye with that in the other eye. If one eye has an optic nerve defect, that eye will see the red object as faded and the other eye will see it as bright red. As a rule, moderate macular lesions do not distort color perception.

Testing with the Amsler Grid

The Amsler grid charts can be helpful in detecting subtle macular lesions in patients complaining of both blurred vision and distorted vision. Small changes in retinal topography, such as caused by central serous retinopathy, can distort the perfect appearance of the grid to the patients. The lines may appear to be distorted the same way the symmetry of a chain link fence is altered by someone's leaning against it.

HEREDITARY CAUSES

Optic atrophy and blurred vision from hereditary causes are rare. Kjer groups them into Leber's disease, recessive congenital optic atrophy, and two forms of dominant optic atrophy—congenital and infantile.

Leber's Optic Atrophy

Leber's optic atrophy is the best known of the hereditary optic atrophies. It begins usually in a person in his teens or twenties, and it is predominantly a disease of males. It begins in one eye, frequently as a papillitis. Shortly after the first eye is involved, invariably the second eye becomes similarly involved. The atrophy of the disc appears weeks later. In genetic classifications, the disease is usually described as sex linked, with recessive inheritance; however, pedigrees of Leber's optic atrophy do not follow strictly the mendelian rules for this type of genetic transmission. Although the male is predominantly affected, he does not transmit the disease to his children. The woman who is heterozygous for the gene can transmit the disease to both her male and her female offspring. Since the gene is recessive, 50% of her sons will have the clinical disease. All her daughters will be carriers, but only about 10% will have the clinical disease.

The patient typically has large central scotomas, which may enlarge to the point that they break out into the periphery and (most commonly) in the upper nasal quadrant. Some patients report improvement after the initial episode, but the "improvement" may represent an increased ability to use the remaining field rather than a real improvement.

Smith, Hoyt, and Susac have reported that in the early phase of optic neuritis there is circumpapillary telangiectatic microangiopathy. This is associated with swelling of the nerve fiber layer around the disc and an absence of staining on fluorescein angiography. Tortuosity of the peripheral retinal vessels was also noted.

Optic neuritis is the only constant symptom of Leber's atrophy. Periodic headaches, ataxic paraplegia, spasticity, and various degrees of mental defects and seizures have been recorded. A review of the cases shows that a significant number of patients have had recurrent convulsions and cramping of the calf muscles.

In advanced cases of Leber's optic neuritis there is no VEP. In less severe cases, the VEP is reduced in size, delayed, and desynchronized. As the time increases from the initial clinical episode, the VEP in Leber's optic neuritis progressively deteriorates, which is not the case in optic neuritis caused by demyelinating disease unless episodes are recurrent. VEP abnormalities have been seen in the fellow asymptomatic eyes of patients with Leber's optic neuritis just as they have been seen in the fellow asymptomatic eyes of patients with demyelinating disease. If the fellow eye is asymptomatic, the greater abnormality is usually found in those patients with demyelinating disease than in those with Leber's optic neuritis. The VEP cannot differentiate in its response Leber's optic neuritis from demyelination caused by multiple sclerosis. The VEP only attests to a conduction defect in the optic nerve.

Recessive Congenital Optic Atrophy

As described by Waardenburg, recessive congenital optic atrophy begins with the onset of optic atrophy, either at birth or during the first few years of life. The patients have poor vision and severe defects in their color vision. Since the poor vision developed before the patients were 4 years of age, nystagmus also developed. (This situation is not true in Leber's optic atrophy, which begins later in life.) Bilateral poor vision developing before age 4 usually is accompanied by nystagmus, whereas after age 6 it is not.

Dominant Juvenile Optic Atrophy

This type of optic atrophy comes on early in the first decade of life, but it is usually not severe and frequently is not discovered until the child goes to school. The decrease in acuity is frequently mild to moderate, with the majority of children maintaining an acuity of 20/200 or better. A defect to blue is particularly evident. Nystagmus is rare and is probably related to an onset late in the first decade of life. Kjer's report mentions that 25% of sufferers had some abnormalities of mentation or personality but rarely other neurologic symptoms. The pallor of the disc is predominantly temporal, not circumferential.

Krabbe's Disease (Familial Infantile Diffuse Brain Sclerosis)

Optic atrophy and blindness are prominent features of this disease. It results from an autosomal recessive inheritance defect in the sphingolipid metabolism. Children with Krabbe's disease are usually normal at birth but rapidly deteriorate, beginning to experience symptoms somewhere between 6 weeks and 6 months of age. They develop progressive rigidity, convulsions, deafness, and blindness, and death occurs usually by the age of 2 years.

Leigh's Disease (Subacute Necrotizing Encephalomyelopathy)

These patients develop blindness owing to optic atrophy. Leigh's is a progressive disease with a course ranging from weeks to years. The diagnosis is rarely made pre-mortem unless there is a family history, which is present in about one half of the infantile cases. The juvenile and adult forms occur sporadically and the diagnosis is not confirmed until the autopsy. In addition to blindness, patients develop somnolence, deafness, and spasticity of the limbs. At postmortem there are bilateral, focal, subacute, necrotic lesions from the thalamus to the pons. The course prior to death varies from weeks to months.

Dominant Congenital Optic Atrophy

This type of optic atrophy exhibits nystagmus, which places the onset of the disease earlier, perhaps before 4 years of age. Besides the decrease in visual acuity, constriction of the peripheral field varies from slight to severe, depending on the family pedigree.

Optic Atrophy Associated with Hereditary Ataxias

Optic atrophy is also associated with certain forms of spinocerebellar atrophy that are more generally referred to as the hereditary ataxias.

Friedreich's disease exhibits ataxia, loss of tendon reflexes, and pes cavus. The patients do not have optic atrophy, but they do have nystagmus. The disease begins in persons between the ages of 6 and 15; clumsiness of the arms and legs is the earliest sign. The clumsiness progresses to incomplete incoordination until the patient is bedridden.

Optic atrophy is an early sign in the spastic types of hereditary cerebellar ataxia (such as Sanger-Brown's ataxia and Marie's ataxia). Since Sanger-Brown's ataxia comes on between the ages of 16 and 35, nystagmus does not accompany the development of optic atrophy. The symptoms are those of lack of coordination of the arms and hands, but the incoordination is caused by spasticity. This fact, as well as the presence of optic atrophy, helps differentiate Sanger-Brown's ataxia from Friedreich's ataxia. The optic atrophy is seen early, is progressive, and is associated with loss of the peripheral field.

DEMYELINATING DISEASE CAUSES

Optic Neuritis

The retrobulbar form, which is the more common, and the papillitis form are the two types of optic neuritis. The causes of both forms are the same; it is the site of origin in the optic nerve that is different. The patient usually reports pain on movement of the affected eye, either immediately preceding or simultaneously with the onset of blurred vision. Then a precipitous drop in vision occurs, with a lessening or cessation of the pain. The vision stays at a low level for several days or weeks and then slowly but steadily improves over several weeks or months. The prognosis for return to normal or near normal vision is excellent with the first attack. The prognosis in subsequent attacks is not as good. Even when full recovery of vision occurs, an obvious temporal or even a generalized optic nerve atrophy is not unusual. This disparity between recovery of acuity and atrophy of the disc is particularly common in optic neuritis owing to multiple sclerosis. In years past, it was said that about 50% of cases of optic neuritis were caused by multiple sclerosis; more recent studies put the figure closer to 18%. Bilateral optic neuritis, even if the two episodes are separate in time, and recurrent optic neuritis are associated with a much higher incidence of multiple sclerosis. The usual field defect is a central scotoma; however, other field defects, such as arcuate scotomas and quadrantic defects, are seen. Some cases of optic neuritis even occur with normal visual acuity but an extrafoveal field defect. In such cases, usually an afferent pupillary defect and a color vision defect exist, as demonstrated by the HRR plates. On rare occasions, the lesion of optic neuritis is located in the nerve just as it enters the chiasm; therefore it also affects the lower nasal fibers crossing over from the other optic nerve. The result is a junction scotoma, which is an ipsilateral central defect in the affected eye, and an upper temporal field cut in the other eye. This type of defect more commonly occurs with chiasmal masses and must therefore be differentiated from optic neuritis.

Occasionally, the patient complains of a fluctuation in his vision when he takes a hot bath or indulges in prolonged and strenuous exercise. The increase in body temperature that results from both types of activity causes a change in the conduction ability of nerves already compromised by the demyelinating process. Such a fluctuation in vision is called Uhthoff's sign.

The usual report of the examination in retrobulbar neuritis is that the patient sees nothing and the physician sees nothing. At the onset of the diseae the patient says he sees nothing or what he sees is blurred. In the retrobulbar form, no fundus or disc changes occur; therefore, the physician sees nothing abnormal. The atrophy comes on later; it is the pupillary signs, the field defect, and the rapid visual loss that suggest the diagnosis. The patient who has a slow and steady visual loss should be regarded as possibly having a condition other than optic neuritis. A mass lesion should be seriously considered in any case of chronic progressive visual loss. In cases of papillitis, the disc is swollen and hemorrhages may be present around the disc. Swelling of the disc in papillitis cannot be differentiated from papilledema owing to increased intracranial pressure solely from the appearance of the disc. The appearance of the disc in papillitis and papilledema is also similar with fluorescein staining, so fluorescein studies are not useful in differentiating the conditions.

The disease usually begins in young people, but rarely in those under 10 years of age. If a child has visual loss in one eye, be suspicious of any report that the onset was sudden. Although the recognition of a chronic process may have been sudden (such as in a school vision-screening test), the onset may not have been. In a child under 10 years of age, the condition may be a slow-growing optic nerve glioma that is followed only weeks or months later by clinically obvious optic atrophy.

Evaluation of optic neuritis includes a carefully taken history—the signs and symptoms must fit the diagnosis. The history taking should also include questions about poor eating habits as possible causes of a nutritional amblyopia, particularly if the patient is a fad dieter.

Ask the patient particularly about possible exposure to toxins at work or at home (for example, lead or mercury). Today, it is especially important to ask about the use of drugs, even the legitimate ones (such as ethchlorvynol [Placidyl], the birth control pills, ethambutol, and isoniazid). Ask too about the use of tobacco and alcohol; they are more commonly associated with nutritional amblyopia than with true optic neuritis, but still they may contribute to the optic neuritis.

Roentgenograms should be made of the optic canal and sphenoid ridge, and bone changes suggestive of tumor should be looked for. (Some of the more important and common bone changes from tumors affecting the optic canal are discussed in greater detail in Chapter 8.)

Ultrasonography and computerized tomography of the retro-orbital space are important in excluding an orbital-mass lesion that may be affecting only the optic nerve and not causing ophthalmoplegia or exophthalmos. The two techniques can show the optic nerve to be swollen in optic neuritis, which helps somewhat to confirm the diagnosis. The enlarged optic nerve may also represent an intrinsic tumor such as glioma or meningioma. The treatment of optic neuritis is either no treatment or removal of the offending agent (such as a drug or toxin). I have found the administration of steroids by either the systemic or topical route to be of no value.

Multiple Sclerosis

Optic neuritis is frequently the presenting sign of multiple sclerosis, particularly, in the young patient. Of the patients in whom optic neuritis is the presenting sign, 17% also develop other signs and symptoms of multiple sclerosis. Of those who present with another symptom, between 27 and 37% develop optic neuritis. Obviously, the length of follow-up will vary the statistics for the course of optic neuritis in these patients. Hutchinson in Ireland, followed his patients with multiple sclerosis for 15 years and found that 78% of them had optic nerve involvement. Similar long-term studies in America report much lesser numbers. Bilateral optic neuritis in the adult has a worse prognosis for the development of multiple sclerosis than either the unilateral or recurrent forms. This is not true in children in whom there is no correlation between bilateral optic neuritis and multiple sclerosis. The optic neuritis in children also has a better prognosis for recovery than in the adult.

If one looks at the functional disability of these patients with multiple sclerosis 15 or more years later, 73% were independent and leading active lives. Because of this, I consider it not in the patients' best interest to tell them that their optic neuritis may be caused by multiple sclerosis.

As mentioned earlier in this chapter, color testing is important in evaluating optic nerve function. Even with visual acuity of 20/40 or better, defects can still be found using the Farnsworth-Munsell 100 HUE test. It is also important, with a history of optic neuritis, to look at these patients in red-free light for the optic nerve drop-out that one sees.

In cases of multiple sclerosis, Charcot's triad of nystagmus, intention tremor, and scanning speech is rarely seen at the onset of optic neuritis. The diagnosis of multiple sclerosis is usually made after both white and gray matter have multiple lesions that are separated in time and location and that are characterized by remissions and exacerbations.

The nystagmus in Charcot's traid is usually nonspecific, and it can take any form, including horizontal, vertical, or ocular dysmetria. The nystagmus of internuclear ophthalmoplegia is more specific. The nystagmus occurs in the abducted eye when the eyes are directed into horizontal gaze. When the internuclear ophthalmoplegia is bilateral, the nystagmus occurs in the abducted eye in both directions and the diagnosis of multiple sclerosis is almost certain. In about 10% of cases of optic neuritis owing to multiple sclerosis, sheathing of the peripheral veins occurs. The sheathing probably represents some degree of periphlebitis, but it is usually so mild that the patient does not have symptoms.

Internuclear ophthalmoplegia, cerebellar ataxia, intention tremor, urinary sphincter problems, sensory changes, motor disturbances, and emotional aberrations are all part of the symptom complex. Electric-shock-like waves moving down the spinal cord, particularly with neck flexion (L'Hermitte's sign) suggest multiple sclerosis, but they can also be seen with spinal cord tumors.

The diagnosis of multiple sclerosis is usually made on the basis of the occurrence of remissions and exacerbations and the presence of widely separated lesions in the central nervous system. Occasionally, laboratory studies can help in making the diagnosis. In 50% of the cases there is a slight increase in the spinal fluid cell count (the count should not exceed 50 cells per cubic millimeter).

Trying to predict which patients with unilateral optic neuritis will be the ones to develop multiple sclerosis is impossible at this state of our knowledge. Examining the spinal fluid of these patients for pleocytosis, IgG or oligoclonal band distribution is a poor prognosticator for the development of multiple sclerosis.

Immersing a patient suspected of having multiple sclerosis in a hot bath is still a good test. A worsening of the patient's symptoms or the development of new symptoms or signs is positive evidence that a conduction defect exists in the affected nerves. Rasminsky and co-workers demonstrated that increases in temperature amounting to as little as 0.5° could induce symptoms. This worsening of nerve function is probably related to a change in the sodium and potassium flux in and around the myelin sheath. This test should not be undertaken lightly since permanent defects have been reported.

In looking for widely separated signs in the central nervous system, the visual evoked potential (VEP) has been a useful tool. The VEP may demonstrate a conduction defect in one optic nerve, suggesting its involvement when the patient has no present symptoms or past history of that nerve being involved. This would then fix the criteria for separation in time and space in a person who was having unexplained paresthesias. In the interpretation of the VEP, not only the absolute latency but also the intraocular differences in latency and the wave form are all diagnostic. In recent years, a constant, reversing checkerboard pattern has produced a more consistent response than the old flash technique. Demyelinating disease is not the only disease that can produce these abnormal changes in the VEP. Similar abnormalities can be seen in glaucoma or in the sector optic atrophy of ischemic optic neuritis. Both of these latter diseases may spare fixation, suggesting that these VEP changes are not specific for the papillomacular bundle but reflect only axonal damage. It is, therefore, not a specific test for multiple sclerosis; however, as an adjunct test in establishing the diagnosis of multiple sclerosis, Halliday, McDonald, and Mushin found conduction delays in one or both optic nerves in many patients in whom there was no history of optic nerve involvement in the disease process.

The latency of the human occipital potential by a light flash depends on the intensity of the light stimulus. The dimmer the flash of light, the longer the latency. The same difference occurs with equal light flashes to both eyes, but with slower conduction of information to the occipital pole in the damaged nerve. The Pulfrich effect is that the central nervous system will not correct for the temporal discrepancy in the arrival of information from the two eyes. This lack of central nervous system correction for temporal discrepancy of sensory stimuli has also been shown clinically by Halliday and McDonald. They conducted experiments in which the toe and index finger of a patient were simultaneously stimulated. Because the finger was closer than the toe to the brain, the finger was perceived by the patient as being stimulated first. If the brain corrected for any visual time lag, sterioscopy could not occur.

A test for evaluating the conduction velocity of one optic nerve versus the other employs the Pulfrich phenomenon. If an object moves from a normal patient's right field to his left and back again in a straight line, it will be perceived as moving in a straight line. If one eye has a conduction time delay owing to an optic nerve disease such as optic neuritis, the retinal images of the involved eye will arrive later at the visual cortex than those of the normal eye. The object, therefore, will be perceived as moving in an elliptical fashion rather than in a straight line. This is an example of the temporal discrepancy mentioned before. The background objects may influence the response to this test and it is best done against a blank background. The experiment should not be performed with a luminous object in a dark room as a technique to decrease visual clues. It should be done in a lighted room so that the retina can be light-adapted. The Pulfrich phenomenon is not meant to replace the VEP, but rather to add another test to the office or bedside armamentarium of the clinician in trying to evaluate subtle decreases in vision. It can help in differentiating subtle macular disease from optic nerve disease, since macular disease does not cause a time delay to the visual cortex. Even patients who apparently have recovered fully from an episode of optic neuritis and who have 20/20 vision, a full visual field, and apparently normal color vision with the pseudoisochromatic plates, may still complain about their vision. Frequently, they will say the vision in the affected eye is dull or different. If there is still a conduction defect in that nerve, they may have symptoms as a variation of the Pulfrich phenomenon. Frisen, Hoyt, Bird, and Weale reported patients who had difficulties knowing what station on the subway to get off because of the induced Pulfrich phenomenon caused by the moving train.

Hoyt, and Van Dalen and Greve, feel that the earliest defects in multiple sclerosis are isolated defects in the Bjerrum area but off center between 15 and 25°. These defects were found in visually asymptomatic patients; however, a central scotoma is the most common field defect in those patients with visual complaints and multiple sclerosis. Hoyt found narrow arcuate defects in the Bjerrum area and correlated them with nerve fiber bundle defects found by the red-free light technique. Patterson and Heron reported a similar experience in patients with multiple sclerosis and no visual symptoms or history of visual system disease.

Vitreous fluorophotometry is one of the new tests for evaluating retrobulbar neuritis. The increased concentration of fluorescein in the posterior vitreous compartment is not specific for retrobulbar neuritis caused by multiple sclerosis. It indicates a disturbance in the vascular-vitreous barrier, which is altered in optic neuritis from any cause. Since most cases of retrobular optic neuritis have normal-appearing nerve heads initially, this test may be of help in cases in which the diagnosis is in doubt.

Neuromyelitis Optica

This disorder is extremely rare today. The sufferer develops bilateral optic neuritis (but both optic nerves are usually not affected simultaneously), which is followed some weeks later by a transverse myelitis at any level of the spinal cord. The transverse myelitis can come first, but it rarely does so. The optic neuritis usually disappears but generally not as fully as in the cases of optic neuritis already discussed. The disc may appear normal, or, more typically, a low-grade edema of the nerve head exists. Nystagmus, which is so prominent in multiple sclerosis, is rare in neuromyelitis optica. Usually, some residual paralysis results from the transverse myelitis, but a significant degree of recovery is the rule.

The cause and treatment of neuromyelitis are not known, and its relationship to multiple sclerosis is questionable at best. Despite some of the obvious similarities (noted previously), marked differences exist between this disease and multiple sclerosis. Bilateral optic neuritis is rare in multiple sclerosis but the rule in neuromyelitis optica. Significant differences also occur in the pathologic findings.

Schilder's Disease (Encephalitis Periaxialis Diffusa)

This disease, although rare, should be considered because of its relationship to vision. Its onset is late in the first decade of life. It is one of the few causes of acquired cortical blindness in children in this age group. Apparent blindness, along with personality changes (unusual crying, irritability, apathy) in a previously healthy child, suggest this disease. Visual problems are not always an early sign, which adds to the difficulty of making the diagnosis. As the disease spreads anteriorly into the internal capsule, spastic paralysis develops. When the frontal lobes become enlarged, intellect and personality further deteriorate.

The fundus may be normal, or it may show papilledema (in about 20% of cases) owing to slightly increased intracranial pressure.

The cause and treatment are unknown, and death usually occurs within a year.

Some cases may have a hereditary component, and such a possibility should be particularly evaluated in every instance.

ISCHEMIC CAUSES

Anterior Ischemic Optic Neuritis

This disorder is a major cause of loss of vision in persons over 60 years of age. (Typically, the patient is younger than one with temporal arteritis.) The loss may first be related to a central scotoma, but altitudinal defects are more common. The optic disc usually shows a low-grade pale edema with a few splinter hemorrhages. No filling of disc vessels occurs as in papilledema owing to increased intracranial pressure. More that 50% of patients have other vascular disease, such as hypertension.

The initial episode is usually acute, but once it stabilizes, it does not recur in the affected eye. About 75% of patients with only a central scotoma show some improvement. Those with altitudinal field losses do not show improvement. Involvement of the second eye, which occurs in about 40% of the cases, may take place weeks or months later. When it occurs, the patient has optic atrophy with visual loss in the previously affected eye and pale edema in the acutely affected eye. This condition can be mistaken for the Foster Kennedy syndrome, which generally is considered to be caused by a frontal lobe tumor and which, as described, is rare. Ischemic edema is generally the cause of the visual loss, and lack of the other signs of increased intracranial pressure should rule out an intracranial mass. Hayreh stated that the basic problem lies in the posterior ciliary arteries located in the disc and the retrolaminar area. In about 30% of cases, patchy atrophied areas appear in the more peripheral parts of the choroid. The atrophy is caused by involvement of other posterior ciliary arteries.

The sedimentation rate (unlike that in temporal arteritis) is normal. According to Hayreh, fluorescein angiography may be of some help; although early in the course of the disease, no optic disc fluorescence is present. About a week after the onset of the first episode, some fluorescein staining of the disc appears, but only late in the fluorescein sequence. Choroidal filling is delayed, particularly in the peripapillary area.

Temporal Arteritis

This disorder presents as a sudden unilateral loss of vision. Most patients, if they review their history, can tell of other signs and symptoms of temporal arteritis that they had either ignored or misinterpreted. Sometimes, however, the patient has no premonitory symptoms (Simmons and Cogan).

Classic temporal arteritis develops as a headache with temporal scalp tenderness. This tenderness is sometimes so pronounced that the patient cannot comb his hair or put on his hat. Erythema and swelling may appear in the area of the temporal arteries. If erythema and swelling are not present, the temporal arteries feel like pipe stems, and they are not comprehensible. Other symptoms, such as stiffness (usually starting in the neck and the shoulder girdle), polymyalgia, jaw pain, weight loss, low-grade fever, anemia, and an elevated sedimentation rate are also found. The disease affects persons 55 years of age or older; most patients are in their seventies and eighties—about 10 years older than persons with anterior ischemic neuritis. Persons with central visual loss owing to temporal arteritis do not recover their vision. (Most people with anterior ischemic optic neuritis recover some of their vision.) In untreated temporal arteritis, the second eye is frequently involved. Involvement of the second eye can occur at anytime, but rarely after 8 weeks. The optic disc does not show the edema seen in arterior ischemic optic neuritis. Despite the severe loss of central vision, the fundus picture of occlusion of the central retinal artery is not present.

The diagnosis should be suggested by the history and the elevated sedimentation rate. A temporal artery biopsy is indicated to establish the diagnosis (see Figs. 14–1 and 14–2). Steroid therapy should be started as soon as the sedimentation rate is reported to be elevated. It is unwise to wait for the confirmation by biopsy, because the other eye may become involved during the delay. Moreover, even if steroid therapy has been started, the biopsy can be done within the next 48 hours without its validity being affected by the steroid therapy.

Transient Ischemic Attacks (Adults)

The word stroke carries with it the same fear as the word cancer. The fear of finality or helplessness associated with the word stroke has been prevalent since the Greeks coined the word apoplexia—to strike down. Throughout all these years, the consensus has been that strokes were caused by vascular accidents to the brain that were neither preventable nor treatable. Gowers was the first to bring to our attention the relationship between retinal emboli and hemiplegia. The emboli that he saw and reported were presumably caused by the patient's heart disease, not concomitant carotid artery disease.

During the last 20 years of intensive research into the cause of stroke and its prevention, it has become apparent that lesions of the intracranial arteries may cause strokes and may be treated surgically. Frequently, the stroke itself may be preceded by focal attacks of cerebral or retinal ischemia that we arbitrarily refer to as transient ischemic attacks (TIA) if they last less than 24 hours and leave no residual neurologic deficit. Many investigators have used the eye as a monitor of carotid blood flow, when these lesions are below the branching off of the ophthalmic artery as it comes off the internal carotid artery. The significance and prognostic value of different types of TIAs is not as clear-cut as we would like in terms of who is more likely to develop a stroke, or specifically, where the lesion is or what it is. We rely, therefore, on different instrumentation such as ophthalmodynamometry and, finally, arteriography.

Arteriography helps to identify the surgical candidates. Even certain types of intracranial ischemic symptoms, particularly along the distribution of the middle cerebral artery, have been treated surgically by the superficial temporal artery anastomosis technique described by Yasargil and his co-workers.

Some studies have tried to review the patients suspected of having TIAs and, based on the types and frequency, make a prognostic evaluation in terms of predicting a stroke. A TIA increases the likelihood of a stroke seventeenfold in the year after the first TIA. The TIA signals the risk of a stroke occurring within 5 years. The risk overall is 40%; half of these will occur in the first month after the initial TIA. The most vulnerable period is the first 18 months after the initial TIA. Angiographic data indicate that 75% of the patients with ischemic strokes have at least one responsible lesion, and in 40% of the cases, the lesions are limited to the extracranial vasculature. These are operable lesions, and hypothetically most of these strokes might be avoided by timely endarterectomy, if demonstrated before the stroke.

How good an indicator are some of the signs of TIA? Consider carotid bruit as one sign of arteriosclerotic disease. A well-localized bruit that extends throughout systole indicates a stenosis of at least 50%. It usually is considered hemodynamically significant since it reduces the cross-sectional area of the artery by 75%, substantially diminishing the blood flow.

Jarett and McHugh studied the natural history of carotid bifurcation plaques by performing serial arteriograms during a period of 1 to 9 years. Notable increases in the size of the plaques were found in 62% of the atheroma, and in one third of the lesions; the plaques increased in size by

more than 25% per year. In a long term follow up study by Thompson and Talkington, almost one half of the 102 patients they studied with asymptomatic bruits became symptomatic; one fourth had TIAs and underwent endarterectomy; while another 19% suffered strokes without any prodromal symptoms. Owing to the development of the state of the art, complications of arteriography are few, but they can, and do, occur and so it is not a procedure to be taken lightly. Reviewing other aspects of the combined university TIA study, Futty and his co-workers evaluated the visual symptoms of TIAs and their significance. The most common transient symptoms of carotid system disease were monocular loss of vision and contralateral sensory or motor symptoms. A third common symptom was dysarthria. Dysarthria occurred as often in vertebral basilar system disease and, therefore, was not a reliable sign of carotid artery disease alone. Since today's vascular surgery is designed primarily for carotid artery disease, it is important to identify carotid artery disease. The only combinations of symptoms that are more predictive of significant carotid system disease than is a single symptom, such as transient loss of vision, are contralateral sensory or motor symptoms for the left carotid artery system and language disturbance, and right arm and leg motor or sensory symptoms and facial weakness. These were in additon to the visual loss. In most cases, the patient had more than one symptom; however, visual loss was the most common single symptom. It seems reasonable to assume that most patients with potentially treatable carotid system disease will be seen by, or present to, an ophthalmologist. It behooves the ophthalmologist to be alert to these patients and to try to develop easy, quick, reliable and nontraumatic tests to identify these patients who require further evaluation.

Classically, carotid artery insufficiency or occlusion is supposed to cause ipsilateral loss of vision and contralateral hemiplegia, but such a syndrome rarely occurs. When the carotid artery is gradually occluded, collateral circulation frequently develops to protect the cerebral hemisphere. Ipsilateral loss of vision does occur, however, and carotid disease must be included in the differential diagnosis of monocular sudden loss of vision. After occlusion of the artery and loss of vision, the fundus may initially appear normal. Clinically obvious optic atrophy usually occurs weeks later. It may occur sooner, if the infarction of the optic nerve occurs just behind the lamina cribrosa. As part of the workup in acute visual loss, ophthalmodynamometry should be performed. If the reading shows a significant decrease in ophthalmic artery pressure, carotid artery occlusive disease with probable ischemia is suggested. Although, by today's techniques, ophthalmodynamometry (ODM) seems crude, it is readily available in the office of any doctor interested in cerebral vascular disease. It requires high-grade obstruction in the carotid artery to cause a significant decrease in blood flow to the eye and be reflected in a drop in ophthalmodynamometry pressure. ODM will not detect moderate or low-grade obstruction or irregularity of the arterial lumen from arteriosclerotic plaques. All of these can cause similar transient visual symptoms, just as if there were high-grade obstruction of the artery. Ischemia of the optic nerve can also give transient, partial, or complete loss of vision to one eye, but with a normal ophthalmodynamometry reading. Decreased pulsations of the ipsilateral carotid artery and the presence of a carotid artery bruit are good evidence of a decreased blood flow to the ipsilateral eye. Since collateral circulation may supply enough blood to give a normal ophthalmodynamometry reading, a negative response does not rule out the possibility of carotid artery insufficiency. The acute loss of vision can be caused by a combination of a drop in pressure with an already decompensated small

vessel circulation in the optic nerve that is caused by hypertension and atherosclerosis. Significant long-term obstruction to a carotid artery may be inferred in patients with significant diabetes or hypertension, in whom the eye ipsilateral with the carotid artery insufficiency shows none of the fundus changes of these diseases. Since carotid artery occlusion is caused by atheromatous disease, embolization from an ulcerated atheromatous plaque may also cause the acute vision loss. As described by Hollenhorst, these plaques lodge at bifurcations or narrowings of vessels (as when they pass through the lamina cribrosa) (Fig. 13–1). The retina should be carefully inspected for the yellow, crystalline plaques, particularly at the bifurcation of vessels. If the plaques occlude a branch, central vision is spared, sector defects occur, and whitish edema of the retina in that sector is easily seen during the acute stage. If the embolization occurs in the central artery, the entire retina is cloudy white and a cherry-red spot appears in the macula. When the embolization occurs some distance behind the lamina cribrosa, the retina may appear normal. Hollenhorst plaques can lodge in vessels without causing an obstruction. Even when the entire vision of the eye is lost, it is worthwhile examining the retina in detail for evidence of these plaques because they may give a clue as to what is causing the loss of vision. Light pressure on the globe as the fundus is viewed causes the vessels to pulsate and the plaques in an artery to move, which may make them more readily visible.

The other embolic phenomenon causing transient symptomatology is called white plugs. These result from increased adhesiveness of the platelets, causing a rouleux effect. They become stacked on one another to form a platelet plug. These temporarily lodge in retinal vessels, causing ischemia and transient loss of vision before passing on into the peripheral circulation. Carotid arteriosclerotic plaques can contribute to increased platelet adhesiveness

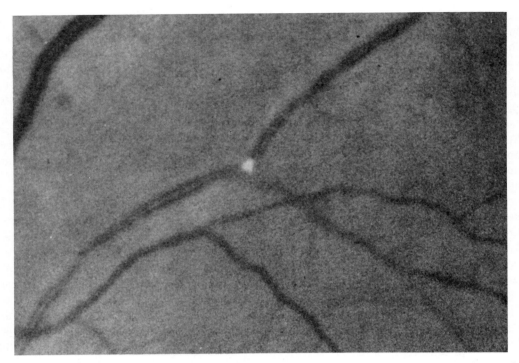

Fig. 13–1. The white area represents a Hollenhorst plaque at the typical place of a bifurcation of a vessel.

owing to changes in laminar flow over these irregular areas. Larger white emboli are considered to originate in the heart.

Venous stasis retinopathy is another sign of vascular insufficiency, representing a more chronic cause of decreased blood flow to the eye. The fundus picture is one of microaneurysm, particularly near retinal veins, hemorrhages, and dilated and tortuous veins. It is usually unilateral, and the findings are more prominent in the midperiphery than at the posterior pole. Diabetic retinopathy with which it has been confused in not usually unilateral and is more concentrated in the posterior pole. Patients who have venous stasis retinopathy on the basis of carotid ischemia can also have ischemic facial pain. Improving blood flow by endarterectomy or by superficial temporal-middle cerebral artery bypass surgery can reverse the fundus changes and facial pain and cerebral symptomatology.

Until recently, noninvasive techniques were never quite adequate for the diagnosis of carotid obstructive disease. If your index of suspicion was high for significant treatable carotid disease, hospital admission was required and arteriography was performed. This was not only expensive and time consuming for all involved, but the test carried some serious risks with it to the patient. Today, with digital subtraction angiography, a test equal in quality to direct arteriography is now available (Fig. 13–2A,B). Performing this test from the venous side of the circulation reduces the morbidity of direct arteriography. It is done as an outpatient procedure. The qualities of the picture from the aortic arch up to the carotid siphon can be as good as standard arteriography. Since most remedial carotid artery disease is at the bifurcation in the extracranial carotid artery, this test is particularly valuable. In view of the natural history of transient ischemic attacks, it is now more important than ever to identify the patients who can be helped by surgery.

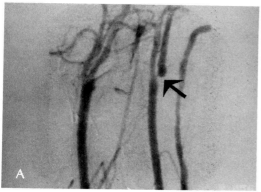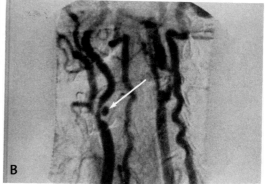

Fig. 13–2. **A.** A digital examination demonstrating a string-like narrowing of the internal carotid artery. **B.** This examination also has a narrowing but a plaque can be seen protruding into the vessel lumen.

The differential diagnosis in the older age group for transient visual ischemia after arteriosclerotic disease is not great. Diseases that affect platelet adhesiveness are rare in this age group and are discussed in the section on transient ischemic attacks in children and young adults. Cardiac arrhythmia should always be high on the list of differential diagnoses. Patients going in and out of atrial fibrillation can cause valvular vegetations to break off and produce embolic symptoms. Postural hypotension causing transient symptoms usually can be suspected from the history. A carotid sinus syndrome may also be suspected from a careful history. A recurrence of migraine is always in the differential diagnosis, but it is much more common in females than in males. The usual migraine presentation is for a female to have had several episodes of classic migraine in her teenage years, and then go into a state of remission for 20 years. As she approaches the menopause, the visual symptoms return without the headache and are interpreted as transient ischemic attacks, secondary to vascular disease, rather than as true migraine. The patient is a little young for significant arteriosclerotic disease, since she is usually in her fifties; this should alert the wary physician that this constellation of symptoms represents something other than carotid vascular insufficiency.

Transient Ischemic Attacks (Children and Young Adults)

It is a general perception in medicine that there is little therapeutic advantage in searching for the cause of a nonhemorrhagic stroke, unless the diagnosis of remedial extracranial arterial disease can be made. This is generally true in the older age group of 60 years or older, described in the previous section. This rule does not apply to children and young adults. Although only 5% of all strokes occur under the age of 45, there is a high incidence of treatable diseases that are not caused by atherosclerotic disease. Since many of these diseases are not found on routine neurodiagnostic procedures, it requires better history taking to uncover the clues that will lead to the proper diagnostic tests and diagnosis. One of the easiest tests to perform is to take the blood pressure in both arms and legs. It is also important to have a proper size cuff, rather than one cuff for all ages. Although hypertension in young people is rare as compared with the older population, it is not that uncommon in young patients with transient ischemic symptoms. Because of the rarity of hypertension in young people, blood pressure is infrequently taken in this age group. The ophthalmologist has an opportunity to make a quick and simple diagnosis of hypertensive vascular disease. A list of the causes of hypertensive vascular disease in this age group would fill several pages. It is not the province of the ophthalmologist to do a work-up on the patient for hypertensive vascular disease and to identify the specific cause, but to be alert enough to identify hypertension as a problem and bring it to the attention of the family physician.

Pure ocular transient ischemic attacks and retinal artery obstructions in young people are even more rare than strokes, if one excludes migraine. This is because the collateral ocular circulation in this nonatheromatous age group is adequate to keep this symptom from occurring. The following discussion briefly reviews the differential diagnosis of transient ischemic attacks and strokes in children and young adults, both with and without visual symptoms. This list is by no means complete but represents the causes that we have seen in our practice.

ATRIAL MYXOMA
MITRAL VALVE PROLAPSE
"THE PILL"
CONSUMPTION COAGULOPATHIES
WALDENSTRÖM'S MACROGLOBULI-
    NEMIA
TROUSSEAU SYNDROME
SICKLE CELL ANEMIA
SUBARACHNOID HEMORRHAGE
MOYA MOYA DISEASE
NEUROFIBROMATOSIS
CAROTID SINUS SYNDROME
TAKAYASU SYNDROME
TALC
CONGENITAL HEART DISEASE
FIBROMUSCULAR DYSPLASIA
POSTICTAL
PORPHYRIA
DYSAUTONOMIA (SHY-DRAGER
    SYNDROME, RILEY-DAY SYN-
    DROME)
PERIARTERITIS NODOSA

Atrial Myxoma. Cardiac tumors occur in about .05% of routine autopsies; 50% of these are atrial myxomas and the vast majority of them are found in the fossa ovalus of the left atrium (Fig. 13–3). These tumors occur in a ratio of about 3 to 1 for women over men, and can be symptomatic at any age. When patients are symptomatic, it is usually between the third and sixth decade of life. They may present with an embolic phenomenon or progressive obstruction of cardiac outflow with progressive failure, or they may have constitutional symptoms suggestive of cardiovascular disease or endocarditis. The murmur these patients develop may mimic that of mitral stenosis or mitral insufficiency and will vary with the position they are placed in. Patients with atrial myxoma will also show a decrease in weight, increases in their sedimentation rate, and in their gamma globulin, fatigue, mild anemia, and embolization phenomenon. Embolic phenomenon may cause an initial infarction. It may also cause weakening of the arterial walls so that aneurysm formation may occur years later after the atrial myxoma has been surgically resected. This aneurysm may then present as a subarachnoid hemorrhage or as a primary intraparenchymal hemorrhage.

The three conclusions that one can draw about atrial myxoma are (1) that it is a preventable cause of cerebrovascular disease if found in time; (2) it is a disease that should be considered even in young patients without cardiac symptoms; and (3) aneurysms can occur late in the disease even after definitive treatment has been undertaken.

Mitral Valve Prolapse Syndrome (Barlow Syndrome). The mitral valve prolapse syndrome is also referred to as the midsystolic click-murmur syndrome. It also occurs more frequently in women than in men, and is present in approximately 6 to 8% of our adult female population. Most patients are asymptomatic, but 30 to 40% may have nonspecific symptoms. Not infrequently, there is a positive family history to help in the diagnosis. The symptoms and signs include fatigue and

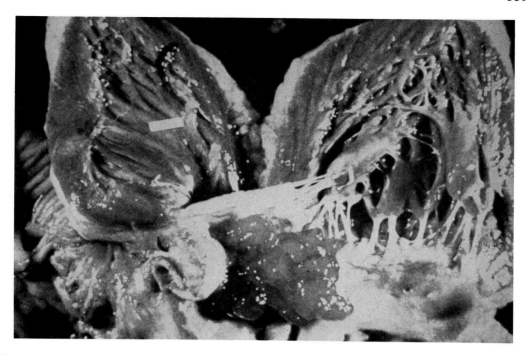

Fig. 13–3. Pathology specimen revealing a gelatinous mass of an atrial myxoma. (From Jampol, L.M., Wong, A., and Albert, D.M.: Atrial myxoma and central retinal artery occlusion. Am. J. Ophthalmol., 75:242, 1973. Published with permission from the American Journal of Ophthalmology. Copyright by the Ophthalmic Publishing Company.)

exertional dyspnea, so that one may consider other forms of cardiac or pulmonary disease. Palpitation and occasional detectable arrhythmias are also part of the picture. Some patients suffer from syncope, frequently with light-headedness, particularly during exercise and, on rare occasions, at rest. Chest pain is usually dull and aching over the precordium without radiating into the arm and is unchanged by exertion or nitroglycerin. The cause of this syndrome is debated and may represent some unusual form of coronary artery spasm or papillary muscle ischemia. On physical examination, there is a mid-systolic click or a later systolic murmur. The click is heard early if the left ventricular volume is decreased, such as in the Valsalva maneuver, or may be heard in late systole if the volume of the left ventricle is enlarged, such as in bradycardia. These patients usually have an asthenic build, with high arched palates and associated thoracic

bony abnormalities such as pectus excavatum, marked scoliosis, and loss of the normal kyphosis. They may also show signs such as hyperextensibility of the skin which bruises easily, and hypermobility of the joints, as one sees in the Ehler-Danlos syndrome. They have an abnormal bifid cardiac pulse, particularly when the patient is in the left lateral position.

The ECG shows inverted T-waves, particularly in lead II. Supraventricular arrhythmias such as atrial fibrillation are seen in about 60% of these patients. They also have conduction disturbances such as the Wolff-Parkinson-White syndrome. For M Mode echocardiography, there is a pansystolic prolapse posteriorly of the mitral valve leaflets, which is seen best in the posterior leaflet (Fig. 13–4A, B, C). A late systolic dipping posteriorly of the leaflets may also be seen. In 2-dimensional echocardiography, one or both leaflets go posteriorly beyond the mitral ring.

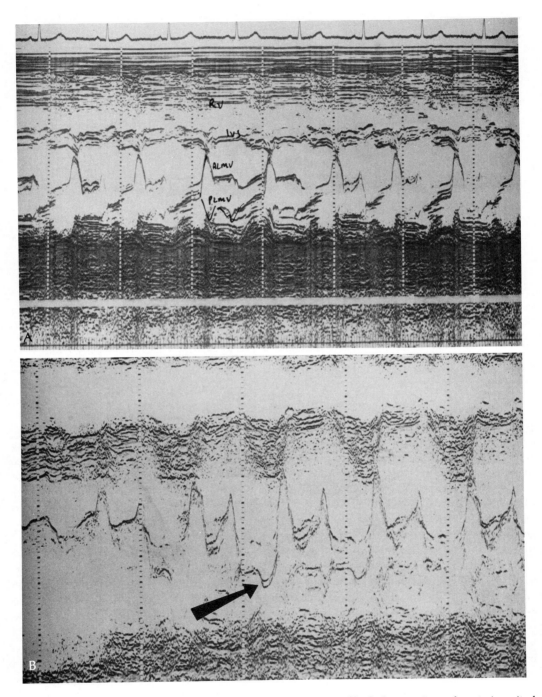

Fig. 13–4. **A.** Echocardiogram of a patient with normal movement of both the anterior and posterior mitral leaflets. **B.** The arrow indicates the hammocking of the posterior mitral leaflet which is characteristic of this syndrome.

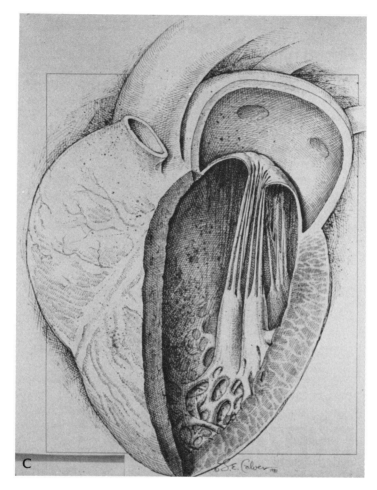

Fig. 13–4. C. Diagrammatic representation of prolapsing mitral valves into atrium. (Courtesy of Lewis E. Calver.)

Complications of this syndrome are progressive mitral regurgitation with failure, infective endocarditis, spontaneous rupture of the chordae tendinae secondary to endocarditis, or myxomatous degeneration of the valve with sudden failure and, rarely, sudden death.

"The Pill." Oral contraception medication or "the pill" has been with us since the mid 1960s. Despite the controversies, it is generally agreed that there is an increased risk of deep vein thrombosis and pulmonary embolism in patients taking the pill. The results are an increased incidence of the migraine syndrome in this group of patients who already have a propensity for migraine. Therefore, it has been recommended that people with problems consistent with congenital heart disease or other vascular abnormalities are probably poor candidates for using this method of contraception; however, the relationship of the pill and the occurrence of stroke in young women is still somewhat controversial. There has not been as significant an increase in stoke since the introduction of the pill as there has been of deep vein thrombosis. In those women developing a stroke-like syndrome, the findings are unusual. About one fourth of these patients

develop a stroke along the distribution of the vertebral basilar arterial system. Just as experimental animals on exogenous steroids develop intimal hyperplasia and secondary thrombosis, so too did the women on oral contraceptives develop these changes demonstrated at postmortem. Until such time as we can identify which patients are at risk for stroke as well as for deep vein thrombosis, we should consider the pill as the potential cause of any cerebral vascular accident in young women.

Consumption Coagulopathies. Consumption coagulopathies represent an abnormal state of the blood coagulation mechanism. This results from an increase in intravascular coagulation factors, often associated with diseases that have a hemorrhagic diathesis. This may be seen in such diseases as abruptio placenta, fat embolism, endotoxin shock, Waterhouse-Friderichsen syndrome, thrombocytopenia purpura, cirrhosis, acute pancreatitis, hemorrhagic shock, extensive surgery, acute leukemia, and carcinomatosis. The common denominator of all of these is a release of thromboplastin or a thromboplastin-like substance into the vascular system. These diseases do not present to the ophthalmologist as a patient's initial complaint, and so are not high on the list of differential diagnoses considered by the ophthalmologist.

Waldenström's Macroglobulinema. This syndrome occurs in mid- to late life, rather than in childhood or very young adulthood, but it generally appears earlier than symptomatic cerebral arteriosclerosis. It occurs mostly in males. It usually has an insidious onset with the patient's experiencing increasing weakness, lassitude, weight loss, pallor, hemorrhagic diathesis (epistaxis, gingival, retinal, and cutaneous hemorrhages). These patients can also demonstrate a painless increase in the size of their lymph nodes and will have hepatosplenomegaly, anemia, relative lymphocytosis, thrombocytopenia, and an increase in their sedimentation rate. About 25% of these patients have neurologic signs, with retinal changes seen in about 30%. Convulsions are uncommon. Strokes or focal brain syndromes, encephalopathies, neuropathies, and subarachnoid hemorrhages are some of the neurologic presentations.

The Sia test is the appropriate one to perform. If a drop of the patient's serum is added to a test tube of distilled water, a white flocculus is formed.

Trousseau Syndrome. This is the syndrome that is familiar to all of us from medical school days with the presentation of thrombophlebitis, associated with neoplasia. The most common neoplastic process is that of cancer of the tail of the pancreas. Cancer of the head of the pancreas presents with other signs and symptoms at a much earlier stage of the development of the cancer. Other abdominal malignancies can also do this, but the pancreas is still the outstanding example.

Sickle Cell Disease. Sickle cell trait occurs in about 8% of black Americans, whereas sickle cell anemia occurs in 0.15% of black Americans, and most of these are children. The reason it occurs more in children is that the life expectancy of these patients is shortened and therefore the incidence drops in the adult age group. Persons who have sickle traits usually have minimal symptoms. The precipitating factor for their becoming symptomatic is a reaction to toxic agents, infections, or severe stress. The organ that is the most frequent target is the renal medulla, which develops small infarcts. As a result, patients have difficulty concentrating their urine and develop painless hematuria, which causes hypertonicity of the intravascular fluid. Any situation that pulls water out of the red blood cells increases the chances of their sickling. The involvement of the renal medulla with sickling usually does not start until after 6 months of life when the HbF is replaced by HbS. Patients who have sickle cell disease usually show an impairment of growth and a failure to thrive during their first few years. They also have difficulty in fighting infection because of recurrent splenic infarcts, which decreases their ability to clear circulating bacteria. The morbity and mortality of this disease usually are caused by recurrent vaso-occlusive episodes. Other, more common, symptoms include abdominal pain suggestive of an acute abdomen, chest pain with a differential diagnosis of infection versus infarction and joint involvement. All of these symptoms may be precipitated and preceded by upper respiratory infections. They may also occur more frequently in cold weather when there is vaso-constriction of vessels. These patients can also have signs and symptoms of central nervous system involvement, with seizures, strokes, and coma. The retinal changes are described in Chapter 7, Retinal Disease, by Dr. Welch. Patients with sickle cell disease can also have central retinal artery occlusions, although this is not common. The conjunctival sickling sign is well known, and one can see it with the magnification of the slit lamp (Fig. 13–5). If one places topical phenylephrine HCl on the conjunctiva, the vasoconstriction it causes may increase the sickling sign. On the other hand, the increased heat of a prolonged observation with the slit lamp may decrease the amount of sickling that one usually sees.

Subarachnoid Hemorrhage. Aneurysms frequently present as a subarachnoid hemorrhage. The differential diagnosis of subarachnoid hemorrhage in children includes syndromes that have a hemorrhage diathesis such as leukemia, idiopathic purpura, hemophilia. These diseases usually show bleeding in other areas as well, which helps in the differential diagnosis. If bleeding occurs only into the central nervous system, then one should consider rupture of an arteriovenous malformation, aneurysm, vascular hamartoma, bleeding associated with a tumor, or extension of an intercerebral hemorrhage into the subarachnoid space, or a spinal cord tumor. If a tumor bleeds into the subarachnoid space directly, it is usually an ependymoma or a tumor of the choroid plexus. Under the age of 30, bleeding from an arteriovenous malformation is much more common than an aneurysm. Most of these patients bleed intracerebrally, rather than into the subarachnoid space. Bruits can be heard in about 20% of these patients and are heard best over an eye or in the temporal fossa.

Moya Moya Disease. Moya Moya disease presents either as motor paresis in the young or as apoplectic stroke in the middle aged. The anatomic findings are occlusion of the carotid arteries in the area of the carotid siphon. This is usually a bilateral disease. Besides this obstruction, there is a bilateral hemangiomatous vascular network which extends across the base of the brain and is easily seen on cerebral angiography. Before the development of sophisticated subtraction techniques, these vessels were not easily seen and only the dye was seen as a misty diffuse pattern in the area of this network. This appearance was the reason for the name of the disease. This fine network of vessels is more easily seen as individual vessels with today's techniques of subtraction and magnification (Fig. 13–6). The cause of this vascular abnormality is not well known but is felt

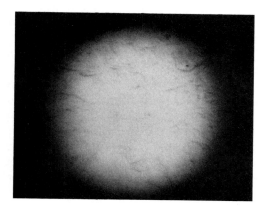

Fig. 13–5. The conjunctival vessel sickling sign is diagnostic of sickle cell anemia. The heat of a prolonged slit-lamp examination may bring this out. (Courtesy of Morton Goldberg.)

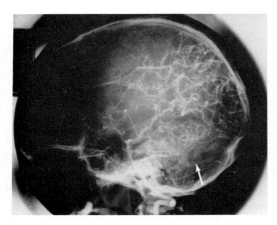

Fig. 13–6. A fine rete mirabile of the vessels off the carotid artery is diagnostic of this disease. In some areas, no individual vessels are seen but only dye because of the small caliber of the vessels.

to be of a congenital nature. Anatomic examination of the vascular development in fetus specimens reveals a similar network prior to the full development of the carotid system. Many investigators feel that this is an example of the lack of development of that carotid system. Moya Moya disease was originally described by the Japanese but has now been seen in all other races and parts of the world. Most of these patients do well, but some of them show progressive changes in their carotid artery on repeat arteriography, and some of them die. In a series of 111 patients reported in Japan, 73 were under the age of 16. Six of these children had progressive neurologic deficit and 4 died. The other 38 patients in this series were over the age of 16, and 19 had subarachnoid hemorrhages with varying results.

Neurofibromatosis. Neurofibromatosis is well known to have associated with it cardiovascular disease, including congenital heart disease, valvular stenosis, and systemic vascular occlusive disease, including renal artery stenosis. Focal neurologic signs are often thought to be caused by tumors, but one should keep an open mind, because they may be related to cerebrovascular disease. It has now been established that neurofibromatosis can cause

a Moya Moya-like syndrome. Patients show gradual development of narrow carotid arteries leading to occlusion in the supraclinoid portion. This obstruction is caused by proliferation of Schwann cells with intimal thickening. If the obstruction is unilateral, then no changes may occur, owing to the gradual development of collateral circulation through the circle of Willis. If the obstruction is bilateral, then the hemangiomatous vascular network develops in the region of the basal ganglia and on the surface of the corpus callosum. This involvement of the cerebrovascular network is not common, but has been reported and should be kept in mind when dealing with patients with neurofibromatosis, rather than ascribing all of their cerebral symptoms to a recurrence of their tumors or to the development of new tumors.

Carotid Sinus Syndrome. Stimulation of a hyperirritable carotid sinus can result in a profound fall in arterial pressure associated with a marked bradycardia. Carotid sinus syndrome tends to be more common in males in the sixth decade of life than in young adults, but it can occur in this age group and should be given some consideration. These patients may experience light-headedness and syncope, and may have an associated decrease in blood flow to the eyes, with a decrease in vision. The most common causes are arteriosclerosis and hypertensive vascular disease, which is not a disease of the young as a rule. Other causes can be local disease such as lymphadenopathy, scars, and carotid artery tumors. Carotid sinus syndrome can also be caused by anatomic changes, such as extreme turning of the head with compression of one of the vertebral arteries, with the other one being incompetent, perhaps congenitally. The condition can also be seen with hyperextension of the neck, constricting neck wear, and carrying heavy weights on the shoulder, which compresses the carotid sinus. It can also be secondary to intravascular causes exciting the carotid baroreceptors; although this is an uncommon cause in the young age group, it should not be totally dismissed. The history of the circumstances under which syncopy occurs each time usually points the alert physician toward the proper diagnosis.

Takayasu's Disease. Takayasu's disease was originally described in young Japanese females, but has been seen in other races throughout the world. It is produced by a slowly progressive obliteration of the major vessels arising from the aortic arch with a decrease in blood flow to the head and the upper extremities. It is primarily a disease of the aorta but can extend down to the renal arteries, with the development of secondary hypertension. The pathologic studies reveal a panarteritis with intimal thickening, fibrosis, and vascularization of the media and fragmentation of elastic tissue. There is also some mild lymphocytic infiltration and thickening of the walls of the vasa vasorum in the adventitia. The symptoms are usually those of amaurosis fugax, which is made worse with standing or with exercise. Ophthalmodynamometry usually shows a decrease in readings, particularly when taken immediately after changing from the lying or sitting to the standing position. The fundus is typically pale in appearance, with dilated retinal vessels. This dilation of vessels is particularly obvious around the disc and forms a caput medusa type of arteriovenous anastomosis around the nerve head. There is also some peripheral retinal artery obliteration, and occasionally, a central retinal artery occlusion may develop with secondary retinitis proliferans and vitreous hemorrhages.

Talc. An uncommon cause of blurred vision seen in private practice is found in association with the injection of foreign materials into the bloodstream which become lodged in the eye. One of the more common substances that we see today is the dilution of narcotics with talc. These pieces of talc can act as emboli in the retinal vessels. They have been reported infrequently but have been documented photographically.

Congenital Heart Disease. The patient with congenital heart disease is usually discovered at an early age and does not normally present initially with an ophthalmologic problem. The congenital heart defects that cause a right-to-left shunt allow emboli from the peripheral veins to bypass the lungs and enter the arterial circulation. It is from this point that they become lodged in arterial vessels, causing the signs and symptoms of thrombosis in the tissue fed by that vessel. Arterial thrombosis is uncommon in young people, but children under 1 year of age with cyanotic congenital heart disease are predisposed to venous thrombosis. This phenomenon can result in focal neurologic signs such as decreased vision, increased intracranial pressure, seizures, and coma. A majority of these children have polycythemia, but they may also have microcytic hypochromic anemia.

Fibromuscular Dysplasia. Fibromuscular dysplasia is a disease caused by irregularly spaced areas of fibrous and muscular hyperplasia of the media, with disruption of the elastic lamina. At these areas of rupture, there is an aneurysm-like appearance. The most common area for this to develop is the middle third of the extracranial carotid artery. Patients with this disorder may also have hypertension; many of them are young women with involvement of the renal arteries and development of secondary hypertension. The arteriogram picture is characteristic and shows a corrugated appearance in the areas where there is spaced fibrous and muscular hyperplasia (Fig. 13–7). This sign has been referred to as the "string of pearls." In women who have this disease, it is more common to find additional aneurysms throughout the vascular system than it is with the population in general. Because these patients are young, with good collateral circulation, decreased vision and defects of the optic nerve or field defects have

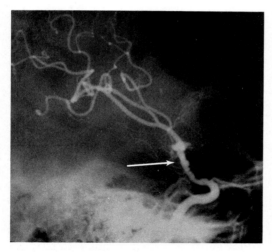

Fig. 13–7. The corrugation or "string of pearls" sign is well represented by this roentgenogram.

been recorded only five times in the literature. This collateral circulation, however, does not protect their renal arteries from the disease, therefore, secondary hypertension is a frequent problem with its associated ocular findings.

Postictal. The hemiparesis and aphasia that may follow a generalized seizure and that clears within 24 hours has been referred to as Todd's paralysis. This decrease in neuronal function can be seen in the visual system as well. Three possible mechanisms have been proposed: one is neuronal exhaustion; another is the vaso-constriction and vasodilation phases of the vascular response, causing ischemia and metabolic exhaustion of the neurons; the third proposes that there is an active inhibitory state of the cells after a seizure. Cells around the active seizure site may discharge an increase of inhibitory substance to the cells that are involved in the active seizure pattern. The symptoms and signs of this postseizure neuronal depression should clear within 24 hours.

Porphyria. The two major forms of porphyria are erythropoietic and hepatic. The usual onset is between the third and the fifth decade of life. It can be precipitated by fasting or starvation or by such drugs

as barbiturates, hormones, and steroids. The acute intermittent variety is hepatic and is inherited as a mendelian dominant trait. It usually presents with recurrent gastrointestinal, psychiatric, and neurologic symptomatology. Parasthesias of the extremities are common initial symptoms. Weakness of the muscles of the trunk and extremities may rapidly advance to complete paralysis. Weakness is usually generated in the distal parts, but occasionally, proximal muscles may be more severely involved. Also, any cranial nerve, including those of the visual system, can be involved. The erythropoietic form is rare and is recessively inherited.

Dysautonomias. One of the more common syndromes of this unusual group of diseases is the Shy-Drager syndrome. Patients with this disorder present with postural hypotension without a change in their pulse rate. This represents adrenergic system failure owing to intermediolateral column cell disease. There are also cases with cholinergic dysfunction involving lacrimal and salivary glands, gastrointestinal, urinary, bladder, and sweat gland signs and symptoms. These patients do not show pupillary dilatation to topical hydroxyamphetamine; there is an absence of the ciliospinal response, and no tachycardia is seen with the postural hypotension. The tests for parasympathetic dysfunction include using dilute pilocarpine to induce pupillary miosis. Also, no change occurs in the heart rate with the Valsalva maneuver. These patients show minimal tachycardia in response to a pharmacologic dose of atropine, suggesting vagal hypoactivity.

The more common childhood form of dysautonomias is the Riley Day syndrome. Children with this disorder exhibit episodic hypertension, excessive sweating, skin blotching, episodic vomiting, insensitivity to pain and absence of taste discrimination. Almost all of these children show an autosomal recessive type of inheritance. They show an increase in homovanillic acid in the urine, which suggests a defect in enzyme dopamine-beta-hydroxylase. There is also a decrease of norepinephrine concentration in the serum of these patients as well as of dopamine-beta-hydroxylase after standing when one compares these levels with those of normal patients. Dysautonomic patients, after standing for awhile, do not have a normal increase in these levels of norepinephrine, which supports the view that the hypo- and hypertension in these patients were related to abnormal rates of norepinephrine release.

These patients usually start their symptoms during the first 5 years of life, showing emotional irritability, insensitivity to pain, absence of taste discrimination, and attacks of severe vomiting. They also have hyperpyrexia, hypo- and hypertensive episodes, and episodes of skin blotching alternating with pallor. They may have seizures, absent deep tendon reflexes, and dysphasia. They frequently have recurrent upper respiratory infections and pneumonias, and may die from pneumonia, hyperpyrexia, or severe dehydration. The physical examination shows absence of fungiform and circumvallate papillae of the tongue. These patients also have impairment of normal lacrimation.

Laboratory studies reveal an increased ratio in urinary excretion of homovanillic acid to vanillylmandelic acid. There is low serum dopamine-beta-hydroxylase activity and impaired norepinephrine release.

Periarteritis Nodosa. This is a disease caused by focal disseminated inflammatory lesions involving the medium and small arteries. The average age of onset for this disease is 47, but may range all the way from age 9 to 77 years. Those who have the severe form, which ends in death, have an active period of signs and symptoms averaging about 12 months. They commonly have neurologic signs, particularly peripheral neuropathy. Laboratory examinations reveals anemia, increase sedimentation rate, reversal of the AG ratio, abnormal urinary findings, leukocytosis, and increased BUN. Roentgenograms may show pulmonary infiltrates suggestive of this type of disease.

Hypotension

No matter what the cause, hypotension can result in acute loss of vision in one or both eyes. Loss of vision related to acute hypotension usually has other signs and symptoms so that the diagnosis is not obscure. One cause of hypotension that is usually not obvious is a too rapid and too ambitious control of hypertensive vascular disease. The following descriptions of three hypothetic patients illustrate this iatrogenic cause of hypotension.

1. Patient 1 has had no symptoms of a visual disorder. He has had known hypertension for years, and his eye is accustomed to a high head of pressure. His well-meaning physician aggressively lowers the patient's blood pressure, so the patient has no systemic symptoms of hypertension. In the course of his hypertensive therapy, he loses vision. The eye that has had a high head of pressure and that has arteriosclerotic changes now experiences ischemia and the optic nerve is infarcted. The ophthalmologist should consider such infarction in a patient who has pronounced hypertensive retinopathy, relatively normal blood pressure, and visual loss.

2. Patient 2 has a hypertensive fundus and normal blood pressure, but has had no recent changes in the medication he is taking for hypertension. His blood pressure may not have been under good control, and now it has dropped because of a silent myocardial infarction. An electrocardiogram is indicated for this patient, as well as for Patient 1.

3. Patient 3 has hypertension and glaucoma. The glaucoma has been well controlled for years, but not the arterial hypertension. The glaucomatous eye, which has perhaps marginal perfusion, is accustomed to a certain head of pressure. When the arterial pressure is dropped for any reason, the glaucomatous eye may suddenly

begin to lose field even though the intra-ocular pressure seems to be at the same level as it was on previous examinations. The drop in this patient's arterial pressure should be evaluated as a possible cause of the change in his glaucoma.

It is well recognized that patients with advanced glaucoma who have small resid-ual central islands of vision can have that remnant snuffed out even when surgery goes smoothly. It probably has to do with a sudden change in the vascular dynamics of the eye. It may result from the pressure being lowered too fast (e.g., by too much filtration). It has now been reported in sim-ilar cases of laser iridotomy for acute-angle closure glaucoma with sudden lowering of intraocular pressure. The central island of vision can also be lost through a secondary but transient rise in intraocular pressure such as may occur after laser trabeculo-plasty. Both extremes of a tenous status of ocular vascular dynamics can produce loss of this small remaining island of vision.

HEMATOLOGIC AND VASCULAR CAUSES

Blood Loss

Acute or chronic blood loss may also cause loss of vision or field in one or both eyes. Acute blood loss rarely causes these defects unless chronic compromise of the ocular circulation already exists or unless the blood loss is severe (as in postpartum hemorrhage and massive gastrointestinal hemorrhage). A day or two after the hem-orrhage, the patient may complain of loss of vision and show a decrease in vision or an altitudinal field loss, particularly in the lower field. The optic disc shows an is-chemic edema.

Chronic Anemia in Pregnancy

This anemia occurred in the past, but is rarely seen today.

Vascular Operation

Vascular or any other kind of surgical procedure in which cardiac arrest or pro-longed hypotension occurs can leave the patient with unilateral loss of vision or even cortical blindness. The degree and duration of hypotension and the status of the vessels in the affected area are factors that contribute to the degree of visual loss.

Blood Dyscrasias

Blood dyscrasias are of several varieties. Optic neuritis with a cecocentral field de-fect is well known in pernicious anemia. This disease usually occurs in persons over the age of 30, and it should be suspected in patients who have optic neuritis with evidence of glossitis and gastrointestinal symptoms. It is a macrocytic anemia with a defect in the gastrointestinal absorption of vitamin B_{12}. The Schilling test, the ac-cepted confirmatory test, measures the body's ability to absorb radioactive vitamin B_{12} over a 24-hour period. Another fre-quently used test involves the injection of histamine and the measurement of hydro-chloric acid secretion in the stomach. (This secretion is severely impaired in pernicious anemia.)

The treatment is to use hydroxycobala-mine rather than the standard form of vi-tamin B_{12}, and thus bypass the enzymatic defect that prevents proper absorption.

Another form of blood abnormality—and an all too common one—is central ret-inal vein occlusion. The patient with this abnormality complains initially of blurred vision; his visual acuity is usually 20/200 or better. The fundus shows hemorrhage, particularly along the veins, which are fat and sausage-like, with a sludging of the blood column. Sometimes, such veins are seen with no hemorrhage, a condition that is referred to as impending venous occlu-sion. Patients with impending venous oc-clusion usually have no symptoms. Some have transient blurring of vision, which leads them to seek an evaluation.

Central retinal vein occlusion is caused by a sludging of the blood column, which may be caused by an elevated pressure in the eye (glaucoma), slowing of the blood column, or a decrease in blood flow into the eye with normal intraocular pressure. It may also occur in known diabetes or as a premonitory symptom of early unsuspected diabetes. Central retinal vein occlusion is caused by a change in blood viscosity, and it can also be seen in the rarer hyperviscosity syndromes, such as Waldenström's macroglobulinemia. These hyperviscosity syndromes, which can be identified by paper electrophoresis of the blood proteins, can also be seen as secondary manifestations of carcinoma. Polycythemia vera can also cause sludging of the blood; it may occasionally be secondary to a hemangioblastoma of the cerebellum.

The diagnosis of central retinal vein occlusion usually presents no problem since the appearance of the retina is dramatic and specific.

Transient Obscurations

This form of blurred vision is occasionally seen with increased intracranial pressure. Because the episodes last only 5 to 15 seconds and occur only a few times a day, the patient usually does not complain of them. He thinks they are insignificant. I happen to have treated several patients who experienced transient obscurations frequently during the day and so did complain of them.)

The obscurations are different from the amaurosis fugax of carotid artery insufficiency, which lasts anywhere from 5 to 25 minutes and which the patient notices and does complain about. Transient obscurations are usually bilateral, and they are always related to increased intracranial pressure. Other causes of disc edema do not cause transient obscurations; thus they are quite specific.

Cortical Blindness

The most common cause of cortical blindness is arteriosclerosis, and it obviously occurs in the older age group. In the young patient, the causes are more protean. They include trauma, poisoning from carbon monoxide and nitrous oxide, neoplasms, infections, such as meningococcal, mumps, rubeola, and syphilitic meningitis. Cortical blindness also occurs after seizures and represents a form of Todd's paralysis. In the days of ventriculography, it would occur occasionally with that procedure. The cause of this loss owing to ventriculography is only speculative. It was felt that it occurred more commonly with multiple passes of the ventriculography needle or was owing to some shift of the brain when the ventricular fluid was withdrawn. Cardiac surgery with cardiac arrest or severe decreased blood pressure during the procedure is also one of the causes implicated in cortical blindness. Rare cases of cortical blindness have been reported with acute intermittent porphyria, blood transfusions, and temporal arteritis.

Aneurysm

Rupture of an aneurysm is either a lethal or, at the least, a devastating disease. Signs of impending rupture are not always easy to detect. Headache, although a common symptom, is infrequently of a severity or type that would suggest an aneurysm and the work-up that it demands. Visual deficits can range from total blindness in one eye to field defects, which are variable from one examiner to another. It is this latter variability that should alert an astute clinician to the possibility of an aneurysm rather than having him suspect that it was the quality of the examiners that was variable. In a recent retrospective survey of aneurysm patients, the highest incidence of warning signs was for those aneurysms located at the junction of the internal carotid and posterior communicating arteries, with those at the bifurcation of the carotid and the middle cerebral arteries running a close second. The older the patient who ruptures an aneurysm, the less warning signs usually occur. The three mechanisms for these premonitory symptoms and signs are (1) vascular disturbances; (2) minor leakage of blood; and (3) ischemic lesions.

Ninety percent of intracranial aneurysms are congenital and average between 0.5 and 1.5 cm in diameter. Those that enlarge up to 3 cm, in size are called giant aneurysms. Aneurysms cause symptoms either by rupture into the subarachnoid space or by slow expansion with compression of nearby structures such as in the carvernous sinus. Those that are less than 5 mm in diameter rarely bleed. This is fortunate since aneurysms 5 mm or more can be seen on today's high quality computer tomography machines if cuts are made in the appropriate place. If they are not seen, that test is not so accurate as to preclude arteriography if the suspicion of aneurysm is high enough. Aneurysms appear in 4% of adult autopsies and are multiple in 20% of cases. The aneurysms usually become symptomatic between 40 and 65 years of age. They account for 10% of all fatal cerebral vascular accidents and for 50% of all fatal cerebral vascular accidents occurring in patients under 45 years of age. Eighty-five percent of aneurysms occur on the anterior circle of Willis. In those 15% that occur in the posterior circulation, the majority occur at the bifurcation of the basilar artery and posterior cerebral artery.

The symptoms can vary from mild to the most severe of headaches. Alterations in consciousness can vary from mild confusion to unresponsiveness even to painful stimuli. Meningeal irritation can be demonstrated by positive Kernig and Brudzinski signs. These patients may also demonstrate photophobia, hyperacusis, and hyperesthesia, mild fever from meningeal irritation or high fever secondary to hypothalmic disturbances. There may be other hypothalamic dysfunctions, such as vomiting, sweating, chills, and irregular heart rate. Focal damage may give a clue as to which artery is affected. Weakness in one or both legs suggests hemorrhage from the anterior communicating artery. Weakness in an arm and the face suggests a mid-

dle cerebral artery location. If a dense hemiplegia occurs, its location is usually in the internal capsule. This involvement is from an aneurysm in the upward extension of the internal carotid or in a middle cerebral artery. Since any of these aneurysms can cause a significant and sudden rise in cerebral spinal fluid pressure, a preretinal hemorrhage may be seen. If the preretinal hemorrhage is in front of the nerve, then no visual symptoms occur; however, if the hemorrhage occurs in a subhyaloid location in front of the macular, there may be a severe decrease in acuity. If the patient survives and the hemorrhage does not break out into the vitreous, the hemorrhage will absorb and good vision be restored.

Not all aneurysms present with the same signs and symptoms. The posterior cerebral artery passes around the cerebral peduncle medial to the temporal lobe, superior to the third nerve and inferior to the optic tract. Aneurysms of this artery cause hemiplegia with involvement of the corticospinal tract in the cerebral peduncle, homonymous field defects, temporal lobe seizures, and third cranial nerve paresis.

The anterior communicating and anterior cerebral arteries are located above the optic nerve and chiasm and below the olfactory nerve. A giant aneurysm of the anterior cerebral artery causes unilateral loss of vision and smell; that on the anterior communicating artery may give a bitemporal field defect.

Those aneurysms located along the middle cerebral artery occur in the sylvian fissure and cause hemiplegia, focal seizures, homonymous field defects, and speech problems.

Aneurysms of the posterior communicating artery occur near the junction of the internal carotid artery, usually between the anterior choroidal and posterior communicating arteries, and rarely, at the junction of the two. These aneurysms present with classic third cranial nerve palsy with pupillary involvement. Discussion of these aneurysms and those of the cavernous sinus are more fully described in the section on the third cranial nerve in Chapter 6, Diplopia.

Aneurysms occurring on the basilar artery, particularly in the interpeduncular fossa, produce third cranial nerve paresis and headaches that are not necessarily caused by rupture of the aneurysm but by the obstruction of the sylvian acqueduct that then causes increased intracranial pressure and autonomic disturbances with hypothalamic pressure. Pressure on the fifth nerve can cause a tic-like syndrome, and pressure on the facial nerve in particular can cause hemifacial spasm. Aneurysms located on the vertebral artery and posterior inferior cerebellar artery cause apraxia and bulbar involvement. If they occur on the anterior inferior cerebellar artery, they may cause hemifacial spasm and can mimic a cerebellopontine angle tumor or Meniere's disease.

INFLAMMATORY CAUSES

Intraocular Inflammations

Those intraocular inflammations that cause blurred vision are numerous enough to compromise a division of ophthalmology. Only some of them are alluded to here. Endophthalmitis is usually a complication of intraocular surgical procedures, so the diagnosis is not usually missed. Blood-borne endophthalmitis is a rarer inflammation, however, and initially the physician may not consider it as a cause of blurred vision. Meningococcal meningitis is a rare disease. Ocular involvement is prominent in some epidemics and rare in others. Its most common ocular involvement is endophthalmitis. In meningitis, ocular pain and a cloudy-yellow pupillary reflex suggest meningococcus as the causative organism. Decreased vision and hazy media always suggest either intraocular infection or uveitis. Retrobulbar optic neuritis and visual cortex involvement occur much more rarely in meningococcal en-cephalitis, but the prognosis in regard to vision is good when the condition is treated promptly.

Uveitis is usually caused by one of the granulomatous diseases. The chorioretinitis that these diseases cause may sometimes be identified from the appearance of the fundus. Histoplasmosis should be considered when macular hemorrhages and peripheral yellow drusen-like choroidal lesions occur without surrounding reactive pigmentary changes. In toxoplasmosis, large punched-out chorioretinal lesions with pigmentary clumping occur, particularly in the macular area. Toxoplasmosis in an adult probably is a recurrent condition, since most cases first occur during the intrauterine period. With each recurrence, new daughter lesions develop that frequently can be followed out along one vessel into the periphery. Serologic confirmatory tests for both histoplasmosis and toxoplasmosis can be done conveniently (that is, without recourse to state laboratories). Sarcoid uveitis is less common than the forms of uveitis already described, but it shows the typical fundus, with the individual white exudates extending from the vessels into the vitreous humor, particularly in the peripheral retina. (These exudates are referred to as candle wax drippings, "en taches de bourgie." The optic disc may also be involved by a localized granuloma (Fig. 13–8 A, B). Sarcoid has protean manifestations beyond ocular involvement. These may be unilateral or bilateral painless swelling of the lacrimal gland with or without involvement of the parotid gland. The symptoms may be minimal with only decreased tearing and mild symptoms of keratitis sicca, or they may progress to the more severe form of Sjögren syndrome. Since lacrimal gland involvement is so common and is often asymptomatic, a gallium scan may be useful in identifying it. Infiltration of the angle can cause obstruction of the trabecular meshwork, with the development of secondary glaucoma. Gonioscopy will easily

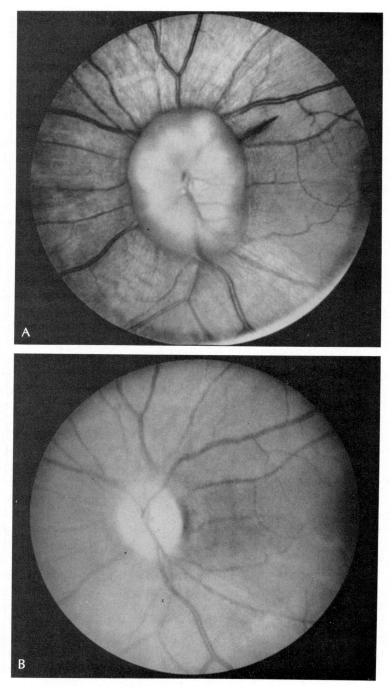

Fig. 13–8. **A.** A sarcoid granuloma involvement of the optic disc. **B.** The disc after systemic steroid therapy. (From Jampol, L.M., Woodfen, W., and McLean, E.B.: Optic nerve sarcoidosis. Arch. Ophthalmol., *87*:355, 1972.)

demonstrate the deposits on the mesh-work and confirm the diagnosis. This inflammatory form of glaucoma should be a serious consideration in the differential diagnosis of unilateral glaucoma. Conjunctival biopsies are useful in establishing a tissue diagnosis even when symptoms of sarcoid occur in other tissues. Nichols reports up to 55% positive biopsies in random conjunctival biopsy specimens.

Recently, there has been interest in the angiotensin-converting enzyme test as a means of identifying sarcoid in the laboratory. This enzyme is usually produced by the endothelial cells of most capillaries and some arteries as well as by the cells of the proximal convoluted tubules of the kidney. It is found elevated in other diseases such as leprosy and Gaucher's disease. It is postulated that this enzyme is produced from monocytic cells that have been transformed from phagocytic into storage or secretory cells.

Since a chest roentgenogram may show signs of pulmonary involvement, one should be done in all cases of suspected sarcoid uveitis. A careful physical examination may also reveal a lymph node (particularly in the supraclavicular area), so a biopsy should be performed. If the patient has signs of diabetes insipidus or a facial paralysis, sarcoid uveitis should be considerred first as the cause of the blurred vision. About 12% of cases of sarcoid uveitis have central nervous system involvement, with diabetes insipidus and facial paralysis being the two most common manifestations. Tuberculosis, usually miliary tuberculosis, is a much less common cause of uveitis but it does not present a diagnostic problem. Coccidioidomycosis and blastomycosis are even rarer causes of uveitis. The chest roentgenogram and the skin tests (and, in the case of coccidioidomycosis, knowing that the patient has lived in the San Joaquin Valley) help to confirm the diagnosis.

Intraocular reticulum cell sarcoma may present as a nonspecific uveitis (Fig. 13–9).

If a patient presenting with this diagnosis also develops a cranial nerve paresis, particularly a seventh cranial nerve paresis, consider reticulum cell sarcoma as well as sarcoid in the differential diagnosis. When the diagnosis remains obscure, a vitreous biopsy may show the presence of a monoclonal immunoglobulin and light chains in the B lymphocytes present in the vitreous inflammatory tissue.

Orbital Inflammations

These inflammations usually show sufficient signs to suggest the diagnosis. The relationship of sinus disease to optic neuritis has been vastly overemphasized. If sinus infections affect the optic nerve, they usually do so when they break through the medial wall and the periosteum into the orbit and create an orbital abscess with marked edema, erythema, pain, and systemic signs of infection. In children, sinus infection generally comes from the ethmoid sinuses, since these sinuses are formed in early life and only a thin wall (the lamina papyracea) separates them from the orbital contents. Frontal sinus disease is not seen until the teenage years since the frontal sinuses do not form until a person is about 12 years of age.

Orbital infection in infants, which occurs rarely, is caused by an infected tooth bud.

Thyroid disease, either the thyrotoxic or the thyrotropic form, can cause optic neuritis, probably as a result of orbital inflammation or an enlarged confluence of muscles at the orbital apex, causing vascular compression (see Fig. 4–5). Most patients can be treated conservatively with steroids; but occasionally, orbital decompression may be required (infrequently, I find). Optic neuritis has also been related to diabetes, but the relationship is on less solid ground.

Optic nerve involvement related to typical herpes zoster ophthalmicus with vesicles over the first division of the trigeminal nerve is rare. If it is of the ischemic variety, it frequently leads to blindness.

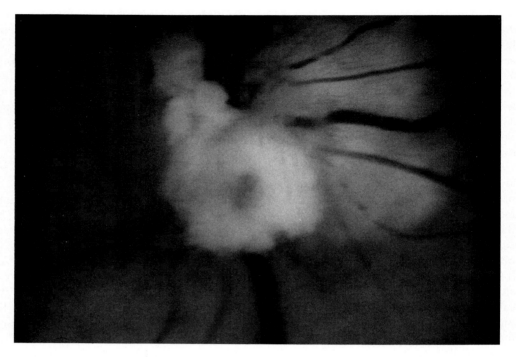

Fig. 13–9. Lymphomatous involvement of the nerve with compromise of the disc circulation and severe loss of vision.

Sarcoid uveitis has been discussed. Orbital sarcoid involvement as a mass lesion can also occur. It requires the same type of evaluation as that for sarcoid uveitis, as well as the evaluation outlined for an orbital mass. Syphilis causes many types of ocular involvement. When the disease involves the optic nerve, it affects the peripheral part of that nerve more than the axial part. The opposite happens in other forms of optic neuritis, such as that owing to multiple sclerosis. Although the central visual acuity is not totally spared. The peripheral field loss is greater. The serologic tests and the other clinical signs should establish the diagnosis. Optic neuritis is usually a form of secondary syphilis. A rare form of ocular involvement is periostitis of the orbit. There is severe pain when the periosteum is palpated. The appropriate serologic tests will confirm the diagnosis.

Pars Planitis

This chronic exudative inflammation of the pars plana area of the retina occurs with gross involvement of the anterior vitreous humor. A chronic inflammation, it causes blurred vision (owing to the presence of cellular debris in the vitreous humor) and, eventually, macular edema. Pars planitis usually occurs in persons between the ages of 20 and 35. It is bilateral in 75% of the cases. Anterior uveal involvement usually occurs, as exhibited by a slight anterior chamber flair and fine keratic precipitates. The most specific sign is the collection of white exudates (referred to as snow banking) on the peripheral retina, particularly inferiorly. The cause is not known. Systemic steroids appear to be of little help.

Radiation Retinopathy

Delayed radiation effects occur 18 to 36 months after the radiation therapy. This may present as progressive bitemporal field loss after radiation for pituitary adenoma, confusing the issue of recurrent tumor versus radiation effect. This can occur even when proper amounts of radiation have been administered. If the brain radiation is anterior, radiation retinopathy may occur even when the eye was properly shielded. The retinal findings are those of small vessel telangiectasis with capillary microaneurysms, hemorrhages, and cotton-wool spots. The resulting exudate frequently takes a circinate pattern. Additional signs of vasculitis include sheathing of vessels. There is a particular predilection for the macular and perimacular areas. Secondary to this ischemic process, papillitis and subsequent optic atrophy may occur.

Intracranial Inflammations

Herpes simplex encephalitis is uncommon but not as rare as we once thought. This is because the diagnosis was only made postmortem. The condition begins abruptly with fever and headache. Convulsions and delerium also occur, which progress to coma and death within 1 week on the average. Frequently, there is cranial nerve involvement, signs of pyramidal tract damage, and an unusual increase in intracranial pressure. The initial and most vital treatment is directed toward equalizing the increased intracranial pressure by steroids or surgical decompression. The cerebral spinal fluid usually shows a lymphocytosis of 175 to 1000 cells per cm^3. Viral cultures are rarely positive, but a rising antibody titer against herpes simplex can help make the diagnosis. A brain biopsy with a demonstration of inflammatory changes consistent with acute encephalitis in association with a Cowdry-type intranuclear inclusion body is helpful in establishing the diagnosis. The disease usually results in death; spontaneous recovery is rare. Type 1 herpes simplex is the usual type in the adult form. Type 2, which is associated with genital herpes, is seen in infants who are infected with the virus as they pass through the vaginal canal. Herpes simplex encephalitis occurs so infrequently that it is hard to associate it with any contributing factors; however, it is slightly more prevelant in patients who have Hodgkin's dis-

ease. This is most likely due in those patients to a reduced or impaired host-immune response.

TUMOROUS CAUSES

Ocular Tumors

These tumors are primarily melanomas or metastatic tumors from the breast or lung. They affect central vision either primarily by way of a solid retinal detachment involving the macula or by the edema around the mass that extends into the macula. A careful fundus examination easily identifies this cause of blurred vision as a mass lesion.

Leukemia

When leukemia occurs with increased blood viscosity owing to an increase in leukemic cells or to the presence of abnormal proteins (such as macroglobulins or cryoglobulins), vascular occlusive disease may be the result. The acute variety of leukemia shows more retinal changes, with mild disc edema and retinal hemorrhages, particularly Roth's spots (Plate 2-IC). A loss of vision may also occur owing to choroidal infiltrates with overlying serous detachment of the retina. The chronic form of leukemia can produce a retrobulbar optic neuritis whose relationship to chronic lymphatic leukemia may go unnoticed because of the time lapse between the onset of leukemia and the appearnce of the optic neuritis. Steroids are particularly beneficial in this type of optic neuritis, which is the reason for identifying the cause.

Optic neuropathy related to carcinoma is becoming more widely understood. Carcinoma can cause optic neuropathy without direct involvement, probably because of the vitamin and other nutritional deficiencies that are caused by the malignancy. If meningeal involvement and secondary involvement of the optic nerve are present, a cerebral spinal fluid examination should be performed. The spinal fluid can be spun down for a cell block examination. The spinal fluid sugar can be decreased as well, suggesting a malignancy is likely.

In some types of carcinoma, particularly carcinoma of the stomach, an increase of the macroglobulins and cryoglobulins causes intravascular coagulability. The vision can be affected also by the hypercoagulability and sludging of the formed elements of the blood in the polycythemia that is secondary to hemangioblastoma of the cerebellum.

Extraocular Tumors

The entire range of orbital and intracranial tumors makes up the extraocular tumors affecting vision. Chronic increased intracranial pressure from whatever cause—tumor or psuedotumor—eventually causes progressive loss of vision and, if not treated, blindness. The discussion that follows is limited to two of the more common orbital tumors—glioma and meningioma.

Glioma of the optic nerve usually has an insidious onset. The diagnosis of poor visual acuity generally is made at a school vision-screening test, or a strabismus is noted. The patient usually does not come to the physician with a specific complaint of loss of vision. Eighty to 90% of optic nerve gliomas occur in persons under 20 years of age, and the majority of these occur in persons under 10 years of age. The central visual acuity is decreased, and occasionally, exophthalmos has already begun.

In a person under 10 years of age who has loss of vision in one eye, optic nerve glioma, rather than optic neuritis, should be ruled out first. Since optic nerve gliomas usually start in the intraorbital part of the optic nerve, vision loss and exophthalmos are the early observable signs. Roentgenography of the optic canal may already show erosion of the canal, a finding that not only confirms that a tumor is present but also indicates its intracranial extension. Observation of the patient for any of the signs of neurofibromatosis is also important; they are present in about 25% of cases of optic nerve glioma. Ultrasonography or computerized tomography of the orbit should show enlargement of the optic nerve. If possible, a careful field examination of the uninvolved eye should be done. Pay particular attention to the presence of a temporal field defect in the upper quadrant of the uninvolved eye, which indicates that the intracranial involvement has reached the chiasm.

The treatment of gliomas is somewhat controversial. Glaser, Hoyt, and Corbett in their review of chiasmal gliomas, and Hoyt and Baghdassarin in their review of cases of optic nerve gliomas, concluded that these tumors represent a hamartoma. They felt that most cases maintain stable vision and do not require radical surgery except for the relief of proptosis in a blind eye. Optic nerve gliomas appear to act differently than do gliomas in other parts of the central nervous system. This may be the result of their high association with neurofibromatosis. In a review of cases in the British literature, a similar conclusion was made that optic nerve gliomas associated with neurofibromatosis act less aggressively than do gliomas of the central nervous system in general. All of these cases, however, must be followed closely for any signs of continued growth into the intracranial cavity.

Meningioma is the most common intracranial tumor and the second most common intracranial tumor that produces neuro-ophthalmologic signs (pituitary tumor is first). Loss of vision is the most common of these signs. The tumor can occur in persons of any age, but it is most common in persons in their forties and fifties. It is more common in women than in men. Meningiomas in children are rare and account for 1.5% of all meningiomas. In adults, menigiomas occur predominantly in the anterior fossa. In children, they occur in all the fossas. The prognosis for meningioma in children is somewhat worse because they undergo sarcomatous changes. The presence of shunt vessels on the disc is an excellent sign that one is dealing with a meningioma of the optic nerve. Although a few cases have been reported in which the tumor was surgically removed from the nerve, leaving good vision, this is not the usual experience of most physicians treating this disease. It is felt that in removing the tumor from the nerve, the fine vessels from the perineurium to the nerve are also destroyed, causing more ischemia to an already compromised nerve. Sphenoid ridge meningiomas commonly affect vision before they cause exophthalmos or extraocular muscle paralysis.

Roentgenograms of the sphenoid ridge usually show changes—for example, diffuse decalcification that has left only a shadowy bony area where the sphenoid bone, with all its landmarks, should be. Hyperostosis of the superior orbital fissure and optic canal is another possible change, and one that is far more suggestive of the diagnosis. If hyperostosis is present, the patient needs to be evaluated by a neurosurgeon and with contrast studies that outline the extent of the lesion. The tumor may spread to surrounding structures to such an extent that removal may be impractical because of the neurologic deficit that an operation would cause.

Craniopharyngioma is another tumor that may be missed because of its symptomatology. Instead of a slow, steady, progressive course, the symptoms are often intermittent and variable. Although these tumors are the result of a congenital variant, they can cause symptoms at any age. They may cause disturbances of growth and sex development in children, both with and without increased intracranial pressure. Progressive loss of vision is common. In adults, dementia and visual loss are the most common signs and symptoms. In children, the roentgenogram shows calcification in the suprasellar region in over 90% of cases. This calcification is rarely seen in the adult form of the disease.

Sometimes it is difficult to differentiate infectious from neoplastic meningitis. Carcinomatous infiltration can take the form of a subacute meningoencephalitis, with headache, associated disturbances in mentation, and sixth cranial nerve paresis. Patients may also develop blindness and deafness from infiltration of those cranial nerves. In cases of carcinomatous meningitis, the deep tendon reflexes are usually decreased or absent, whereas in the infectious form, the reflexes are usually intact or accentuated. There is no fever in the neoplastic form. In carcinomatous infiltration, the cerebral spinal fluid has an increase in intracranial pressure, usually with 100 per mm^3 or less white blood cells, predominantly of the lympocytic and, to a lesser degree, the polymorphocytic type. There is also an increase in protein and a decrease in the glucose level of the fluid. These laboratory findings can also be seen in cryptococcal, Candida, and sarcoid involvement of the meninges. The cerebral spinal fluid cytology, India-ink preparations, and culture of the spinal fluid should make the differential diagnosis. The spinal fluid cytologic examination of bacterial meningitis usually contains 1000 to 10,000 cells with polymorphocytic cells predominating. One exceptiion to this is that in about 20% of patients with meningococcal meningitis, the count is less than 100 cells per mm^3.

TOXIC CAUSES

Tobacco-Alcohol Amblyopia

This syndrome has been misnamed; the condition appears to be the result of a biochemical defect related to thiamine deficiency. The clinical syndrome can be seen in nutritonally deprived persons who do not use tobacco or alcohol as well as in persons who use excessive amounts of tobacco and alcohol and thus have poor appetites and poor nutrition). In tobacco-alcohol amblyopia—and in all the toxic amblyopias—the involvement is bilateral. Usually one eye is involved for several weeks or months before the other eye is affected. The typical field defect in tobacco-alcohol amblyopia is the cecocentral defect, which serves to quickly differentiate the condition from other causes of optic nerve or chiasmal disease. Kearns and Rucker have reported one case of a chiasmal tumor that caused a cecocentral field defect, but such an occurrence is extremley rare. In the toxic amblyopias, the fundus appears normal for a long time before temporal disc atrophy develops. The treatment, if any, is usually a proper diet with a multivitamin supplement. Foulds and his co-workers believe that cyanide plays a role in tobacco-alcohol amblyopia, and they report success in treating the condition with hydroxycobalamine. My limited experience with hydroxycobalamine in treating the condition has been uniformly unsuccessful.

Lead

Lead intoxication is more rare today than it was previously because of the decreased use of lead-based paints. Children who are exposed to such paints, especially children with a pica, develop lead poisoning after eating paint chips from walls, toys, and other objects. But lead can be absorbed through the skin and respiratory tract as well, so it is important to question the adult patient carefully about his job and hobbies. It has been reported that toll takers at bridges and tunnels have had increased blood lead levels because of their exposure to the exhaust fumes from automobiles, but I am not aware of any cases of associated optic nerve disease.

In acute lead intoxication, particularly in children, convulsions may be the presenting sign. In the chronic form, colic, constipation, headache, and muscle weakness are more common. Since the lead is stored primarily in the bones and liver, a ready store may be present after the initial period of absorption. During infections that cause some degree of acidosis, lead is released from the bone storage depots, and the signs and symptoms of lead poisoning occur.

Vision is commonly affected; the more severe the lead poisoning, the worse the optic nerve involvement and the prognosis in regard to vision. Extraocular muscle involvement in association with the visual deficits indicates a poor prognosis in regard to vision.

The laboratory findings in lead intoxication include anemia with punctate basophilia and stippled red blood cells. A blood lead level greater than 0.1% is required for a diagnosis of lead poisoning.

Roentgenograms of the lower end of the femur and upper end of the humerus show a lead line. In lead encephalitis, the spinal fluid has an increase in globulin that is disproportionately high for the increase in cells, which rarely exceed 100 per mm^3.

Prompt use of a chelating agent is the treatment of choice.

Methyl Alcohol

Even in small amounts, methyl alcohol is particularly harmful to the retinal ganglion cells. The history and associated symptoms usually suggest methyl alcohol poisoning. Blindness is a common result. No treatment exists.

Digitalis

This poisoning may be acute, or it may represent a chronic buildup, over months, caused by inadequate utilization and excretion. In toxic conditions, serious cardiac problems (such as heart block) occur, and these problems take precedence over the visual complaints. The usual visual complaint is of a change in color vision; for example, the patient may say that everything looks yellow. Regulation of the digitalis dosage reverses the visual symptoms.

Isoniazid

Taking isoniazid in small doses rarely causes ocular symptoms. With larger doses, particularly when the drug is given in combination with a salicylate or alcohol, the ocular symptoms appear. The symptoms are optic neuritis, optic atrophy, vertigo, paresthesias, and convulsions. These symptoms are similar to those of pyridoxine deficiency, so the treatment is administration of pyridoxine as well as reduction of isoniazid.

Ethambutol

Visual toxicity from ethambutol, one of the newer antituberculosis drugs, is usually an early sign of drug intoxication. Loss of color vision is the first sign of this toxicity, and all patients taking the drug should be screened periodically with the HRR plates. After he develops a color defect, the patient develops a cecocentral field defect. Even these defects should be reversible if they have not progressed to an advanced stage.

Favism

For years favism was thought to occur only among people living in Mediterranean areas and eating fava beans. It is now known to occur also in the United States. In susceptible persons, ingestion of fava beans causes hemolytic anemia. The retinal signs of favism are those of hemorrhage secondary to increased coagulation. The increased hemolysis of the red blood cells causes a thromboplastin-like activity in the blood that leads to increased coagulation.

Iodochlorhydroxyquin (Entero-Vioform)

This drug is commonly used outside the United States for treatment of diarrhea. In recent years frequent reports have detailed the toxic effects of this drug, including optic neuritis. A carefully taken history of patients who have traveled outside the United States may reveal exposure to this medication.

Antimetabolic Agents

Antimetabolic agents have many undesirable side effects, which are all too common. Ocular side effects are rare except for the secondary cataracts and secondary glaucoma associated with steroid therapy. Vincristine not uncommonly causes peripheral neuropathies with paresthesias of the extremities and a decrease of the deep tendon reflexes. It also causes abdominal pain and convulsions. Eye signs are rare, but optic neuritis has been reported with this drug in particular.

Ketogenic Diets

The ketogenic diet has become a popular adjunctive form of therapy in children with inadequate control of epilepsy. The mechanism of this diet is thought to be through the production of ketone bodies which help to decrease the excitability of cerebral tissues. This diet is much more effective in children since their cerebral cortex has a greater ability to oxidize ketone bodies as the metabolic substrate than does the adult cortex. The systemic reactions are usually minimal and limited to occasional vomiting, diarrhea, and abdominal pain. Ketone diets are deficient in vitamin B. As the carbohydrate intake decreases, there is a concomitant decrease in thiamine requirement. Therefore, we do not see the usual thiamine deficiency syndrome of Wernicke's encephalopathy in these children. Infrequent cases of optic neuritis have been reported; however, optic neuritis and Wernicke syndrome can be seen in any prolonged diet regimen without vitamin supplements, particularly, in the adult population, who do not handle ketones as well as do children.

OPACITIES OF THE MEDIA

Most opacities of the media involve the lens, with cataract leading the list. It is amazing that most people with nuclear sclerosis cataract and a decrease in acuity rarely notice their loss unless it is severe, whereas persons with a small degree of posterior subcapsular cataract complain bitterly of it.

Dislocation of the lens can result from trauma. It also occurs in congenital syphilis, homocystinuria, and Marfan syndrome.

Vitreous degeneration is almost as common a problem as cataract. The degeneration causes parts of the vitreous humor to become visible to the patient, and if the degeneration is extensive, the patient's vision is slightly blurred. The prime cause of the degeneration is age. Myopia and chronic inflammations are the next most common causes.

Hemorrhages into the vitreous humor may herald the onset of retinal tears and detachment. If diabetes or angiomas are present, the hemorrhages come from abnormal vessels. A detailed look at the retina will readily identify the cause. Frequently, the hemorrhages are so severe that the retina is obscured. Continued observation of the patient as the hemorrhages clear eventually affords an adequate view of the fundus. If an earlier decision is desired as to whether a retinal detachment is present, ultrasonography can be employed. Examination of the fellow eye may reveal signs of diabetes or peripheral retinal degeneration that is most likely caused by retinal detachment.

Corneal opacities may be caused by corneal dystrophy, bullous keratopathy, or band keratopathy. Band keratopathy may be seen in defects of calcium metabolism, chronic uveitis with secondary corneal decompensation, or juvenile rheumatoid arthritis.

Numerous retinal causes of blurred vision also exist. Unsuspected diabetes or hypertension, conditions that the ophthalmologist may be the first to diagnose, are among them.

REFRACTIVE ERRORS

The person who experiences normal changes in refractive errors usually does not complain to the ophthalmologist about acute loss of vision. In some diseases associated with a slow change in visual acuity, however, the person interprets the problem as a sign that he needs a change in his prescription. The following paragraphs describe the diseases that cause hyperopic, myopic, and astigmatic changes.

In my experience, hyperopic changes caused by disease are the least common ones, usually because the retinal rods and cones are moved into a more anterior plane, without their ability to function being materially affected. This situation occurs in posterior scleritis or with retrobulbar masses that indent the posterior part of the globe. A refraction of both eyes shows a difference in refractive error, which indicates the reasons for the blurred vision (although it is not absolute proof). Horizontal striae at the posterior pole are more commonly seen in tumors of the muscle cone, but may also occur with the edema of posterior scleritis. (see Fig. 4–6).

Retinal edema is not always easily observed. Central serous retinopathy with some degree of hyperopia can be one of the more difficult forms of retinal edema to identify. Patients with this condition usually have only modest decreases in vision. Because of the slight retinal elevation, they may complain of distortion, which can best be evaluated by means of the Amsler grid. The retinal edema in central serous retinopahty is not as easily seen with the opthalmoscope as it is in branch artery occlusion. The slit lamp and the fundus contact lens must be used. With the ophthalmoscope, it is difficult to differentiate central serous retinopathy from detachment of the pigment epithelium. I often use fluorescein angiography in making the differential diagnosis.

Myopic changes occur more commonly. Spasm of accommodation is frequently a cause in young women. A comparison of the manifest refraction and the cycloplegic refraction establishes the diagnosis. Diabetes also causes myopia owing to the lens changes characteristic of this disease. Cataracts from whatever cause, particularly nuclear sclerosis cataracts, cause myopia. Chronic use of the sulfonamides can cause myopia, by a mechanism that is not understood. The mechanism is not ciliary muscle spasm because atropine does not relieve the condition. Diamox and the thiazide compounds, closely related to the sulfonamides, may also cause myopia. As mentioned, patients with Marfan syndrome have increased curvature of the lens, which causes myopia. A partially anteriorly subluxated lens, as in Marfan syndrome or homocystinuria, shows a myopic shift. Trauma to the globe can also cause shallowing of the anterior chamber with anterior displacement of the lens-iris diaphragm and a myopic change.

Astigmatism is associated with corneal diseases, such as keratoconus and peripheral corneal dystrophy (for example, furrow dystrophy), which place unequal stresses on the cornea. Keratometer readings, Placido's disc testing, and careful slit lamp evaluations will identify the cause. Cataract formation, as well as the healing of incisions for cataract operations, can result in astigmatism. Lid tumors and, occasionally, chalazions can press on the eye and create astigmatism. Increase in accommodation from the rest position to the reading distance at near increases astigmatism by 10%. Ciliary muscle spasm can also cause astigmatism because of the unequal pull on the ciliary muscles in the lens.

BIBLIOGRAPHY

Anderson, D., and Khalil, M.: Meningioma and the ophthalmologist. Ophthalmology 88:1004, 1981.

Archambeau, P.L., Hollenhorst, R.W., and Rucker, C.W.: Uveitis a manifestation of multiple sclerosis. Proc. Mayo Clin. 40:544, 1965.

Balkan, R.J., et al.: Loss of central visual acuity after laser peripheral iridectomy. Ann. Ophthalmol. 14:721, 1982.

Berger, J.R., and Sheremata, W.A.: Persistant neurological deficit precipitated by hot bath test in multiple sclerosis. JAMA 249:1751, 1983.

Bicknell, J.M., and Holland, J.V.: Neurologic manifestations of Cogan's syndrome. Neurology 28:278, 1978.

Bilchik, R.C., Muller-Bergh, H.A., and Frishman, M.E.: Ischemic retinopathy due to CO poisoning. Arch. Ophthalmol. 86:142, 1971.

Bird, A.C., Nolan, B., and Gargano, F.P.: Unruptured aneurysm of the supraclinoid carotid artery. Neurology 20:445, 1970.

Bodian, M.: Transient loss of vision following head trauma. N.Y. State J. Med. 64:916, 1964.

Bradley, W.G., and Whitty, C.W.M.: Acute optic neuritis: prognosis for development of multiple sclerosis. J. Neurol. Neurosurg. Psychiatry 31;10, 1968.

Brown, G.C., Shields, J.A., and Goldberg, R.E.: Congenital pits of the optic nerve head. II. Clinical studies in humans. Ophthalmology 87:51, 1980.

Brucker, A.J.: Disk and peripheral retinal neovascularization secondary to talc and cornstarch emboli. Am. J. Ophthalmol. 88:864, 1979.

Brunt, P.W., and McKusick, V.A.: Familial dysautonomia. Medicine (Baltimore) 49:343, 1970.

Caltrides, N.C., et al.: Retinal emboli in patients with mitral valve prolapse. Am. J. Ophthalmol. 90:534, 1980.

Carroll, F.D.: Alcohol amblyopia, pellagra, polyneuritis: report of ten cases. Arch. Ophthalmol. 16:919, 1936.

Carroll, F.D.: The etiology and treatment of tobacco-alcohol amblyopia. Am. J. Ophthalmol. 27:713, 1944.

Carroll, W.M., and Mastaglia, F.L.: Leber's optic neuropathy. Brain 102:559, 1979.

Casey, E.B., Jellife, A.M., LeQuesne, P.M., and Millet, Y.L.: Vincristine neuropathy. Brain 96:69, 1973.

Chumbley, L.C., and Kearns, T.P.: Retinopathy of sarcoidosis. Am.J. Ophthalmol. 73:123, 1972.

Cogan, D.G., and Wray, S.H.: Vascular occlusions in the eye from cardiac myxoma. Am. J. Ophthalmol. 80:396, 1975.

Cohen, D.N., and Smith, T.R.: Skip areas in temporal arteritis: myth versus fact. Trans. Am. Acad. Ophthalmol. Otolaryngol. 78:772, 1974.

Collins, R.C., Hamid Al-Mondhiry, M.B., and Chernick, M.L.: Neurologic manifestations of intravascular coagulation in patients with cancer. Neurology 25:795, 1975.

Coppeto, J., and Lessell, S.: Retinopathy in systemic lupus erythematosus. Arch. Ophthalmol. 95:794, 1977.

Corbett, J.J., Butler, A.B., and Kaufman, B.: Sneeze syncope, basilar invagination and Arnold-Chiari Type I malformation. J. Neurol. Neurosurg. Psychiatry 39:381, 1976.

Cowan, C.L., and Knox, D.L.: Migraine optic neuropathy. Ann. Ophthalmol. 14:164, 1982.

Crouse, S.K., and Berg, B.O.: Intracranial meningiomas in childhood and adolescence. Neurol. 22:135, 1972.

Daroff, R.B., and Smith, J.L.: Intraocular optic neuritis with normal visual acuity. Neurology 15:409, 1965.

Davis, L.E., Harms, A.C., and Chin, T.D.Y.: Transient cortical blindness and cerebellar ataxis associated with mumps. Arch. Ophthalmol. 85:366, 1971.

Dodge, P.R., and Griffith, J.F.: Some transient ocular manifestations of neurologic disease in children. Neuro-ophthalmology Symposium of the University of Miami and Bascom Palmer Eye Institute. Vol. III. Edited by J. L. Smith. St. Louis, C.V. Mosby Co., 1967, p. 316.

Dougal, M.A., Evans, L.S., McClellan, K.R., and Robinson, J.: Central retinal artery occlusion in systemic lupus erythematosus. Ann. Ophthalmol. 15:38, 1983.

Douglas, A.C., and Maloney, A.F.: Sarcoidosis of the central nervous system. J. Neurol. Neurosurg. Psychiatry. 36:1024, 1973.

Drance, S.M. et al.: Studies of factors involved in the production of low tension glaucoma. Arch. Ophthalmol. 89:457, 1973.

Drance, S.M., Morgan, R.W., and Sweeney, V.P.: Shock-induced optic neuropathy. A cause of nonprogressive glaucoma. N. Engl. J. Med. 288:392, 1973.

Dugdale, M., and Masi, A.T.: Hormonal contraception and thromboembolic disease: effects of the oral contraceptives on hemostatic mechanism. J. Chron. Dis. 23:775, 1971.

Edwards, W.C., and Layden, W.E.: Optic nerve hypoplasia. Am. J. Ophthalmol. 70:950, 1970.

Efron, R.: An extension of the Pulfrich stereoscopic effect. Brain 86:295, 1963.

Ellenberger, C., Keltner, J.L., and Burde, R.M.: Acute optic neuropathy in older patients. Arch. Neurol. 28:182, 1973.

Emery, J.M., Green, W.R., and Huff, D.S.: Krabbe's disease. Am. J. Ophthalmol. 74:400, 1972.

Enos, W.F., Pierre, R.V., and Rosenblatt, J.E.: Giant cell arteritis detected by bone marrow biopsy. Mayo Clin. Proc. 56:381, 1981.

Feinsod, M., and Hoyt, W.F.: Subclinical optic neuropathy in multiple sclerosis. J. Neurol. Neurosurg. Psychiatry 38:1109, 1975.

Finelli, P.F.: Sickle cell trait and transient monocular blindness. Am. J. Ophthalmol. 81:850, 1976.

Ford, R.G., and Siekert, R.G.: Central nervous system manifestations of periarteritis nodosa. Neurology 15:114, 1965.

Foulds, W.S., Cant, J.S., and Chisholm, I.A.: Hydroxycobalamin in the treatment of Leber's hereditary optic atrophy. Lancet 1:896, 1968.

Frisen, L., and Hoyt, W.F.: Insidious atrophy of retinal nerve fibers in multiple sclerosis. Arch. Ophthalmol. 92:91, 1974.

Frisen, L., Hoyt, W.F., Bird, A.C., and Weale, R.: Implications of the Pulfrich phenomenon. Lancet 2:385, 1973.

Fukado, Y.: Decompression of the optic nerve. Neurol. Surg. (Tokyo) 4:1137, 1976.

Futty, D.E., et al.: Cooperative study of hospital frequency and character of transient ischemic attacks: V. Symptoms Analysis. JAMA 238:2386, 1977.

Galligoni, F., Iraci, G., and Marin, G.: Fibromuscular hyperplasia of the extracranial internal carotid artery. J. Neurosurg. 34:647, 1971.

Gardner, H.B. and Irvine, A.R.: Optic nerve hypoplasia with good visual acuity. Arch. Ophthalmol. 88:255, 1972.

Gass, J.D.M.: Serous detachment of the macular secondary to congenital pit of the optic nerve head. Am. J. Ophthalmol. 67:821, 1969.

Gay, A.J., and Rosenbaum, A.L.: Retinal artery pressure in asymmetric diabetic retinopathy. Arch. Ophthalmol. 75:758, 1966.

Glaser, J.S.: Clincal evaluation of optic nerve function. Trans. Ophthalmol. Soc. U.K. 96:359, 1976.

Glaser, J.S., Hoyt, W.F., and Corbett, J.: Visual morbidity with chiasmal glioma. Arch. Ophthalmol. 85:3, 1971.

Goldstein, J.E., and Cogan, D.G.: Exercise and the optic neuropathy of multiple sclerosis. Arch. Ophthalmol. 72:168, 1964.

Gowers, W.R.: Simultaneous embolism of central retinal and middle cerebral arteries. Lancet 2:794, 1875.

Griffen, J.F. and Wray, S.H.: Acquired color vision defects in retrobulbar neuritis. Am. J. Ophthalmol. 86:193, 1978.

Griffiths, J.D., and Smith, B.: Optic atrophy following Caldwell Luc procedure. Arch. Ophthalmol. 86:15, 1971.

Hackett, E.R., et al.: Optic neuritis in systemic lupus erythema*osus. Arch. Neurol. 31:9, 1974.

Halliday, A., and McDonald, W.: Pathophysiology of demyelinating disease. Br. Med. Bull. 33:21, 1977.

Halliday, A., McDonald, W. and Mushin, J.: Visual evoked responses in diagnosis of multiple sclerosis. Br. Med. J. 4:661, 1973.

Hart, R.G., and Carter, J.E.: Pseudotumor cerebri and facial pain. Arch. Neurol. 39:440, 1982.

Hayreh, S.S.: Anterior ischemic optic neuropathy. I. Terminology and pathogenesis. Br. J. Ophthalmol. 58:955, 1974.

Hayreh, S.S.: Anterior ischemic optic neuropathy. 2. Fundus on ophthalmoscopy and fluorescein angiography. Br. J. Ophthalmol. 58:964, 1974.

Hayreh, S.S.: Anterior ischemic optic neuropathy. 3. Treatment, prophylaxis and differential diagnosis. Br. J. Ophthalmol. 58:981, 1974.

Hedges, T.R.: Retinal atheromatous plaques; their recognition by elevating the intraocular pressure. Trans. Am. Ophthalmol. Soc. 74:172, 1976.

Hedges, T.R., McAllister, R., and Coriell, L.L.: Metastatic endophthalmitis as a complication of meningococci meningitis. Arch. Ophthalmol. 55:503, 1956.

Henkind, P.: Sarcoidosis: an expanding ophthalmic horizon. J. Roy. Soc. Med. 75:153, 1982.

Hirsowitz, S., and Saffer, D.: Hemiplegia and the billowing mitral leaf syndrome. J. Neurol. Neurosurg. Psychiatry 41:381, 1978.

Hoden, H.C.: Metastatic endophthalmitis associated with epidemic cerebro-spinal meningitis. Am. J. Ophthalmol. 1:647, 1918.

Hoeppner, T., and Lolas, F.: Visual evoked responses and visual symptoms in multiple sclerosis. J. Neurol. Neurosurg. Psychiatry 41:493, 1978.

Hoff, J.T., and Patterson, R.H.: Craniopharyngiomas in children and adults. J. Neurosurg. 36:299, 1972.

Hollenhorst, R.W.: Carotid and vertebral-basilar arterial stenosis and occlusion: neuroophthalmologic considerations. Trans. Am. Acad. Ophthalmol. Otolaryngol. 66:166, 1962.

Hollenhorst, R.W.: Effect of posture on retinal ischemia from temporal arteritis. Trans. Am. Ophthalmol. Soc. 65:94, 1967.

Hollenhorst, R.W., Jr., Hollenhorst, R.W., Sr., and MacCarty, C.S.: Visual prognosis of optic nerve sheath meningiomas producing shunt vessels of the optic disk: the Hoyt-Spencer syndrome. Trans. Am. Ophthalmol. Soc. 75:140, 1977.

Hollenhorst, R.W., and Wagener, H.D.: Loss of vision after distant hemorrhage. Am. J. Med. Sci. 218:209, 1950.

Hoyt, C.S., and Billson, F.A.: Optic neuropathy in ketogenic diet. Br. J. Ophthalmol. 63:191, 1979.

Hoyt, W.F.: Funduscopy of the retinal nerve fiber layer in neurosurgical practice. Neurol. Med. Chirurg. 13:3, 1973.

Hoyt, W.F., and Baghdassarian, S.A.: Optic glioma of childhood. Br. J. Ophthalmol. 53:793, 1969.

Hoyt, W.F., Fresin, L., and Neuman, N.M.: Funduscopy of nerve fiber layer defects in glaucoma. Invest. Ophthalmol. 12:814, 1973.

Hutchinson, W.M.: Acute optic neuritis and the prognosis for multiple sclerosis. J. Neurol. Neurosurg. Psychiatry 39:283, 1976.

Hyam, J.W.: Oculomotor palsy following dental anesthesia. Arch. Ophthalmol. 94:1281, 1976.

Jampol, L.M., Wong, A.S., and Albert, D.M.: Atrial myxoma and central retinal artery occlusion. Am. J. Ophthalmol. 75:242, 1973.

Jarrett, F., and McHugh, W.: Transient ischemic attacks, asymptomatic bruits and carotid endarterectomy. JAMA 239:2027, 1978.

Kalendovsky, Z., Austin, J., and Steele, P.: Increased platelet aggregability in young patients with stroke. Arch. Neurol. 32:13, 1975.

Kalina, R.E., and Mills, R.P.: Acquired hyperopia with choroidal folds. Ophthalmol. 87:44, 1980.

Kearns, T.P.: Changes in the ocular fundus in blood diseases. Med. Clin. North Am. 40:1209, 1956.

Kearns, T.P.: Ophthalmology and carotid artery. Am. J. Ophthalmol. 88:714, 1979.

Kearns, T.P., Younge, B.R., and Piepgras, D.G.: Resolution of venous stasis retinopathy after carotid artery bypass surgery. Mayo Clin. Proc. 55:342, 1980.

Kennedy, C., and Carroll, F.D.: Optic neuritis in children. Arch. Ophthalmol. 63:747, 1960.

Ketz, E., and Gaspar, B.: Intracerebral fibromuscular dysplasia (second case of involvement of the posterior cerebral artery). Neuro-ophthalmology 1:281, 1981.

Khurana, R.K., et al.: Shy-Drager syndrome: Diagnosis and treatment of cholinergic dysfunction. Neurology 30:805, 1980.

Kjer, P.: Hereditary infantile optic atrophy with dominant transmission. Dan. Med. Bull. 3:135, 1956.

Klatte, E.C., Franken, E.A., and Smith, J.A.: The radiographic spectrum in neurofibromatosis. Semin. Roentgenol. 11:17, 1976.

Klein, R.G., et al.: Skip lesions in temporal arteritis. Proc. Mayo clin. 51:504, 1976.

Klewin, K.M., Appen, R.E., and Kaufman, P.L.: Amaurosis and blood loss. Am. J. Ophthalmol. 86:669, 1978.

Knight, C.L., and Hoyt, W.F.: Monocular blindness from drusen of the optic disk. Am. J. Ophthalmol. 73:890, 1972.

Kosnik, E., Paulson, C.W., and LaGuna, J.F.: Postictal blindness. Neurology 26:248, 1976.

Kothandaram, P., Dawson, B.H., and Kroyt, R.C.: Carotid-ophthalmic aneurysm. J. Neurosurg. 34:544, 1971.

Krill, A.E., and Fishman, G.A.: Acquired color vision defects. Trans. Am. Acad. Ophthalmol. Otolaryngol. 75:1095, 1971.

Levisohn, P.M., Mikhael, M.A., and Rothman, S.M.: Cerebrovascular changes in neurofibromatosis. Dev. Med. Child Neurol. 20:789, 1978.

Lyle, T.K., and Wybar, K.: Retinal vasculitis. Br. J. Ophthalmol. 45:778, 1961.

Malhotra, A.S., and Goren, H.: The hot bath test in the diagnosis of multiple sclerosis. JAMA 246:1113, 1981.

Masi, A.T., and Dugdale, M.: Cerebrovascular diseases associated with the use of oral contraceptives. Ann. Intern. Med. 72:111, 1970.

McDonald, W.I.: Conduction in the optic nerve. Trans. Ophthalmol. Soc. U.K. 96:352, 1976.

McLeod, J.G., and Penny, R.: Vincristine neuropathy: an electrophysiological and histological study. J. Neurol. Neurosurg. Psychiatry 32:297, 1969.

Meadows, S.P.: Temporal or giant cell arteritis. Proc. R. Soc. Med. 59:329, 1966.

Meadows, S.P.: Temporal or giant cell arteritis. Neuro-opthalmology Symposium of the University of Miami and Bascom Palmer Eye Institute. Vol. 4. Edited by J.L. Smith. St. Louis, C.V. Mosby Co., 1968, p. 148.

Meadows, S.P.: Retrobulbar and optic neuritis in childhood and adolescence. Trans. Ophthalmol. Soc. U.K. 89:603, 1969.

Michelson, J.B., Michelson, P.E., Bordin, G.M., and Chesari, E.V.: Ocular reticulum cell sarcoma. Am. J. Ophthalmol. 73:431, 1972.

Miller, G.R., and Smith, J.L.: Ischemic optic neuropathy. Am. J. Ophthalmol. 62:103, 1966.

Morganroth, J., Deisseroth, A., and Winokur, S.: Differentiation of carcinomatosis and bilateral meningitis. Neurology 22:1240, 1972.

Mustonen, E., and Varonen, T.: Congenital pit of the optic nerve head associated with serous detachment of the macula. Acta Ophthalmologia 50:689, 1972.

Nagpal, K.C., et al.: Conjunctival sickling sign, hemoglobin S and irreversibly sickled erythrocytes. Arch. Ophthalmol. 95:808, 1977.

Neelon, F.A., Gorel, J.A., and Lebovitz, H.E.: The primary empty sella: clinical and radiographic characteristics and endocrine function. Medicine 52:73, 1973.

Neetens, A., Hendratay, Y., and VanRompaey, J.: Pattern and flash evoked responses in disseminated and selective optic pathway damage. Trans. Ophthalmol. Soc. U.K. 99:103, 1979.

Neupert, J.R., Brukaer, R.F., Kearns, T.P., and Sundt, T.M.: Rapid resolution of venous stases retinopathy after carotid endarterectomy. Am. J. Ophthalmol. 81:600, 1976.

Nichols, C.W., et al.: Conjunctival biopsy as an aid in the evaluation of the patient with suspected sarcoidosis. Ophthalmology 87:287, 1980.

Nikoskelainen, E.: symptoms, signs and early course of optic neuritis. Acta Ophthalmologica 53:254, 1975.

Nikoskelainen, E., Sogg, R.L., and Rosenthal, R.: The

early phase in Leber's hereditary optic atrophy. Arch. Ophthalmol. *95*:969, 1977.

Nilsson, B.Y.: Visual evoked responses in multiple sclerosis: comparison of two methods for pattern reversal. J. Neurol. Neurosurg. Psychiatry *41*:499, 1978.

Obrador, S.: The empty sella and some related syndromes. J. Neurosurg. *36*:162, 1972.

Okawara, S.H.: Warning signs prior to rupture of an intracranial aneurysm. J. Neurosurg. *38*:575, 1973.

Oliver, M., Beller, A.J., and Behar, A.: Chiasmal arachnoiditis as a manifestation of generalized arachnoiditis in systemic vascular disease. Br. J. Ophthalmol. *52*:227, 1968.

Page, L.K., Tyler, H.R., and Shillito., J.: Neurosurgical experiences with herpes simplex encephalitis. J. Neurosurg. *27*:346, 1967.

Palacios, E., and MacGree, E.E.: The radiographic diagnosis of trigeminal neurenomas. J. Neurosurg. *36*:153, 1972.

Palestine, A.G., Younge, B.R., and Piepgras, D.G.: Visual prognosis in carotid cavernous fistula. Arch. Ophthalmol. *99*:1600, 1981.

Patterson, V.H., and Heron, J.R.: Visual field abnormalities in multiple sclerosis. J. Neurol. Neurosurg. Psychiatry *43*:205, 1980.

Pellock J.M., et al. Childhood hypertensive stroke with neurofibromatosis. Neurology *30*:657, 1980.

Percy, A.K., Nobrega, F.T., and Kurland, L.T.: Optic neuritis and multiple sclerosis: an epidemiologic study. Arch. Ophthalmol. *87*:135, 1972.

Perkins, E.S.: Ocular sarcoidoses. Arch. Ophthalmol. *99*:1193, 1981.

Peterson, K.A.: Optic nerve hypoplasia with good visual acuity. Arch. Ophthalmol. *95*:254, 1977.

Rasminsky, M.: The effects of temperature on conduction in demyelinated single nerve fibers. Arch. Neurol. *28*:287, 1973.

Rucker, W.C.: Sheathing of the retinal veins in multiple sclerosis. Proc. Mayo Clin. *19*:176, 1944.

Rucker, W.C., and Kearns, T.P.: Mistaken diagnosis in some cases of meningioma. Clinics in Perimetry, No. 5. Am. J. Ophthalmol. *51*:15, 1961.

Sack, G. H., Levin, J., and Bell, W.R.: Trousseau's syndrome and other manifestations of chronic disseminated coagulopathy in patients with neoplasm. Clinical pathophysiologic and therapeutic features. Medicine (Baltimore) *56*:1, 1977.

Sandberg-Wollkeim, M.: Optic neuritis: studies with cerebrospinal fluid in relation to clinical course in 61 patients. Acta Neurol. Scandinav. *52*:167, 1975.

Sandersen, P.A., and Kuwabara, T.: Optic-neuropathy presumably caused by vincristine therapy. Am. J. Ophthalmol. *81*:146, 1976.

Sartwell, P.E., et al.: Thromboembolism and oral contraceptives: an epidemiologic case-control study. Am. J. Epidemiol. *90*:365, 1969.

Sauer, C., and Levinsohn, M.U.: Horner's syndrome in childhood. Neurology *26*:216, 1976.

Scott, G.I.: Neuromyelitis optica. Am. J. Ophthalmol. *35*:755, 1952.

Sears, M.L.: Choroidal and retinal detachments associated with scleritis. Am. J. Ophthalmol. *58*:764, 1964.

Sengupta, R.P., Gryspeerdt, G.L., and Hankinson, J.: Carotid-ophthalmic aneurysm. J. Neurol. Neurosurg. Psychiatry *39*:837, 1976.

Severin, S.L., Tour, R.L., and Kershaw, R.H.: Macular function and the photostress test 1. Arch. Ophthalmol. *77*:2, 1967.

Severin, S.L. Tour, R.L., and Kershaw, R.H.: Macular function and the photostress test 2. Arch. Ophthalmol. *77*:163, 1967.

Sharpe, J.A., et al.: Methanol optic neuropathy: a histopathological study. Neurology. *32*:1093, 1982.

Simmons, R.J., and Cogan, D.G.: Occult temporal arteritis. Arch. Ophthalmol. *68*:8, 1962.

Slagsnold, J.E.: Pulfrich pendulum phenomenon in patients with a history of acute optic neuritis. Acta Ophthalmologica *56*:817, 1978.

Smith, J.L.: Central retinal and internal carotid artery occlusion. Arch. Ophthalmol. *65*:550, 1961.

Smith, J.L.: Cortical blindness in congenital hydrocephalus. Neuro-ophthalmology Symposium of the University of Miami and Bascom Palmer Eye Institute. Vol. III. Edited by J.L. Smith. St. Louis, C.V. Mosby Co., 1967, p. 211.

Smith, J.L., Hoyt, W.F., and Susac, J.C.: Ocular fundus in acute Leber optic neuropathy. Ophthalmol. *90*:349, 1973.

Sorr, E.M., and Goldberg, R.E.: Traumatic central retinal artery occlusion with sickle cell trait. Am. J. Ophthalmol. *80*:648, 1975.

Spencer, W.F., and Hoyt, W.F.: A fatal case of giant cell arteritis (temporal or cranial arteritis) with ocular involvement. Arch. Ophthalmol. *64*:862, 1960.

Stansbury, F.C.: Neuromyelitis optica (Devic's disease) (review). Arch. Ophthalmol. *42*:292, 1949.

Sypert, G.W., Luffman, H., and Ojemann, G.A.: Occult normal pressure hydrocephalus manifested by parkinsonism-dementia complex. Neurology *23*:234, 1973.

Taub, R.G., and Rucker, C.W.: Relationship of retrobulbar neuritis to multiple sclerosis. Am. J. Ophthalmol. *37*:494, 1954.

Taugher, P.J.: Visual loss after cardiopulmonary bypass. Am. J. Ophthalmol. *81*:280, 1976.

Thompson, J.E., and Talkington, C.M.: Carotid endarterectomy. Ann. Surg. *184*:1, 1976.

Tso, M.O.: Pathology and pathogenesis of drusen of the optic nervehead. Ophthalmology *88*:1066, 1981.

Van Dalen, J.T.W., and Greve, E.L.: Visual field defects in multiple sclerosis. Neuro-ophthalmology *2*:93, 1981.

Victor, M.: Tobacco-alcohol amblyopia. A critique of current concepts of this disorder, with special reference to the role of nutritional deficiency in its causation. Arch. Ophthalmol. *70*:313, 1963.

Waardenburg, P.J.: Leber's optic-atrophy and the opinions of Ruth Lundsgaard. Ophthalmologica *115*:369, 1948.

Wald, G., and Burian, H.M.: The dissociation of form and light perception in stabismic amblyopia. Am. J. Ophthalmol. *27*:950, 1944.

Walsh, F.B., Clark, D.B., Thompson, R.S., and Nicholson, D.H.: Oral contraceptives and neuro-opthalmologic interest. Arch. Opthalmol. *74*:628, 1965.

Walsh, T.J., Smith, J.L., and Shipley, T.: Neurologic blindness in infancy. Neuro-ophthalmology Symposium of the University of Miami and Bascom Palmer Eye Institute. Vol. III. Edited by J.L. Smith. St. Louis, C.V. Mosby Co., 1967, p. 200.

Weber, M.B.: The neurological complications of consumption coagulopathies. Neurology *18*:185, 1968.

Welch, R., and Maumanee, A.E.: Pars planitis. Arch. Ophthalmol. *64*:540, 1960.

Weleber, R.G., and Shults, W.T.: Digoxin retinal toxicity. Arch. Ophthalmol. *99*:1568, 1981.

Wertham, F.: The cerebral lesions in purulent meningitis. Arch. Neurol. Psychiatry *26*:549, 1931.

Wilkinson, I.M.S., and Russell, R.W.R.: Arteries of the head and neck in giant cell arteritis. A pathological study to show the patterns of arterial involvement. Arch. Neurol. *27*:378, 1972.

Wilson, R.S., and Ruiz, R.S.: Bilateral central retinal artery occlusion in homocystinuria. Arch. Ophthalmol. *82*:267, 1969.

Woldoff, H.S., Gerber, M., and Desser, K.B.: Retinal vascular visions in two patients with prolapsed mitral valve leaflets. Am. J. Ophthalmol. *79*:382, 1975.

Womack, L.W., and Liesegang, T.J.: Complications of herpes zoster ophthalmicus. Arch. Ophthalmol. *101*:42, 1983.

Yasargil, M.G.: Diagnosis and indications for operations in cerebrovascular occlusive disease. *In* Microsurgery applied to Neurosurgery. Edited by M.G. Yasargil. Stuttgart, George Theime Verlag, 1969.

Yasargil, M.G., Kraginbuhl, H.A., and Jacobson, J.H.: Microsurgical arterial reconstruction. Surgery *67*:221, 1970.

Zalka, K.A., et al.: Opticociliary veins in a primary optic nerve sheath meningioma. Am. J. Ophthalmol. *87*:91, 1979.

Zeki, S.M.: Colour coding in Rhesus monkey prestriate cortex. Brain Res. *53*:422, 1973.

Chapter 14

Headache

THOMAS J. WALSH

Headache is one of the most common complaints that the physician hears, particularly the ophthalmologist. Many patients are referred to the ophthalmologist because of the belief that pain in and around the eye represents purely ocular disease or that refractive errors are a frequent cause of headaches.

Since headache is so frequent a complaint, most physicians treat it with various analgesics or tranquilizers, without even asking the patient the most basic of questions to identify the cause. The vast majority of headaches are psychogenic in origin, but even the tension headache may be made up of factors that, if identified, could be treated or eliminated. A carefully taken history can often identify these factors (among them, diet, allergy, sinus disease).

A complete review of all causes of headache is not the intent of this chapter, but rather discussions of (1) the pain-sensitive anatomic structures pertinent to headache, (2) the evaluation of the patient with headache, and (3) the types of headache, including the symptoms and physical findings peculiar to each. The discussions are confined to those types of headaches that are common and easily identified or that have a specific treatment.

PAIN-SENSITIVE ANATOMIC STRUCTURES

The skin that covers the cranium and a limited number of intracranial structures are the pain-sensitive structures related to headache. (The cranium itself is insensitive.) The periosteum has varying sensitivity to pain.

All the pain-sensitive structures in the anterior fossa and the middle fossa are supplied by the fifth cranial nerve, which is also the sensory nerve for the ocular structures.

The middle meningeal artery, a branch of the internal carotid artery, is the primary vascular supply to the supratentorial dura, except over the floor of the anterior fossa. The floor of the anterior fossa and the anterior pole of the brain are supplied by branches of the anterior and posterior ethmoidal arteries, as well as by the cavernous portion of the internal carotid artery. These arteries, which are particularly pain-sensitive, frequently refer pain to the forehead above the ipsilateral eye or in and behind that eye, thus suggesting an ocular cause for the condition being investigated.

The dura also varies in its sensitivity to pain. Stimulation of the floor of the anterior fossa sometimes causes pain in the ocular region. The dura of the orbit and sphenoid ridge is only moderately pain sensitive. Pressure to the superior surface of the tentorium, as well as to the dura of the sella, causes pain over the ipsilateral forehead and eye.

The great venous sinuses, which are reflections of the dura, are also pain-sensitive structures. The superior sagittal sinus, especially, refers pain to the ipsilateral eye.

The third ventricle and both lateral ventricles refer pain to the ocular region or to the forehead when they are suddenly distended or decompressed.

The ninth through twelfth cranial nerves and the upper cervical nerves refer pain to the vertex and suboccipital area. The ninth and tenth cranial nerves, which supply part of the sensory innervation to the posterior fossa, occasionally refer pain to the throat and ear.

EVALUATION OF THE PATIENT

The physician must use all his history taking skill in evaluating the patient with headache. He must be complete in his history taking, skilled in evaluating the patient's responses, and alert to avenues of exploration that might open up during the history taking. Investigating a complaint of headache is time consuming and challenging.

History of Headache

Severity and Duration of Headache

In taking the patient's history, the logical first questions are: How severe is the headache and how long has it been present? The severity of the headache is probably less important than its duration, since the degree of seriousness and the degree of pain are not necessarily related. However, a sudden and severe onset followed by alterations in consciousness or some other neurologic sign or symptom suggests subarachnoid hemorrhage. A severe headache preceded by a neurologic symptom (such as a visual aura) suggests migraine. A

headache that has not changed its severity or character for many years suggests a more benign cause. A change in the type or the character of the patient's headache is a cause for concern and further investigation.

Quality of Headache

A generally less helpful feature is the quality of the headache. A pulsating headache suggests a vascular origin. The tension headache is usually a dull constant ache that varies in intensity according to the daily pressures but not to the pulse. The patient with a tension headache may describe it in particular terms—as a band around the head or a pressure inside that pushes against the bones of the skull.

Location of Headache

A valuable clue to the cause of a headache may be its location. Tenderness of the scalp in the temporal region may result from an inflamed tender temporal artery suggestive of cranial arteritis, or the area may be the site of an infection or another local disease process. Jaw pain (particularly on movement) radiating to the ear or side of the skull suggests temporal arteritis or a temporomandibular joint disorder or even a dental problem. Tic douloureux causes severe pain in the region of the eye. Cluster headache may have signs and symptoms similar to those of tic douloureux, but it also has unilateral nasal symptoms and no trigger zone. As mentioned, the site of the pain is not always the site of the problem; many diverse intracranial sites refer pain to the ocular region. Wolff's review of the relationship of pain site and tumor site reveals that only about one third of brain tumors have pain over the region of the tumor.

There is an overlapping territory of sensory supply between the fifth, seventh, ninth, and tenth cranial nerves. There is also some common ground between these four cranial nerves and the upper cervical nerves. The lowest portion of the trigeminal nerve subserving sensation to the eye is adjacent to the sensory portion of the upper cervical nerves and may account for the ocular pain associated with diseases in the region of the neck. Tumors of the posterior fossa can produce bifrontal headaches, and this can occur before there is any increased intracranial pressure or displacement of intracranial structures. The tentorial nerves arise from the first or ophthalmic division of the trigeminal nerve and run along the superior edge of the tentorium. Since these nerves run on the superior surface, it would take considerable pressure and stretching from a mass lesion below to cause any pain. If ocular frontal pain occurs from tumors of much less severity in this area, another cause must be postulated. Experimental interest has shifted to the upper cervical dorsal rootlets. Stimulation of C2 does not evoke frontal or ocular pain. The dorsal root of C1, which was once considered nonexistent by anatomists, is now found to be absent in only 8% of patients. When this dorsal root is stimulated, pain in the orbital region and the midfrontal area occurs. Since a peripheral association with trigeminal nerves to the orbit is unknown, a central association with the descending tract and nucleus of the trigeminal nerve is postulated. For example, tumors of the cerebellum commonly cause the cerebellar tonsils to be displaced through the foramen magnum; frequently, they may be displaced as far down as the level of C2 and thus catch the dorsal roots of C1 as they are displaced. Supratentorial lesions, on the other hand, cause the hyppocampal gyrus to herniate through the tentorial notch, where it can easily impinge on the nerves running along the superior edge of the tentorium.

Time of Onset and Frequency of Headache

The next factors to be evaluated are the time of onset and the frequency of the headache. Is the headache—even one that waxes and wanes—constant? If it is constant and also tends to worsen with the cares of the day, such as those related to the patient's job or family or school, tension is a likely cause. Migraine and cluster headaches tend to have periods when the patient has pain and periods when he is pain free. Cluster headaches, particularly, tend to come on at the same time of day. Headaches related to hypertension are present when the patient awakens and they may improve through the day. The tension headache rarely awakens the sufferer from a sound sleep although it may prolong getting to sleep or shorten the sleeping period. It is not uncommon for the person with migraine headache or cluster headache to go to bed pain free only to be aroused from deep sleep by severe pain.

Features of Onset of Headache

Significant features of the onset should be investigated. Does pain come on with a certain action (for example, touching a trigger zone, as in tic douloureux)? Do premonitory phenomena (such as scintillating scotoma or other aura) herald the onset? The migraine headache may not always be typical. The premonitory signs of migraine may not always be visual; they may be gastrointestinal, with nausea and vomiting or an acute awareness of noisome smells. Persons with cluster headache frequently have an associated Horner syndrome and prominent unilateral nasal stuffiness. Ask the patient whether the onset of the headache is associated with some feature of his job or with a social habit (such as smoking).

Sudden irregular onset of severe headache associated with a sixth cranial nerve paralysis suggests intermittent and sudden blocking of the aqueduct of Sylvius with acute rise in intracranial pressure, such as occurs with a colloid cyst of the third ventricle. I had a patient who had been admitted to the psychiatric service because, when he had a headache, he would hit his head against a wall to relieve the pain. During one such headache episode he was noted to have bilateral lateral rectus muscle paralysis. The paralysis was not present when the headache was absent. On investigation, he was found to have a colloid cyst of the third ventricle. At some point the patient had discovered that jarring his head relieved the headache pain. The banging dislodged the colloid cyst from the aqueduct opening; the patient did not understand the mechanism, only that his technique worked. A ventricular shunt was performed on the patient, and he had no further symptoms.

Associated findings in the form of a change in consciousness, seizures, or focal neurologic conditions are much more ominous signs and call for a more detailed investigation. Ask the patient's spouse or other family members about changes in the patient's personality or habits that might not be obvious in ordinary conversation with the patient. Occasionally, ophthalmoplegia occurs in migraine headache, bringing the concern that the patient is harboring an aneurysm. Headache after a severe ear infection that is followed by a lateral rectus muscle paralysis suggests Gradenigo syndrome or, more rarely, a brain abscess.

Ask the patient about any factors that relieve the headache. Headaches associated with increased intracranial pressure can be worsened by coughing or by the Valsalva maneuver. The worsening is not exclusively a sign of increased intracranial pressure; vascular headache occasionally may be made worse by the same mechanism. Dietary factors, such as the ingestion of certain foods or drinks, may precipitate an attack. There is some evidence that tyramine may be an exciting factor in migraine. The substance is found in cheese, vinegar, yogurt, beer, red wine, gin, vodka, and bourbon. A liberal use of monosodium glutamate, such as in Chinese cooking, may result in a recognizable headache syndrome.

People who are exposed to nitrites (for example, munitions workers) may develop headaches, even true migraine headaches. The physician should consider factors that raise the vascular pressure. Among these are sexual intercourse, the use of diet pills, and repeated performance of Valsalva maneuver (as in weight lifting), which causes intermittent decreased venous return from the cranial vault.

Some headaches, particularly those with nasal or sinus symptoms or with a history that suggests a sinus origin, may be related to changes in the weather. Headache often occurs with sudden changes in barometric conditions, such as in rapid airplane descents and rapid elevator rides. A person who lives for brief periods of time at an altitude different from his usual one (for example, the New Yorker who vacations for a week in Mexico City or Denver) or who moves from a dry climate to a moist or humid one may suffer from a headache of sinus origin.

Neck pain may be caused by tenseness of the neck muscles. The cause of the tension may be psychogenic; or, the person may be guarding against the pain of moving the neck because he has cervical disc disease or arthritis or meningeal irritation.

Knowing any factors that relieve the headache may be helpful in making a diagnosis. Examples of palliative factors are (1) avoiding touching a trigger zone and (2) avoiding eating so that the temporomandibular joint is not moved. The response of the headache to analgesics is of varying importance.

General Review of Health

Accompanying a general review of the patient's health should be a systematic review of the various body systems. Chronic loss of weight, particularly in an adult, suggests a malignancy. Loss of weight and anemia may also suggest a chronic infection, such as pyelonephritis, which may lead to hypertension and headache. Investigate the possibility of a past operation, particularly for a malignancy, that the patient may not have mentioned, perhaps because he believes—or would like to believe—that he has been cured. A recent head trauma suggests a potential for a subdural hematoma or cervical disc disease. Ask the patient whether he is being treated for a chronic disease. Medications for any treatment or any recent changes in dosage or type of therapy may be the cause of the headache.

Noting the patient's general appearance may give some valuable clues. The patient may have a hypometabolic appearance; that is, his skin may be smooth, he may be slightly obese, and he may have hair loss— all factors that suggest a pituitary gland dysfunction. On the other hand, the patient may have one of the cutaneous signs of the phakomatoses that are associated with intracranial masses. Café-au-lait spots may also suggest pheochromocytoma, with its intermittent hypertension.

Most diseases are at some stage associated with headache. To discuss all such diseases is not possible here. Suffice it to say that a careful inspection of abnormalities not immediately related to the complaint of headache may provide an important clue to the diagnosis and treatment.

Review of Body Systems

Since many headaches are located in the ocular region, it is important to review initially the complete ocular history. A history of intermittent pain with or without blurred vision or halos may represent intermittent attacks of narrow-angle glaucoma. Steady pain and redness of an eye may be signs of iritis. Pain only when the patient is reading suggests presbyopia, convergence insufficiency, or an incorrect prescription (if the prescription change has been made recently). A change in prescription that incorporates a new feature, such as correction for astigmatism, may be the cause of the headache. A change in the size of the lens, base curve, or type of bifocal may cause ocular problems. Most of these errors cause aching of the eyes, not true headaches; but the patient does not make a distinction when he presents his complaint.

Blurring of vision for a few seconds suggests the transient obscurations of increased intracranial pressure. Episodes lasting 5 to 20 minutes suggest carotid artery or vertebral basilar insufficiency. Progressive loss of vision may mean a retrobulbar mass with or without obvious exophthalmos. Decreased acuity associated with pain on movement of the eyes is consistent with optic neuritis.

Next, review the ear, nose, and throat system, searching for symptoms of chronic nasal obstruction or sinus disease or a seasonal allergic phenomenon. Has there been nasal or sinus operation, particularly a surgical procedure followed by irradiation therapy? Such a history may point to a malignancy.

In evaluating the endocrine system, ask the patient about unusual loss or gain of weight, brittleness or loss of hair, impotence, amenorrhea, polyuria, polydipsia, and changes in tolerance to temperature changes. These symptoms suggest pituitary or thyroid malfunction just as changes in skin pigmentation suggest adrenal disease. The genitourinary system should be evaluated by asking the patient questions about chronic urinary infection and kidney stones, which can lead to kidney failure and to hypertension. Symptoms of renal obstruction in men suggest prostatic carcinoma that could metastasize to the brain. Malignancy should also be suspected in women who have irregular menses or excessive and irregular vaginal bleeding.

In regard to the cutaneous system, presence of the stigmata of the phakomatoses suggests intracranial tumors.

In the cardiopulmonary system, chronic obstructive respiratory disease may cause retention of carbon dioxide with secondary headache. Intermittent hypertension suggests pheochromocytoma. Cardiac disease of many kinds may be associated with hypertension.

Family History

Knowing the family history may help to positively identify a familial type headache in the patient who does not have a fully typical headache. The migraine headache, which frequently has a familial tendency, is a case in point. A family history of phakomatoses suggests an associated intracranial mass, even if the cutaneous signs alone are not sufficient in the patient himself to point to this cause for the headache.

Personal History

This history should include questions about possible problems with the patient's marriage, children, in-laws, sexual satisfaction, finances, and use of drugs, including tobacco and alcohol. Ask the patient about his job. Is he satisfied or not with his work? Are younger persons about to displace or pass over him? Has a change in company management brought more than the usual pressure? Even if the patient is an executive, ask whether he is exposed to toxic substances. The headache may occur only when he makes a trip to the plant.

Physical Examination

This examination should be more than an examination for eyeglasses, for intraocular tension, for intraocular inflammations (using the slit lamp), and for papilledema (using the ophthalmoscope). It should include a painstaking examination for mild (perhaps asymptomatic) motility disturbances and for subtle pupillary changes, as in Horner syndrome. The physician may miss Horner syndrome in bright illumination; he should remember, too, that the patient may be masking a ptosis by furrowing his brow. The physician should evaluate all three divisions of the fifth cranial nerve, as well as corneal sensitivity. Subtle exophthalmos may be discovered only by measuring for it. Pulsations of the globe are best seen from the side rather than by looking at the eye straight on. Palpation of the orbit, which is easily performed, may reveal an orbital mass. Listen for bruits. Look for disturbances of up-gaze movements, which suggest an aqueduct of Sylvius lesion with sec-

ondary hydrocephalus and headache. Disturbances of horizontal gaze suggest a pontine location of the disease with secondary hydrocephalus owing to obstruction of the cerebrospinal fluid flow at that level. The nose and the sinuses should be examined next. The frontal and maxillary sinuses can easily be transilluminated with the Finnoff head illuminator to look for opacification. The Finnoff head illuminator with or without a nasal speculum may reveal a nasal mass that was not suspected but is now causing orbital signs and symptoms.

Next, examine the skull, looking for local signs of disease, such as the tender artery of temporal arteritis, the cranial bruits of carotid cavernous sinus fistula, or an unusual bony configuration that suggests a cranial dysostosis or acromegaly. In infants palpate open fontanelles to evaluate any increased intracranial pressure. Palpate the neck muscles for spasm. To test for weakness of the facial nerve, have the patient wrinkle his brow, smile, and keep his eyelids closed against pressure from your finger.

The eighth cranial nerve can be tested grossly by having the patient listen to the ticking or humming of a wristwatch. If he cannot hear the watch on one side, this inability, coupled with another ocular sign (such as a decreased corneal reflex and a facial and lateral rectus muscle weakness), suggests a cerebellopontine angle tumor.

Test the twelfth cranial nerve by asking the patient to stick out his tongue. Deviation of the tongue to one side indicates some involvement of the ipsilateral nerve. The combination of pain in the second division of the trigeminal nerve and twelfth nerve involvement suggests a nasopharyngeal tumor.

WEATHER VANES OF SERIOUS HEADACHES

The following signs suggest a more serious cause for the headache:

1. History of neurologic signs accompa-

nying each headache or persisting after it (for example, weakness, diplopia, or seizure).

2. Change in mentation or personality.

3. Onset of a headache different from the regular headache or onset of headache in a person usually headache-free.

4. Sudden resistance of headache to medications that had previously relieved the pain.

5. Headache that never changes location.

6. Headache associated with a fever.

7. History of a chronic or recent illness with associated headache; such a combination indicates a worsening or a complication of the illness.

8. Recurring severe headache in a child, particularly one that changes the child's play or sleeping habits.

VASCULAR HEADACHE

This type of headache comprises three groups: migraine, migraine-equivalent, and nonmigraine.

Migraine Group

It is difficult, at best, to formulate a definition of migraine headache that covers all the types of headache that, in my opinion, belong to one group. The following definition was proposed by the research group in migraine and headache of the World Federation of Neurology.

> Migraine is a familial disorder characterized by recurrent headaches that vary widely in intensity, frequency, and duration. Migraine headaches are commonly unilateral, and they are usually associated with anorexia, nausea, and vomiting. They are sometimes preceded by or associated with neurologic and mood disturbances.

Migraine comes in many forms. Many patients diagnose their headaches as migraine when in reality the headaches have nothing in common with migraine. Perhaps they use the term migraine because migraine headaches are usually considered to be severe and thus bring the sufferer more sympathy and other psychologic gain than an ordinary tension headache might.

On the other hand, many patients with true migraine have the visual aura but only a mild headache or none at all and thus feel they do not have migraine because the headache is not prostrating.

Classic Migraine

This migraine is the variety that most physicians are familiar with. The incidence of classic migraine in the general population is said to be between 6 and 15%. The patient usually has some prodromata, which may vary from severe depression and fatigue to hyperactivity and excitement that precedes the headache by up to 24 hours.

The patient usually has a family history of migraine, the trait being transmitted in a dominant fashion. Discovering the family history may be difficult because the migraine headache in the other family members may never have been diagnosed. Frequent attacks of colic or carsickness or other gastrointestinal disturbances in the patient's childhood may represent a variant of migraine that developed into the classic form in the patient's teens or twenties. Gastrointestinal and vestibular symptoms are twice as common in patients with classic migraine as in those who suffer from tension headaches. The migraine attacks may be precipitated by stress, such as that related to examinations or a new job or a family problem. They may also be triggered by mild to moderate head trauma, which can cause syndromes such as temporary blindness. Haas, Pineda, and Lourie reported the onset of classic migraine in British football players who used their heads to return a football in motion. This can occur even without a period of unconsciousness, but it usually stuns the patient momentarily. More severe periods of unconsciousness, such as occur with a contusion of the brain, can naturally be expected to produce more significant neurologic symptoms and signs either permanently or transiently.

Migraine occurs in both sexes, but the

incidence is three times greater in women than in men. The incidence may be increased in early pregnancy. Other changes in endocrine status (such as one brought about by the use of birth control pills) may also cause an increased incidence. Menopause, on the other hand, may cause the migraine headaches to cease. A not infrequent change at the menopause is that the sufferer has the visual phenomena but not the headache pain. In such a patient the physician may be led astray. He may not think of the condition as migraine because the pain is absent, or he may consider the cause to be the transient amaurosis of vertebral basilar insufficiency, even though the patient's age and sex militate against such a diagnosis.

Persons suffering from migraine have a certain personality pattern. They are highly productive, aggressive, and, frequently, obsessive compulsive. A striking characteristic of migraine patients is that they describe the attacks in great detail.

Migraine attacks are sometimes triggered by stress although attacks can come also when stress is reduced and the person is about to relax.

Immediately before the headache, the scotoma appears. It is hemianopic although the patient may not realize this fact, saying that the phenomenon occurred in one eye. The scotoma is described in many ways. Commonly the patient notices a shimmering or waviness in front of his vision, usually just off center. The waviness expands toward the periphery, leaving behind a negative scotoma. The waviness may progress to the zigzag-lines (fortifications) phenomenon. The size of the fortifications remains the same, but their number increases to fill up the larger peripheral field. The entire visual episode lasts about 20 to 30 minutes. This spreading of neural depression moves at the rate of 2 to 3 mm per minute, and it covers an area of occipital cortex of about 67 mm. The scotoma sometimes moves from the periphery toward the center, and it may be associated more commonly with permanent visual defects, as in the bilateral hemianopic form. Some people experience a burst of light with general blurring of vision and then a gradual clearing from the center toward the periphery.

Other forms of visual phenomena can be experienced, and some have been recorded in history and literature. The visions of Hildegard and, particularly, the scotoma of Lewis Carroll are examples. Carroll experienced micropsia (Lilliputianism) and macropsia (Brobdingnagianism) according to Wolff.

A particularly interesting visual phenomenon is that referred to as the completion of geometric figures. In the area of the scotoma, a portion of the head of a person the patient is looking at may be blurred or absent, but a geometric pattern completed on the wall behind the area of blurring is not blurred. This was first described by Poppelreuter, who referred to it as Vorstellungsmässige Ergänzung (imaginative completion). Not all patients with migrainous field defects will do this and so it cannot be interpreted as a normal physiologic response to a field defect. Warrington's analysis of their cases concluded that this phenomenon of completion was related to simultaneous involvement of the parietal lobes.

Photophobia is a common complaint. Many migraine sufferers prefer to be in a darkened room during a migraine attack in order to avoid visual stimulation and a worsening of photosensitivity. The photosensitivity may be caused by irritation of the fifth cranial nerve (the headache is transmitted over this nerve), or it may be caused by the abnormal increase in awareness that occurs in all the senses during a migraine attack.

Migraine headache is unilateral in about two thirds of sufferers and bilateral in about one third. When it is unilateral, the headache is on the side opposite the scotoma. In 80% of sufferers the headache will, at one time or another, affect the other side. This change is helpful in establishing a diagnosis of migraine. All migraine headaches do not eventually change sides, but if they do not, it is worrisome. The condition may represent a more serious local disease process that is mimicking migraine.

The migraine headache usually begins as a dull unilateral ache that progresses to a throbbing or pulsating pain and then perhaps becomes a steady pain that spreads over the entire skull. The duration is several hours (usually) to 24 hours (rarely). The sufferer tries to relieve the pain by pressing the scalp and underlying arteries in the area of the pain. The same effect can be obtained by compression of the ipsilateral carotid artery, which reduces the pulsations in the scalp.

The attack may be resolved in one of three ways: (1) the patient becomes exhausted and sleeps off the headache, or (2) a lysis type of solution occurs, with nausea and vomiting followed by relief or (3) (more rarely) by crisis exhibited by a sudden increase in physical and mental activity. Even after the acute symptoms of an attack have disappeared, fatigue, even exhaustion, may remain for several days.

Associated symptoms and signs occur often enough to be considered part of the migraine fabric. Frequently, a noticeable increase in weight occurs before the onset of an attack, with oliguria preceding the attack and diuresis following it. Gastrointestinal symptoms are prominent in most attacks of migraine. Most sufferers experience nausea and some vomiting, with mild diarrhea during the attack and, perhaps, constipation after the attack. The severity of these symptoms is not related to the severity of the headache; these symptoms are simply part of the total body effect of the migraine complex. The gastrointestinal complaints are more common in children, and they may be the most prominent feature of the attack (as in cyclic infantile colic). As the patient gets older, the gastrointestinal symptoms are less prominent,

and the headache and visual symptoms make up the new migraine pattern.

Common Migraine

This migraine is not as easily identified as is the classic variety. As in the classic variety, a strong family history is evident and is helpful in making the diagnosis; the patients often have had the same childhood gastrointestinal symptoms as well as the association of the symptoms with stress. The common migraine, however, tends to occur at less predictable and more irregular intervals than does the classic variety. Pregnancy frequently brings relief from the attacks, a characteristic that differentiates common migraine from classic migraine. The menopause also brings relief from common migraine.

The premonitory symptoms are not as dramatic and specific as the periods of excitement or depression seen in classic migraine. The sufferers tend to be drowsy or have a general feeling of not being well. No visual scotomas are present, but photophobia may occur.

Headache is frequently present when the person awakens, and it builds hour by hour. It lasts longer than in the classic variety, and it may persist for several days. It is usually unilateral, but it may spread over the entire cranium.

Nausea and vomiting, polyuria, and diarrhea may follow shortly after the onset of headache. Nasal symptoms, such as stuffiness or a watery nasal discharge, often occur. The headache ends with sleep rather than by lysis or crisis.

Migraine-Equivalent Group

Hemisensory and Hemiplegic Forms

Fortunately, these two varieties of headache are rare. The visual phenomenon of fortifications spreads in one direction at a set rate (as described for migraine), but the usual sensory symptoms do not spread in a similar manner. Numbness may begin in an arm and then involve the ipsilateral face and tongue. Transient aphasia and agraphia do occur, but rarely. Their presence casts doubt on the migraine designation. If the sufferer has a speech defect, it is of the motor variety; that is, he has difficulty in finding the correct motor pathway for what he wants to say. The defect is transient, but it may last up to several days. Angiography might be considered in these headaches since they comprise an unusual form of migraine; however, if an established history of migraine exists and the effects are transient or if other signs typical of migraine occur with hemisensory or hemiplegic deficit, angiography should be avoided. Studies concerning the use of angiography in the evaluation of migraine patients were conducted when angiography was performed by direct carotid artery injection. There have been no studies of angiography by the femoral catheter technique to evaluate migraine patients. In any event, the decision concerning whether to do an angiogram should be made by the neurologist or neurosurgeon. The literature has ample evidence that the incidence of morbidity, with some permanent defects, is higher in patients with migraine than in other patients undergoing angiography. In patients with a typical migraine history, the search for an angioma or arteriovenous malformation is usually futile. Occasionally, a vascular malformation is found, but usually one that is surgically inaccessible. (In some instances, had the history been better evaluated, the diagnosis of migraine would not have been considered.) On rare occasions, a pial vessel may bleed, with the result that blood is found in the subarachnoid space. This finding, plus the patient's history and the physician's experience, can guide the physician as to how far to work up the patient with contrast studies.

Basilar Artery Form

This form of vascular headache may affect both sides of the cerebral cortex, causing bilateral scintillating scotoma. Vertigo, dysarthria, tinnitus, bilateral paralysis, and diplopia may be seen. Nausea and vomiting may also occur in this form of headache, as well as in the common and classic varieties. In this headache, the nausea and vomiting may result from brain stem dysfunction. Unconsciousness or syncope may be mistaken for an epileptic seizure, but it is probably caused by depression of the reticular formation in the brain stem. When it occurs, it is usually brief and akinetic.

Ophthalmoplegic Form

If this rare form of headache occurs as an isolated entity, it is difficult to distinguish from ophthalmoplegia secondary to a carotid artery aneurysm. Involvement of the third cranial nerve is more common than is involvement of the sixth or fourth cranial nerve, and total ophthalmoplegia is rarest of all. The background for the establishment of the diagnosis is a typical migraine attack, with the visual phenomenon just preceding the ophthalmoplegia.

The rationale for the ophthalmoplegia has not been definitely established, but Parkinson's theory is persuasive. He feels that some of the small nutrient arteries from the intracavernous portion of the carotid artery that supply the third cranial nerve are the site of the problem. Parkinson believes that, since the walls of the arteries become edematous and narrow during an attack of migraine, the same phenomenon could happen in these small intracavernous arteries, causing ischemia to the third cranial nerve. It has been reported that up to 10% of ophthalmoplegic migraine patients may not recover fully or at all—a finding that further calls into question the migraine designation. In addition, the ophthalmoplegia is not necessarily on the same side as the headache.

Retinal Form

When this variety is associated with a vascular headache, it may also exhibit the scintillating scotoma but not the fortifications phenomenon that occurs in the occipital cortex. Retinal and conjunctival hemorrhages, ischemic papillitis, and even hemorrhages of the vitreous humor may be associated with the retinal form. If repeated ocular episodes occur, retinal pigmentary changes may occur, presumably secondary to repeated retinal ischemia.

Meniere Syndrome

This syndrome, with episodes of vertigo, may be caused by paroxysmal labyrinthine hydrops. Since the attacks occur in groups, the patient is symptom-free for months or years. The history is similar to that of cluster headache. The arterial supply to the labyrinth is from the caroticotympanic plexus of the internal carotid artery. When the vertigo and nausea result from basilar artery migraine, they occur because of the effect of small penetrating basilar artery branches on the pontine tegmentum. Usually, other signs also indicate basilar artery involvement, such as hemiplegia or visual scotomas.

Carotodynia

Patients with carotodynia experience pain over the common carotid artery that radiates to the face and ear. The pain is increased by touching the common carotid artery, yawning, swallowing, or coughing.

The cause of this syndrome is a painful dilatation of the carotid artery, usually found in the region of the carotid bulb. The pain radiates along the course of the external carotid artery to the postauricular area. The pain is usually not as severe as a typical migraine headache, but it may be more chronic and be present for days to weeks. It is more common in women in the fifth decade of life but has been reported in patients ranging from age 10 to age 80.

Melkersson Syndrome

This syndrome has several specific features that usually set it apart from other facial pain. The headache is periodic and usually begins in early adult life. Painful facial swelling, recurrent facial nerve paralysis, and congenitally fissured tongue are present.

Lower Hemifacial Pain

This pain is different from cluster headache in that it does not have the associated migraine features, such as Horner syndrome and gastrointestinal symptoms. It lasts longer than cluster headache, with pain radiating from an area of the lower face (such as the palate) up the face to the ear. It is also different from cluster headache in that it is not frequent and the attacks do not come in groups.

Horner Syndrome

This syndrome occurs in migraine attacks, but it is usually transient. It may be caused by edema of the internal carotid artery, with a secondary effect on the sympathetic chain, which runs in the adventitial sheath of the carotid artery. In other forms of migraine, such as cluster headache, other autonomic signs appear, such as nasal stuffiness, watery nasal discharge, chemosis, hyperemia of the globe, and bradycardia. In such cases, the episode may represent an abnormal autonomic discharge.

Cluster Headache

This headache is included in the migraine spectrum even though it has significant differences. A family history is not as common in cluster headache as it is in migraine. Cluster headache is predominantly a disease of men, whereas true migraine is predominantly a disease of women. The onset varies, but it is usually in the third or fourth decade of life. The pain is unilateral, and it rarely changes to the other side of the head. It is usually more severe and incapacitating than is the pain of the usual migraine headache. Unlike the patient with migraine, who tries to sleep off the headache, the patient with cluster headache tends to be active, as if to walk off the headache. The attacks occur up to several times a day, starting and stopping abruptly. They may last from several minutes to several hours, but rarely longer. The episodes occur over several weeks or months and the condition then goes into spontaneous remission, only to recur several months or years later.

There are three types of cluster headaches: the periodic form, in which there are multiple or single daily attacks which last for weeks or months and then abruptly stop; the chronic form, which shows no sign of remission; and the chronic paroxysmal hemicrania type, which occurs more frequently in middle-aged women and responds to aspirin and indomethacin. In the first two types, a short course of prednisone is effective rather than the beta-blocker class of drugs so effective in other migraine syndromes. Lithium carbonate has been effective in chronic cluster headaches, but the effective dosage may cause gastrointestinal side effects, tremors, and nephrotoxicity, which makes its use unacceptable.

Of the associated features, the most striking one is ipsilateral Horner syndrome, usually with the sweating mechanism intact. Conjunctival hyperemia and chemosis are prominent. The nasal symptoms are also prominent, running the gamut from nasal discharge to nasal obstruction. Extreme hyperalgesia of the face and scalp is common, as is tenderness over the dilated and pulsatile temporal artery. Although no true tactile trigger zone exists (as it does in tic douloureux), the use of alcohol is frequently a precipitating factor.

The patients are said to have a distinctive facial appearance, with a deeply furrowed forehead, vertical skin creases on the forehead, particularly at the glabella, and coarse skin on the cheeks. Peptic ulcers are rather common in cluster headache, but they are not always associated.

Raeder's Paratrigeminal Neuralgia

This disorder is characterized by severe ocular pain associated with miosis, ptosis, and a preserved ipsilateral sweating mechanism. It is almost exclusively a disease of middle-aged men, who have a significant history of recurrent morning headaches, with nausea and vomiting.

The initial reports of this syndrome were associated with multiple parasellar cranial nerves and a middle fossa mass. As a result of this, Raeder syndrome can be separated into several categories. The first group of patients are those with a painful Horner syndrome and other cranial nerve involvement. These patients require detailed neuroradiologic investigation for a mass lesion. Those without cranial nerve involvement fall into two groups: those who have the cluster type of headache and those with a noncluster type, who have a single sustained episode of hemicrania lasting hours to weeks. These latter two have a benign course, and the pain eventually resolves itself. These patients do not usually require neuroradiologic investigation unless their pain does not resolve. During the course of the disease, it is important to follow and reevaluate the patients for any new signs of cranial nerve involvement. If they occur, then these patients would move into the first group of Raeder's and require neuroradiologic investigation. The pain of this syndrome occurs over the first division of the trigeminal nerve. If the second and third divisions are involved, this should be considered as though one of the other parasellar nerves were involved, and these patients then investigated accordingly, rather than interpreting this expansion of sensory nerve involvement as a typical benign Raeder syndrome. A few patients in the benign group have been reported to have fibromuscular dysplasia and other local changes along the internal carotid artery. If the pain and the Horner's does not remit, then I would consider, at the least, digital venous arteriography, since this is safer and easier than direct arteriography and gives the same information from the carotid arch up to the carotid syphon.

The headaches should be considered ominous if they are accompanied with any neurologic deficit no matter how minor or transient.

Nonmigraine Group

Headache Associated with Aneurysm

The onset of a ruptured aneurysm with subarachnoid hemorrhage is dramatic and usually clear-cut. A sudden and severe supraorbital pain is associated with a partial or complete third cranial nerve paralysis, with the pupil involved in well over 95% of cases. The patient's level of consciousness may vary from normal to (more commonly) some degree of obtundation. The real problem in diagnosing some cases of aneurysm occurs when the aneurysm leaks slowly. Recurrent headache, photophobia, and stiff neck are present, but not the dramatic identifying signs of subarachnoid hemorrhage. The aneurysm that produces the signs of subarachnoid hemorrhage and isolated third cranial nerve paralysis is almost always located at the junction of the internal carotid and posterior communicating arteries. Uncommonly, an aneurysm may occur on the vertebral basilar arterial systems, as the third nerve passes between the junction of the posterior cerebral and superior cerebellar arteries, and cause the patient to have a third cranial nerve paralysis. The usual posterior circulation symptomatic aneurysm, however, generally does not affect only the third cranial nerve. It produces some degree of hemiparesis. The headache associated with the posteriorly located aneurysm is not referred to the ocular region. The pain caused by a ruptured aneurysm on the internal carotid artery is referred to the supraorbital region, because the first division of the fifth cranial nerve serves the area of the internal carotid artery and ipsilateral forehead.

Headache Associated with Diabetic Neuropathy

Persons with diabetes usually have a third cranial nerve paralysis with minimal pain and no involvement of the pupil; however, as many as 50% of patients have some pain, and as many as 25% have some pupillary involvement. When the pupil is involved, the condition is difficult to distinguish from an aneurysm. If the pupil is totally uninvolved, the likelihood that the pain and paralysis are secondary to an aneurysm is extremely small. If the pupil is involved, the physician must consider an aneurysm. Clearness of the spinal fluid does not rule out an aneurysm since not all aneurysms bleed grossly into the subarachnoid space. Fifty percent of cases of diabetic third cranial nerve neuropathy occur in patients who had not been known to have diabetes, and establishing the diagnosis may require a formal glucose tolerance test. The pain of diabetic neuropathy is probably related to occlusive small vessel disease causing ischemia to the fifth cranial nerve just as it causes ischemia to the third cranial nerve. If the pupil is not involved, it is because the pupillary fibers in the superior peripheral part of the nerve receive a secondary blood supply from surrounding pial vessels that maintains the pupil's integrity despite the ischemia from the primary vascular supply. In spite of secondary vascular supply, about 50% of diabetic third cranial nerve paralyses show some pupillary involvement. The pain is referred to the forehead or retrobulbar area as it is in other causes of involvement of the first division of the fifth cranial nerve.

Headache Associated with Angioma and Arteriovenous Malformations

The signs and symptoms caused by angiomas and arteriovenous malformation depend on their location, size, rapidity of growth, and degree of suddenness of subarachnoid hemorrhage. The symptoms may be mistaken for migraine if the headaches are intermittent and any neurologic signs are transient. Recurrence of the headache is usually not as predictable as it is in migraine. The association of seizures is a more ominous sign, pointing to a mass lesion, such as an angioma or an arteriovenous malformation, rather than to migraine. Occasionally, cranial bruits can be heard, but their presence is not necessary for diagnosis. The ocular or neurologic signs may suggest the location of these entities, but only an arteriogram fully outlines their extent.

Headache Associated with Hypertensive Vascular Disease

The patient with hypertension is usually not bothered by headache, and frequently he is not aware that he has hypertension. Headache is more likely to occur when hypertensive encephalopathy occurs with cerebral edema and increased intracranial pressure. The paroxysmal form of hypertension and the hypertension that has a sudden and severe onset (such as is seen with pheochromocytoma and eclampsia) frequently exhibit headache. The location and character of the pain are not specific. Any patient complaining of headache should have his blood pressure taken in both arms because of the possible presence of coarctation of the aorta, which causes hypertension and asymmetric blood pressure in the arms.

Caffeine-Induced Headache

This headache may occur from overindulgence in coffee or certain soft drinks. The patient's history should point to a diagnosis. A caffeine-induced headache may also occur after a sudden decrease in the usual amount of caffeine ingested, the headache being a withdrawal symptom. Severe overdose of caffeine can cause mental confusion, vomiting, tremors, and diarrhea. Caffeine taken orally is a vasoconstrictor. It produces ischemic changes that in turn probably produce the headache. The treatment is slow withdrawal of the caffeine.

Postconcussion Headache

The duration of the headache that follows a cranial injury is variable. If the initial injury did not result in a period of unconsciousness or transient neurologic deficit, the headache usually lasts less than 2 months. A psychiatric history or a history of chronic headache probably alters this timetable significantly, as may any insurance litigation. The patient may not have had any neurologic deficit but he may have sustained extensive soft tissue injury to the face or scalp. Local injury to scalp vessels owing to contusion or associated with skin lacerations and secondary scarring may cause pain in the distribution of those vessels. The intracranial portion of the headache results from the postconcussion dilatation of intracranial vessels. Further jarring of the head or a sudden increase in intracranial pressure such as caused by Valsalva maneuver increases the pain. A single type of post-concussion headache does not exist. The headache may be generalized, with varying intensity, or it may be episodic. The patient may have associated complaints of vertigo, poor memory, poor concentration, or insomnia. On careful examination, he may be found to have some degree of vertical nystagmus, particularly in up gaze, which suggests a posterior fossa dysfunction. Severe blows, particularly to the vertex area, can cause a decrease in convergence and accommodation, even without obvious ocular muscle weakness. The decrease usually clears after many months, but the patients may have to wear eyeglasses for a time for near work. Some patients may even show a transient or permanent Horner syndrome, which attests to the severity of the trauma.

Besides the intracranial and extracranial causes of headache, spasm of the neck muscles may be a cause. The spasm may result from some injury to the cervical vertebrae or from a protective mechanism against moving the neck.

The emotional factors bearing on the degree and duration of headache are many, and they must be considered. Is the patient using the headache as a socially acceptable reason for not returning to a job he dislikes or cannot handle? Is the headache his way of managing an unhappy home situation? Does he have a history of hypochondriasis? Cranial trauma is an ideal scapegoat, giving the patient a specific episode on which to blame all his problems. The patient who is looking for financial gain from his illness probably will not want to get better until a legal settlement has been made. Such a patient may be the loser in the long run, however, in that he may have developed such a habit of pain and an attachment to the secondary gain that his pain has brought that he cannot do without his headache crutch.

Headache Associated with Increased Intracranial Pressure

The pain of increased intracranial pressure is not always helpful in localizing or even identifying the problem. Tumors may cause headache without an increase in intracranial pressure merely by traction on pain-sensitive structures. If the changes are not local to the tumor but are in another part of the brain, it is not uncommon for the pain not to be over the area of the mass lesion. On the other hand, not all patients with increased intracranial pressure have headache, an observation that has been demonstrated experimentally. Although the sign is not specific, an increase in headache caused by changes in position or by coughing, straining, or performing the Valsalva maneuver suggests increased intracranial pressure. Projectile vomiting without nausea is even stronger evidence of increased intracranial pressure.

PSYCHOGENIC HEADACHE

This headache, including the tension headache, accounts for most cases. The psychogenic headache differs from the migraine headache in that it is usually bilateral or hatband-like in distribution. It also has no aura or focal neurologic signs. The psychogenic headache recurs much more often than does migraine. In about 50% of cases, the headache is present all the time to some degree. Migraine sufferers tend to get relief with sleep, whereas persons with psychogenic headache have difficulty with sleep. Unlike the situation in migraine headache, puberty, pregnancy, or menopause does not seem to affect the character of the psychogenic headache.

The tension headache is not associated with nausea or vomiting, but it may be associated with anorexia. The pain of tension headache is considered to be owing to contraction of the muscles of the head and neck. The pain may be caused also by muscle ischemia from severe prolonged contraction that causes changes in the blood flow to the muscle. Tenderness of the muscles of the neck on palpation may be an important diagnostic clue.

The psychiatric history may give information about any headache pattern. Is there a time of day or a day of the week when the headache is worse? Is it worse when the patient is at work or when he is at home? What is his work situation? Is he constantly passed over for promotion? Are technologic changes getting to be too much for him? Is a younger person out to get his job or about to be promoted over him? Do his financial commitments exceed his earning capacity?

Ask the patient about home life. Are there many arguments or fights? Does the spouse nag or constantly put the patient down? Is the patient's sex life satisfactory? If an extramarital relationship exists, does the patient feel anxiety and guilt?

These questions are only a few of the ones that need to be asked. Some patients may resent such questioning and not answer truthfully because they think the physician is simply prying. The physician who hopes to gain the patient's confidence and cooperation must be tactful. He must also be alert. Sometimes even an untruthful answer may be important because of its inflection or the certainty with which it is given. Return to a sensitive subject later—

when a trusting doctor-patient relationship has been established.

HEADACHE CAUSED BY INFECTIONS

Sinus Disease

Sinus infection is the most common infection that causes headache (although headaches are blamed far too often on sinus infections). Since the sinuses surround the eye, it is understandable that the patient with sinus disease may consult an ophthalmologist.

A severe upper respiratory tract infection may precede the sinus infection. The respiratory tract infection may lead to nasal congestion, with secondary blocking of the osteum of the sinus and then secondary sinusitis. Any cause of osteum obstruction can result in sinusitis, including obstructive malformation of the nasal septum and turbinates, as well as nasal polyps and constant allergic conditions that keep the nasal mucosa edematous. Tumor of the sinuses or nasal passages can also cause sinusitis.

The pain in frontal and maxillary sinusitis is usually steady and over the affected sinus. Percussion of the area may elicit an increase in pain. Pain from ethmoid sinusitis is felt over the bridge of the nose or in the retro-orbital area. Pain from the sphenoid sinus is located deep in the head or at the vertex of the skull. One type of frontal sinusitis is the result not of infection but of the closing of the orifice of the nasofrontal duct. The closing causes the air inside the sinus to be absorbed, resulting in a partial vacuum and pain owing to traction on the pain-sensitive sinus mucosa.

Many persons with sinusitis have nasal symptoms, such as a discharge or an alteration in their capacity to smell.

Transillumination of the frontal and maxillary sinuses may be done with the Finnoff head illuminator in a darkened room, but the procedure should not be looked on as a substitute for good quality roentgenograms and expert evaluation of them.

Orbital Cellulitis

The usual cause of orbital cellulitis is extension of an infection from one of the paranasal sinuses. In children, the infection more commonly originates from the ethmoid sinuses, whereas in teenage and adult patients the frontal sinuses are the more common site. The patient's main symptoms and signs often are orbital, and the sinus origin may not be discovered until roentgenograms are taken. Untreated orbital cellulitis can lead to loss of vision or cavernous sinus thrombosis, ending possibly in death.

I have treated two persons with intense local pain on the nasal aspect of the orbit that I felt represented subperiosteal abscess that had not broken out into the orbit. These patients did not exhibit the usual signs of orbital abscess. Both patients recovered after treatment with antibiotics, and no sequelae occurred.

Gradenigo Syndrome

This syndrome has rarely been seen since the beginning of the antibiotic era. The syndrome begins as a middle ear infection that travels unabated to involve the petrous bone, including Dorello's canal. Pain and paralysis of the sixth cranial nerve are the presenting features. The condition can progress to brain abscess formation. Since the petrosal dural sinus is very close to Dorello's canal, it too may become inflamed, with progression to a lateral sinus thrombosis and pseudotumor cerebri.

Periostitis

Severe orbital pain is present in periostitis. The pain is worse on palpation of the periosteum along the orbital rim. Roentgenographic examination shows periosteal thickening. The cause of the infection is generally considered to be syphilis.

Herpes Zoster

The pain in herpes zoster precedes the development of typical vesicles of the first division of the trigeminal nerve. Once these vesicles appear, the diagnosis is obvious. (Thus a full description of herpes zoster ophthalmicus and its signs and complications need not be given here.)

As a result of the healing of the vesicles and of scarring, an area of anesthesia may be present, and patients may find this complication as intolerable as the severe postherpetic neuralgia. The anesthesia sometimes persists for months after an acute herpes episode. On the other hand, lancinating pain suggests tic douloureux (but no trigger zone exists). The post-herpetic neuralgia may last for years, and it may be so severe that the patient even threatens suicide. A history of herpes zoster is the all-important clue in diagnosing prolonged facial neuralgia of obscure cause.

Ramsay Hunt Syndrome

This syndrome is a rare form of herpes zoster infection in the ear with typical vesicles in the external canal and involvement of the geniculate ganglion. Ear pain, facial paralysis, and deafness are the important features, but as a rule they disappear spontaneously. As in other types of herpes zoster, the pain precedes the vesicle formation by several days. The main differential diagnoses are tic douloureux and glossopharyngeal neuralgia. Tic douloureux has a trigger zone, and glossopharyngeal neuralgia is more prominent in the throat area. Neither condition has the vesicles that eventually develop in and positively identify the Ramsay Hunt syndrome.

HEADACHE CAUSED BY INFLAMMATIONS

Temporal Arteritis

This disease generally occurs in people over 55 years of age. The patient complains of headache, malaise, and arthralgia, but his condition frequently goes undiagnosed. If the symptoms are severe enough and if the patient loses weight, the physician should consider an occult malig-

nancy. The headache may become more specific, and the temporal artery is found to be hard, tender, and incompressible (Figs. 14–1 and 14–2).

The major complication of untreated temporal arteritis is irreversible blindness. Headache in an elderly patient, particularly a steady headache that is located in the temporal region, suggests temporal arteritis. In taking the history, the ophthalmologist should ask specifically about arthralgia, jaw claudication, weight loss, myalgia, and fever. The patient may not volunteer information about such symptoms because he may feel that they are not pertinent.

Tolosa-Hunt Syndrome

This syndrome (superior orbital fissure syndrome) is caused by a nonspecific granulomatous inflammation that involves any or all of the nerves of the superior orbital fissure or anterior cavernous sinus. Gross inflammation is not common (it is common in pseudotumor of the orbit), but it does occasionally occur, as does mild exophthalmos. The diagnosis is made by exclusion. The disease is self-limited, but the pain may be too severe for the patient to wait for spontaneous remission. Moderate doses of systemic steroids usually relieve the pain within 24 hours. The ophthalmoplegia responds much more slowly. Despite the rapid and excellent response to steroids, often it takes many months before the patient can completely stop using steroids. If the signs of Tolosa-Hunt syndrome do not disappear completely, the patient should be worked up again, with the physician looking for a tumor or some other cause.

HEADACHE CAUSED BY CERVICAL DISEASES

Cervical Vertebral Degenerative Disease

This disease usually involves some degree of pain. To avoid the pain, the sufferer restricts movement of the neck by contract-

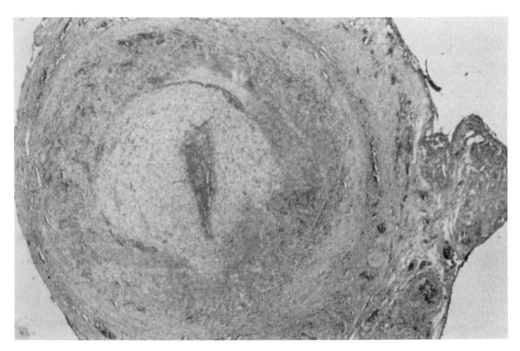

Fig. 14–1. Totally occluded artery from temporal arteritis. (Courtesy of Douglas McCrae.)

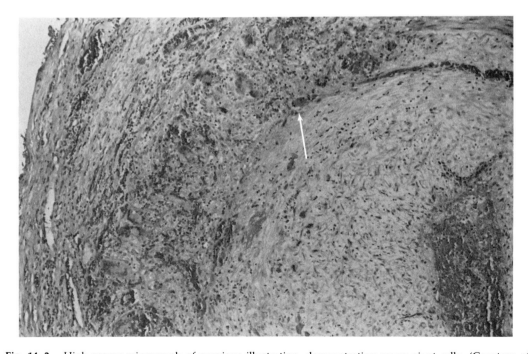

Fig. 14–2. High-power micrograph of previous illustration, demonstrating many giant cells. (Courtesy of Douglas McCrae.)

ing the head and neck muscles. This prolonged contraction can cause headache. The pain is located in the neck and suboccipital area; it is steady and it radiates to the shoulders. After a prolonged period of pain, the muscles may be tender to touch. Osteoarthritic changes may be seen—and should be looked for—on the roentgenogram.

Cervical Vertebral Disc Disease

Posterior displacement of the intervertebral disc causes pressure on the cervical nerve roots and results in pain. Even stretching the ligaments can cause pain. In addition, muscle pain may occur owing to the splinting action of the muscles. A tearing of the annulus, with further protrusion of the disc, causes further compression of the nerve roots in the intervertebral canals. Except when it is the result of trauma, the disease occurs most commonly in persons from 40 to 60 years of age. The usual roentgenograms for cervical disease should be ordered; in particular, the anteroposterior and open-mouth views and the lateral views in flexion and extension. Prolonged compression of the cervical nerves can cause neurologic deficits, and this compression should be looked for.

Cervical Rib Syndrome

This syndrome (the scalenus anticus syndrome) affects the last cervical root and the first dorsal root. Headache can occur, but more commonly, pain is referred to the ulnar side of the arm. If the condition is severe, sensory and motor symptoms may occur. The arm may feel cold and the pulse may be markedly reduced in that arm. The pain is usually unilateral, and muscle spasm may occur as a result of the patient's effort to avoid unnecessary movement. Surgical removal of the rib is the treatment.

Cervical Root Syndrome

This syndrome is more frequently caused by poor posture. The poor vertebral alignment causes compression of the nerve roots, particularly with forward protrusion of the head, a posture that straightens the normal lordotic cervical curve. The trouble may be aggravated by preexisting conditions, such as compression of the cervical disc or arthritic spurs. Secondary contraction of cervical roots or contraction of neck muscles leads to the development of local and suboccipital headaches.

HEADACHE CAUSED BY REFERRED PAIN

Temporomandibular Joint Syndrome

The temporomandibular joint is almost constantly moving with eating and talking. A deformity or malalignment of the jaw causes pain. The normal jaw alignment is governed by the position of the teeth; absence of teeth or a poor bite causes the jaw alignment to change, putting tension on the temporomandibular ligaments and resulting in secondary pain. Since most of the chewing is done posteriorly with the molars, any loss of these teeth is a particular problem. Poorly fitting dentures cause the same problem. The poor fit may be owing to incorrectly designed dentures or to a change in jaw size, such as occurs in acromegaly.

The pain is usually local to the jaw, but it may spread over the ipsilateral face. Occasionally, pain may be of the claudication type rather than pain on movement. Claudication-type pain in persons in their sixties or seventies suggests temporal arteritis.

Dental Disease

Dental pain and dental disease are not always localized to the affected tooth. The pain may radiate to one side of the jaw or to the ipsilateral temporal area or over the entire mandibular and maxillary division of the trigeminal nerve, which supplies that area. The area over the tooth may also be sensitive, and the sensitivity is increased when the sufferer chews or bites or when he eats or drinks foods that are extremely hot or extremely cold.

HEADACHE CAUSED BY BONE DISEASES

Paget's Disease

In this chronic disease, headache is a prominent feature. The bones of the head enlarge and encroach on the nerves that traverse the bones, causing local pain. Skull roentgenograms usually supply enough information to establish a diagnosis.

Oxycephaly

This congenital defect involves cranial suture closure. Owing to premature closure of the sagittal and coronal sutures, the cranial vault is smaller than usual and growth of the brain is restricted. Besides the peculiar appearance of the head, headache, progressive exophthalmos, and optic nerve compression are the most prominent signs. Treatment is by operation. Without operation oxycephaly can end in blindness.

HEADACHE CAUSED BY TUMORS

Nasopharyngeal Tumors

These tumors comprise a group rather than one specific type. They are sarcomas, which are relatively radiosensitive, squamous cell carcinomas, or endotheliomas, which generally are not radiosensitive. The tumors tend to occur in persons from 20 to 60 years of age. The incidence is slightly higher in men than in women. For some reason, in China nasopharyngeal tumor is the leading malignancy in men. This statistic is not true of Chinese people whose families have lived in the United States for several generations. The most common site of nasopharyngeal tumors is Rosenmüller's fossa. Because the tumors tend to grow submucosally, routine inspection of this site usually reveals a normal appearance. If the physician has a strong suspicion of the diagnosis, a biopsy of material from this area may be confirmatory, even if the gross appearance is normal.

Although persons with nasopharyngeal tumors usually do not have nasal symptoms, such symptoms are sometimes present when the soft palate is infiltrated and bulges into the nasopharynx. Unilateral deafness is usually present, but it is frequently unnoticed. Thus the physician should test for any hearing defect. Other ear symptoms are chronic serous otitis and tinnitus owing to obstruction of the eustachian tube. The physician should ask the patient about any frequent popping of the ears. Ear popping is caused by obstruction of the eustachian tube.

Pain or dysesthesia over the second division of the trigeminal nerve is one of the most prominent symptoms of nasopharyngeal tumor. Occasionally, pain spills over into the third division, but it is not a common or presenting sign. Nodes in the neck are fairly common. If situated near the sympathetic chain, they may cause Horner syndrome.

In most series, the most common presenting cranial nerve involvement has been that of the sixth cranial nerve. The combination of pain in the distribution of the second division of the trigeminal nerve and a sixth cranial nerve paralysis is highly suggestive of nasopharyngeal tumor. If pain accompanies a twelfth cranial nerve paralysis, a nasopharyngeal tumor is almost certainly present. The vidian nerve is closer to Rosenmüller's fossa than are the fifth and sixth cranial nerves. Some authors find that, as a result, tear function significantly decreases although keratitis sicca is not a clinical problem. The Schirmer test shows tear production to be significantly decreased. Other orbital nerves may be involved if the tumor invades the superior orbital fissure, and loss of function of the third and fourth cranial nerves may result. More extensive invasion produces a brawny exophthalmos.

A nasopharyngeal tumor may go undiagnosed as it affects one cranial nerve after another. Nasopharyngeal tumors grow intracranially but in the extradural space, producing the phenomenon described as the march of cranial nerves unilaterally across the base.

The roentgenograms to obtain are stereoscopic views of the basal foramina and fissures. These roentgenograms will show erosion (which is the clue to the diagnosis), but routine skull roentgenograms will not. Next, a biopsy of any nodes in the neck or a biopsy of tissue in Rosenmüller's fossa should be done. In some types of tumors (for example, sarcomas), irradiation prolongs life but does not usually effect a cure.

HEADACHE CAUSED BY CRANIAL NEURITIS

Tic Douloureux (Trigeminal Neuralgia)

The pain in tic douloureux is excruciating and lancinating, and it usually last a few seconds or minutes. Several pain episodes may occur in a short period of time. The pain is over any one or all of the three divisions of the trigeminal nerve. The second division is the one most commonly affected, followed by the third division, and, last, the first (or ophthalmic) division. The ophthalmic division is rarely affected alone. The presence of a trigger zone sets this pain apart from all others. Stimulation of the trigger zone, which is usually a small area, by touching, chewing, or swallowing can bring on these spasms of pain. Even such a minimal stimulus as a breeze can trigger the pain. After an attack there is a refractory period when stimulation of the trigger zone does not bring on the pain. Persons with tic douloureux will not wash or shave the trigger area or brush their teeth for fear of setting off an attack. During the attack, the face may be contorted with pain. The sufferer does not touch his face or try to compress the pain area as do persons with other forms of facial pain. The attacks begin in middle life, occur in a series, and then go into spontaneous remission. If the pain is steady or if it is not associated with a trigger zone, tumor, particularly one in the posterior fossa, should be considered. About 4% of cases of tic

douloureux occur as the presenting sign of multiple sclerosis. The cause of tic douloureux is not well understood. Recently a "vascular anomaly" theory was proposed. According to this theory, as the afflicted person ages, a vessel of the posterior circulation comes to lie on the trigeminal nerve and intermittently stimulates it.

In the past, the pain of tic douloureux would drive some people to suicide. Until recently, our treatment either was not effective or would cause as many disagreeable side effects as the treatment attempted to cure. Many drugs have been tried and initially hailed with great enthusiasm but with time, have fallen by the wayside. The drug that we started to use in 1964 is carbamazepine. It has been found useful in the treatment of tic douloureux but of no value in atypical facial pains or post herpes zoster. It has continued to be a useful drug over these last 20 years and has been estimated to control the condition in two thirds of afflicted patients, with varying doses up to 1600 mg a day. Periodic evaluation of the blood count and liver function test is mandatory to monitor the adverse effects of this medication.

Phenytoin has also been used in the treatment of tic douloureux, with doses up to 600 mg a day, but it is much less effective overall than carbamazepine. Phenytoin, as well as carbamazepine, has side effects of nausea and dizziness which may require discontinuation of therapy.

Nerve block with alcohol is useful if well performed but is of limited value since pain almost always recurs after 1 year. Repeat alcohol blocks are less effective. The dense anesthesia from the alcohol block may be as much of a discomfort for the patient as the pain of tic douloureux.

Surgical therapy has also been used. Previous surgical operations attacking the fifth nerve directly in the posterior fossa were frequently associated with complications of all sorts, including damage to other cranial nerves. Janetta has revamped the old operations, using microsurgical techniques.

He felt that tic douloureux was caused by a mechanical distortion of the nerve by tumor, blood vessels, or bone. If one were to relieve this pressure on the nerve, it was felt that the tic douloureux syndrome would disappear. Janetta identifies the offending anatomic structure with microsurgical techniques and screens the structure from the trigeminal nerve by a nonabsorbable sponge. Besides the excellent success rate with this procedure, he has lowered the morbidity by his surgical techniques. In addition, by protecting the nerve from the offending structure rather than cutting the nerve, he spared the patient the significant discomfort of the anesthesia produced by previous procedures or by an alcohol block.

A less formidable procedure is percutaneous radiofrequency trigeminal gangliolysis. As with alcohol, this is not a permanent cure, but success rates of 80% up to 1 year and 50% up to 5 years have generally been reported. This technique has the advantage of being able to be used on elderly, debilitated patients who could not otherwise undergo intracranial surgery. Since tic douloureux often occurs in the older age group, this situation is not uncommon. If all else fails, then a tractotomy of the descending trigeminal tract at the cervico medullary junction can be performed. This type of procedure has the added problem of severe anesthesia, which may be equally unacceptable to the patient as is his level of medical control. In order to assess the patient's ability to cope with this anesthesia, a long-acting local injection of an anesthetic followed later by an alcohol block might be tried. If the alcohol block fails, but the patient does not mind the anesthesia as compared with the pain, then a tractotomy could be done with the beforehand knowledge of the patient's reaction to the anesthesia.

Syndrome of the Nasal Nerve

The nasociliary nerve serves as the pain fibers for the eye as well as for the nose.

If the anterior ethmoidal area is involved, the pain may be felt not only on the side of the nose but also in the forehead over the ipsilateral eye. Besides the pain, there may be a unilateral nasal discharge, keratitis, conjunctivitis, and iritis. The severity of these three infections is usually not in proportion to the severity of the pain. Swelling of the inferior turbinate usually occurs; application of cocaine to this turbinate promptly relieves the pain of this condition.

Glossopharyngeal Neuralgia

Although the pain of glossopharyngeal neuralgia is not easily confused with pain of ocular origin, it is discussed here because of its special characteristics. The pain begins in the posterior part of the throat. (The patient describes the pain as located just to the side of the Adam's apple.) It then radiates to the ear. The attacks come in groups (as do the attacks of tic douloureux), but the condition does not eventually go into remission (as does tic douloureux). If medication such as carbamazepine fails, intracranial sectioning of the nerve is the treatment of choice.

Sphenopalatine Neuralgia (Sluder's Neuralgia)

The pain of sphenopalatine neuralgia is severe, and it may be on one or both sides. It is located at the root of the nose, around the eyes, upper teeth, and jaws, or in the temporal and zygomatic areas. After an attack, a moderate amount of residual tenderness may be present in the neck muscles.

The ocular signs and symptoms are photophobia, conjunctivitis, and lacrimation. The nasal complaints are of stuffiness, watery discharge, and itchiness. The oral symptoms are pain on swallowing, anesthesia of the soft palate, itching of the hard palate, and tonsillar pillars. Application of cocaine to the area of the nose in proximity to the sphenopalatine ganglion provides temporary relief. If the cocaine application does not work, instillation of the anesthetic into the sphenoid sinus may give the desired relief. The pain may also arise from the vidian nerve in the floor of the sinus. If anesthesia of this nerve gives relief, the condition is described as vidian neuralgia.

Greater Occipital Nerve Neuralgia

The pain of greater occipital nerve neuralgia is located in the neck region all the way to the coronal suture, and a general stiffness of the neck muscles occurs. The pain may spill over into any or all of the divisions of the trigeminal nerve. An alcohol block of this nerve gives relief that is frequently permanent.

HEADACHE CAUSED BY OCULAR DISEASES

A full description of ocular diseases that cause pain is beyond the scope of this book; however, a brief discussion of the more common entities is in order.

Since iritis is not often related to a specific disease, investigation for an underlying cause is usually unproductive. The pain of iritis is steady, is located in or above the eye, and is aggravated by light. Redness of the eye is particularly noticeable in the circumcorneal area. The definitive diagnosis is made with the slit lamp.

A foreign body in the cornea or under the upper lid should be observable with the naked eye and proper lighting. A loupe or slit lamp may be needed to see tiny foreign bodies or those that blend with ocular tissues.

Keratitis from any cause can be very painful, particularly with blinking. Some of the most common causes are arc welding accidents, overexposure to ultraviolet sunlamps, and overwearing of contact lenses. Fluorescein staining of the cornea will demonstrate any keratitis. The slit lamp is invaluable in the examination for keratitis because the fluorescein staining may be minimal and not visible with the naked eye or loupe.

Intermittent narrow-angle glaucoma should be considered a possible diagnosis,

even if the intraocular pressure measures as normal. Gonioscopy of the angle is mandatory. Episcleritis, which appears as a patchy red area of dilated vessels in a raised edematous area, can be painful, particularly the nodular variety of scleritis. Muscle balance problems, particularly high-grade phorias, may cause headache. Convergence insufficiency, the most common problem, is symptomatic during the school years, when a lot of prolonged reading is done. Measuring the vergences with prisms is the diagnostic method of choice. The traditional pencil "push up" exercises are probably as valuable as (and certainly less expensive than) other forms of treatment.

Refractive errors, particularly those associated with astigmatism correction, cause the most problems. Separation of the optical centers secondary to the wearing of large frames is a problem of more recent origin. If the patient has a significant refractive error, a separation of the optical centers, of even several millimeters, causes symptomatic prismatic displacement. It is true that the refractive problems may be present without causing symptoms. It is also true that these problems cause ocular discomfort, not severe headache. But in the evaluation of headaches, every stone should be turned.

HEADACHE CAUSED BY OTHER CONDITIONS

Hypoglycemia

The headache secondary to hypoglycemia is not specific in character and is probably vascular in origin. It frequently begins before meals, often before breakfast. Strenuous exercise that lowers the blood sugar level may bring it on, as may a starvation diet. More serious causes are hyperinsulinism owing to a functioning tumor of the pancreas and hyperplasia with hypersecretion. Besides headache, hunger, nausea and vomiting, fatigue, irritability, tremor, and sweating may occur.

The treatment of hypoglycemia is varied, and it depends on the cause. An adjustment in the patient's eating habits or an operation to remove a functioning tumor of the pancreas may be required.

Acute Alcoholism

The headache of acute alcoholism usually comes on the day after overindulgence, as the other symptoms—mental confusion and lack of coordination—are clearing. The headache is constant, moderately severe, and throbbing, and is usually made worse by any movement of the head. Since headache is caused by vascular dilatation, any increase in intracranial pressure makes it worse. Sufferers frequently notice that lying flat increases the headache, whereas a slight elevation, which lowers the intracranial pressure, gives some relief. The history of alcoholism, which is usually enough to make the diagnosis, is not always easy to elicit. The signs of acute alcoholism are a flushed face, slow respiration, pounding pulse, and a telltale breath. Still, the diagnosis should not be made facilely. Persons suffering from alcoholism are prone to trauma, and more than one such patient has turned out to have headache secondary to subdural hematoma.

Poisoning

Bromide poisoning used to be a more common cause of headache than it is today because many old-time headache remedies contained bromides. The bromide headache is dull and aching, and it usually begins in the morning. In more severe cases of bromide poisoning, the patient has loss of appetite, constipation, unsteadiness of gait, tremor, sleep disturbances, and ataxia. The treatment is obvious—stop the bromides.

Lead poisoning occurs primarily in children who ingest chips of lead-based paints, perhaps from old toys or furniture or from the walls of their houses, schools, or other institutions. Headache of a nondescript na-

ture is prominent. Convulsions, colic, and optic neuritis are frequently present. A blue gum line, stippling of the red blood cells, a lead line in the bones, and lead blood level are signs of lead intoxication. The treatment is to stop the ingestion and to institute medical treatment by chelating the lead, with excretion through the kidneys.

Phenytoin poisoning should be considered in anyone taking this drug (even in therapeutic doses) and experiencing headache. Determination of phenytoin blood levels can now be easily obtained. Besides headache, the symptoms are nausea, vomiting, hyperplasia of the gums, reflex changes, nystagmus, and ataxia. Proper adjustment of the dosage relieves these symptoms. Hyperplasia of the gums usually persists since it is related to chronic use of phenytoin rather than to overdosage.

Hematologic Diseases

The extremes of too little blood (anemia) and too much blood (polycythemia) can each cause headache. The headache is usually generalized, constant, and nonspecific. The diagnosis is easily made by a complete blood count, which should be part of any workup of headache of obscure cause.

Sexual Activity

In time, the "not-tonight-dear-I-have-a-headache" headache may develop into a real one. The reluctant partner who actually does have pain feels less guilty than the reluctant partner who feigns a headache to avoid intercourse.

The headache that occurs during or after coitus may be ominous. Although it is not unusual for the blood pressure to be elevated during intercourse, normally the elevation does not cause a severe headache. The sufferer may have unsuspected hypertension, which is aggravated during intercourse, or this type of headache may represent a more serious form of paroxysmal hypertension. Rupture of an unsuspected aneurysm should also be considered as a cause. If the person dies during coitus, the circumstances of death are often difficult to establish because the partner usually feels somewhat at fault.

After Spinal Tap

Headaches after spinal tap, particularly on assuming the upright position, are common. The cause is felt to be leakage of fluid through the tap site with secondary displacement of the brain and traction on sensory nerves. One theory postulates that the size of the needle as well as the angle of entry into the epidural space can decrease the incidence of spinal fluid leakage and subsequent headache. It is a twofold argument: If one uses a smaller bore needle, the smaller hole is more likely to self seal and less likely to leak. Secondly, a tangential approach from a lateral approach is not as likely to have the dura and arachnoid openings overlap and, therefore, is easier to close.

BIBLIOGRAPHY

Anthony, M., and Lance, J.: Histamine and serotonin in cluster headache. Arch. Neurol. 25:225, 1971.

Anthony, M., and Lance, J.: Monamine oxidase inhibition in the treatment of migraine. Arch. Neurol. 21:263, 1969.

Berger, J.R., and Sheremata, W.A.: Persistent neurological deficit precipitated by hot bath in multiple sclerosis. JAMA 249:1751, 1983.

Bickerstaff, E.: Basilar artery migraine. Lancet 1:15, 1961.

Boniuk, M., and Schlezenger, N.: Raeder's paratrigeminal syndrome. Am. J. Ophthalmol. 54:1074, 1962.

Brennan, J., and McCrary, J.A.: Diagnosis of superficial temporal arteritis. Ann. Ophthalmol. 7:1125, 1975.

Brenner, C., et al.: Post traumatic headache. J. Neurosurg. 1:379, 1944.

Campbell, H.: Discussion of headache, its cause and treatment. Br. Med. J. 2:578, 1914.

Connolly, J.F., Gawel, M., Clifford Rose, F.: Migraine patients exhibit abnormalities in the visual evoked potential. J. Neurol. Neurosurg. Psychiatry 45:464, 1982.

Costen, J.: Neuralgias and ear symptoms associated with disturbed function of the temporomandibular joint. JAMA 107:252, 1936.

Diamond, S.: Diagnosing the life threatening cause of headache. Diagnosis July-Aug.:40, 1979.

Doggart, J.: Herpes zoster ophthalmicus. Br. J. Ophthalmol. 17:513, 1933.

Dugan, M., Locke, S. and Gallagher, J.: Occipital neuralgia in adolescents and young adults. N. Engl. J. Med. 267:1166, 1962.

Every, R.: The significance of extreme mandibular movements. Lancet 2:37, 1960.

Ford, F.: A clinical classification of vestibular disorders with differentiation of three syndromes and discussions of a common form of vertigo induced by sudden movement of the head. Bull. Johns Hopkins Hosp. 87:299, 1950.

Ford, F.: The carotid pain syndrome: report of two cases which suggest that, in some instances, migraine is responsible. Bull. Johns Hopkins Hosp. 114:266, 1964.

Ford, F., and Walsh, F.: Raeder's paratrigeminal syndrome: a benign disorder possibly a complication of migraine. Bull. Johns Hopkins Hosp. 103:296, 1958.

Forsman, B., et al.: Propanolol for migraine prophylaxis. Headache 16:238, 1976.

Friedman, A., and Merritt, H.: Migraine and tension headaches, a clinical study of 2,000 cases. Neurology 4:773, 1954.

Fromm, G.H., Terrence, C.F., and Chattha, A.A.: Baclofen in the treatment of refractory trigeminal neuralgia. Neurology 29:550, 1979.

Graham, J.R.: Migraine headache: Diagnosis and management. Headache 19:133, 1979.

Grimson, B.S., and Thompson, H.S.: Raeder's syndrome: a clinical review. Surv. Ophthalmol. 24:199, 1980.

Haas, D.C., Pineda, G.S., and Lourie, H.: Juvenile head trauma syndromes and their relationship to migraine. Arch. Neurol. 32:727, 1975.

Hachinski, V.C., Porchawka, J., and Steele, J.C.: Visual symptoms in the migraine syndrome. Neurology 23:570, 1973.

Hatfalvi, B.I.: The dynamics of post spinal headache. Headache 17:64, 1977.

Henderson, A., and Raskin, N.: Hot-dog headache: individual susceptibility to nitrite. Lancet 2:1162, 1972.

Hitchings, R.A.: The symptom of ocular pain. Trans. Ophthalmol. Soc. U.K. 100:257, 1980.

Horton, B.: Histamine cephalgia: differential diagnosis and treatment. Proc. Staff Meet. Mayo Clin. 31:325, 1956.

Horton, B.: The use of histamine in the treatment of specific types of headache. JAMA 116:377, 1941.

Hunt, J.: The sensory system of the facial nerve and its symptomatology J. Nerv. Ment. Dis. 36:321, 1909.

Janetta, P.J.: Arterial compression of the trigeminal nerve at the pons in patients with trigeminal neuralgia. J. Neurosurg. 26:159, 1967.

Jannetta, P.J.: Observations of the etiology of the trigeminal neuralgia in 100 consecutive operative cases. Definitive microsurgical treatment by relief of compression distortion of the trigeminal nerve at the brain stem. Neurosurg. Congress, Tokyo, Sept., 1973.

Janetta, P.J.: Microsurgical approach to the trigeminal

nerve for tic douloureux. Prog. Neurol. Surg. 7:180, 1976.

Jonasson, F., Cullen, J.F., and Elton, R.A.: Temporal arteritis. Scot. Med. J. 24:111, 1979.

Kerr, F.W.I.: A mechanism to account for frontal headache in cases of posterior-fossa tumors. J. Neurosurg. 18:605, 1961.

Kligon, G., and Smith, W.: Raeder's paratrigeminal syndrome. Neurology 6:750, 1956.

Kudrow, L.: Cluster headache: diagnosis and management. Headache 19:142, 1979.

Kunkel, R.S.: Evaluating the headache patient: history and workup. Headache 19:122, 1979.

Lance, J.W.: Headaches related to sexual activity. J. Neurol. Neurosurg. Psychiatry 39:1226, 1976.

Lance, J., and Anthony, M.: Migrainous neuralgia or cluster headache? J. Neurol. Sci. 13:401, 1971.

Lance, J., Curran, D., and Anthony, M.: Investigations into mechanism and management of chronic headache. Med. J. Aust. 2:909, 1965.

Lees, F.: The migrainous symptoms of cerebral angiomata. J. Neurol. Neurosurg. Psychiatry 25:45, 1962.

Loeser, J.D.: What to do about tic douloureux. JAMA 239:1153, 1978.

Lovshin, L.L.: Carotidynia. Headache 17:192, 1977.

McDonald, W.I.: Pain around the eye: inflammatory and neoplastic causes. Trans. Ophthalmol. Soc. U.K. 100:260, 1980.

Meadows, S.P.: Temporal or giant cell arteritis. Neuro-ophthalmology Symposium of the University of Miami and Bascom Palmer Eye Institute. Vol. 4. Edited by J.L. Smith. St. Louis, C.V. Mosby Co., 1968, p. 148.

Medina, J.L., and Diamond, S.: The clinical link between migraine and cluster headaches. Arch. Neurol. 34:470, 1977.

Moffett, A., Swash, M., and Scott, D.: Effect of chocolate in migraine: a double blind study. J. Neurol. Neurosurg. Psychiatry 37:445, 1974.

O'Connell, J.E.A.: Trigeminal false localizing signs and their causation. Brain 101:119, 1978.

Olafson, R., Rushton, J., and Sayre, G.: Trigeminal neuralgia in a patient with multiple sclerosis: an autopsy report. J. Neurosurg. 24:755, 1966.

Parkinson, D.: Collateral circulation of cavernous carotid artery anatomy. Can. J. Surg., 7:251, 1964.

Paulson, G., and Klawans, H.: Benign orgasmic cephalgia. Headache 13:181, 1974.

Pearce, J.: Insulin induced hyperglycaemia in migraine. J. Neurol. Neurosurg. Psychiatry 34:154, 1971.

Pickering, G., and Hess, W.: Observations on the mechanism of headache produced by histamine. Clin. Sci. 1:77, 1933.

Raeder, J.: Paratrigeminal paralysis of oculopupillary sympathetic. Brain 47:149, 1924.

Raskin, N.H., and Schwartz, R.K.: Icepick-like pain. Neurology 30:203, 1980.

Ray, B., and Wolff, H.: Experimental studies on headache. Pain sensitive structures of the head and their significance in headache. Arch. Surg. 41:813, 1940.

Roseman, D.: Diagnosis of carotidynia. N.Y. State J. Med. 63:2651, 1963.

Ross Russell, R.W.: Vascular causes of ocular pain. Trans. Ophthalmol. Soc. U.K. 100:251, 1980.

Ryan, R.E., and Facer, G.W.: Sphenopalatine ganglion neuralgia and cluster headache: comparisons, contrasts and treatment. Headache 17:7, 1977.

Schott, G.D.: Neurogenic facial pain. Trans. Ophthalmol. Soc. U.K. 100:253, 1980.

Selby, G., and Lance, J.: Observations on 500 cases of migraine and allied vascular headaches. J. Neurol. Neurosurg. Psychiatry 23:23, 1960.

Sluder, G.: Etiology, diagnosis, prognosis and treatment of sphenopalatine ganglion neuralgia. JAMA 61:1201, 1913.

Somerville, B.: The role of progesterone in menstrual migraine. Neurology 21:853, 1971.

Smith, J.: Raeder's paratrigeminal syndrome. Am. J. Ophthalmol. 46:194, 1958.

Smith, J. and Taxdal, D.: Painful ophthalmoplegia: the Tolosa-Hunt syndrome. Am. J. Ophthalmol. 61:1466, 1966.

Swanson, J.W., and Vick, N.A.: Basilar artery migraine. Neurology 28:782, 1978.

Vardi, Y., et al.: Migraine attacks. Neurology 26:447, 1976.

Warrington, E.K.: The completion of visual forms across hemianopic field defects. J. Neurol. Neurosurg. Psychiatry 25:208, 1962.

Wiley, R.G.: The scintillating scotoma without headache. Ann. Ophthalmol. 11:581, 1979.

Wolff, H.G.: Headache and Other Head Pain. New York, Oxford University Press, 1948.

Chapter *15*

Conjugate and Disjugate Eye Movements

PATRICK J.M. LAVIN

CONJUGATE EYE MOVEMENTS (VERSIONS)

Versions are conjugate eye movements; the eyes move together. Vergence eye movements are disconjugate; the eyes do not move together.

Gaze is most frequently used in reference to conjugate eye movement in the head, although technically it refers to conjugate eye movement in space; i.e., gaze = combined head and eye movement.

Saccades are fast eye movements (up to 800°/sec) that change the direction of gaze to fixate new targets. Once the eyes have fixed on a target, optimal visual acuity is maintained by several ocular motor reflex mechanisms that stabilize the image of the target on the fovea, especially during head movement and target pursuit. These reflexes are controlled by several ocular motor mechanisms: The *pursuit system* enables the eye to track slowly moving targets; if the target moves too quickly (>50°/sec), the eye falls behind and the image moves off the fovea, producing a retinal error that signals a fast (catch-up) saccade to refixate the target. The *vestibular eye movement system*, driven by the semicircular canals in response to changes in head position, maintains eye position in space during head movement; this slow eye movement is a vestibulo-ocular reflex (VOR).

The *optokinetic system* utilizes both fast and slow eye movements to stabilize images of fixed objects or reference points in the environment during head rotations of amplitude greater than the range of the VOR arc, as when turning or spinning, and results in optokinetic nystagmus (OKN).

The *vergence system* enables the eyes to move disconjugately to maintain the visual axis of both eyes aligned on a target moving towards or away from the subject. It is essential for binocularity and stereoscopic depth perception.

Horizontal

When the direction of gaze changes from primary position to a new target—say, to the left—the eyes deviate conjugately with a saccade, the left eye abducts as the right adducts. The initiating stimulus may be volitional, auditory, or peripheral retinal. A surge of innervation (pulse) to the appropriate muscles (left lateral rectus and right medial rectus) moves the eyes to the left with a saccade (Fig. 15–1A), while at the same time, the antagonist muscles are inhibited (Sherrington's law of reciprocal innervation).

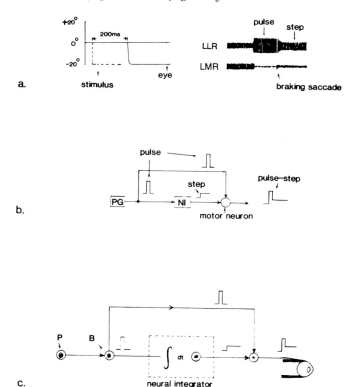

Fig. 15–1. Ocular motor events on left gaze. **A.** Following the appearance of a stimulus 20 ° to the left (− 20 °), the eyes move to the target, with a saccade, after a latency of 200 milliseconds (ms). Electromyography of the left extra-ocular muscles shows the activity in the agonist, the left lateral rectus (LLR), and the antagonist, the left medial rectus (LMR), muscles. **B.** The pulse originates from the pulse generator (PG) and is mathematically integrated by the neural integrator (NI); both signals are summed to produce the pulse-step of innervation to the ocular motor neuron. **C.** The pause cells (P) discharge continuously, suppressing the burst cells (B), except during a saccade when they "pause," allowing the burst cells to discharge, resulting in a pulse.

The neurons that initiate the horizontal saccade are the burst cells (pulse generator) in the ipsilateral gaze center in the paramedian pontine reticular formation (PPRF) and are almost constantly suppressed by the tonically discharging pause cells, also in the PPRF. The burst cells are thus silent, except at the initiation of a saccade, to the ipsilateral side, when the pause cells stop discharging momentarily (Fig. 15–1C). The burst neurons in the PPRF project to the ipsilateral sixth nerve nuclei neurons, approximately 50% of which are interneurons with a different neurotransmitter than the neurons subserving the sixth cranial nerve; these interneurons relay to the contralateral third nerve subnucleus for the medial rectus, via the medial longitudinal fasciculus (MLF) (Fig. 15–2).

To maintain gaze in the eccentric position, the muscles involved maintain a new level of tone achieved by integrating the pulse signal (velocity command) mathematically to a step signal (position command) (Fig. 15–1B). The pulse signal from the burst cells is also relayed to the neural integrator, thought to be partly in the perihypoglossal nuclear complex, the PPRF, and the vestibulocerebellum where it is integrated to a tonic signal in order to maintain the eyes in the eccentric position. The cerebellum and PPRF control the gain, and therefore the output, of the neural integrator (Fig. 15–3). The gain of a system is the

GAZE LEFT

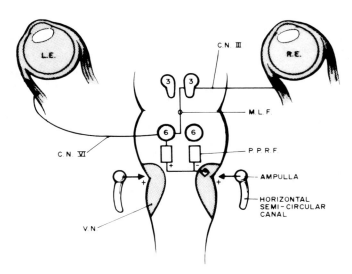

Fig. 15–2. Stimulation of the semicircular canals, by movement of the endolymph towards the ampula, excites the contralateral and inhibits the ipsilateral gaze centers in the paramedian pontine reticular formation (PPRF) via the vestibular nuclei (VN). Each PPRF drives the ipsilateral sixth cranial nerve and the contralateral subnucleus for the medial rectus (part of CN III) via the medial longitudinal fasciculus (MLF).

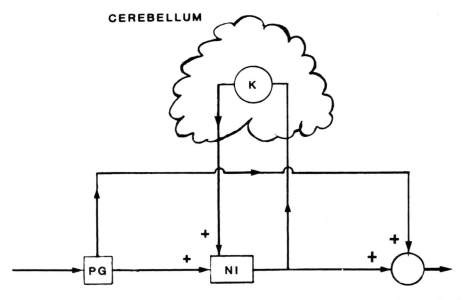

Fig. 15–3. The gain of the brain stem neural integrator (NI) and therefore its output (innervation for gaze holding) is controlled predominantly by the cerebellum. Dysfunction of the gain control (K) may cause the integrator output to fall (the signal decays because of a shortened time constant), allowing the eyes to drift off target. Conversely, an increase in K would result in an unstable integrator, causing an increasing velocity drift off target.

ratio of its output to its input, e.g., the gain of the VOR $= \dfrac{\text{eye movement}}{\text{head movement}}$, e.g., $\dfrac{30°}{30°}$ $= 1$. The PPRF receives commands for voluntary saccades, predominantly from the contralateral frontal lobe. Commands for pursuit come predominantly from the ipsilateral hemisphere, most likely from the posterior parietal lobe.

Each vestibular apparatus has an input to the PPRF via the vestibular nuclei; e.g., for horizontal vestibular reflex eye movements, signals from the ipsilateral horizontal semicircular canal are inhibitory, while those from the contralateral canal are excitatory—in a push-pull fashion (Fig. 15–2). This is the basis for both the vestibulo-ocular and the oculocephalic reflex (doll's eyes).

Vertical

The midbrain reticular formation (MRF) contains neurons involved in vertical eye movements. Burst and tonic cells are scattered throughout the MRF, and burst-tonic cells in the interstitial nucleus of Cajal relay to the rostral interstitial nucleus of the medial longitudinal fasciculus (riMLF). The riMLF (also known as the prerubral fields of Forel) is a well-defined nucleus in monkeys and probably the principle pre-motor relay for vertical saccades in man (Fig. 15–4). The riMLF also receives input from the PPRF, which has some influence on the generation of vertical saccades, but its significance is unknown, as a persistent paralysis of vertical gaze does not result from lesions of the PPRF. The riMLF projects bilaterally (dorsally and caudally) to the third and fourth nerve nuclei. Bilateral lesions of the riMLF or its efferents produce a down-gaze paralysis (Fig. 15–4A). In man such isolated lesions rarely occur except with vascular occlusion of the posterior thalamo-subthalamic branch of the posterior cerebral artery. More commonly, bilateral lesions occur as part of a more diffuse disorder such as progressive supranuclear palsy or neurovisceral lipid storage disease (e.g., the DAF syndrome—down-gaze palsy, ataxia, and foamy macrophages).

Disorders of vertical gaze, particularly down-gaze palsy, and also combined up-and-down-gaze palsy, may be overlooked in patients with brain stem vascular disease because of the more dramatic impairment of consciousness that results from damage to the reticular activating system.

The riMLF also projects dorsally and decussates through the posterior commissure before supplying both third- and fourth-nerve nuclei to mediate up gaze. Lesions at or near the posterior commissure or bilateral pretectal lesions result in paralysis of up gaze (Fig. 15–4B).

DISJUGATE EYE MOVEMENTS (VERGENCE)

A group of cells just lateral to the third nerve nuclei, whose firing rate is related to the angle of convergence, have recently been identified. The stimuli for convergence, relayed from the occipital cortex, are accommodative retinal blur and fusional disparity.

DISORDERS OF GAZE

Clinical Evaluation of Gaze Palsies

The examination should determine that the palsy is conjugate and not an ocular motor nerve disorder, or a muscle disorder such as myasthenia or entrapment. The presence of the oculocephalic (doll's eyes maneuver), vestibulo-ocular reflexes (caloric), and Bell's phenomenon (an ocular deviation, usually upward, on forced closure of the eye lid) point to a supranuclear disorder. In most supranuclear palsies, saccades are affected initially, followed by disorders of pursuit. If the gaze centers in the brain stem become involved, reflex eye movements will also be lost.

Causes of gaze palsies and ophthalmoplegia are listed in Table 15–1 and some are described in detail in the following discussions.

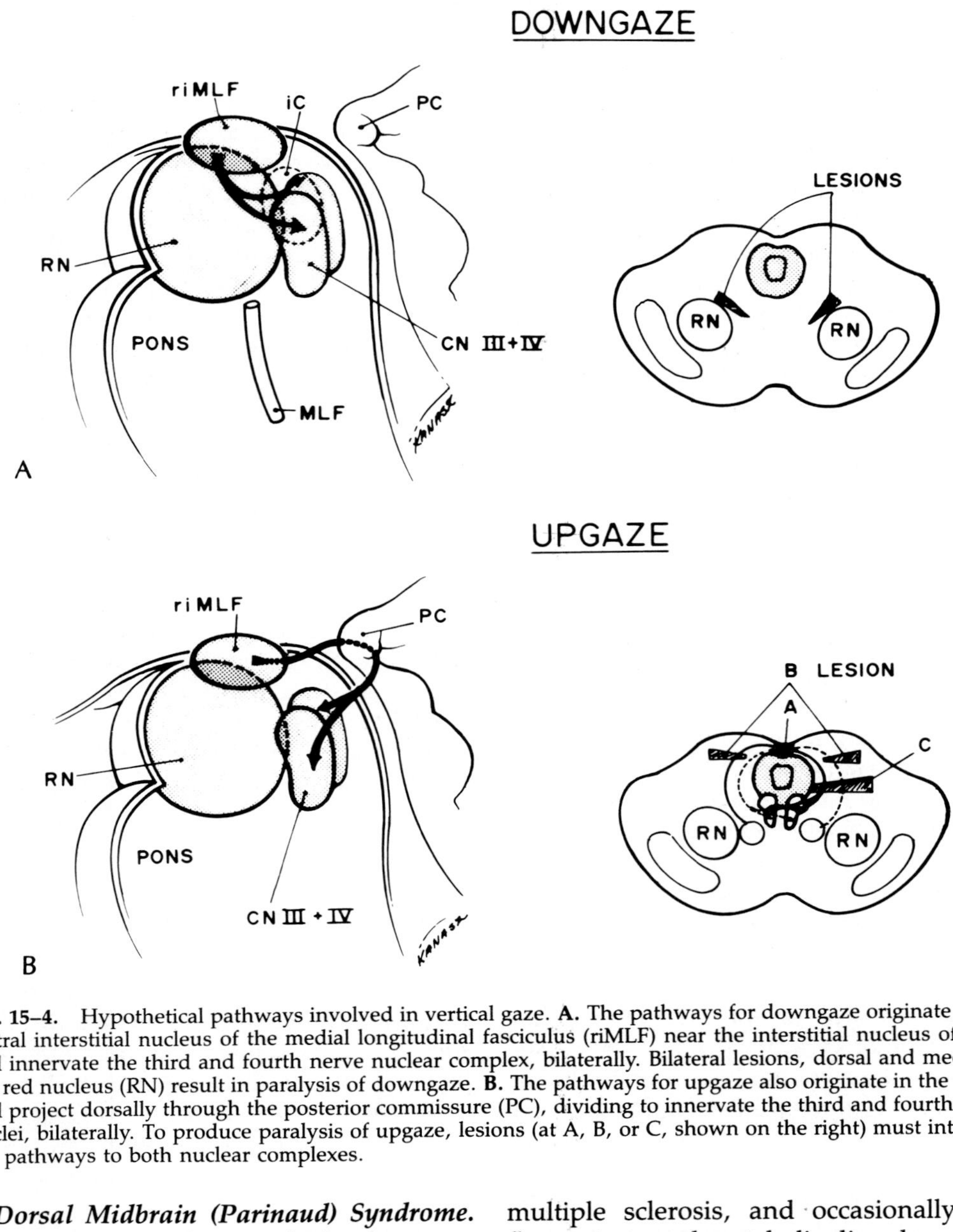

DOWNGAZE

A

UPGAZE

B

Fig. 15–4. Hypothetical pathways involved in vertical gaze. **A.** The pathways for downgaze originate in the rostral interstitial nucleus of the medial longitudinal fasciculus (riMLF) near the interstitial nucleus of Cajal and innervate the third and fourth nerve nuclear complex, bilaterally. Bilateral lesions, dorsal and medial to the red nucleus (RN) result in paralysis of downgaze. **B.** The pathways for upgaze also originate in the riMLF and project dorsally through the posterior commissure (PC), dividing to innervate the third and fourth nerve nuclei, bilaterally. To produce paralysis of upgaze, lesions (at A, B, or C, shown on the right) must interrupt the pathways to both nuclear complexes.

Dorsal Midbrain (Parinaud) Syndrome. This is a supranuclear paralysis of up gaze that may later involve down gaze. Impaired convergence, lid retraction, convergence retraction "nystagmus," and large pupils with light-near dissociation are also part of the syndrome. Early on, the ocular movement reflexes are preserved. This syndrome occurs with tumors in the pineal region, hydrocephalus, vascular disease, multiple sclerosis, and occasionally, inflammatory and metabolic disorders.

Monocular Supranuclear Elevator Palsy. Monocular supranuclear elevator palsy is a limitation of elevation of one eye despite orthotropia in primary position and normal down gaze. It results from a lesion in the contralateral pretectal region, usually vascular or neoplastic.

Ocular Motor Apraxia. Apraxia (from

Table 15–1.   Causes of Gaze Palsies and Ophthalmoplegias

Muscle	Myopathies (CPEO)
	Congenital (e.g., nemaline, multicore)
	Metabolic (carnitine deficiency)
	Kearns syndrome (may be neuropathic)
	Myotonia
	Trauma (orbital entrapment)
	Infiltrative (thyroid and amyloid disease, metastases, congenital familial fibrosis)
	Inflammatory (giant cell arteritis, orbital pseudotumor)
Neuromuscular Junction	Ocular myasthenia
	Eaton-Lambert syndrome (rare)
Ocular Motor Nerve and Nuclei	Chapter 6
Gaze Palsies	Nuclear and paranuclear
	Brain stem injury (vascular, MS, tumor)
	Spinocerebellar degeneration
	Möbius syndrome (agenesis of cranial nerve nuclei)
	Familial congenital gaze palsy
	Internuclear ophthalmoplegia
	Supranuclear (suprapontine)
	Acutely, following hemispheric stroke
	Ocular motor apraxia
	Progressive supranuclear palsy
	Spinocerebellar degeneration
	DAF syndrome
	Whipple's disease
	Wilson's disease
	Maple syrup urine disease
	Jacob Creutzfeld disease
	Alzheimer's disease (1 case autopsied)

the Greek, inaction) means the inability to perform purposeful skilled movements in the absence of obvious paralysis, sensory deficit or incoordination (i.e., random and reflex activities are preserved). Ocular motor apraxia is the inability to perform voluntary saccades. Saccades reflexly induced by peripheral visual and auditory stimuli, as well as the fast phases of OKN and caloric-induced nystagmus, may also be impaired. Pursuit may or may not be affected. The slow phases of caloric-induced nystagmus and OKN are preserved, as are random eye movements.

Congenital ocular motor apraxia, a condition more common in boys, is characterized by impairment of horizontal pursuit and saccades but preservation of vertical eye movements. The child uses head movements to compensate for impaired eye movements, but because of the preserved VOR, the gaze direction does not change when he turns his head. To over-come this VOR response, he closes his eyes to reduce the degree of reflex eye movement (the gain falls from 1.0 to 0.6) while thrusting his head beyond the range of the VOR arc until the eyes are on target; then with the eyes open he slowly straightens his head as the VOR, in the opposite direction, keeps the eyes on target. This explains the characteristic "head thrust" of the disorder. Strabismus, psychomotor developmental delay (particularly reading difficulty), clumsiness, and gait disturbance are often associated with this syndrome. Occasionally, a structural lesion may be present (e.g., porencephalic cyst, agenesis of the corpus callosum, or rarely, hydrocephalus secondary to a medulloblastoma), but usually there is no abnormality found on CT. Ocular motor apraxia also tends to occur in approximately 80% of children with ataxia telangiectasia. The condition improves with age in patients with the idiopathic variety of oculomotor apraxia.

Progressive Supranuclear Palsy. This disorder was first described as a clinicopathologic entity by Steele, et al. in 1964. It has many of the features of Parkinson's disease but is characterized by supranuclear gaze palsy (particularly down gaze), pseudobulbar palsy, axial dystonia, a disturbance of balance and postural reflexes, and a pseudodementia. The VOR is preserved, making fixation even more difficult for the patient. In the later stages, there may be total ophthalmoplegia with loss of the VOR. About one third of these patients improve with dopaminergic medication (e.g., L-dopa, bromocriptine, pergolide) although there is little change in the eye movement disorder.

Familial Gaze Palsy (with or without Scoliosis). Horizontal gaze palsies occasionally occur in families. Affected members have impaired OKN and VORs, but intact convergence and preservation of vertical eye movements; they may also have fine horizontal pendular nystagmus. Individuals in some of these families also have progressive scoliosis, facial myokymia, and facial twitching. Forced ductions are normal. The mode of inheritance is probably autosomal recessive. Hemifacial atrophy and situs inversus of the optic discs is occasionally associated with this disorder. The pathogenesis of familial gaze palsy may be related to developmental failure of the pontine gaze centers or the sixth nerve nuclei.

Internuclear Ophthalmoplegia (INO). When gaze is directed laterally, the pulse of innervation from the PPRF is relayed to the ipsilateral sixth nerve, which innervates the lateral rectus, and via the interneurons in the ipsilateral sixth nerve nucleus and the MLF to the contralateral third nerve subnucleus, which innervates the medial rectus (Fig. 15–2). A lesion of the MLF between the third and sixth nerve nuclei impairs transmission of the signal for the adducting saccade to the ipsilateral eye; adduction will consequently be impaired or slow. With a typical INO, there is also nystagmus of the abducting eye. With bilateral INO, there is almost always upward beating nystagmus. Convergence may be preserved with an INO, but because this maneuver depends on the attention and effort of the patient, its value in localizing the lesion to either the midbrain or pons is not helpful.

A subtle INO may be demonstrated clinically by having the patient make repetitive horizontal saccades (rapid refixations), which will disclose a slow adducting and a normal abducting saccade; there may be overshoot dysmetria of the abducting eye. Similarly, the induction of optokinetic nystagmus (Chapter 16) demonstrates that the amplitude of the abducting saccade is smaller than that of the adducting saccade.

The existence of Lutz posterior INO (supranuclear palsy of abduction) has been disputed, but if its presence is suspected, in an acute situation, cerebellar hemorrhage should be considered in the differential diagnosis.

Convergence Paralysis. Convergence paralysis is usually associated with other features of the dorsal midbrain syndrome discussed earlier. Patients with functional convergence paralysis may be distinguished from those with organic disease by the absence of pupillary constriction (part of the near triad) and preservation of upward gaze. Lack of effort is the most common cause of poor convergence. Convergence becomes more difficult with age. *Convergence insufficiency* is an idiopathic condition that occurs most commonly in women between the ages of 15 and 40 and appears to be an imbalance between accommodation and convergence. It may cause frank diplopia, although eye strain and headache are more common. It responds to orthoptic exercises; less commonly, minus lenses may be required.

Divergence Paralysis. Electromyography of the extraocular muscles during divergence demonstrates activity in the lateral recti, showing that it is not a passive movement; a divergence center has not yet been identified, however. Patients with divergence paralysis are orthotropic for near but have a concomitant esotropia at distance despite a full range of extraocular movement. The condition usually occurs in patients with raised intracranial pressure. The existence of divergence paralysis is controversial and some feel that many of these patients, in fact, have bilateral partial sixth-nerve palsies. Having seen such a patient with bilateral post-traumatic complete sixth-nerve palsy go through a stage resembling divergence paralysis, and having reviewed the relevant literature, I favor the sixth-nerve palsy theory.

Tonic Downward Deviation of Gaze (Forced Down Gaze). This condition occurs in patients with impaired consciousness who have medial thalamic hemorrhage, acute obstructive hydrocephalus, severe metabolic or hypoxic encephalopathy, or diffuse subarachnoid hemorrhage. Downward deviation of the eyes, with preservation of the vertical vestibulo-ocular reflexes (doll's eyes), occurs as a transient phenomenon in otherwise healthy neonates.

Tonic Upward Deviation of Gaze (Forced Up Gaze). With the exception of oculogyric crises and petit mal seizures, in which it may be associated with eyelid flutter, forced up gaze is a rare sign seen only in unconscious patients. Keane has described a series of 17 comatose patients with sustained up gaze following a diffuse insult to the brain (shock, cardiac arrest, heat stroke); postmortem evidence pointed to cerebral and cerebellar hypoxic damage, with relative sparing of the brain stem. Some of those patients went on to develop myoclonic jerks (a recognized accompaniment of anoxic encephalopathy) and large-amplitude downbeat nystagmus, as the upward deviation resolved. Downbeat nystagmus and impaired vertical oculocephalic reflexes, tested in a few patients, suggest a disorder of the vertical vestibulo-ocular reflex pathways (probably in the vestibulocerebellum). The prognosis in Keane's series was very poor.

Skew Deviation. Skew deviation, a vertical divergence that may be noncomitant, is usually seen in patients with brain stem and cerebellar lesions (vascular, demyelinating, tumor) and rarely with peripheral vestibular lesions. It should be distinguished from isolated vertical muscle palsies and dissociated vertical deviation. Skew deviation occurs most commonly with vascular lesions of the lateral medulla (Wallenberg syndrome), presumably because of involvement of the vertical vestibular nuclei. Recently Warren, et al., suggested that a partial third-nerve palsy involving the vertical extraocular muscles caused skew deviation.

Alternating Skew Deviation. This is a rare cyclical vertical divergence of the eyes that usually results from vascular or demyelinating lesions at the pretectal and mesodiencephalic junction (interstitial nucleus of Cajal), although it has recently been associated with periodic alternating nystagmus in a patient with cerebellar degeneration. The skew may alternate with the direction of gaze or alternate spontaneously either in a regular or an irregular manner over a period of seconds or minutes, respectively. Features of the dorsal midbrain syndrome may also be superimposed.

Ocular Tilt Reaction. The ocular tilt reaction is a synkinetic movement that allows us to maintain horizontal orientation of the environment during head tilt. When tilting the head to the left, the left eye rises and intorts as the right eye falls and extorts; when the range of the ocular tilt reflex is exceeded, beyond 15° from the vertical, one loses horizontal orientation and becomes aware of looking at the horizon from a tilted position. With peripheral labyrinthine lesions (particularly of the utricle or its nerve) a spontaneous ocular tilt reaction may occur (ocular counter-rolling) and is associated with a paradoxic head tilt. With central lesions (MS, abscess) of the rostral midbrain, specifically the interstitial nucleus of Cajal and the zona incerta (implicated in the pathogenesis of see-saw nystagmus), a paroxysmal ocular tilt reaction has been described and there is a report of successful treatment with baclofen.

Dissociated Vertical Deviation. This deviation occurs when, during the cover test for phoria or tropia, the covered eye rises without a corresponding fall in the uncovered eye, which may intort, however. This phenomenon, which may be unilateral or bilateral, is a congenital disorder often associated with amblyopia and esotropia. It has no other neurologic significance.

Alternating Gaze Deviation. This is a rare disorder in which the direction of gaze alternates every few minutes. Lateral deviation may be sustained for up to 15 minutes, then gaze returns to the midline where it remains for 10 to 20 seconds before proceeding to the other side. Occasionally, structural lesions are found (pontine vascular lesions, Arnold-Chiari malformations, spinocerebellar degeneration, occipital encephalocele). This disorder is grouped with a number of cyclical ocular phenomena, including cyclical esotropia, cyclical oculomotor palsy, springing pupil, alternating skew deviation, and periodic alternating nystagmus.

Ping Pong Gaze. Ping pong gaze is a conjugate horizontal gaze deviation, which alternates every few seconds, seen in patients (usually comatose) with bilateral cerebral dysfunction or vermal hemorrhage. It is probably a variant of "roving eyes" and suggests that the brain stem (pons) is intact.

Spasm of the Near Reflex (Convergence Spasm). This disorder is characterized by intermittent spasm of convergence, miosis, and accommodation. It is sometimes found during examination of lateral gaze. The patient may complain of blurred or double vision. The condition may mimic unilateral or bilateral sixth nerve paresis but extreme miosis is the diagnostic clue. If the patient looks to one side while converging, an ipsilateral sixth nerve paresis may be simulated (Fig. 15–5). This can be done easily with "a little practice"—which says a lot. Although it occurs in patients with convincing disease (during seizures, head

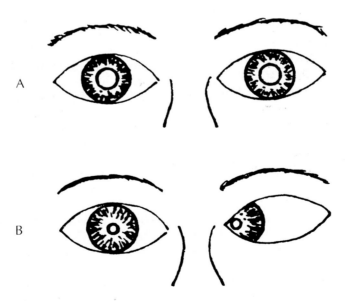

Fig. 15–5. Spasm of the near reflex. **A.** Gaze straight into the distance. **B.** Attempted gaze to the right shows asymmetric convergence while looking to the right, giving the appearance of weakness of the right lateral rectus. Note the clue—constriction of the pupils.

trauma, posterior fossa lesions), it is often found in "hystrionic" patients with no other objective signs.

Mirror Test (Troost's test). Patients may have psychogenic ophthalmoplegia with no eye movements in response to command or pursuit stimuli. Use of a full-field mirror can confirm that the ophthalmoplegia is not organic. The examiner moves the mirror in front of the patient, causing the reflected environment to move, thus stimulating a reflex optokinetic slow eye movement.

The mirror test is also useful in patients with psychogenic total blindness.

BIBLIOGRAPHY

Büttner-Ennever, J.A., et al.: Vertical gaze paralysis and the rostral interstitial nucleus of the medial longitudinal fasciculus. Brain 105:125, 1982.

Cogan, D.G., et al.: Spasm of the near reflex. Arch. Ophthalmol. 54:752, 1955.

Cogan, D.G.: Congenital ocular motor apraxia. Can. J. Ophthalmol. 1:253, 1966.

Cogan, D.G., et al.: The DAF syndrome. Neuro-ophthalmology 2(11):7, 1981.

Corbett, J.J., et al.: Slowly alternating skew deviation. Description of a pretectal syndrome in three patients. Ann. Neurol. 10:540, 1981.

Daroff, R.B.: "See saw nystagmus." Neurology 15(9):874, 1965.

Daroff, R.B., et al.: Supranuclear disorders of eye movements. In Neuro-ophthalmology. Edited by J.S. Glaser. New York, Harper & Row, 1978. (Also In Clinical Ophthalmology. Vol. 2. Edited by T. D. Duane. New York, Harper & Row, 1983.)

Daroff, R.B.: Chronic progressive external ophthalmoplegia. Neurol. Neurosurg. Update Series, 4(7):1, 1983.

Dell'Osso, L.F., et al.: Eye movement characteristics and recording techniques. In Neuro-ophthalmology. Edited by J.S. Glaser. New York, Harper & Row, 1978. (Also In Clinical Ophthalmology. Vol. 2. Edited by T.D. Duane. New York, Harper & Row, 1983.)

Drachman, D.A.: Ophthalmoplegia plus: The neurodegenerative diseases associated with progressive external ophthalmoplegia. Arch. Neurol. 18:654, 1968.

Glaser, J.S.: Myasthenic pseudo-internuclear ophthalmoplegia. Arch. Ophthalmol. 75:363, 1966.

Halmagyi, G.M., et al.: Ocular tilt reaction with peripheral vestibular lesion. Ann. Neurol. 6:80, 1979.

Hedges, T.R., III.: Ocular tilt reaction due to an upper brain stem lesion. Paroxysmal skew deviation, torsion and oscillation of the eyes with head tilt. Ann. Neurol. 11:537, 1982.

Jampel, R.S., et al.: Monocular elevation paresis caused by a CNS lesion. Arch. Ophthalmol. 80:45, 1968.

Keane, J.R.: Sustained upgaze in coma. Ann. Neurol. 9:409, 1981.

Kirham, T.H., et al.: Divergence paralysis with raised intracranial pressure. Br. J. Ophthalmol. 56:776, 1972.

Leigh, R.J., and Zee, D.S.: The diagnostic value of abnormal eye movements: A pathophysiological approach. Johns Hopkins Med. J. 151:122, 1982.

Leigh, R.J., and Zee, D.S.: The Neurology of Eye Movements. Philadelphia, F.A. Davis, 1983.

Lessell, S.: Supra paralysis of monocular elevation. Neurology 25:1134, 1975.

Lewis, J.M., and Kline, L.B.: Periodic alternating nystagmus associated with periodic alternating skew deviation. J. Clin. Neuro-ophthalmol. 3:115, 1983.

Lyle, D.J.: Ocular motor apraxia. Trans. Am. Ophthalmol. Soc. 59:274, 1961.

Mitchell, J.M.: Periodic alternating skew deviation. J. Clin. Neuro-ophthalmol. 1:5, 1981.

Plum, F., and Posner, J.B.: Diagnosis of Stupor and Coma, 3rd Ed. Philadelphia, F.A. Davis, 1980.

Pierrot-Deseilligy, C., et al.: Parinaud's syndrome. Brain 105:667, 1982.

Sharpe, J.A., et al.: Familial paralysis of horizontal gaze. Neurology 25(11):1035, 1975.

Smith, J.L., et al.: Skew deviation. Neurology 14:96, 1964.

Spector, R.H., et al.: The ocular motor system. Ann. Neurol. 9:517, 1981.

Staudenmaier, C., et al.: Periodic alternating gaze deviation with dissociated secondary face turn. Arch. Ophthalmol. 101:202, 1983.

Steele, J.C., et al.: Progressive supranuclear palsy. Arch. Neurol. 10:373, 1964.

Tijssen, C.C., et al.: Spasm of the near reflex: functional or organic disorder? Neuro-ophthalmology 3(1):59, 1983.

Troost, B.T., et al.: The ocular motor defects in progressive supranuclear palsy. Ann. Neurol. 2:397, 1977.

Troost, B.T., et al.: Functional paralysis of horizontal gaze. Neurology 29:82, 1979.

Warren, W., et al.: Atypical oculomotor paresis. J. Clin. Neuro-ophthalmol. 2:13, 1982.

Yee, R.D., et al.: Familial congenital paralysis of horizontal gaze. Arch. Ophthalmol. 100:1449, 1982.

Zee, D.S., et al.: Congenital ocular motor apraxia. Brain 100:581, 1977.

Chapter 16

Nystagmus

PATRICK J.M. LAVIN

GENERAL ASPECTS

Nystagmus is an involuntary rhythmic biphasic ocular oscillation, in which at least one phase is always slow (both phases are slow in pendular nystagmus). The slow phase is pathologic and is responsible for the initiation and generation of the nystagmus; the fast phase (saccade) is merely corrective, bringing the fovea back on target. The longer the fovea is on target (foveation time) the better the acuity (Fig. 16–1).

The word nystagmus comes from the Greek *nustagmos* meaning drowsiness, which in turn comes from "nustazein" meaning to nod in sleep—a good analogy illustrating the initial slow drooping movement of the head as the tonic neck muscles relax during drowsiness and the fast corrective movement that follows.

Clinically, nystagmus may be divided broadly into pendular and jerk forms. Ac-

curate oculographic recordings often reveal that nystagmus, which appears pendular clinically, has in fact a jerk (pseudopendular or pseudocycloid) waveform (Fig. 16–2).

Nystagmus may be associated with poor visual acuity, oscillopsia, and vertigo.

When examining a patient for nystagmus, the following features should be determined:

1. Presence in primary position or on eccentric gaze (gaze-evoked).
2. Conjugate or dissociated.
3. A change in intensity (amplitude by frequency) with direction of gaze.
4. Pendular or jerk.
5. If jerk, direction of fast phase.
6. Spontaneous alteration of direction (PAN)?
7. Provocation by head positioning.

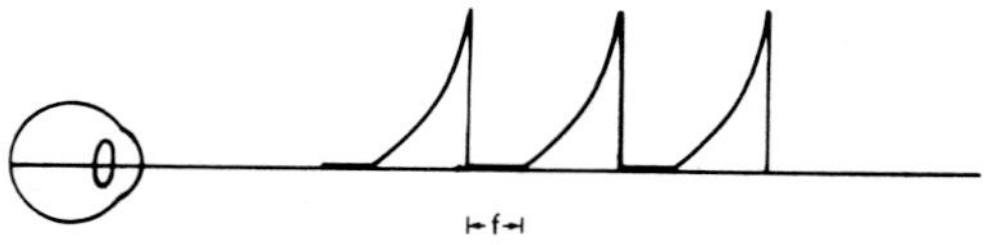

Fig. 16–1. During jerk nystagmus, the fovea remains on target for short periods of time (f); this is referred to as foveation strategy. (After L.F. Dell'Osso)

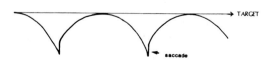

Fig. 16–2. A pseudocycloid waveform, demonstrating a slow drift off target with an increasing velocity slow-phase interrupted by a braking saccade to the right; the saccade is of insufficient amplitude to refoveate the eye and is followed by a decreasing velocity movement returning the eye to target.

8. Presence of a null zone (angle of gaze where nystagmus is minimal or absent).

9. Suppression with convergence.

Pendular Nystagmus. Pendular nystagmus, also called sinusoidal because of its wave form (Fig. 16–3), may be congenital or acquired. The most common causes of acquired pendular nystagmus are multiple sclerosis and brain stem vascular disease affecting the deep cerebellar nuclei or their efferent connections in the brain stem. Vertical pendular nystagmus closely resembles the vertical ocular oscillation associated with *palatal myoclonus* (the oculopalatal syndrome) and may indeed be a restricted form of the same disorder, which is also thought to result from lesions of the cerebellar nuclei or their connections. Brain stem (pontine) infarction, followed by spinocerebellar degeneration, is the most common cause of the oculopalatal syndrome, which is usually confined to the muscles of branchial origin.

Jerk Nystagmus. Jerk nystagmus is designated conventionally by the direction of the fast phase (e.g., with right-beating nystagmus, the fast phase is to the right) and is usually accentuated by gaze in the direction of the fast phase (Alexander's law, which states that the intensity of nystagmus increases with gaze in the direction of the fast phase). Jerk nystagmus may be subdivided into three groups based on the shape of the slow phase, determined by oculographic recordings (Fig. 16–4). The slow phase may have (a) constant velocity (linear slope), as a result of imbalance between the right and left vestibular (and possibly pursuit) input to the pontine gaze

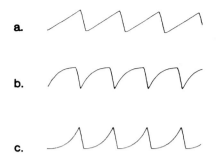

Fig. 16–4. Types of jerk nystagmus (left beating). (**A.**) Linear (constant) velocity slow phase; (**B.**) decreasing velocity slow phase; (**C.**) increasing velocity slow phase.

centers; (b) a decreasing velocity, caused by a defect in the gaze-holding mechanism, i.e., a leaky integrator (Chapter 15); and (c) an increasing velocity, caused by high-gain instability of the slow eye movement subsystem, as a result of dysfunction of the cerebellar or PPRF influence on the gain control of the neural integrator (see Fig. 15–3).

The clinical significance of nystagmus often depends on the accompanying signs. In the past decade, however, better definition and classification of nystagmus have enabled the physician to be more specific clinically. This advance is based largely on oculographic recordings that determine the waveform of the nystagmus.

Optokinetic Nystagmus (OKN). OKN is a natural ocular motor reflex used to stabilize the images of still objects or reference points in the environment, during head movements beyond the range of the vestibulo-ocular reflex arc (Chapter 15). It is tested clinically by having the subject look at repetitively moving stripes. True OKN is stimulated by moving the entire environment, achieved artificially by rotating a large striped drum at a constant velocity around the stationary subject. While the striped drum or tape used in the office does not test true OKN, but rather foveal pursuit followed by refixation saccades, it is still a useful clinical test in the following situations:

1. Patients with homonymous hemiano-

R
↕
L

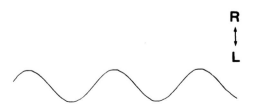

Fig. 16–3. Pendular nystagmus, also called sinusoidal because of its waveform.

pias owing to vascular lesions involving either the parietal or occipital lobe usually have preserved OKN. If a patient with the homonymous hemianopia has an absent OKN response, then a large, deep lesion, involving both the parietal and occipital lobes, should be suspected. Such a lesion is likely to be a neoplasm because two separate vascular territories are involved (Cogan's dictum).

2. Patients with complete organic blindness or ophthalmoplegia do not have an OKN response, whereas patients with psychogenic disease do have such a response.

3. With congenital nystagmus, the direction of the fast phases may be paradoxic; i.e., in the direction of rotation of the drum, said to be a result either of inverted pursuit or shifting of the null zone.

4. Use of the OKN drum/tape may demonstrate a subtle internuclear ophthalmoplegia (Chapter 15).

5. Convergence retraction "nystagmus" may be elicited by rotating the drum downward in an attempt to induce upward saccades.

CLINICAL SYNDROMES

Congenital Nystagmus (CN). Although present from birth, CN may not be noticed for the first few weeks or even years of life. CN may be accompanied by a severe visual deficit, but is not a result of poor vision. Clinically, CN often appears pendular; however, accurate oculographic recordings show that jerk forms are more frequent. Titubation (head tremor) often accompanies CN. CN may be hereditary (autosomal recessive, X-linked dominant, or X-linked recessive). Clinically, the waveform appears horizontal and pendular, becoming jerk on lateral gaze; the intensity may diminish with age. Clinical features that help to differentiate CN from the acquired forms of nystagmus include history of nystagmus in infancy; good visual acuity; titubation; paradoxic response to OKN; damping with convergence; null zone, usually equal in both eyes; latent superimposition (the nystagmus amplitude changes when one eye is occluded); and no oscillopsia. In difficult cases, eye movement recordings help distinguish CN from acquired nystagmus by demonstrating an increasing exponential or a pendular waveform (important for medical/legal reasons). The important clinical points concerning CN are as follows:

1. Convergence damps the nystagmus and may improve acuity.
2. There is usually a null zone where the intensity of the nystagmus is minimal; this may be 5 to 15° laterally, or even upward, and produces a compensatory head turn or tilt that often annoys teachers and parents.

Both 1 and 2 above may be utilized to improve acuity by using prisms to converge the eyes or to direct gaze to the null zone. Surgery on the extraocular muscles may also achieve the same purpose when prisms are too thick for a good visual resolution or too heavy for comfort.

3. Differentiating CN from acquired nystagmus may avoid unnecessary and invasive tests and may also settle potential litigation cases where nystagmus is claimed to be the result of injury.
4. Amblyopia may be present, in the absence of an obvious tropia, and can be detected by the use of plus lenses, which will blur the image of the good eye enough to make the child use the other eye; this will determine the acuity of that eye. It is important not to blur the image too much, as this may produce latent superimposition, which would make the nystagmus worse. This technique may also be used in patients with spasmus nutans and latent nystagmus.

Latent Nystagmus (LN) and Manifest Latent Nystagmus (MLN). LN is brought out by monocular fixation (covering one eye); the slow phase is directed towards the covered eye. With MLN, oscillation is present with both eyes open, but only one is being used for vision; the other is being suppressed because of strabismus or amblyopia.

Dell'Osso's group, using ocular motility recordings, found that even in LN there is a micronystagmus with both eyes open; they feel there is probable suppression of vision in one eye. While LN and MLN are usually congenital, the waveform has a decreasing velocity slow phase, thus differing from true CN.

Spasmus Nutans. Spasmus nutans is a transient form of high-frequency, low-amplitude nystagmus. Its direction may be horizontal, vertical, or torsional, and there may be associated torticollis, titubation, and tropia. Spasmus nutans is not present at birth but occurs most commonly at 6 to 12 months of age, and lasts 18 months to 2 years, although occasionally, as long as 5 years. Spasmus nutans is usually a benign and transient disorder; however, recent reports of its association with other neurologic abnormalities (gliomas of the anterior visual pathways, Leigh's disease), which may be coincidental, suggest that a CT scan should be performed in patients with spasmus nutans.

Vestibular Nystagmus. Vestibular nystagmus, which has a linear slow phase (Fig. 16–4A) is often associated with vertigo and vegetative symptoms (nausea and vomiting), which are more severe with peripheral (end organ) disease. It may result from damage to the labyrinth, vestibular nerve, central vestibular nuclei, or vestibular connections in the brain stem or cerebellum. Vestibular nystagmus may be present in primary position, with the fast phase contralateral to the side of the lesion. The intensity of the nystagmus increases with gaze in the direction of the fast phase. With peripheral vestibular damage, there is also a torsional (rotary) component because of involvement of more than one of the semicircular canals (each canal subserves a different plane); whereas with central disease, a small lesion affecting the

large vestibular nuclei in the brain stem may produce nystagmus in one plane only. Pure vertical nystagmus, although less common than pure horizontal, occurs almost exclusively with central lesions, with the exception of peripheral positional nystagmus. Subtle vestibular nystagmus may be elicited by positioning the head; indeed, the patient may then complain of vertigo.

Central and peripheral nystagmus may be distinguished in the majority of cases by the following (Table 16–1): Peripheral vestibular lesions are associated with severe vertigo and nausea. The nystagmus has a mixed horizontal and torsional component and is never vertical except in the head down position, when the posterior semicircular canal is stimulated (as in benign positional vertigo). Both nystagmus and vertigo, are suppressed by visual fixation. Symptoms are often paroxysmal and recurrent, whereas central vestibular symptoms tend to be chronic and persistent. Peripheral vestibular nystagmus may be associated with deafness and tinnitus and results from trauma, labyrinthitis, Meniere's disease, degenerative inner ear disease, vestibular neuropathy (vestibular "neuronitis"), vascular disease, and drug toxicity. Central lesions result from brain stem ischemia, demyelination, and tumor, and are usually associated with other neurologic signs.

Observations of nystagmus produced by positioning the patient may also help differentiate peripheral from the less common central type. Positional nystagmus (and vertigo) resulting from a peripheral lesion has a latency (interval between positioning the head and onset of nystagmus), is transient, and adapts with repetition of the test.

It is important to be aware that central vestibular lesions may mimic peripheral disease clinically, but the reverse is not the case.

Caloric Testing. The semicircular canals have a steady tonic input to the gaze centers in the PPRF. Via connections through

Table 16–1. Features that Distinguish Central and Peripheral Nystagmus

	Central	Peripheral
Vertigo	mild	severe
Autonomic (e.g., nausea, vomiting, sweating)	mild	severe
Deafness ± tinnitus	rare	frequent
Duration of nystagmus (and vertigo)	persistent (chronic)	short (minutes–weeks), may be recurrent
Vector of nystagmus	uniplanar (horizontal, vertical or torsional), often bidirectional	mixed (horizontal–torsional), unidirectional—fast phase to opposite side
Effect of fixation	none	reduces nystagmus (and vertigo)
Positional changes	no latency, persistent, reproducible, uniplanar	Latent interval, fatigues, adapts, mixed vector (rarely vertical—see text)
Illusion of enviromental movement	variable	towards fast phase
Direction of past pointing	variable	towards slow phase
Direction of Rhomberg (falling)	variable	towards slow phase
Effect of head turn	no effect	changes direction of fall
Other neurologic findings	usually present	absent
Incidence	uncommon	frequent

the vestibular nuclei, the left horizontal canal excites the right PPRF and simultaneously inhibits the left PPRF (see Fig. 15–2). Cold water irrigation of the left ear lowers the tonic firing rate from the left semicircular canal. This reduces excitation to the right PPRF and disinhibits the left PPRF, which are also under steady state inhibition and excitation, respectively, from the nonirrigated right side. The resulting imbalance to the gaze centers drives the eyes to the left. In the unconscious patient, the eyes remain deviated to the ipsilateral side for a couple of minutes, but in the conscious patient with a normal vestibular system, corrective saccades attempt to return the eyes to the primary position, producing a vestibular nystagmus with the fast phase to the opposite side. (COWS, the mnemonic for direction of caloric-induced nystagmus, Cold Opposite, Warm Same, is also a reminder that the horizontal semicircular canals, like the horns of a cow, are inclined at an angle of 30° to the horizontal [Fig. 16–5].) Gross abnormalities of the reflex arc (semicircular canals, vestibular nerve, ipsilateral pontine gaze center) result in either a weakened or absent response. For more subtle findings, quantitative caloric testing is required.

To stimulate the horizontal semicircular canal (Fig. 16–5) and thus test the horizontal vestibular apparatus, cold water is instilled into the external auditory meatus, provided there is no wax, drum perforation, or active infection in the middle or external ear. The test is best performed with the patient's head inclined, on a pillow, at 30° to the horizontal, because of the anatomy of the semicircular canals (Fig. 16–5). Frenzel lenses (+20 diopter), if available, help eliminate fixation and magnify the fine nystagmus for the observer.

Gaze-Evoked Nystagmus. Gaze-evoked nystagmus is not present in primary position, but appears on horizontal eccentric gaze. When it is physiologic or the result of vestibular disease, the waveform has a linear slow phase (Fig. 16–4A). When it occurs as the result of a leaky integrator in patients with diffuse brain stem or cerebellar disease (MS, vascular, drug intoxication, tumor), the waveform has a decreasing velocity slow phase (Fig. 16–4B). In the latter situation, the evoked nystagmus may be upward on up gaze and occasionally downward on down gaze, particularly when the MLF is affected bilaterally. Gaze-evoked nystagmus with a

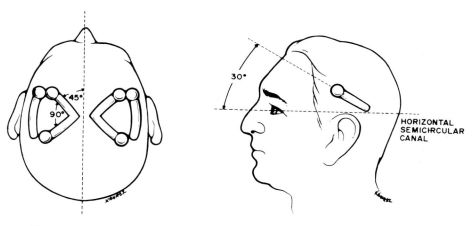

Fig. 16–5. The vestibular apparatus showing the horizontal semicircular canals inclined at an angle of 30° (right).

decreasing velocity slow phase is also referred to as gaze-paretic nystagmus.

Physiologic Nystagmus. Physiologic nystagmus may be sustained or unsustained. When sustained, it may be confused with pathologic nystagmus, but can be identified by certain features. It is present symmetrically at the extremes of horizontal and, occasionally, of vertical gaze. Although it may be unequal in each eye, the nystagmus is of small amplitude and has a linear slow phase (Fig. 16–4A); it may be produced by fatigue. A reasonable clinical guideline is to regard fine symmetrical nystagmus, detected beyond 30° of gaze or beyond the range of binocular vision, as physiologic unless there is a good reason to suspect otherwise.

Dissociated (Disjunctive) Nystagmus. Dissociated nystagmus occurs when the eyes are out of phase with each other and is most often seen with lesions of the medial longitudinal fasciculus (MLF), which produce internuclear ophthalmoplegia and a gaze-evoked nystagmus greater in the abducting eye (Chapter 15). Dissociated nystagmus may also be seen with acquired pendular nystagmus, spasmus nutans, and occasionally, with CN. Dissociated nystagmus can occur with myasthenia when there is an apparent internuclear ophthalmoplegia (pseudo-INO).

Upbeat Nystagmus. Upbeat nystagmus is a spontaneous jerk nystagmus with the fast phase upwards while the eyes are in primary position. It occurs with acquired structural disease of the brain stem or cerebellum, particularly the medulla or anterior vermis of the cerebellum. It may also occur in Wernicke's encephalopathy.

Downbeat Nystagmus. Downbeat nystagmus is a spontaneous jerk nystagmus with the fast phase downwards while the eyes are in primary position or in lateral gaze. The amplitude of the oscillation is usually greatest when the eyes are directed slightly downward and laterally (Daroff's rule). Downbeat nystagmus is frequently associated with structural disease at the craniocervical junction (e.g., Chiari malformations or basilar invagination) (Fig. 16–6); however, it also occurs with alcoholic and familial cerebellar degeneration, vascular and demyelinating disease of the brain stem, and rarely, with anticonvulsant toxicity. Downbeat nystagmus has recently been reported in a patient with Wernicke's encephalopathy and in two patients with magnesium depletion who, however, also had Wernicke's encephalopathy. Baloh and Spooner make the point that even when downbeat nystagmus is not spontaneous but occurs only with rapid positional changes in the sagittal plane (head hanging

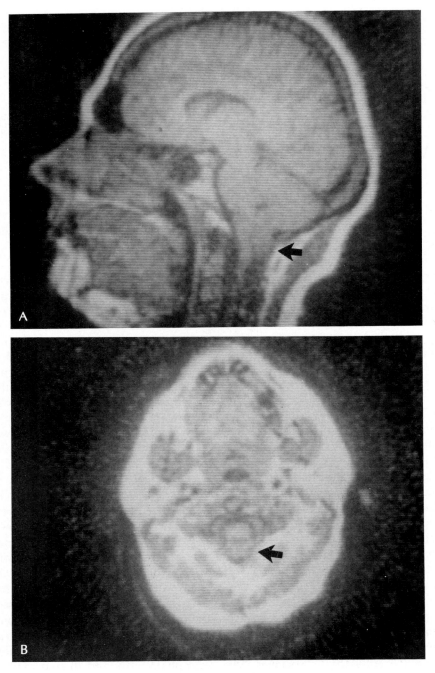

Fig. 16–6. A magnetic resonance imaging (MRI) scan showing a Chiari malformation in a patient with "midline" cerebellar ataxia and downbeat nystagmus. **A.** Herniation of the cerebellar tonsils through the foramen magnum. **B.** Extra-axial mass (tonsils) dorsal to the upper cervical cord at the level of the foramen magnum. (Courtesy of Benjamin Kaufman, University Hospitals of Cleveland, and of Technicare Inc., Solon, Ohio.)

position), it has the same diagnostic significance as when spontaneous. Recently, a young patient of ours with disequilibrium but no other physical findings had downbeat nystagmus only when placed in the head hanging position; midline cerebellar atrophy was demonstrated on CT (Fig. 16–7).

Few patients with acquired nystagmus have had successful suppression of the nystagmus with treatment. Chambers, et al., had some success in one patient, using clonazepam, although spontaneous improvement may have played a part. A patient of ours had downbeat nystagmus (associated with Wernicke's encephalopathy) that suppressed during voluntary convergence; oscillopsia and visual acuity improved with the use of base-out prisms added to the patient's spectacles. Downbeat nystagmus may be associated with periodic alternating nystagmus.

Periodic Alternating Nystagmus (PAN). PAN is associated with disorders of the vestibular nuclei and vestibulocerebellum. It is one of the enigmatic cyclical neuroophthalmologic phenomena (Chapter 15) in which a horizontal jerk nystagmus present in primary position changes direction periodically; i.e., a right-beating nystag-

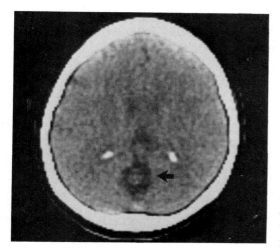

Fig. 16–7. A CT scan showing midline cerebellar atrophy.

mus damps, may become pendular or disappear, and then begins to beat to the left. The whole cycle takes approximately 3 minutes.

PAN may be congenital; however, the acquired form has the same clinical significance as downbeat nystagmus and should focus attention at the craniocervical junction. Acquired PAN has been successfully treated with baclofen. PAN should be distinguished from rebound nystagmus.

Rebound Nystagmus. Rebound nystagmus is a horizontal gaze-evoked jerk nystagmus that changes direction with sustained lateral gaze and that, on return to the primary position, may beat transiently in the opposite direction. It occurs in patients with cerebellar disease.

Convergence-Evoked Nystagmus. This is a rare disorder occurring only during the act of voluntary convergence (fixation and tracking of near targets). It may be congenital or acquired (e.g., MS), conjugate or dissociated, and is usually pendular.

Convergence Nystagmus (Dissociated). This is an extremely rare disorder in which the oscillation of each eye is 180° out of phase. This form of nystagmus, which is usually pendular, may be congenital or acquired. It is to be distinguished from convergence retraction "nystagmus" (discussed later in this chapter), which occurs with the dorsal midbrain syndrome. The anatomic substrate and mechanism are unknown.

Divergence (Dissociated) Nystagmus. Divergence nystagmus occurs when each eye beats outward simultaneously. This rare form of nystagmus is occasionally seen in patients with posterior fossa disease. It may be associated with other forms of nystagmus, particularly downbeat. A patient with spinocerebellar degeneration, referred to our clinic because of an irregular alternating nystagmus (beating right, left, up and down, haphazardly—unlike the regularly rotating vector of windmill nystagmus described by Sanders), had ocular motility recordings that revealed intermittent divergence nystagmus, not detected clinically.

See-Saw Nystagmus. See-saw nystagmus is a spectacular ocular oscillation with two main components at work simultaneously. It occurs with disease in the region of the mesodiencephalic junction, more specifically, the zona incerta and the interstitial nucleus of Cajal. The first component is a pendular vertical oscillation of the eyes. The second component is a torsional movement: one eye rising and intorting at the same time the other eye is falling and extorting. This oscillation represents disordered control of the ocular tilt reflex, which allows horizontal orientation of the environment on the retina during head tilt (Chapter 15). The congenital variety may be associated with a superimposed horizontal pendular nystagmus. The acquired variety occurs with lesions in the region of the third ventricle (sellar and parasellar tumors) and may be associated with a bitemporal hemianopia. See-saw nystagmus may also result from upper brain-stem vascular disease and head trauma. A Japanese group has reported successful treatment of a patient with see-saw nystagmus and of a number of patients with torticollis, following stereotactic destruction of the interstitial nucleus of Cajal.

Lid Nystagmus. A rhythmic, upward jerking movement of the upper eyelids, lid nystagmus occurs in three situations: (1) synchronously with vertical ocular nystagmus; (2) synchronously with the fast phases of gaze-evoked horizontal nystagmus in some patients with the lateral medullary syndrome; (3) during voluntary convergence (said to result from disease of the rostral medulla).

Monocular Nystagmus. Monocular nystagmus may be pendular or jerk, horizontal, vertical, or oblique. It may be seen occasionally in patients with amblyopia, strabismus, monocular blindness, spasmus nutans, internuclear ophthalmoplegia, or rarely, with seizures.

OTHER OCULAR MOVEMENTS THAT ARE NOT NYSTAGMUS

Voluntary "Nystagmus" (Flutter). This condition, more correctly called voluntary flutter, (Fig. 16–8) is in fact a series of fast eye movements (back-to-back saccades) without slow phases or intersaccadic intervals. Subjects may have to converge slightly to initiate the oscillation, but are unable to sustain it for longer than 30 seconds. The ability to perform this "party trick" tends to run in families and was found by Zahn to occur as frequently as in 8% of a student-age population. Occasionally, the phenomenon can cause diagnostic difficulty if the subject claims to have symptoms (e.g., blurred vision), especially if the subject is involved in litigation or seeking emotional gain. The condition should, however, be easily recognized.

Ocular Flutter. A sign of brain stem or cerebellar disease, ocular flutter consists of conjugate horizontal back-to-back saccades that occur spontaneously in intermittent bursts and may be aggravated by attempts at fixation. Flutter may be associated with ocular dysmetria and may progress to opsoclonus.

Opsoclonus. This is a spontaneous chaotic, multivectorial, conjugate, saccadic eye-movement disorder that is aggravated by attempts at fixation and may be associated with myoclonic jerks of the limbs (dancing eyes–dancing feet syndrome) and cerebellar ataxia. Opsoclonus occurs with disorders of the cerebellum and brain stem, such as encephalitis, metabolic and toxic

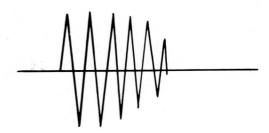

Fig. 16–8. Voluntary nystagmus (flutter). Back-to-back saccades without intersaccadic intervals.

encephalopathy, and as a remote manifestation of malignancy.

Adults with remote carcinoma (breast, lung, uterus) may develop parenchymal cerebellar degeneration and opsoclonus; whereas children with neuroblastomas may have a reversible opsoclonus-myoclonus syndrome (disordered serotonergic neurotransmission), which is responsive to ACTH.

Nutritional deficiency has been implicated in a number of paraneoplastic syndromes including opsoclonus. Nausieda, et al., reported opsoclonic cerebellopathy in a patient with bronchogenic carcinoma, in whom the opsoclonus, but not the ataxia, responded to the administration of *thiamine* before removal of the tumor. Although Wernicke's encephalopathy may have been coexistent, this report certainly opens up a possible line of therapy. *Biotin* replacement has been reported to reverse opsoclonus-myoclonus in a patient with biotin deficiency.

Ocular Dysmetria. Ocular dysmetria occurs with refixation saccades when the eye either overshoots or undershoots the target, and is followed by a brief series of saccadic oscillations of decreasing amplitude (Fig. 16–9). It is a sign of cerebellar disease.

Flutter Dysmetria. Following refixation on a target a brief burst of flutter occurs; this is also a sign of cerebellar disease.

Flutter and opsoclonus are thought to result from disordered control of the pause cells in the PPRF, which tonically suppress the burst cells—the pulse generator (Chapter 15). The pause cells are controlled by the cerebellum; consequently, cerebellar and brain stem dysfunction affecting these cells or their connections may result in unwanted saccadic outbursts.

Convergence Retraction "Nystagmus." Convergence retraction "nystagmus" (and convergence "nystagmus" without retraction) is not true nystagmus but in fact an ocular oscillation initiated by a fast eye movement (nystagmus is initiated by slow eye movement). Clinically, there appears to be a fast convergent movement with synchronous retraction of both globes caused by simultaneous co-contraction of the extraocular muscles (disruption of reciprocal innervation), followed by a slow divergent movement. If the medial recti contract a little more than the other muscles, there is an apparent convergent movement. Less commonly, there may be a divergent movement if the lateral recti are dominant. This oscillation occurs on attempted saccades upward and may be brought out by use of downward-moving OKN stimuli, which induce attempted upward saccades. Convergence retraction "nystagmus" occurs as part of the dorsal midbrain syndrome (Chapter 15).

Ocular Bobbing. This is a rapid downward eye movement followed by a slow drift back to the primary position; the frequency is 2 to 15 per minute. Horizontal gaze is usually impaired. With extensive disease, there may be asymmetric third nerve involvement, resulting in monocular bobbing. In atypical bobbing, horizontal eye movements are preserved. Ocular bobbing occurs with extensive destruction of the central pons (by hemorrhage or infarct), and usually implies a poor prognosis. Such patients are comatose because of involvement of the reticular activating system. There are, however, reports of ocular bobbing in conscious patients; I have seen one such patient with brain stem

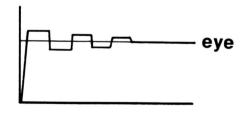

Fig. 16–9. Ocular dysmetria (hypermetria, i.e., overshoot, shown here). A large saccade overshooting the target is followed by a series of smaller saccades, of diminishing amplitude. In hypometria, the eye undershoots the target and is followed by one or more corrective saccades.

multiple sclerosis. Ocular bobbing occasionally occurs with encephalitis, severe metabolic encephalopathy, cerebellar hemorrhage, and hydrocephalus.

Recently, two variants of ocular bobbing have been described: (1) *reverse bobbing*, in which the initial fast phase is upward, followed by a slow drift downward; (2) *inverse bobbing* (dipping), in which the initial deviation is a slow phase downward, followed by a rapid return to the primary position. Patients with both of these variants are usually comatose and have severe structural or metabolic disorders affecting the mesodiencephalic region.

Superior Oblique Myokymia. More correctly termed intermittent uniocular microtremor by Hoyt and Keane, this is a rapid monocular torsional-vertical oscillation of small amplitude, resulting from intermittent contraction of the superior oblique muscle. Some patients may have a slower large-amplitude torsional oscillation, termed microrotary deviation by Rosenberg and Glaser, which causes oscillopsia.

Superior oblique myokymia is best seen with the ophthalmoscope. This condition, which usually has a remitting–relapsing course, occurs in otherwise healthy adults. It may respond dramatically to carbamazepine (Tegretol) and rarely requires tenotomy.

Periodic Ataxia. This is a disorder in which the patient suffers bouts of vertigo, ataxia, and nystagmus (torsional, vertical, or dissociated), lasting up to a day; the frequency varies from daily to a few times per year. It occurs with MS, hereditary inborn errors of metabolism, and in families without any detectable metabolic defect. Acetazolamide (Diamox) has been used successfully to prevent attacks in familial cases.

There are many other involuntary ocular movements (e.g., square-wave jerks, macro-saccadic oscillations, and glissades), descriptions of which can be found in the excellent textbooks on ocular motility that are listed in the bibliography.

BIBLIOGRAPHY

Abel, L.A., Parker, L., Daroff, R.B., and Dell'Osso, L.F.: End point nystagmus. Invest. Ophthalmol. Vis. Sci. 17(6):539, 1978.

Anthony, J.H., Ouvrier, R.A., and Wise, G.: Spasmus nutans: A mistaken identity. Arch. Neurol. 37:373, 1980.

Aschoff, J.C., Conrad, B., and Kornhuber, H.H.: Acquired pendular nystagmus with oscillopsia in multiple sclerosis: a sign of cerebellar nuclei disease. J. Neurol. Neurosurg. Psychiatry 37:570, 1974.

Baloh, R.W., and Spooner, J.W.: Downbeat nystagmus: a type of central vestibular nystagmus. Neurology, 31:304, 1981.

Chambers, B.R., et al.: Case of downbeat nystagmus influenced by otolithic stimulation. Ann. Neurol. 13:204, 1983.

Daroff, R.B., and Dell'Osso, L.F.: Periodic alternating nystagmus and the shifting null. Can. J. Otolaryngol. 33:367, 1974.

Daroff, R.B., Troost, B.T., and Dell'Osso, L.F.: Nystagmus and other ocular oscillations. In Neuro-ophthalmology. Edited by J.S. Glaser. New York, Harper & Row, 1978.

Dell'Osso, L.F., Flynn, J.T., and Daroff, R.B.: Hereditary congenital nystagmus: an intrafamilial study. Arch. Ophthalmol. 92:366, 1974.

Dell'Osso, L.F., and Daroff, R.B.: Congenital nystagmus waveforms and foveation strategy. Docum. Ophthalmol. (Den Haag) 39:155, 1975.

Dell'Osso, L.F., Schmidt, D., and Daroff, R.B.: Latent, manifest latent, and congenital nystagmus. Arch. Ophthalmol. 97:1977, 1979.

Dell'Osso, L.F., and Flynn, J.T.: Congenital nystagmus surgery: a quantitative evaluation of the effects. Arch. Ophthalmol. 97:462, 1979.

Dell'Osso, L.F.: Nystagmus and other ocular motor oscillations. In Neuro-ophthalmology. Vol. 3. Edited by S. Lessell and J.T.W. van Dalen. Amsterdam, Excerpta Medica, 1984.

Donat, J.R., et al.: Familial periodic ataxia. Arch. Neurol. 36:568, 1979.

Ellenberger, C., Campa, J.F., and Nelsky, M.G.: Opsoclonus and parenchymatous degeneration of the cerebellum. Neurology 18:1041, 1968.

Fisher, C.M.: Ocular bobbing. Arch. Neurol. 11:543, 1964.

Halmagyi, G.M., Gresty, M.A., and Leech, J.: Reversed optokinetic nystagmus (OKN): mechanism and clinical significance. Ann. Neurol. 7:429, 1980.

Halmagyi, G.M., et al.: Treatment of periodic alternating nystagmus. Ann. Neurol. 8:609, 1980.

Hoyt, W.F., and Keane, J.R.: Superior oblique myokymia. Arch. Ophthalmol. 84:461, 1970.

Knobler, R.L., Somasundarum, M., and Schutta, H.: Inverse ocular bobbing. Ann. Neurol. 9:126, 1981.

Lavin, P.J.M., Smith, D., Kori, S.H., and Ellenberger, C., Jr.: Wernicke's encephalopathy: A predictable complication of hyperemesis gravidarum. Obstet. Gynecol. 62(3):13S, 1983.

Lavin, P.J.M., Traccis, S., Dell'Osso, L.F., and Abel, L.A.: Downbeat nystagmus with a pseudocycloid waveform: Improvement with base-out prisms. Ann. Neurol. *13*(6):621, 1983.

Leigh, R.J., and Zee, D.S.: The Neurology of Eye Movements. Philadelphia, F.A. Davis, 1983.

Nausieda, T.A., et al.: Opsoclonic cerebellopathy: a paraneoplastic syndrome responsive to thiamine. Arch. Neurol. *38*:770, 1981.

Norton, E.W.D., and Cogan, D.G.: Spasmus nutans. Arch. Ophthalmol *52*:442, 1954.

Parker, W.D., et al.: Biotin responsive opsoclonus-myoclonus syndrome. Neurology, *33* (Suppl. 2):153, 1983.

Pierrot-Desceilligny, C., et al.: Parinaud's syndrome. Brain *105*:667, 1982.

Rosenberg, M.L., and Glaser, J.L.: Superior oblique myokymia. Ann. Neurol. *13*:667, 1983.

Sanders, M.D., Hoyt, W.F., and Daroff, R.B.: Lid nystagmus evoked by ocular convergence: An ocular electromyographic study. J. Neurol. Neurosurg. Psychiatry *31*:368, 1968.

Sanders, M.D.: Alternating windmill nystagmus in neuro-ophthalmology: Symposium of the University of Miami and the Bascom-Palmer Eye Institute. Vol. VII. Edited by J.L. Smith and J.S. Glaser. St. Louis, C.V. Mosby Co., 1973.

Sandok, B.A., and Kranz, H.: Opsoclonus as the initial manifestation of occult neuroblastoma. Arch. Ophthalmol. *86*:235, 1977.

Saul, R.F., and Selhorst, J.B.: Downbeat nystagmus with magnesium depletion. Arch. Neurol. *38*:605, 1981.

Schott, G.D.: Familial cerebellar ataxia presenting with downbeat nystagmus. J. Med. Genet. *17*:115, 1980.

Sedwick, L.A., Burde, R.M., Hodges, F.J.: Leigh's subacute necrotizing encephalomyelopathy manifesting as spasmus nutans. Arch. Neurol., *102*:1046–1048, 1984.

Susac, J.O., Hoyt, W.F., Daroff, R.B., and Lawrence, W.: Clinical spectrum of ocular bobbing. J. Neurol. Neurosurg. Psychiatry *33*:771, 1970.

Troost, B.T.: An overview of ocular motor physiology. Ann. Otol. Rhinol. Laryngol. (Suppl.) *86*:90(4):29, 1981.

Zahn, J.R.: Incidence and characteristics of voluntary nystagmus. J. Neurol. Neurosurg. Psychiatry *41*:617, 1978.

Chapter 17

Visual Field Defects

THOMAS J. WALSH

EXAMINATION TECHNIQUES

To get as much information as possible from a field examination, the physician must make some adjustments for the type of field defect he expects to see and for the ability of the patient to perform a particular test. The patient who has neuro-ophthalmologic problems may be a difficult subject for perimetry. He may be ill, slightly obtunded, frightened that he has a terrible disease, or simply apprehensive about having his first field examination. Such factors tend to affect the test results.

In a patient who is slightly obtunded, a good confrontation field test may be more revealing than a formal Goldmann field test in which the patient performs poorly because of his lowered level of consciousness. The patient with headaches and skull roentgenograms that show a sella turcica at the upper limits of normal in size probably has a bitemporal defect. Thus the physician who spends an inordinate amount of time mapping a blind spot or looking in the Bjerrum area succeeds only in fatiguing such a patient. He does not find the subtle bitemporal field defect, which starts at the vertical meridian peripherally.

Recorded Fields

The tangent screen test is a sensitive one, and it can be relied on to identify any cen-

tral field defect. I use it most of the time initially because it permits me to observe the patient closely and to evaluate his degree of alertness and his speed of response. Later on we obtain Goldmann fields. Many neuro-ophthalmologic patients are ill, and it is more satisfactory to seat them in the examining chair than to have them balance on a stool with their head on a small stand in a fishbowl. The tangent field method also allows the physician more intimate contact with the patient so that he can question him when needed. I find this contact lacking when I see the patient only through the observer tube of the Goldmann perimeter. I prefer to start with a 2-mm white object and then vary the size and color and technique as the situation demands.

When doing a peripheral field examination, I use the Aimark perimeter for many of the same reasons that I gave for selecting the tangent screen. The real value of this projection perimeter is that it helps keep the patient unaware of the direction from which the test object is coming. The Aimark instrument is particularly useful in examining children, whose fixation span is short even before adding a confusing instrument to the already difficult examination. The Goldmann perimeter is useful in following the progress of the patient if the patient is alert and cooperative. The large number of variables that can be used with the Goldmann perimeter makes it a valuable instrument for identifying the presence and extent of subtle defects and their progress or resolution.

Automated perimetry is a significant step forward in quantitating field testing. My experience is solely with the octopus instrument, which displays the almost 3000 points in a series of symbols and shades of gray to black, much like the gray scale of a CT scan. Certain qualifications should be made, however. This display of almost 3000 points is mostly interpolation of less than 3% of those points being tested. If you are looking for defects in a certain area, it is, therefore, important to select the appropriate program. It is a useful instrument in long-term follow-up of patients who can be expected to show subtle and slow changes in their fields. As an initial testing technique for many neuro-ophthalmologic patients, I find it too prolonged a test for the attention span of sick patients who may also have cerebration problems owing to their disease and who have never had any experience with field testing (Figs. 17–1, and 17–2).

Nonself Recorded Fields

Several other types of field testing are important and should be considered for the patient who cannot perform when one of the more formal testing techniques is used. The techniques discussed in the following sections may help to identify a field defect that would be missed with more formal testing techniques if the patient is not alert or is uncooperative.

Confrontation Field Tests

These techniques are much maligned but helpful if they are done properly and used when indicated. They are not a substitute for formal field tests, but they are useful

as screening devices or in bedside examinations.

The confrontation method involves the following three steps.

Step 1. The patient is asked to fixate with one eye on the physician's nose. The physician then uses the field of his right eye as a standard for measuring the field in the patient's left eye, and the field in his left eye for measuring the field in the patient's right eye. Instead of using the wiggling finger method, the physician asks the patient to count the number of fingers on the hand that the physician presents successively to each of the four quadrants of the patient's eye. The number of fingers may be one, two, five, or none. Thus four choices are given rather than the two choices of the wiggling finger method. If the patient fixates poorly, a variation on the finger-counting method may be substituted. The physician presents the finger(s) to the patient quickly—before the patient has a chance to shift his fixation.

Step 2. The physician uses his two hands simultaneously, presenting stimuli to both the nasal and temporal fields of one eye. The combination of fingers presented are (1) one finger of one hand and one finger of the other hand, (2) one and two, (3) two and two, or (4) one and five. The patient is asked to tell the number of fingers he sees. Besides evaluating the fields, this step tests both the patient's ability to calculate, which is a parietal lobe function, and the existence of the extinction phenomenon. The patient with parietal lobe disease may miss one-half of the field because of the extinction phenomenon rather than because of a true field defect.

The physician should consider the extinction phenomenon in the patient who consistently misses seeing objects in one field with bilateral stimulation but who has no trouble counting fingers accurately when only one half of the field is tested at a time. Therefore, when a patient who is reported to have a field defect turns out not to have one, the physician should test

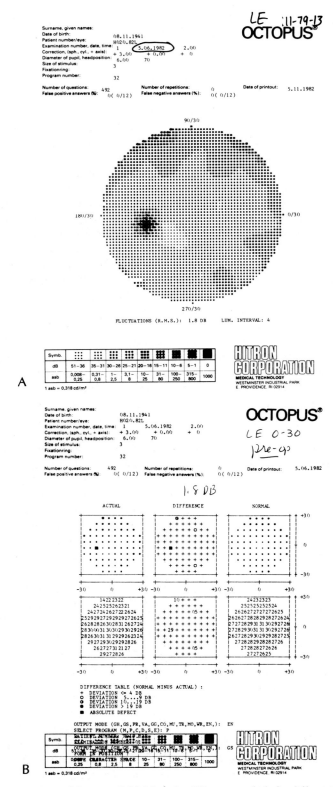

Fig. 17–1. A. Typical printout of Octopus field. Note the different symbols for different densities of the field. The symbols are interpreted in scale at bottom. **B.** Same field but with a digital printout. (From the Hitron Corporation; Westminster Industrial Park, E. Providence, RI.)

436

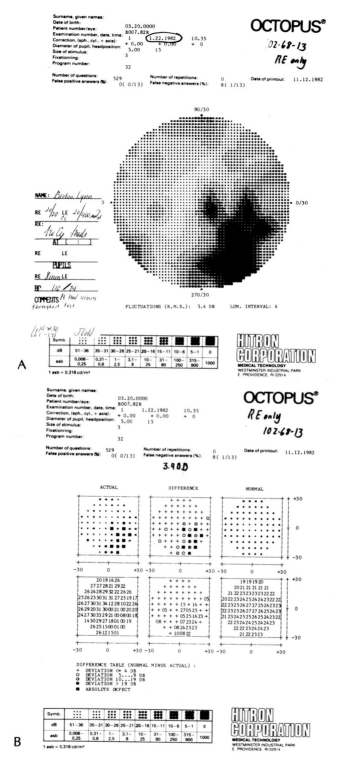

Fig. 17–2. **A.** Abnormal Octopus field with homonymous quadrant defective. Note difference in this one eye versus the normal field in Fig. 17–1A. **B.** Note difference here in digital readout as compared with Fig. 17–1B. (From the Hitron Corporation; Westminster Industrial Park, E. Providence, RI.)

for the extinction phenomenon by bilateral field testing using confrontation. In this instance, a gross technique may pick up a defect that a more sophisticated method has missed using a single test object.

Step 3. The physician presents his fingers to the patient's nasal and temporal fields as he did in Step 2. This time, however, the patient is asked to compare the appearance of the fingers. Are pieces of a finger missing? Is one finger faded compared to the other? Although this test requires that the patient make a subjective judgment, it may be valuable, when the results are compared with those in the other eye, in detecting a bitemporal or homonymous defect.

After all three steps are completed with one eye, they are repeated for the other eye.

A more subtle confrontation test involves presenting identically colored test objects to the patient's nasal and temporal fields. (The red tops of two plastic mydriatic bottles can be used.) If the defect is subtle, the patient may say that one cap is not colored or is a faded-red or pink color compared with the other cap. Such a response indicates the presence of a subtle hemianopic defect. In optic nerve disease, the patient's response is usually uniform in that one eye sees the color the same in all four quadrants, and the caps may only look different when compared with the way the other eye sees them. A more subtle defect in optic nerve disease may be suggested when the color of the cap is more faded when the patient looks at it directly than when the cap is held in a para-central position.

Projection Light Test

This test can also be used with the patient who cannot be tested with more formal techniques because he is bedridden, but who needs a more critical examination than the confrontation field test. The physician uses a battery-operated flashlight that has a small focused beam of light (of the type used as a pointer during lectures). The physician asks the bedridden patient to cover one eye and then to look at a fixation point on the wall or on the ceiling. The physician, standing out of the patient's view, shines the light on the wall or ceiling and looks for and identifies the patient's blind spot. Using the field of his right eye as a point of reference, the physician explores the limits of the field of the patient's right eye. Each time he moves the light, the physician covers the light with his hand so that the patient has no idea in what direction the physician is next going to move it. The physician should shine the light frequently into the patient's blind spot to determine whether the patient still sees the light. If the patient consistently does not see the light when it is in the blind spot he must be fixating accurately; if he consistently sees the light, he must not be fixating accurately. To increase the sensitivity of the test, the physician can partially cover the light with his hand and thus make the light less intense. The background illumination in the room also influences the test sensitivity.

HRR Plates

Using the HRR plates can be more valuable than simply examining the patient for congenital defects in red-green color vision. Patients with optic nerve disease, even those with excellent visual acuity, frequently miss most of the HRR plates. On the other hand, a patient with severe macular degeneration usually does not miss any—at most one or two—of the more subtle plates. Identifying optic nerve disease versus macular disease with the use of the HRR plates is easier than trying to plot a central scotoma in a patient with minimal decrease in acuity to the 20/30 level.

Amsler Grid

This test can be valuable, but in my experience it is difficult for the patient to perform. The patient is asked to look at the center of a grid system and to say whether any of the lines are faded, distorted, or missing (Figs. 17–3, 17–4). I find that most patients have a hard time fixating centrally and simultaneously appreciating the surrounding area. Most patients, regardless of instructions, tend to explore the surrounding area with their fovea, a maneuver that defeats the point of the test. Also, by the time I have explained to the patient what I want him to see or not to see, I have almost suggested the defect to him. This test requires considerable understanding and patience from both the physician and the patient. If it is used correctly and if the patient is intelligent, the test can be valuable for detecting subtle defects. I have found a useful variation in the standard format. One of the standard test plates is made up of red lines on a black background. The red lines are so dark that frequently even the normally intelligent patient misses them. I have made up grids of

the same size but with red lines on a white background. With such a grid, the patient can easily detect lines that are faded red or missing or completely lacking in color.

A specific response to the Amsler grid test is seen in patients with serous detachments of the macula. Even small amounts of serous macular disease result in symptomatic central defects that cause a patient to complain. These macular changes are often missed on routine ophthalmoscopy. The patient with serous macular disease sees the Amsler grid as distorted rather than as having pieces missing. The distortion is similar to that caused in a chain link fence when somebody leans against it (Fig. 17–5). When the patient reports such a distortion in the Amsler grid, the physician should study the fundus carefully with a fundus contact lens in order to identify the cause of the complaint.

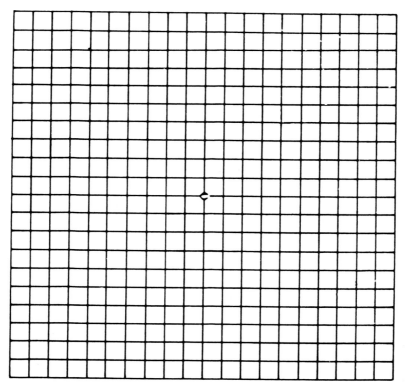

Fig. 17–3. All lines in the Amsler grid chart are straight and equally clear when no central defect exists.

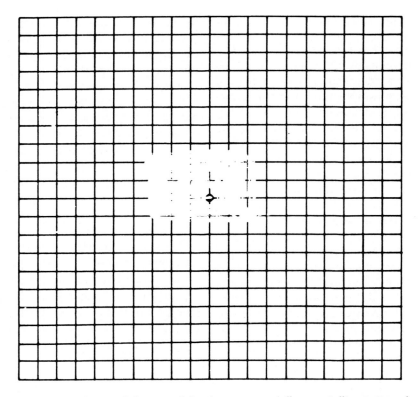

Fig. 17–4. Parts of the grid around the central fixation spot are dull or partially missing when a central scotoma exists.

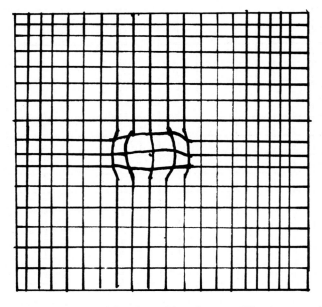

Fig. 17–5. Serous elevation of macula with bending of foveal area as if leaning on a chain link fence.

Use of Color

The use of color in testing for field defects appears in the literature as a controversial and confusing procedure; however, the physician who does a number of field tests knows the value and the many uses of color. The most important use of color is in the detection of subtle central scotomas. In optic nerve disease in the patient who has reasonably good visual acuity, identifying a central field defect with even small white test objects may be difficult. The defect that can be observed when a small red test object is used is generally so pronounced and easy to map that it is hard to believe how difficult it was to find with a small white test object. A common mistake of the beginner is to go from the smallest white test object to the smallest red test object. It is usually better to go from the 1-mm white test object to a 6- or 9-mm red test object. The patient is able to see the test object but not its color. He describes the test object as either faded red or black. The physician then moves the test object out from that area where the color of the object is abnormal in all directions until it reaches the area in which the patient can perceive the proper color. This technique delineates the scotoma area, and the information obtained can be used for comparison on subsequent field examinations.

Color as a reduced stimulus for measuring subtle field defects has just been discussed; however, lack of appreciation of colored stimuli can take several other forms. This lack may also be caused by a greater effect of the disease on fibers sensitive to color, such as we see in early optic nerve disease. Another form of color defect is the congenital variety, which is seen to various degrees in about 6% of the male population. This latter type of color defect is through the entire visual field and should not cause a localized field defect. These defects in color testing are known by any perimetrist. A more rarely encountered form is a color loss secondary to a

lesion of the central nervous system. Central loss of color can be subdivided into two broad groups. Persons in one group have an intellectual problem in recognizing or naming colors but have no specific color defect. The second group is comprised of persons who are intellectually intact, with excellent acuity to perceive color, but who have a central color defect (cerebral dyschromatopsia) in the cerebral cortical area that appreciates colored information.

A specific aphasia for naming colors does exist, but more commonly, it is associated with other forms of aphasia. We can demonstrate that this color-naming aphasia exists by testing the patient with the pseudoisochromatic plates. He will see even the most subtle plates if he has no congenital color defect, thus attesting to the fact that his defect is not in seeing colors, but in naming the colors, and that it is acquired. Yet, he will miss naming the bright green color of a large watermelon. This defect appears to be more common with left hemisphere lesions, according to Benson and Greenberg and Geschwind who feel that the lesion is in the left occipital lobe with a secondary defect in the splenium of the corpus callosum. Another category in the intellectual color-defect group is in the naming of colors and is referred to as a visual agnosia. There is some controversy concerning the existence of this particular phenomenon but there have been several excellent cases to support its existence. If there is such a separate category, there are patients who cannot recognize the object and thus cannot name the appropriate color. There is nothing wrong with the patient's ability to see the object (acuity) or his color appreciation, since he sees the subtle, hidden symbols in the color plates; he can name the correct color if given other sensory stimuli, such as touching the object. If he feels the banana and knows it is a fruit that is long and slim, he can recognize it as a banana and make the appropriate association.

Zeki has done experimental studies in

monkeys who have demonstrated color responsive cells in the fourth visual area. This may be considered to be comparable to an area in the human occipital cortex that has been implicated in cerebral dyschromatopsia. In the few cases studied postmortem, the comparable area in humans involves the fusiform and lingual gyri.

One area of confusion in interpreting an individual case is whether the patient has had a congenital color defect or is a case of acquired cerebral dyschromatopsia. Green and Lessell made the following differential points between the two types of patients. In cerebral dyschromatopsia, the color defect is random and does not follow any pattern such as protanopia or deutanopia. If patients with cerebral dyschromatopsia are tested with the pseudoisochromatic plate, they do not see the confusion numbers. Patients with cerebral dyschromatopsia have field defects. These field defects, however, can not account for their extensive loss of color appreciation. The most common cause of cerebral dyschromatopsia has been vascular, but Green and Lessell reported two cases secondary to a tumor.

The disproportionate loss of color function versus loss of acuity, field, or other cerebral function may be secondary to selective loss of certain groups of cells. Zeki identified in monkeys columns of cortical cells that were responsive to certain color stimuli. Although it is hard to suggest that a vascular episode or even less, a mass lesion, would disproportionately affect such a small population of cells, nevertheless, it occasionally occurs. One explanation may be suggested from experiments demonstrating a decrease in color function at high altitudes where there is lower oxygen saturation. In these altitude experiments, color was affected before vision and fields. This may also be the case in cerebral ischemia.

Chamlin pointed out that homonymous bitemporal field defects, when the defect is subtle, are really owing to hemiretinal suppression rather than to a defect involving just a few peripheral fibers. Chamlin's testing technique is to compare the retinal sensitivity of the two halves of the field. The following paragraph describes a variation of Chamlin's technique that uses small white test objects and colored test objects.

It is sometimes difficult to evaluate small peripheral contractions of a field. Do they represent early but definite intracranial pathology? A slow response from the patient? A big eyebrow? A peripheral retinal degeneration? The correct answer can be discovered in several ways. The first and most common method is to take two identical white test objects, small enough to show up the peripheral contraction. The physician should bring these two test objects down from above on either side of the vertical meridian (Figs. 17–6 and 17–7). If the patient sees the test object on the side of the peripheral contraction later than on the other side, the previous peripheral contraction may represent an intracranial hemianopic defect. There must be a 10° difference from one side to the other in recognizing the 2 test objects. In many cases, a consistent difference is shown, but not one that is as much as 10°. But in these cases, color again can be of use. Using 2 identical red test objects that are 6 or 9 mm in size, the physician should ask the patient to report when he can recognize the color. (He will first see the test objects as white or as colorless.) If a hemianopic defect is present, the patient will see color in the test object presented to the nonaffected side before he sees it in the test object presented to the abnormal side.

In patients who show an equivocal response to a small white test object, a big difference may be found when red test objects are used. It is not uncommon for a patient who shows a 7° difference to a small white test object to then show an absence of color in an entire quadrant. Occasionally, even this technique may not be consistently reproduced. If it cannot be repro-

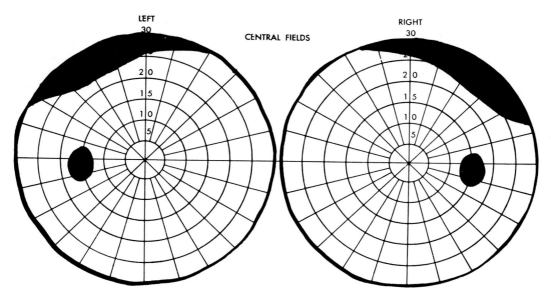

Fig. 17–6. Chamlin step—If the test objects are presented only every 15° and the nearest isopter to the vertical meridian is 15° away, the difference on either side of the vertical meridian is not appreciated.

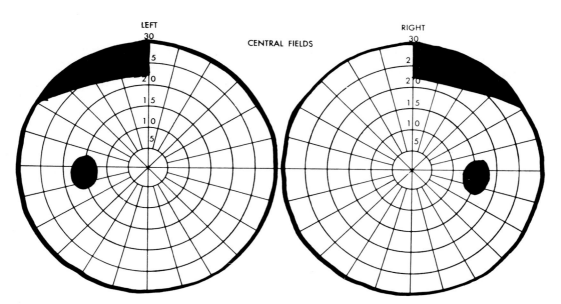

Fig. 17–7. Chamlin step performed with a test object presented just on either side of the vertical meridian reveals a significant step defect.

duced, the physician should move the red test objects horizontally rather than vertically. Then the red test object should be brought from the area where the color is lacking across the vertical meridian into the area where the patient can appreciate the color normally. Each time the test object crosses the vertical meridian, the patient quickly perceives the color. The vertical meridian effect identifies the difference between the nasal and temporal fields and establishes the significance of the defect and its intracranial location.

Pumpkin Test

As mentioned, a central scotoma in a patient with reasonably good visual acuity is difficult to plot. I find that cecocentral defects are even more difficult to identify. It is essential to establish that a defect is cecocentral and not just central, because if the defect is cecocentral, the diagnostic possibilities are three, whereas a central scotoma can be caused by many more diseases. Cecocentral defects are more commonly caused by nutritional amblyopia; occasionally they are caused by pernicious anemia and rarely by Leber's disease.

To establish the cecocentral nature of the defect, I have used a variation on the color technique described for central scotomas. I have found that when small colored test objects are used, it is difficult to plot the cecocentral defect and to be sure that the defect is not just a central scotoma. These patients seem to fixate more poorly than the usual patient does, which obscures the validity of the test. There are also varying degrees and islands of different density in the area between fixation and the blind spot that keep varying the patient's response. Therefore, instead of pursuing the usual technique of moving a test object from a nonseeing to a seeing area of the field, I make the entire central field a colored test object. I then ask the patient to point out any color defects. The color field is created by using a standard-size orange poster board which easily covers fixation

and the blind spot. (Orange proved, by trial and error, to be the best color because red poster board is so dark a red that it is hard for the patient to differentiate an area of dark red from one that is simply dark or is black.) A fixation object is attached about one third of the way in from one edge of the cardboard. The fixation object so placed allows the cecocentral area to be more easily and completely covered by the cardboard than would a central spot on the cardboard. The patient is instructed to delineate with a long dowel rod the area(s) where the orange color is missing while he looks at the fixation target. If the patient does not fixate steadily, the area he is trying to delineate seems to him to move, and he cannot outline it. This difficulty encourages him to fixate more steadily. With this method, he can tell the physician that the defect is worse between fixation and the blind spot and not in front of him. He can also show the physician that the defect is not equidistant around fixation (as it is in a central scotoma) but that it extends more toward the blind spot (Figs. 17–8 and 17–9).

TOPICAL DIAGNOSIS

Retinal Defects

Optic Nerve Defects Contrasted with Retinal Defects

The diagnosis of monocular field defects can be difficult. The appearance of the fundus frequently does not identify whether the defect arises from a retinal lesion or an optic nerve lesion. If a retinal defect is very recent, obvious changes shown on ophthalmoscopy may establish the site of the lesion, but days or weeks after the defect has occurred, the retina returns to normal and the ophthalmoscopic sign is gone. One feature of field testing, however, usually does distinguish a retinal site of origin from an optic nerve one. Optic nerve quadrantic or hemianopic field loss begins at fixation (Fig. 17–10). If the defect is caused by a retinal vascular lesion, the apex of the

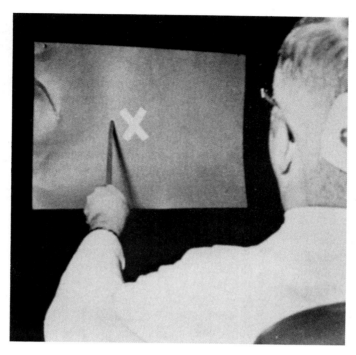

Fig. 17–8. Orange board covers cecocentral area and has large fixation device placed eccentrically in order to locate more of cecocentral area on the board.

defect is at the blind spot (Fig. 17–11). The retina is separated into quadrants vascularly by the vessels coming off the disc, not off the fovea. Therefore, in defects that are less than a quadrant, smaller and smaller test objects should be used to enlarge the defect so that the location of the apex can be identified.

Cecocentral scotomas involve not only the central part of vision but extend temporally to involve the blind spot. In testing fields, it is important to differentiate pure central scotomas from cecocentral, since the cecocentral scotomas have a much more limited differential diagnosis. One additional feature of cecocentral versus central scotoma is that the densest part may not be at the center of the defect, but located between fixation and the blind spot. Once the diagnosis of cecocentral scotoma is made, the differential diagnosis becomes more limited. Cecocentral scotomas most commonly present bilaterally and the

most common cause is tobacco-alcohol-nutritional amblyopia, Bilateral cases have been reported on a congenital as well as a demyelinating basis but are not as common as are the ones caused by tobacco-alcohol. Unilateral cases are much less commonly seen. A large series of this type of defect was reviewed by Shaw and Smith. In their series of 13 unilateral cases, they found inflammatory, idiopathic, and demyelinating causes. He also adds one other cause and that is optic nerve pits. The field defect in this case usually is denser above the horizontal meridian, corresponding to the usual inferotemporal location of the pit on the optic nerve head. In my experience, one other cause can be confusing if one is not careful in performing the fields. I have seen four cases in which there was aqueduct stenosis with enlargement of the third ventricle, pressing down on the chiasm. This produced bitemporal defects, which were paracentral and initially interpreted

Visual Field Defects

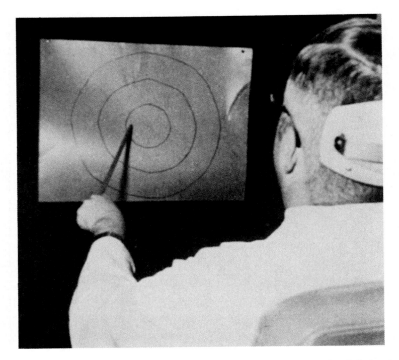

Fig. 17–9. The patient is now using dowel rod to point areas where orange color faded out or is missing, representing scotoma.

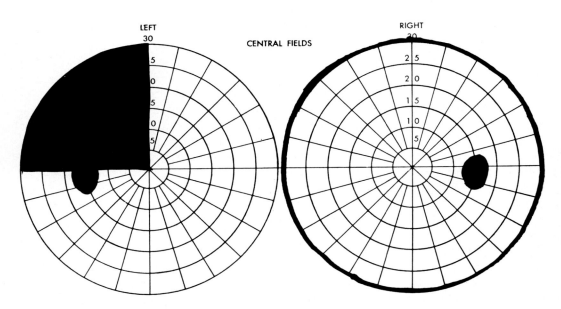

Fig. 17–10. A defect with the apex at fixation locates the defect behind the globe in the optic nerve.

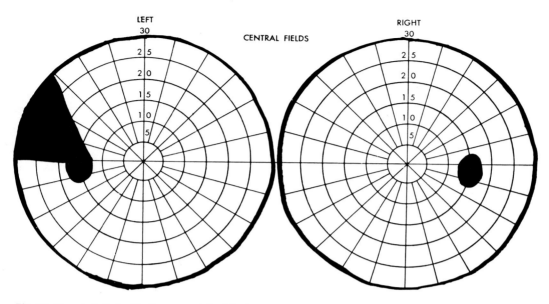

Fig. 17–11. A defect with the apex at the blind spot represents retinal vascular disease.

as cecocentral defects since they extended more temporally than nasally. Careful observation of the patient's fixation and identification of the shape of the defect and where the densest part of the defect is will usually clarify any confusion.

Gun Barrel Fields

These fields (tubular fields, severe peripheral contraction) are usually considered to indicate hysteria or malingering; however, organic causes of small central fields should also be considered. Glaucoma is probably the most common one. It is easily diagnosed at this stage by inspection of the disc. By the time the field is reduced to 5°, the cupping of the nerve head should be so extensive as to be obvious.

The next most common organic cause of gun barrel fields is retinitis pigmentosa. Patients with this condition, who have 5° fields, do not have the central acuity that persons with glaucoma have. Occasionally, the retinal pigmentary changes are minimal, and they may be missed when only the posterior pole of the retina is seen through a small pupil, and if there is no family history to suggest the diagnosis.

The atrophy of the disc is frequently interpreted as optic atrophy, the cause of which is unknown. Therefore, in persons with contracted fields, examination of the fundus when the pupils are dilated is mandatory. Particular attention should be paid to the equatorial region, where the pigmentation usually begins and is more likely to be seen.

Patients with cerebral vascular disease may develop bilateral hemianopia owing to occipital lobe infarction. Some of these patients have sparing of the macular projection in the occipital lobe, and are thus left with 2 to 5° of field and good central acuity in both eyes. Such patients have a normal fundus and normal pupils.

This type of field defect may be seen in one eye if a central retinal artery occlusion occurs but the cilioretinal artery is spared. The cilioretinal artery supplies the fovea and preserves a small central field and good acuity. In such cases, optic atrophy is present. It is different since in occipital cortical infarction, the fundus has a normal appearance.

Severe contraction of the fields can also occur in extensive chorioretinitis. The condition is obvious on ophthalmoscopic examination.

Arcuate Scotomas

These scotomas are usually associated with glaucoma. Any patient with an arcuate scotoma should be investigated first, and exhaustively, for glaucoma. Other diseases and conditions occasionally cause an arcuate scotoma (Table 17–1).

Optic Nerve Disease

Peripheral Loss and Central Loss

The usual field defect in optic nerve disease is a central scotoma with or without peripheral field loss. Sometimes relative sparing of central acuity and pronounced loss of peripheral field are seen (as seen, occasionally, in syphilitic optic neuropathy). The leading known cause of axial optic nerve disease with sparing of the peripheral field is demyelinating disease. (Other causes of axial—as opposed to periaxial—optic nerve disease are discussed elsewhere.)

Junction Scotoma

Usually, if the lesion causing the loss of vision is located in the optic nerve, no features exist to identify what part of the nerve is affected; however, a lesion in one area of the optic nerve does have a sign that is of localizing value. This lesion occurs where the optic nerve joins the chiasm. The lower nasal fibers coming across the chiasm dip up into the opposite optic nerve for about 1 mm before they turn into the optic tract. A lesion so located causes not only a central scotoma in one eye but also an upper temporal field defect in the other eye (Fig. 17–12). The patient who has a central scotoma should have the upper temporal quadrant of his other eye examined carefully for an upper temporal field defect. The patient is usually unaware of such a field defect since he has no central visual loss in that eye.

A lesion at the posterior aspect of the chiasm damages the posterior knee of Wilbrand. The expected defect is a lower temporal field defect in the ipsilateral eye, but it is rarely seen. An incongruous hemianopia is the most common defect. The location of the defect usually depends on whether the tract or the chiasm sustains more damage. Occasionally, there is encroachment on the macular crossing fibers, and a paracentral homonymous defect occurs in the other eye and a temporal defect occurs in the ipsilateral eye owing to involvement of the posterior knee of Wilbrand.

Chiasmal Field Defects

The usual chiasmal defect is the bitemporal hemianopia that begins in the upper

Table 17–1.   Some Causes of Arcuate Scotomas

When Lesion is at Disc	When Lesion is of Anterior Nerve	When Lesion is in Posterior Nerve and Chiasm	When Blind Spot is Enlarged
Juxtapapillary choroiditis	Ischemic infarct and segmental atrophy	Meningioma at optic foramen	Papilledema
Colobomas and pits of optic nerve	Cerebral arteritis	Meningioma of dorsum sellae	Peripapillary atrophy
Drusen of optic nerve	Retrobulbar neuritis	Pituitary adenoma	Drusen
Papillitis		Opticochiasmatic arachnoiditis	Juxtapapillary choroiditis
Arteriosclerotic plaque in vessel on the disc			Myelination
			Tilted discs
			Colobomas
			Slow patient response

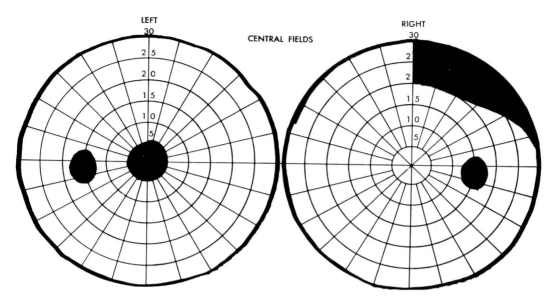

Fig. 17–12. A junction scotoma of the left optic nerve with a central scotoma in the field of the left eye and an upper temporal field defect in the right eye field.

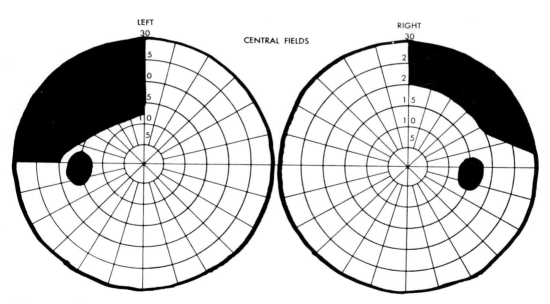

Fig. 17–13. Bitemporal hemianopia that is asymmetric and typically begins in the upper quadrants.

quadrant (Fig. 17–13) and occasionally in the lower quadrants (Fig. 17–14). Cushing tried to divide diseases that cause this type of field defect into two groups. Cushing's first group shows bitemporal hemianopia, optic atrophy, and roentgenographic changes, particularly enlargement of the

sella turcica. This group is made up primarily of pituitary adenomas with an enlarged sella turcica, as shown on the roentgenogram. The second group shows bitemporal hemianopia, optic atrophy, and normal roentgenograms. This group is made up of meningiomas, craniopharyn-

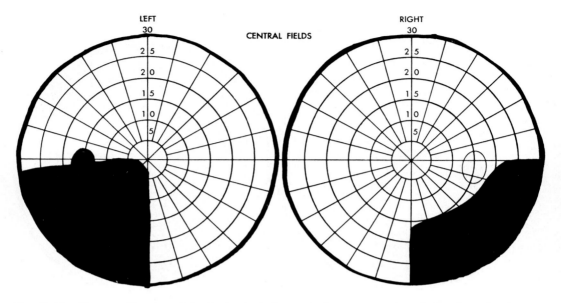

Fig. 17–14. Bitemporal hemianopia beginning in the lower quadrants, suggesting a lesion above the chiasm.

giomas, and aneurysms. The second group does not have as negative an appearance on the roentgenogram as was once thought. Eighty-five percent of childhood craniopharyngiomas show suprasellar calcification. Occasionally, long-standing aneurysms have a curvilinear calcification that may be seen on routine roentgenograms. Suprasellar meningiomas are still difficult to visualize on plain roentgenograms, and the use of techniques that examine the suprasellar space, such as a CT scan with contrast material, is required. The majority of J-shaped sellars are caused by gliomas of the chiasm; however, they can also be seen in patients with achondroplasia, osteogenesis imperfecta, Morquio syndrome, Hurler syndrome, Turner syndrome, hydrocephalus, and chondroectodermal dysplasia.

Bitemporal Hemianopia

For years it was thought that the macular fibers crossed exclusively in the posterior chiasm and that a lesion in that area affected the macular fibers primarily. In the textbooks, such a lesion was described as causing a bitemporal paracentral defect. A common cause of such a field defect is enlargement of the third ventricle that causes the ventricle to press on the posterior chiasm from above and posteriorly when the chiasm is anteriorly placed. I have seen only one such paramacular bitemporal field defect. My experience with lesions so located in the posterior chiasm is that they cause the usual bitemporal hemianopia or, occasionally, an optic tract defect.

One of the more useful advances in chiasmal disease has been the finding of elevated prolactin levels in the blood of patients with diseases involving the pituitary-hypothalamic axis. This elevation of prolactin is not specific for these organs, but in the context of bitemporal visual field defects or an enlarged sella, it is certainly compatible and highly suggestive of tumors affecting these organs. Other causes of elevated prolactin can be stress, pregnancy, nursing mothers, intercourse, estrogen administration, some cases of primary hypothyroidism, occasionally secondary ammenorrhea, renal failure, and some drugs such as thyrotropin-releasing hormone, phenothiazines, methyldopa (Aldomet), reserpine and "the pill." It has also been reported in diseases of the hypothalamus such as sarcoidosis, Schüller-Christian disease, and craniopharyngioma. The mechanism by which these diseases of the hypothalamus cause an elevated prolactin is an interference with the pituitary-hypothalamic axis. The hypothalamus secretes a prolactin-inhibitory factor (PIF), which regulates the level of prolactin in the blood stream. When this inhibitory factor is not secreted in sufficient amounts owing to some local disease, then the prolactin level can rise. It is important to say that a lack of an elevated prolactin level does not rule out a pituitary tumor; however, in view of a patient's signs and symptoms with or without field defects an elevated prolactin level is certainly confirmatory evidence of such a tumor being present.

In the past, many surgical procedures involving the pituitary gland were difficult to do without encountering some further damage to the chiasm that was overlying it. The transsphenoidal approach using microsurgery has been a tremendous step forward in managing these tumors and reducing the morbidity to the patient and to his visual status. A review by Laws, Teautmann, and Hollenhorst of a fairly large series of tumors managed by this surgical approach shows that the visual result has been at least as good if not better, and that the patients in general have been immeasurably better, than by the subfrontal craniotomy approach. There are some limitations, however, as to the patients for whom this procedure is selected. This surgical approach is best selected for patients with an adenoma confined to the sella turcica, those with cerebrospinal fluid rhinorrhea, and tumors with sphenoid sinus extension. It also is indicated for tumors with paracentral scotomas. This latter field defect indicates either retrochiasmal extension, a prefixed optic chiasm, and a tumor that is difficult to remove by means of the standard subfrontal approach. Some tumors with suprasella extension can also be removed by this technique, but this is more difficult and is related to the experience of the surgeon. Several groups of patients are not candidates for this approach. Those patients with a dumbbell type of adenoma in which there is tumor not only in the fossa, but extending through the diaphragma sella would not be good candidates for this approach. Lateral suprasellar extension or massive suprasellar tumor or an incompletely pneumatized sphenoid sinus would all preclude this surgical approach. The greatest advantages of this procedure are that the optic nerves are directly visualized through the microscope, and therefore, less surgical damage can result during the extirpation of the tumor. This approach through the sphenoid sinus rather than through a craniotomy is much less stressful for patients and many of them are up and around comfortably the next day.

False Localizing Hemianopia

Bitemporal hemianopia has always been associated with a chiasmal location; however, there are cases of falsely localizing bitemporal hemianopia. Third ventricle enlargement from any cause results in compression of the posterior chiasm. Sylvian aqueduct stenosis causes enlargement of the third ventricle and secondary compression of the chiasm. In such a case, the disease is somewhat remote from the chiasm proper. Associated signs of the sylvian aqueductal syndrome, such as paralysis of up gaze, retraction nystagmus, and light-near dissociation of the pupils, should help establish the true location of the primary lesion. Another cause of falsely localizing bitemporal field depression is tilted optic discs, which may be confused with the bitemporal hemianopia of chiasmal lesions.

The symptoms of lesions in the chiasmal area usually develop slowly. The field defect is often not noticed nor does the patient complain about it. If the patient has any visual complaints, he makes them when the central acuity fails, a defect that is interpreted as a need for different eyeglasses. In children, loss of vision that cannot be corrected by glasses may signify a glioma. When a bitemporal hemianopia is found in a patient who has had a sudden onset of symptoms (including severe headaches), change in his level of consciousness, and ophthalmoplegia, pituitary apoplexy must be considered. Most of these patients require prompt neurosurgical intervention.

Binasal Field Defects

These field defects are infrequently seen, but it is important that they be recognized (Fig. 17–15). The most common cause of binasal field defects is glaucoma, not a chiasmal lesion. Other causes of binasal defects are drusen and chronic increased intracranial pressure. The internal carotid arteries are located just lateral to the chiasm, and compression of the chiasm by arteriosclerotic carotid arteries allegedly causes compression of the crossing temporal fibers and thus produces a binasal field defect. A more plausible explanation of the binasal field defect is that the arteriosclerotic process that affects the internal carotid arteries also affects the nutrient arteries to the lateral chiasm.

Tilted Disc Syndrome

This syndrome is a rare cause of bitemporal field depression. Characteristically there is a situs inversus of the disc, with a tilting of its vertical axis in an oblique direction. In about 80% of the cases, the condition is bitemporal. A temporal hemianopia also exists; if bilateral, it gives the impression of a bitemporal hemianopia owing to chiasmal disease (Fig. 17–16). The hemianopia is peripheral, and it is not progressive. The patient may have a large increase in his myopic correction in the lower fundus compared with the upper fundus. If such is the case, repeating the field examination with an increase in the myopic correction may cause the bitemporal defect to decrease or disappear.

Besides tilting of the disc and myopia, thinning of the retinal pigment epithelium and of the choroid is also present.

Optic Tract Defects

Lesions of the optic tract characteristically give rise to incongruous homony-

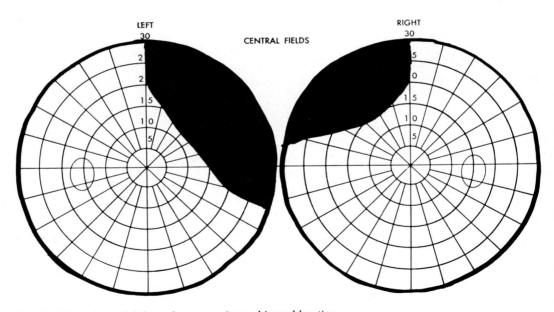

Fig. 17–15.   A binasal defect, also suggesting a chiasmal location.

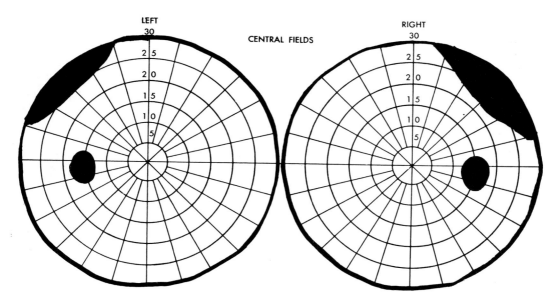

Fig. 17–16. A bitemporal defect owing to tilted disc syndrome. This defect does not come to vertical meridian as does true chiasmal disease.

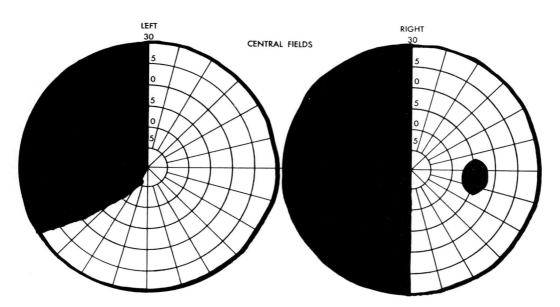

Fig. 17–17. Homonymous hemianopia that is incongruous and suggests an optic tract location.

mous hemianopia (Fig. 17–17). If the defect is gross in both the patient's eyes, the incongruous nature easily identifies it as an optic tract lesion. If the defect is subtle and highly incongruous, however, the homonymous nature of the defect may be missed. In a field defect that involves a hemianopia in one eye, a careful search should be made for a homonymous defect in the other eye. It is in just such a situation that use of the Chamlin step defect, perhaps using color, is of great value.

Newman and Miller also demonstrated an afferent pupillary defect in some of their cases. In general, the denser or more complete the optic tract lesion, the more likely was the presence of an afferent pupillary defect. Therefore, in cases of a complete homonymous hemianopia in which the anatomic location in the visual pathway is not immediately obvious, an afferent pupillary defect confirms the location in the tract.

Lateral Geniculate Body Defects

The lateral geniculate body derives its blood supply from the anterior and posterior choroidal arteries. These two arteries, in turn, send perforating branches into the lateral geniculate body, following the columnar architecture of the cells; they generally do not anastamose. One would then expect that occlusion of the main choroidal arteries or of one or more of their branches would produce defects consistent with that anatomic arrangement, which defects would be dense, sharp, and congruous. The denseness would be expected because of the lack of anastamosis. This vascular arrangement was demonstrated in monkeys by Fujino many years ago. Frisen, Holmegaard, and Rosenkrantz reported two clinical patients with homonymous sector defects consistent with an area supplied by the lateral choroidal arteries. They also demonstrated sector atrophy of the retinal nerve fiber layers. In one case, a review of the arteriogram revealed a vascular malformation of the choroidal arteries, and in a second case, a CT scan revealed a defect in the area of the lateral geniculate body. Hoyt and Newton reported several cases of incongruous field defects owing to lesions of the lateral geniculate body; however, in view of the anatomic arrangement of fibers and blood supply, I think that congruous defects are the rule and incongruous ones the exception.

Optic Radiation Field Defects

Temporal Lobe

These field defects are homonymous, and they always begin at the vertical meridian. Therefore, in a patient suspected of having a temporal lobe disease, the vertical meridian is the field area to concentrate on. Since a large area in the tip of the temporal lobe has no fibers of Meyer's loop, tumors in this area will not produce a field defect. If the tumor encroaches on these fibers and causes an early defect (which often is subtle), the mass may be large. Use of color can also be of value in detecting minimal temporal lobe field defects as well as chiasmal and optic nerve defects.

Presence of other neurologic symptoms, such as seizures and formed visual hallucinations, suggests possible temporal lobe disease and calls for prompt and careful inspection of the field. Since the fibers of Meyer's loop spread out, the field defect progresses through the upper quadrant of the field in a stepwise fashion. The fibers of the lower field, which are in a tight bundle, are affected as a group. Therefore, the field in the lower quadrant is lost as a unit, a phenomenon that differentiates the defect from one in the upper quadrant, in which the field is lost progressively from the vertical meridian down to the horizontal raphe (Figs. 17–18, 17–19, 17–20). The pace of loss of the lower quadrant is different from the pace of loss of the upper quadrant because of a difference in anatomy rather than a difference in the growth of the tumor.

The question of whether temporal lobe field defects are congruous or incongruous is still a matter of controversy. In my experience, the majority of temporal lobe field defects are congruous; however, some are definitely incongruous. This finding has also been the experience of others. The reason for the variation is not clear, but the presence of these two different types of field defects in the same area is a clinical fact. One proposed explanation of

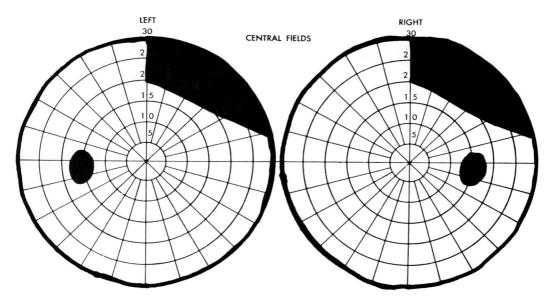

Fig. 17–18. Early temporal lobe homonymous hemianopia that is congruous and densest at the vertical meridian, suggesting an anterior temporal lobe lesion.

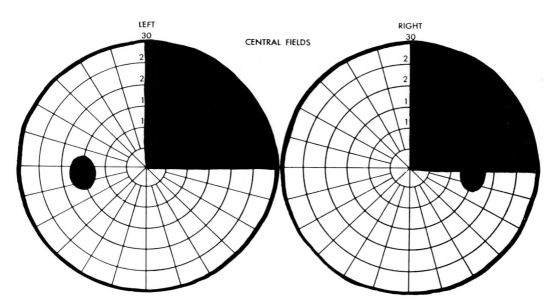

Fig. 17–19. Progression of a temporal lobe defect to a full quadrantanopsia.

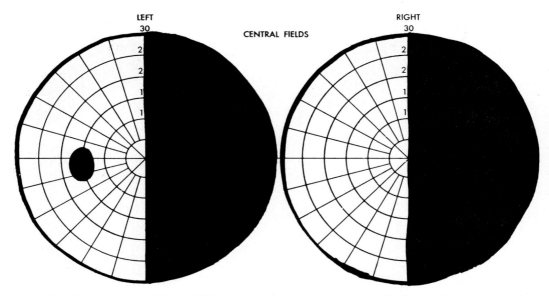

Fig. 17–20. In the temporal lobe, a full homonymous hemianopia occurs after the quadrantanopsia rather than progressing down the lower field.

the incongruous nature of some temporal lobe field defects is that the temporal lobe tumor exerts pressure medially and compresses the tract.

Parietal Lobe

These field defects are described as homonymous hemianopias that have the densest part of the defect in the lower field (Fig. 17–21). Patients with a parietal lobe field defect may also have a defect in the horizontal optokinetic response as well as right-left confusion, finger agnosia, dysgraphia, dyscalculia, or dyslexia. These signs, which can be easily tested by the perimetrist, help in the interpretation of any field defect that he finds.

Two signs of parietal lobe field defects are of particular interest and require further comment—the extinction phenomenon and the motor impersistent sign. If the ophthalmologist cannot find a field defect in a patient who has been referred for the evaluation of a field defect, the ophthalmologist should not assume that the referring physician made an error. The patient may have the extinction phenomenon, which can be detected only when the nasal and temporal fields are examined simultaneously. Such an examination can best be done with the confrontation field technique. Simultaneous stimulation of both fields is not routinely or easily done with most of the instruments used for performing field examinations, so the extinction phenomenon is usually missed.

The motor impersistent sign is also frequently missed. Patients with the motor impersistent sign cannot maintain a willed motor act, a condition that manifests itself by the patient's inability to maintain fixation. Because the patient cannot maintain fixation, it is almost impossible to do an accurate field examination. Such a patient seems intelligent enough to perform the test, but he also seems cantankerous, a combination that brings the physician close to frustration and even anger. The physician who has a right-handed patient who fits this description should consider the possibility that the patient may have right-sided parietal disease and may thus be unable to maintain fixation. A good confrontation field examination done

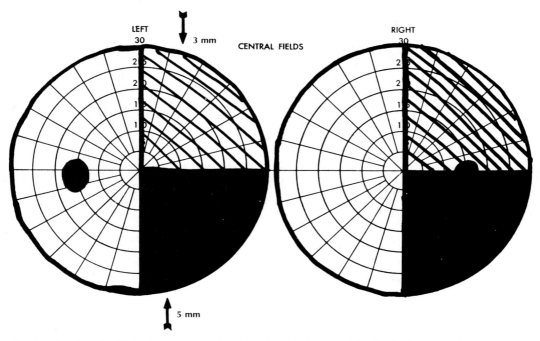

Fig. 17–21. A parietal lobe homonymous hemianopia with densest defect in the lower quadrants.

quickly—before the patient can shift fixation—may readily demonstrate a large degree of hemianopia, at which point the physician should examine the patient for the other signs of parietal lobe defects (described previously).

Occipital Lobe

These field defects are varied; they include homonymous hemianopias, homonymous quadrantanopsias, altitudinal defects, paracentral and midzone defects, as well as cases of splitting and sparing of fixation (Figs. 17–22, 17–23, 17–24, 17–25, 17–26).

The Riddoch phenomenon is an infrequent but valuable sign of occipital lobe disease. In occipital lobe infarction with hemianopia, perception of motion before perception of form is indicative of the Riddoch phenomenon and of some recovery in the occipital lobe. The patient does not perceive a steady nonmoving light that has been projected into the blind field until the light moves. The Riddoch phenomenon

does not indicate full recovery from the field defect, but it is a sign of improvement. The phenomenon occurs only in occipital lobe field defects. The patient often complains about paracentral defects because they are located near the center of vision and thus interfere with reading. On examination, the vision and the peripheral field are found to be normal. Many physicians feel that, when visual acuity is normal, no central defect exists, and therefore no need exists to examine the central field; however, presence of the paracentral field defect belies this conclusion (Fig. 17–26).

Homonymous hemianopia occurring in the calcarine cortex can, on rare occasions, be a false localizing sign. In such a case, the true disorder lies in the frontal lobe. Frontal lobe tumors can cause displacement of the brain, which compresses the posterior cerebral arteries as they cross over the tentorial edge and causes an occipital lobe field defect. Therefore, what initially was considered a vascular cause appears on the radioisotope brain scan to

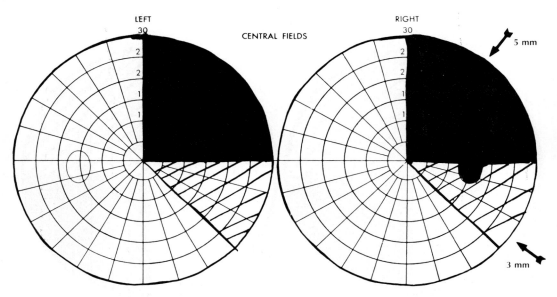

Fig. 17–22.   Homonymous defect that is congruous and suggests an occipital lobe location.

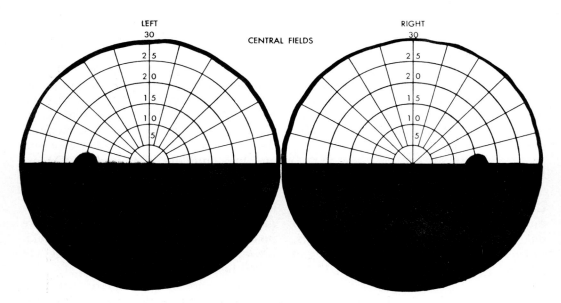

Fig. 17–23.   An altitudinal hemianopia that involves both sides of the upper calcarine cortex and is located in the occipital lobe.

be 2 lesions and can be misinterpreted as metastatic disease because of the multiple defects; however, only 1 tumor (one that is probably surgically accessible) exists in the frontal lobe. A brain scan repeated 6 weeks later will show a resolution of the occipital lobe defect that essentially rules out an occipital lobe tumor. The frontal lobe defect would show no change on the scan—a fact that suggests the diagnosis to the physician. A CT scan will show a difference in tissue density on the initial scan, suggesting that one side is a tumor and that one is an infarction. This scan provides im-

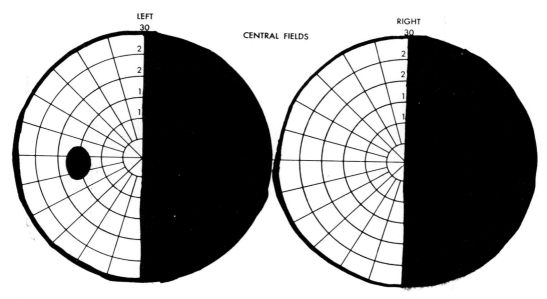

Fig. 17–24. Homonymous hemianopia that splits right through fixation.

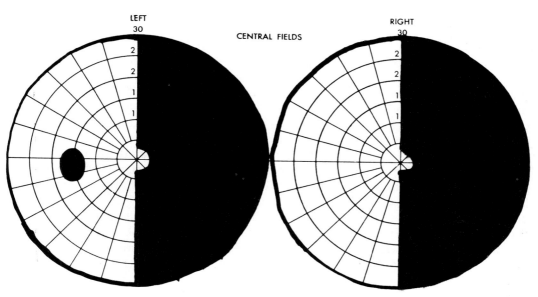

Fig. 17–25. Homonymous hemianopia that spares 3° around fixation is called sparing and indicates an occipital lobe location.

mediate evidence as opposed to the comparison scan, which requires a 6-week waiting period.

Sometimes, the time of onset of the homonymous hemianopia is inaccurately reported. The patient may say that the onset was acute (an acute onset suggests a vascular cause), but he may be referring to the time that he first noticed the condition, not to when the condition first occurred. Simmons and Cogan have suggested the use of the optokinetic test for identifying tumors from a vascular cause of occipital lobe homonymous hemianopia. They have

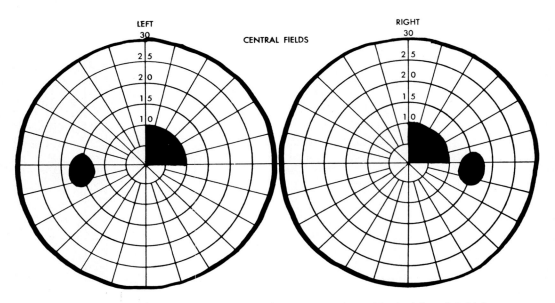

Fig. 17–26. A paracentral homonymous congruous hemianopia is located in the left occipital lobe.

stated that, if the horizontal optokinetic response is normal in an occipital lobe homonymous hemianopia, the cause is most likely vascular. If the optokinetic response is abnormal, a tumor is more likely to be the cause. The rationale behind this distinction is that a tumor will not readily localize to the occipital lobe, but it will encroach on the parietal lobe and the optokinetic pathway.

The occurrence of macular sparing versus macular splitting as a sign of occipital lobe lesions has raged for years. One form of this sparing occurs when the patient fixes eccentrically and moves the entire hemianopic line over. He does not spare just the 2 to 5° around fixation but all up and down the vertical meridian. There are examples, however, of occipital lesions that do spare the central 2 to 5° even when there is a total homonymous hemianopic defect around this area. As precise an anatomic idea as it is that vision is cut down the middle evenly and exactly in every person, it probably is not so. Young, in his examination of visual field defects in the radiations, postulated that there is no sharp vertical line exactly at the vertical me-

ridian but rather that it may be off by several degrees on either side. Morax proposed that the foveal area of the retina of each eye is composed of a mixture of both crossed and uncrossed fibers. This overlapping of crossed and uncrossed fibers, at least in the foveal area, has been shown to be present in cats and in the primate monkey. Cowey's experiments are the most interesting in this regard. In monkeys who had undergone occipital lobectomies, Cowey performed single-cell recording in the foveal receptor area of the other occipital lobe. When he stimulated a single retinal foveal cell, he got responses in the foveal area corresponding to the area served by the extirpated occipital lobe from the other side. The assumption then is that the surviving occipital lobe has projections to both sides of the vertical meridian of the fovea. McIlwain's studies came to a similar conclusion doing experiments on the lateral geniculate body.

Perversion of Visual Fields

Alterations in vision or field may be negative or positive. Decreases in visual acuity or hemianopic field defects are examples of negative alterations in the visual field. Hallucinations, allesthesia, perseveration, and palinopsia are examples of positive alterations in the visual system.

Visual perseveration is a continuation or repetition of a visual stimulus after it is no longer present and actively stimulating the retina. Visual perseveration occurs as a normal phenomenon, such as the afterimage of a strobe light shone in an eye. The length of time the phenomenon lasts is related to the intensity of the stimulus and the length of time of the exposure. That is why a bright light such as a strobe light has a longer afterimage than a weak flashlight or a table top. All stimulate the retina and may do so for the same interval of time, but all do not have the same intensity effect on the retina.

Palinopsia is an abnormal extrapolation of the normal phenomenon of perseveration. The patient may see a face on television and at different times have that face appear as though it was on the TV at that moment. This differs from hallucinations since this visual phenomenon actually occurred as the initial episode. It also differs from the visual phenomena of patients with migraine, retinal detachment, or posterior vitreous detachment, which constitute abnormal stimulation of the visual system. Tumors, vascular lesions, and occasionally, trauma have been reported to cause palinopsia. Palinopsia occurs with other defects in the visual system and usually means involvement of the occipital parietal area.

Visual allesthesia is the transference of images from one half field to the other, with palinopsia of those images. Studies on a small number of patients with visual allesthesia reported EEG abnormalities also in the parietal occipital area. These patients not only had field defects but other evidence of seizure activity.

FUNCTIONAL VISUAL LOSS

Hysteric and malingering types of visual loss are similar; only the underlying psychologic reasons for the loss vary. This discussion, therefore, treats only the types of functional visual loss and the tests used to establish the functional nature of the conditions. Needless to say, the physician must make every effort to rule out organic disease, no matter what the patient's personality is.

Loss of Central Visual Acuity

The loss of central vision is a common functional complaint. If the loss is related to emotional gain rather than to financial gain, it is usually bilateral. Bilateral loss of vision allows the person to become completely dependent and to retreat from whatever it is that he feels he can no longer cope with emotionally. A person who has loss of vision in only one eye would still be expected to cope with his problems. Monocular functional loss of vision does occur, however, and the condition is usually related to accidental trauma to or around the eye. Frequently, the patient is involved in litigation concerning an insurance claim. In organic monocular loss of vision, some clinical findings should exist in support of the patient's complaints, for example, changes in the fundus (such as destructive lesions), changes in the macula, optic atrophy, and cataract. A common exception to this rule occurs in retrobulbar neuritis, in which nothing is shown initially on ophthalmologic examination except the afferent pupillary defect.

Cases with bilateral organic loss of vision are more difficult to diagnose. Organic lesions at the chiasm may not show optic atrophy for some time. Persons with occipital cortical blindness do not show any changes on ophthalmoscopy, and their pupils are essentially normal.

Patients who complain of loss of central vision but who have a full peripheral field should be considered as having an organic lesion. Those with functional loss of central vision usually have severe contraction of the field. The person with retrobulbar neuritis has loss of central vision, a normal fundus, and usually a full peripheral field; however, it cannot be inferred that the opposite clinical finding—loss of central vision with severe contraction of the field—is always functional.

Testing of Visual Acuity

A painstaking examination of only the visual acuity may be all that can be accomplished on the patient's first visit. The examination may take an inordinate amount of time. (In such an examination, the patient's vision has been referred to as iron maiden vision since the physician seems to be like the torturer of old, applying repeated pressure until the "correct" answer is forthcoming from the patient.) As the physician uses different techniques to measure acuity, the patient's vision may slowly improve from 20/200 to close to 20/20; however, the fact that normal acuity eventually results does not change the fact that the initial loss of acuity was functional. Thirty minutes of testing does not improve organic loss of vision.

Another form of acuity testing involves comparing near and distance acuity. In organic disease, both types of acuity are either the same or within one Snellen line of each other.

In monocular loss of vision in which an obvious cause cannot be determined by ophthalmoscopy, the use of the afferent pupillary defect may be of value in establishing organic optic nerve disease. The method of eliciting this sign is discussed elsewhere.

Acuity testing can be done at distances other than 20 feet or 14 inches. For instance, have the patient walk 10 feet to the chart and then have him read the letters. The letters that were 20/100 at 20 feet will then be equal to 20/200, a relationship that can be applied proportionately to all the other lines of letters.

Cycloplegic Test

A carefully done refraction with and without a pinhole test is always the first step in evaluating decreased vision. The second step is cycloplegic refraction, which can rule out such problems as spasm of accommodation and latent hyperopia.

In monocular functional visual loss, a cycloplegic refraction can also be of value. Both eyes should be completely corrected for distance, and the acuity of each eye then tested separately. Since the patient is aware when the eye with the poor vision is being tested, he gives the same response about poor vision as before. The physician then puts a plus 2.50 sphere in the Phoroptor before the eye with the alleged decreased acuity. The sphere blurs that eye for distance. The patient's visual acuity is then tested with both his eyes uncovered behind the Phoroptor, and he reads the distance chart again. The patient does not usually resist this test since he can explain a correct reading of the chart by the fact that he was reading the chart with just the good eye. The physician should then flip down the near card at 16 inches and ask the patient to read it, again with both eyes. Since the normal eye is under cycloplegia without an appropriate add, the affected eye, which has the proper add, is the only eye capable of reading the chart at 16 inches. Since the patient knows that the eye he is complaining about was blurred at a distance with both eyes open, he assumes that it will be blurred at 16 inches. If the test is done quickly—before the patient thinks to close each eye separately to check which eye is seeing at close range—he falls into the obvious mistake.

Red-Green Test

Another useful test of functional loss of vision that can be done with the Phoroptor involves the red-green filters. To do this test, the physician seats the patient behind the Phoroptor and does the same refraction with the proper correction for distance. He puts a red filter in front of one eye and a green filter in front of the other eye. Then the physician puts the red-green slide in the projector so that the letters projected on the screen are green on one side and red on the other side. The patient sees the red letters with the eye with the red filter and the green letters with the eye with the green filter. This test is usually not very effective because the patient can easily check which eye sees which set of letters. When a battery of tests is being done, however, any one of them may give the clue the physician seeks.

Polarizing Test

In a clever variation of the red-green filter test, polarizing lenses are used. The red-green slide is taken out of the projector and is replaced by a polarizing lens, which orients half the line of letters at 90 degrees to the other half. Then the polarizing lenses are placed in front of each eye so that one eye sees the half of the chart that has its letters similarly polarized. At first glance, this test would seem to present the same problem as the red-green test. The patient can close each eye separately to check which eye sees which half of the chart. The difference between the tests, however, is that the polarization of the projected letters can be switched by changing the direction of the polarizing lenses with a silent twist of a knob. As a result, the patient's right eye can be seeing the right half of the line of letters one instant and the left eye the right half of the line of letters the next instant. If the polarization is changed quickly and quietly and if the physician remembers which eye saw which half of the line of letters, the patient with a functional loss can be led into reading with his affected eye.

Optokinetic Test

Use of the optokinetic tape may be of value in examining the patient who complains of monocular or binocular loss of vision of such a severe degree that he cannot even count accurately fingers placed directly in front of him. The patient should be instructed to look steadily ahead, even if he cannot see an object on which to fix-

ate. The optokinetic drum or tape should be moved in the horizontal direction and any response sought. If a response occurs, the test should be repeated at different distances until no response occurs. Obviously, a response with small targets (like the stripes on the drum at 10 feet) and an inability to count fingers at even 6 inches are incongruous findings. The physician cannot give a Snellen evaluation of the patient's vision, but he can certainly say that doubt exists as to the degree of the patient's visual loss.

Sometimes, if the patient shows no response to horizontally displayed optokinetic targets, changing the targets so that they move in a vertical direction may catch the patient off guard; he may forget to ignore the optokinetic target and give a positive response.

Mirror Test

This test is also helpful. It too is used for patients complaining of extremely poor vision in one or both eyes. The patient is asked to look straight ahead and not to move his eyes. The physician holds a 12-by 12-inch mirror about 2 feet in front of the patient's eyes. When the patient says that he cannot see the mirror, the physician reassures him that it is not necessary to see the mirror but it is necessary that he hold his eyes still. While talking to the patient about something other than the test, the physician moves the mirror very slowly from side to side. If the patient's eyes move, he is able to see better than he admits, and the defect can therefore be considered functional.

As in most branches of medicine, in ophthalmology the most difficult patient to evaluate is the one who has an organic disorder with a lot of functional overlay. Therefore, in every patient in whom a functional loss of vision is suspected, every effort must be made to rule out organic disease; and the patient must be reexamined at regular intervals to check the clinical findings.

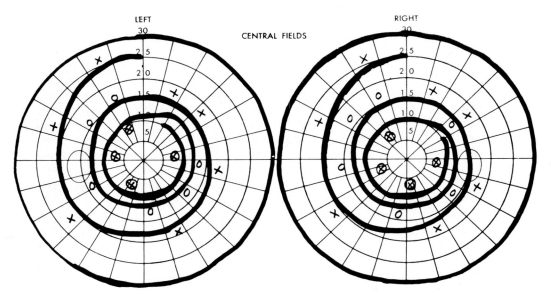

Fig. 17-27. Spiral field of hysteria—all points marked are with the same test object. X represents first time field is performed. O is second time, and ⊗ is third time field is performed.

Peripheral Field Loss

The traditional field defect of hysteria is the spiral field defect (Fig. 17–27). The spiral field gets progressively smaller as the peripheral isopters are reexamined—a phenomenon that can also be a sign of fatigue, particularly in very ill patients. The same phenomenon is frequently seen in patients subjected to a protracted field examination. The length of time a patient can be expected to submit to a field examination varies from patient to patient, but the problem must be kept in mind as the perimetrist does the field tests.

Contraction of the peripheral field is a much more common finding in functional field loss than is spiral field defect. The organic causes of gun barrel fields have been discussed earlier. To distinguish functionally small fields from organically small fields, the examination should be done at 2 different distances. If the field defect at 1 m is 10° with a 1-mm test object, it should be 10° at any distance with a comparable test object. Therefore, to duplicate the testing circumstances, the patient should be

moved back to 2 m from the tangent screen and a 2-mm test object used (Fig. 17–28, 17–29). The patient should again show a 10° field defect; however, the area in the tangent screen that was the 10° isopter is now the 5° isopter at 2 m, and the isopter that previously was 20° is now the 10° isopter. The field of vision, therefore, covers a larger area on the screen. The patient who does not see the 2-mm test object until it comes into the original 10° isopter on the tangent screen has a functional field loss. He is reporting that his field is smaller at 2 m than it was at 1 m.

A mistake the perimetrist may make in doing this test is to forget to double the size of the test object when he doubles the testing distance. If the physician does not double the size of the test object, he is not duplicating the test. The 1-mm test object at 2 m is one-half the size of the 1-mm test object at 1 m on the retina; therefore, the test is not the same. A less sophisticated but effective and dramatic way to illustrate this fact is as follows. The patient demonstrates a 10° field to a 3-mm white test object at 1 m. The physician then backs

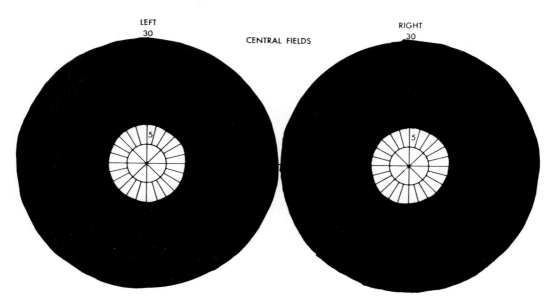

Fig. 17–28. Contracted field done with 5-mm white test object at 1 m shows a 10° field.

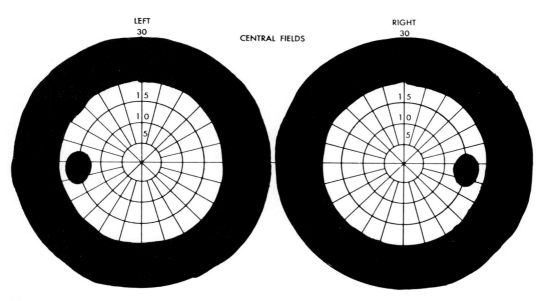

Fig. 17–29. Contracted field performed at 2 m on same screen with a 10-mm white test object shows normal enlargement. The 20° meridian is really 10° now that the subject is twice the distance from the screen.

away about 16 feet and asks the patient to cover one eye and to fix on the physician's nose with the other eye. The physician uses his hand as a test object and asks the patient to tell him when he sees the hand. Obviously, the physician's hand is larger than 36 mm, which is the size of the test object that would have to be used to duplicate the test performed at 1 m. The physician then brings his hand in from the periphery until the patient sees it. The area in which the patient sees the hand is no larger than the area the patient saw on the tangent screen at 1 m. This test establishes more firmly that the defect is a functional one.

The usual testing technique involves going from nonseeing to seeing. In patients with very small fields, it may be of value to go from seeing to nonseeing. The physician should ask the patient to tell him when he does not see the test object. A considerably larger field may be found by this technique. The physician must judge whether it is a true field or whether the "larger" field has resulted from a slow response from a dull or obtunded patient.

Color has its use in testing for peripheral field loss. The size of fields in response to colored test objects is not only different but also sequential, appearing in a certain order in regard to which is a larger and which is a smaller field. The test checks color recognition and is not a reduced color intensity test. When the test is used this way, the smallest field is green, the next larger field (to the same size test object) is red, and the next larger is blue. If any reversal of this order occurs, the defect should be considered functional. (However, the test may not be reliable if the patient has some degree of red-green color blindness.)

Cortical Blindness

Three types of cortical blindness occur, and one of these types is frequently considered functional by the unwary physician. The site of all three types is the visual cortex of the occipital lobe. In one type of cortical blindness, the patient has an infarction of both occipital lobes, and he sees little or nothing. This patient says that he cannot see, and he acts accordingly. In a second type of cortical blindness, the patient has the same field loss, but he denies that he is blind. He probably has disturbances not only in visual cortex area 17 but in association area 18 as well. If this patient has Anton syndrome, he also has a Korsakoff-type reaction in that he confabulates

about his blindness. He has not learned from his experiences that he is blind, and he confabulates to justify his poor visual performance.

It is the person with the third type of cortical blindness who frequently is said to have functional blindness. Such a person has the bilateral hemianopia owing to bilateral occipital lobe involvement, but has sparing of the tip of the occipital lobe, where the macular projection is located. In about 20% of people studied by arteriography, this area of the visual cortex has a secondary blood supply from the carotid system, a phenomenon that is analogous to the secondary blood supply to the fovea from the cilioretinal artery. In vascular infarction of both occipital lobes, the accessory blood supply from the carotid system may preserve the macular projection. As a result, the patient has a preserved central acuity but only a small field, usually measuring 2 to 3°. The patient acts blind, stumbling into things because of the small peripheral field. Since the patient tells the physician that he is blind, he is usually tested first with the 20/200 letters, which he cannot see because of his small field. Since the patient cannot see the large letters, he is not tested with the smaller letters, and he is called blind. However, if the examiner notices that the patient can see very small objects, he assumes, logically enough, that the patient has a functional disorder. The patient can see small objects (but not the 20/200 letters) because his central vision is intact. The physician should test the patient with small letters, preferably with the near card. As the patient holds the near card, the proprioception phenomenon involved in holding it helps the patient to direct his small field to the card and find the appropriate size of print. The patient can also see letters at 20 feet, but with more difficulty because he would have to direct his small field to exactly the point in space that the physician indicates. For distance testing, the physician should direct the patient to sight down his arm, with the physician pointing the patient's arm as an aiming stake. I have examined patients whose field was so small that they could not see 20/200 letters but could see 20/50 letters.

Once this type of field defect is discovered, the usual tests (such as doubling and tripling the testing distance) can be performed to determine whether the defect is functional or organic. The bilaterality of the defect establishes that the lesion is located in the occipital lobe.

BIBLIOGRAPHY

Albert, M.L., Reches, A., and Silverberg, R.: Hemianopic colour blindness. J. Neurol. Neurosurg. Psychiatry 38:546, 1975.

Albert, M.L., et al.: The anatomic basis of visual agnosia. Neurology 29:876, 1979.

Alexander, G.L.: Diagnostic value of colour fields in neurosurgery. Trans. Ophthalmol. Soc. U.K. 76:235, 1956.

Amsler, M.: Earliest symptoms of disease of the macula. Br. J. Ophthalmol. 37:521, 1953.

Arden, G.B., and Gucukoglu, A.G.: Grating test of contrast sensitivity in patients with retrobulbar neuritis. Arch. Ophthalmol. 96:1626, 1978.

Balagura, S., Frantz, A.G., Housepian, E.M., and Carmel, P.W.: The specificity of serum prolactin as a diagnostic indicator of pituitary adenoma. J. Neurosurg. 51:42, 1979.

Barbur, J.L., Ruddock, K.H., and Waterfield, V.A.: Human visual responses in the absence of the geniculocalcarine projection. Brain 103:905, 1980.

Bender, M.B.: Phenomenon of visual extinction in homonymous fields and psychologic principles involved. Arch. Neurol. Psychiatry 53:29, 1945.

Bender, M.B., and Battersby, W.S.: Homonymous macular scotoma in cases of occipital lobe tumor. Arch. Ophthalmol. 60:928, 1958.

Bender, M.B., Feldman, M., and Sobin, A.J.: Palinopsia. Brain 91:321, 1968.

Bender, M.B., and Strauss, I.: Defects in visual field of one eye only in patients with a lesion of one optic radiation. Arch. Ophthalmol. 17:765, 1937.

Benson, D.F., and Greenberg, J.D.: Visual form agnosia. Arch. Neurol. 20:82, 1969.

Benton, A.L., and Hecaen, H.: Stereoscopic vision in patients with unilateral cerebral disease. Neurology 20:1084, 1970.

Benton, S., Levy, I., and Swash, M.: Vision in the temporal crescent in occipital infarction. Brain 103:83, 1980.

Bjork, A., and Kugelberg, E.: Visual field defects after temporal lobectomy. Acta Ophthalmol. 35:210, 1957.

Block, M.A., Goree, J.A., and Jeminez, J.P.: Craniopharyngioma with optic canal enlargement simulating glioma of the optic chiasm. J. Neurosurg. 39:523, 1973.

Braude, L.S., et al.: Diagnosing acute retrobulbar neuritis by vitreous fluorophotometry. Am. J. Ophthalmol. 91:764, 1981.

Bunt, A.H., and Minckles, D.S.: Foveal sparing. Arch. Ophthalmol. 95:1445, 1977.

Bunt, A.H., Minckles, D.S., and Johnson, G.W.: Demonstration of bilateral projection of the central retina of the monkey with horseradish peroxidase neuronography. J. Comp. Neurol. 171:619, 1977.

Burde, R.M., and Gallin, P.F.: Visual parameters associated with recovered retrobulbar optic neuritis. Am. J. Ophthalmol. 70:1034, 1975.

Chamlin, M.: Minimal defects in visual field studies. Arch. Ophthalmol. 42:126, 1949.

Chamlin, M., and Davidoff, L.: The 1/2000 field in chiasmal interference. Arch. Ophthalmol. 44:53, 1950.

Chamlin, M., and Davidoff, L.: Choice of test objects in visual field studies. Am. J. Ophthalmol. 35:381, 1952.

Chamlin, M., and Davidoff, L.: Ophthalmologic changes produced by pituitary tumors. Am. J. Ophthalmol. 40:353, 1955.

Cowey, A.: Projection of the retina onto striate and prestriate cortex in the squirrel monkey Saimiri sciureus. J. Neurophysiol. 27:366, 1964.

Critchley, M.: Types of visual perseveration: "Palinopsia" and "illusory visual spread." Brain 74:267, 1951.

Critchley, M.: Acquired anomalies of colour perception of central origin. Brain 88:711, 1965.

Damasio, A., et al.: Central achromatopsia: behavioral anatomic and physiologic aspects. Neurology. 30:1064, 1980.

Damgaard-Jensen, L.: Vertical steps in isopters at the hemiopic border in normal and glaucomatous eyes. Acta Ophthalmologica 65:111, 1977.

Ellenberger, C.: Modern perimetry in neuro-ophthalmic diagnosis. Arch. Neurol. 30:193, 1974.

Ellenberger, C., and Ziegler, S.B.: Visual evoked potentials and quantitative perimetry in multiple sclerosis. Ann. Neurol. 1:561, 1977.

Enoksson, P.: A study of the visual fields with white and coloured objects in cases of pituitary tumors with especial reference to early diagnosis. Acta Ophthalmol. 31:505, 1953.

Falconer, M.A., and Wilson, J.L.: Visual field changes following anterior temporal lobectomy; their significance in relation to "Meyer's loop" of the optic radiation. Brain 81:1, 1958.

Feldman, M., Todman, L., and Bender, M.: Flight of colours in lesions of the visual system. J. Neurol. Neurosurg. Psychiatry 37:1265, 1974.

French, L.: Studies on the optic radiations; the significance of small field defects in the region of the vertical meridian. J. Neurosurg. 19:522, 1962.

Frisen, L.: A versatile color confrontation for the central visual field. Arch. Ophthalmol. 89:3, 1973.

Frisen, L., Hoyt, W.F., Bird, A.C., and Weale, R.: Implications of the Pulfrich phenomenon. Lancet 2:385, 1973.

Frisen, L., Holmegaard, L., and Rosencrantz, M.: Sectorial optic atrophy and homonymous, horizontal sectoranopia; a lateral choroidal artery syndrome. J. Neurol. Neurosurg. Psychiatry 41:374, 1978.

Fujino, T.: The intrastitial blood supply of the lateral geniculate body. Arch. Ophthalmol. 74:815, 1965.

Gassel, M.M., and William, D.: Visual function in patients with homonymous hemianopia. Part III. The completion phenomenon: insight and attitude to the defect and visual functional efficiency. Brain 86:229, 1963.

Gazzaniga, M.S., and Freedman, H.: Observations in visual processes after posterior callosal section. Neurology. 23:1126, 1973.

Geschwind, N.: Disconnection syndromes in animals and man. Brain 88:237, 1965.

Geschwind, N., and Fusillo, M.: Color-naming defects in association with alexia. Arch. Neurol. 15:137, 1966.

Goldhammer, Y., and Smith, J.L.: Bitemporal hemianopia in chloroquine retinopathy. Neurology 24:1135, 1974.

Goldstein, M.N., et al.: Word blindness with intact central visual fields. Neurology 21:873, 1971.

Gramberg-Danielsen, B.: Die Doppelversorgung des Macula. Graefe Arch. Ophthalmol. 160:534, 1959.

Green, G.J., and Lessell, S.: Acquired cerebral dyschromatopsia. Arch. Ophthalmol. 95:121, 1977.

Greenblatt, S.: Posttraumatic transient cerebral blindness associated with migraine and seizure diatheses. JAMA 225:1073, 1973.

Gunderson, C. and Hoyt, W.: Geniculate hemianopia; incongruous homonymous field defects in two patients with partial lesions of the lateral geniculate nucleus. J. Neurol. Neurosurg. Psychiatry 34:1, 1971.

Halliday, A.M., McDonald, W.I., and Mushin, J.: Delayed visual evoked responses in optic neuritis. Lancet 1:982, 1972.

Harms, H.: Role of perimetry in assessment of optic nerve dysfunction. Trans. Ophthalmol. Soc. U.K. 96:363, 1976.

Harrington, D.: Visual field character in temporal and occipital lobe lesions. Arch. Ophthalmol. 66:36, 1961.

Hedges, T.R.: Preservation of the upper nasal field in the chiasmal syndrome: an anatomic explanation. Trans. Am. Ophthalmol. Soc. 67:131, 1969.

Hoff, J., and Patterson, R.: Craniopharyngiomas in children and adults. J. Neurosurg. 36:299, 1972.

Horrax, G.: Visual hallucinations as a cerebral localizing phenomenon. Arch. Neurol. Psychiatry 10:532, 1923.

Hoyt, W.F., and Newton, T.H.: Angiographic changes with occlusion of arteries that supply the visual cortex. N.Z. Med. J. 72:310, 1970.

Hoyt, W.F., and Walsh, F.: Cortical blindness with partial recovery following acute cerebral anoxia from cardiac arrest. Arch. Ophthalmol. 60:1061, 1958.

Hoyt, W.F., Rios-Montenegro, E., and Behrens, M.: Homonymous hemioptic hypoplasia; funduscopic features in standard and red free illumination in three patients with congenital hemiplegia. Br. J. Ophthalmol. 56:537, 1972.

Hoyt, W.F., Schlicke, B., and Eckelhoff, R.: Fundus-

copic appearance of a nerve fibre bundle defect. Br. J. Ophthalmol. 56:577, 1972.

Hubel, D.H., and Wiesel, T.N.: Sequence regularity and geometry of orientation columns in the monkey striate cortex. J. Comp. Neurol. 158:267, 1974.

Hughes, E.: Some observations on the visual fields in hydrocephalus. J. Neurol. Neurosurg. Psychiatry 9:30, 1946.

Ikeda, H., and Wright, M.: Differential effects of refractive errors and receptive field organization of central and peripheral ganglion cells. Vision Res. 12:1465, 1967.

Jacobs, L.: Visual allesthesia. Neurology 30:1059, 1980.

Kaul, S., DuBoulay, G., and Kendall, B.: Relationship between visual field defect and arterial occlusion in the posterior cerebral circulation. J. Neurol. Neurosurg. Psychiatry 37:1022, 1974.

Kearns, T., and Rucker, C.: Arcuate defects in the visual fields due to chromophobe adenoma of the pituitary gland. Am. J. Ophthalmol. 45:505, 1958.

Kearns, T., Wagener, H., and Millikan, C.: Bilateral homonymous hemianopia. Arch. Ophthalmol. 53:560, 1955.

Kinsbourne, M., and Warrington, E.K.: A study of visual perseveration. J. Neurol. Neurosurg. Psychiatry 26:468, 1963.

Laws, E.R., Trautmann, J.C., and Hollenhorst, R.W.: Transsphenoidal decompression of the optic nerve and chiasm. J. Neurosurg. 46:717, 1977.

Manor, R.S., et al.: Nasal visual field loss with intracranial lesions of the optic nerve pathway. Am. J. Ophthalmol. 90:1, 1980.

Marino, R., and Rasmussen, T.: Visual field changes after temporal lobectomy in man. Neurology 18:825, 1968.

Matthews, W.D., et al.: Patterns reversal evoked visual potential in the diagnosis of multiple sclerosis. J. Neurol. Neurosurg. Psychiatry 40:1009, 1971.

McIlwain, J.T.: Receptive fields of optic tract axons and lateral geniculate cells. Peripheral extent and barbiturate sensitivity. J. Neurophysiol. 27:1154, 1964.

Meadows, J.C.: Disturbed perception of colours associated with localized cerebral lesions. Brain 97:615, 1974.

Meienberg, O.: Sparing of the temporal crescent in homonymous hemianopia and its significance for visual orientation. Neuro-ophthalmology 2:129, 1981.

Mills, D., and Willis, N.: Visual field defects in pregnancy. Can. J. Ophthalmol. 5:16, 1970.

Morax, V.: Discussion des hypothèses faites sur les connexion corticales des faisceaux maculaires. Ann. Oculist 156:103, 1919.

Newman, S.A., and Miller, N.R.: Optic tract syndrome. Arch. Ophthalmol. 101:1241, 1983.

Patterson, V.H., and Heron, J.R.: Visual field abnormalities in multiple sclerosis. J. Neurol. Neurosurg. Psychiatry 43:205, 1980.

Poppel, E., Held, R., and Frost, D.: Residual visual function after brain wounds involving the central visual pathways in man. Nature 243:295, 1973.

Pulfrich, Von C.: Die Stereoskopie im dienste des isochromen und heterochromen Photometrie. Na-lurwissenschafter *10*:553, 1922.

O'Connell, J.E.A.: The anatomy of the optic chiasma and heteronymous hemianopia. J. Neurol. Neurosurg. Psychiatry 36:710, 1973.

Regan, D., Silver, R., and Murray, T.J.: Visual acuity and contrast sensitivity in multiple sclerosis—hidden visual loss. Brain *100*:563, 1977.

Regan, D., et al.: Contrast sensitivity, visual acuity and the discrimination of Snellen letters in multiple sclerosis. Brain *104*:333, 1981.

Renaldi, I., Bolton, J., and Troland, C.: Cortical visual disturbance following ventriculography and/or ventricular decompression. J. Neurosurg. *19*:568, 1962.

Riddoch, G.: Dissociation of visual perception due to occipital injuries with especial reference to appreciation of movement. Brain 40:15, 1917.

Rushton, D.: Use of the Pulfrich pendulum for detecting abnormal delay in the visual pathway in multiple sclerosis. Brain 98:283, 1975.

Salmon, J.: Transient postictal hemianopia. Arch. Ophthalmol. 79:523, 1968.

Shaw, H.E., and Smith, J.L.: Cecocentral scotomas: neuro-ophthalmologic consideration. Neuro-ophthalmology Focus 1980. Edited by J.L. Smith. p. 165.

Simmons, R.J., and Cogan, D.G.: Occult temporal arteritis. Arch. Ophthalmol. 68:8, 1962.

Smith, J.: Homonymous hemianopia; a review of 100 cases. Am. J. Ophthalmol. 54:616, 1963.

Spalding, J.: Wounds of the visual pathway. Part I. The visual radiations. J. Neurol. Neurosurg. Psychiatry 15:99, 1952.

Spalding, J.: Wounds of the visual cortex. Part II. The striate cortex. J. Neurol. Neurosurg. Psychiatry 15:169, 1952.

Spector, R.H., et al.: Occipital lobe infarctions: perimetry and computed tomography. Neurology 31:1098, 1981.

Stensaar, S.S., Eddington, D., and Dobelle, W.: The topography and variability of the primary visual cortex in man. J. Neurosurg. 40:747, 1974.

Stone, J.: The naso temporal division of the cats' retina. J. Comp. Neurol. 126:585, 1966.

Stone, J., Leicester, J., and Sherman, S.M.: The naso temporal division of the monkeys' retina. J. Comp. Neurol. 150:333, 1973.

Symonds, C., and MacKenzie, I.: Bilateral loss of vision from cerebral infarction. Brain 80:415, 1957.

Teuber, H.L.: Alteration of perception and memory in man. *In* Analysis of Behavioral Change. Edited by L. Weiskrantz. Harper and Row, 1968.

Trevarthen, C.B.: Double visual learning in split-brain monkeys. Science *136*:258, 1962.

Trobe, J.D.: Chromophobe adenoma presenting with

a hemianopic temporal arcuate scotoma. Am. J. Ophthalmol. 77:388, 1974.

Trobe, J.D., and Glaser, J.S.: Quantitative perimetry in compressive optic neuropathy and optic neuritis. Arch. Ophthalmol. 96:1210, 1978.

Trobe, J.D., Lorber, M., and Schlezenger, N.: Isolated homonymous hemianopias; a review of 104 cases. Arch. Ophthalmol. 89:377, 1973.

Van Buren, J., and Baldwin, M.: The architecture of the optic radiation in the temporal lobe of man. Brain 81:15, 1958.

Van Dalen, J.T.W., and Greve, E.L.: Visual field defects in multiple sclerosis. Neuro-ophthalmology 2:93, 1981.

Walsh, T.: Paracentral scotoma testing. Ophthalmol. Surg. 4:72, 1973.

Walsh, T.: Temporal crescent or half-moon syndrome. Ann. Ophthalmol. 6:501, 1974.

Welsh, R.: Finger counting in the four quadrants as a method of visual field gross screening. Arch. Ophthalmol. 66:678, 1961.

William, D., and Gassel, M.M.: Visual function in patients with homonymous hemianopia. Part I: The visual field. Brain 85:175, 1962.

William, D., and Gassel, M.M.: Visual function in patients with homonymous hemianopia. Part III: The completion phenomenon: insight and attitude to the defect and visual functional efficiency. Brain 86:229, 1963.

Wilson, T.M.: Quantitative perimetry in the assessment of optic nerve conduction defects. Trans. Ophthalmol. Soc. U.K. 89:67, 1967.

Wilson, C.B., and Dempsey, L.C.: Transsphenoidal microsurgical removal of 250 pituitary adenomas. J. Neurosurg. 48:13, 1978.

Wilson, P., and Falconer, M.: Patterns of visual failure with pituitary tumors; clinical and radiological correlations. Br. J. Ophthalmol. 52:94, 1968.

Wolter, J.R.: The centrifugal nerves in the human optic tract, chiasm, optic nerve and retina. Tr. Am. Ophthalmol. Soc. 63:678, 1965.

Young, S., Walsh, F., and Knox, D.: Tilted disc syndrome. Am. J. Ophthalmol. 82:16, 1976.

Younge, B.R.: Midline tilting between seeing and nonseeing areas. Mayo Clin. Proc. 51:562, 1976.

Zappia, R., Enoch, J., and Stamper, R.: The Riddoch phenomenon revealed in non-occipital lobe lesion. Br. J. Ophthalmol. 55:416, 1971.

Zeki, S.M.: Colour coding in Rhesus monkey prestriate cortex. Brain Res. 53:422, 1973.

Zihl, I., and Von Cramon, D.: Colours anomia restricted to the left visual hemifield after splenial disconnexion. J. Neurol. Neurosurg. Psychiatry 43:719, 1980.

Zimmern, R.I., Campell, F.W., and Wilkinson, I.M.S.: Subtle disturbances of vision after optic neuritis elicited by studying contrast sensitivity. J. Neurol. Neurosurg. Psychiatry 42:407, 1979.

Index

Numbers followed by "f" indicate illustrations; numbers followed by "t" indicate tables.

Neoplasms
  brain. *See* Brain tumors
  brain stem, 281
  cardiac, 358, 359f
  in cavernous sinus, 100
  cerebellopontine angle, 107
  eye movement disorders due to, 64
  of eyelid, 82-83
  facial paralysis due to, 281
  Horner syndrome due to, 50-51
  intracranial. *See also* Brain tumors
    exophthalmos due to, 73
  inverting papilloma of sinuses, 266, 271f
  meningitis due to, 377
  metastatic to orbit, 237, 244
    CT scan in, 241-243f
  nasopharyngeal, 108-109, 266, 269-270f
  optic disc edema due to, 28-29
  orbital, 67-71. *See also* Orbit, neoplasms
    carcinoma, 70
    CT scans of, 234-236f, 237-243f, 244
    dermoid, 70
    glioma, 69-70
    lymphoma, 67
    melanoma, 67
    meningioma, 70
    mucocele, 70-71
    palpation of, 62
    retinoblastoma, 67-68
    rhabdomyosarcoma, 67
  of paranasal sinuses, 266, 267-268f
  on superior orbital fissure, 100
  third cranial nerve paralysis due to, 99
  vision loss in, 375-377
Neostigmine, in testing for myasthenia gravis, 118
Nervus intermedius of Wrisberg, 274. *See also* Facial nerve
Neuralgia
  eye pain due to, 7
  glossopharyngeal, 407
  greater occipital nerve, 408
  in herpes zoster, 401-402
  Raeder's paratrigeminal, 397-398
  sphenopalatine, 407-408
  trigeminal, 406-407
Neuroblastoma, orbital involvement in, 67
Neurocutaneous syndromes. *See* Phakomatoses
  of eyelid, 82-83
  in orbit, 69
Neurofibromatosis, 132, 135-139
  bone in, 139
  brain involvement in, 137
  cerebrovascular disease in, 364
  clinical manifestations, 135-136
  diagnosis, 53
  differential diagnosis, 139
  eye involvement in, 137-138
  of eyelid, 82-83
  genetics, 137, 139
  heterochromia in, 53
  historical background, 136
  notable points in, 139
  optic glioma related to, 225, 376
  in orbit, 69
  pathology, 136-137

peripheral organ involvement in, 139
pheochromocytoma associated with, 139
radiographic evaluation, 190, 194f, 195f
skin in, 138-139
tuberous sclerosis distinguished from, 135
Neurologic disorders, retinitis pigmentosa associated with, 322
Neurologic examination, 11-16
  caudal cranial nerves, 15
  cranial nerves, 11-15
    accessory, 15
    facial, 12-13
    glossopharyngeal, 15
    hypoglossal, 15
    trigeminal, 11-12
    vagus, 15
    vestibulo-acoustic, 13-15
  facial nerve, 12-13
  general observations, 16
  mental functions, 16
  muscles, motor functions and reflexes, 15-16
  sensation, 16
  trigeminal nerve, 11-12
  vestibuloacoustic nerve, 13-15
Neuroma, of eyelid, 82-83
Neuromyelitis optica, 351-352
Neuro-ophthalmology, definition, 127
Neuropathy, diabetic, headache in, 398
Neutral density filter test, 344
Nevus flammeus, 156, 159f
Newborn, myasthenia gravis in, 116
Nose, abnormalities associated with neuro-ophthalmic diagnoses, 11
Nuclear magnetic resonance
  future prospects, 272-273
  of optic nerve, 272f
Nucleosome, 287, 288f
Nucleotide, structure, 286-287, 287f
Nutritional disorders, in opsoclonus, 431
Nystagmus, 422-432
  ataxia associated with, 432
  in brain tumors, 211
  caloric testing in, 425-426
  in chromosomal abnormalities, 298t
  clinical syndromes, 424-430
  congenital, 424
    head position for best visual acuity in, 345
  convergence, 429
  convergence retraction, 431
  convergence-evoked, 429
  definition, 422
  dissociated, 427, 429-430
  distinguishing central from peripheral, 425, 426t
  distinguishing congenital from acquired, 424
  divergence, 429-430
  downbeat, 427, 429
  examination for, 14-15, 422-423, 426t
  eye movements simulating, 430-432
  gaze-evoked, 426-427
  in internuclear ophthalmoplegia, 418
  jerk, 423
  latent, 424-425
  lid, 430
  manifest latent, 424-425
  monocular, 430